Harrison's
Principles of
Internal Medicine

PreTest®
Self-Assessment
and Review

Thirteenth Edition

For use with the 13th edition of
HARRISON'S PRINCIPLES OF INTERNAL MEDICINE

Edited by

Richard M. Stone, M.D.
Dana-Farber Cancer Institute
Brigham and Women's Hospital

Assistant Professor of Medicine, Harvard Medical School
Boston, Massachusetts

McGraw-Hill, Inc.
Health Professions Division
PreTest Series

New York   St. Louis   San Francisco   Auckland
Bogotá   Caracas   Lisbon   London   Madrid
Mexico City   Milan   Montreal   New Delhi
San Juan   Singapore   Sydney   Tokyo   Toronto

Harrison's Principles of Internal Medicine
PreTest® Self-Assessment and Review

23456789MALMAL9987654

ISBN 0-07-052013-5

The editors were Gail Gavert and Bruce MacGregor.
The production supervisor was Gyl A. Favours. Malloy was printer and binder.
This book was set in Times Roman by Compset, Inc.

This book is printed on acid-free paper.

The Appendix, Color Plate B, and the figures accompanying questions 177 and 600 are from Isselbacher et al: *Harrison's Principles of Internal Medicine,* 13/e, New York, McGraw-Hill, 1994, with permission.

Color plates N, O, P, Q, R, S, and T are from Fitzpatrick, et al: *Color Atlas and Synopsis of Clinical Dermatology,* 2/e, New York, McGraw-Hill, 1992, with permission.

Library of Congress Cataloging-in-Publication Data

Harrison's principles of internal medicine—PreTest self-assessment
and review / edited by Richard M. Stone.—13th ed.
    p.   cm.
    "For use with the 13th edition of Harrison's principles of
internal medicine."
    Includes bibliographical references.
    ISBN 0-07-052013-5
    1. Internal medicine—Examinations, questions, etc.   I. Harrison,
Tinsley Randolph,   II. Stone, Richard M.   III. Harrison's
principles of internal medicine.   IV. Title: Principles of internal
medicine—PreTest self-assessment and review.
    [DNLM: 1. Internal Medicine—examination questions.   WB 115 H322
1994 Suppl.]
RC46.H333   1994 Suppl. 2
616'.0076—dc20
DNLM/DLC
for Library of Congress   94-6046

Contents

Introduction

Harrison's Principles of Internal Medicine: PreTest Self-Assessment and Review has been designed to provide physicians with a comprehensive, relevant, and convenient instrument for self-evaluation and review within the broad area of internal medicine. Although it should be particularly helpful for residents preparing for the American Board of Internal Medicine (ABIM) certification examination and for board-certified internists preparing for recertification, it should also be useful for internists, family practitioners, and other practicing physicians who are simply interested in maintaining a high level of competence in internal medicine. Study of this self-assessment and review book should help to (1) identify areas of relative weakness; (2) confirm areas of expertise; (3) assess knowledge of the sciences fundamental to internal medicine; (4) assess clinical judgment and problem-solving skills; and (5) introduce recent developments in general internal medicine.

This book consists of 850 multiple-choice questions that (1) are representative of the major areas covered in *Harrison's Principles of Internal Medicine,* 13th ed., and (2) parallel the format and degree of difficulty of the questions on the examination of the ABIM. Questions have been appropriately updated and chosen to reflect important recent developments in internal medicine, such as the importance of the AIDS epidemic and the increasing contributions of molecular biology to the understanding, diagnosis, and treatment of many disorders. Each question is accompanied by an answer, a paragraph-length explanation, and a reference to a specific chapter in *Harrison's.* In some cases references to more specialized textbooks and current journal articles are also given. A list of normal values used in the laboratory studies in this book can be found in the Appendix, following a Bibliography listing all the sources used for the questions. As in the current edition of *Harrison's,* the system of international units (SI) appears first in the text and the traditional units follow in parentheses. All color plates referred to in the text are found at the back of the book.

We have assumed that the time available to the reader is limited; therefore, this book has been designed to be used profitably a chapter at a time. By allowing no more than two and a half minutes to answer each question, you can simulate the time constraints of the actual board examinations. When you finish answering all the questions in a chapter, spend as much time as necessary verifying answers and carefully reading the accompanying explanations. If after reading the explanations for a given chapter, you feel a need for a more extensive and definitive discussion, consult the chapter in *Harrison's* or any of the other references listed.

Based on our testing experience, on most medical examinations, examinees who answer half the questions correctly would score around the 50th or 60th percentile. A score of 65 percent would place the examinee above the 80th percentile, whereas a score of 30 percent would rank him or her below the 15th percentile. In other words, if you answer fewer than 30 percent of the questions in a chapter correctly, you are relatively weak in that area. A score of 50 percent would be approximately average, and 70 percent or higher would probably be honors.

We have used three basic question types in accordance with the format of the ABIM certification and recertification examinations. In accordance with the changing format of these examinations, the number of matching and true/false questions has been reduced in this edition. Considerable editorial time has been spent trying to ensure that each question is clearly stated and discriminates between those physicians who are well prepared in the subject and those who are less knowledgeable.

This book is a teaching device that provides readers with the opportunity to evaluate and update their clinical expertise, their ability to interpret data, and their ability to diagnose and solve clinical problems.

Infectious Diseases

DIRECTIONS: Each question below contains five suggested responses. Select the **one best** response to each question.

1. A 14-year-old boy has a history of recurrent respiratory infections with *Staphylococcus aureus* and *Aspergillus fumigatus*. When he was 7 years old he had a hepatic abscess that was drained surgically; no organism was cultured, but the problem responded to drainage and prolonged antibiotic therapy. His parents and two younger siblings are healthy, but an older brother died in infancy of infection.

   The laboratory study most likely to assist in establishing the diagnosis is

   (A) determination of leukocyte myeloperoxidase level
   (B) quantitative determination of serum immunoglobulin levels
   (C) T-lymphocyte functional and subpopulation assessment
   (D) nitroblue tetrazolium reduction test
   (E) bone marrow aspiration and biopsy

2. A 23-year-old, previously healthy female letter carrier works in a suburb in which the presence of rabid foxes and skunks has been documented. She is bitten by a bat, which then flies away. Initial examination reveals a clean break in the skin in the right upper forearm. She has no history of receiving treatment for rabies and she is unsure about vaccination against tetanus. The physician should

   (A) clean the wound with a 20% soap solution
   (B) clean the wound with a 20% soap solution and administer tetanus toxoid
   (C) clean the wound with a 20% soap solution, administer tetanus toxoid, and administer human rabies immune globulin intramuscularly
   (D) clean the wound with a 20% soap solution, administer tetanus toxoid, administer human rabies immune globulin intramuscularly, and administer human diploid cell vaccine
   (E) clean the wound with a 20% soap solution and administer human diploid cell vaccine

1

3. During the summer, a previously healthy 10-year-old boy living in rural Louisiana presents with a brief illness characterized by 2 days of fever, headache, and vomiting that progresses to lethargy, disorientation, and most recently a grand mal seizure. Laboratory examination is remarkable for peripheral blood leukocytosis and a normal CSF examination except for the presence of 35 monocytes per microliter. An IgM enzyme–linked immunoassay for the LaCrosse virus returns positive. Anticonvulsive medicine has been administered. At this point the physician should

   (A) tell the family that there is a high likelihood of improvement during the coming week and a good chance for discharge within 2 weeks
   (B) order a brain biopsy to exclude herpes encephalitis
   (C) administer empiric acyclovir
   (D) administer empiric chloramphenicol and ampicillin
   (E) share with the parents your concern that this illness, for which there is no specific therapy, is often fatal

4. A 23-year-old graduate student complains of burning on urination and a vaginal discharge. On physical examination, a bilateral groin rash, generalized vaginal erythema, and a whitish vaginal discharge are observed; the remainder of the physical examination is negative. The laboratory test most likely to detect a specific host-defense defect as a cause of this clinical problem would be

   (A) blood glucose concentration
   (B) blood urea nitrogen concentration
   (C) serum immunoglobulin A concentration
   (D) serum immunoglobulin E concentration
   (E) serum complement concentration

5. The most common source of bacterial infection of intravenous cannulas is

   (A) contamination of fluids during the manufacturing process
   (B) contamination of fluids during insertion of the cannula
   (C) contamination at the site of entry through the skin
   (D) contamination during injection of medications
   (E) seeding from remote sites due to intermittent bacteremia

6. A 73-year-old previously healthy man is hospitalized because of the acute onset of dysuria, urinary frequency, fever, and shaking chills. His temperature is 39.5°C (103.1°F), blood pressure is 100/60 mmHg, pulse is 140 beats per minute, and respiratory rate is 30 breaths per minute. Which of the following interventions would be the most important in the treatment of this acute illness?

   (A) Catheterization of the urinary bladder
   (B) Initiation of antibiotic therapy
   (C) Infusion of Ringer's lactate solution
   (D) Infusion of dopamine hydrochloride
   (E) Intravenous injection of methylprednisolone

7. Infection with *Pseudomonas* organisms is frequently associated with each of the following EXCEPT

   (A) osteomyelitis after a nail puncture wound of the foot
   (B) ecthyma gangrenosum
   (C) both a mild and an invasive form of otitis externa
   (D) meningitis in neonatal infants
   (E) endocarditis in drug addicts

8. A 65-year-old Greek woman visiting her children in New York City complains of upper abdominal pain. The patient is brought to the family physician who notices ecteric sclera and a mass in the right upper quadrant. A CT scan reveals a 10-cm multiloculated cyst with mural calcification that is compressing the common bile duct. Which of the following statements is correct concerning this clinical situation?

   (A) Treatment with the antiamebic agent chloroquine is indicated
   (B) Treatment with an antiechinococcal agent such as albendazole is sufficient
   (C) The adult parasite resides in the patient's intestine
   (D) Infection was probably caused by exposure to infected dogs
   (E) Surgery is contraindicated because of the risk of anaphylaxis from dissemination of infectious material

9. Diagnostic accuracy has been enhanced by the ability to detect specific DNA sequences in all the following infecting microorganisms EXCEPT

   (A) cytomegalovirus (CMV)
   (B) *Staphylococcus aureus*
   (C) *Mycoplasma pneumoniae*
   (D) *Legionella*
   (E) human immunodeficiency virus (HIV)

10. The most common cause of "traveler's diarrhea" ("turista") in Americans traveling abroad is

    (A) *Staphylococcus aureus*
    (B) *Clostridium perfringens*
    (C) *Escherichia coli*
    (D) *Bacillus cereus*
    (E) rotavirus

11. All the following vaccines are recommended for use in immunocompromised adults EXCEPT

    (A) bacille Calmette-Guerin (BCG) vaccine (against tuberculosis)
    (B) inactivated influenza vaccine for current year
    (C) 23-valent pnemococcal vaccine
    (D) quadrivalent meningococcal vaccine
    (E) inactivated polio vaccine

12. A 38-year-old gay man who is known to be infected with the HIV virus presents with a week of fever and tachypnea. Chest x-ray reveals bilateral alveolar infiltrates. Arterial blood gas determination reveals a Pa_{O_2} of 55 mmHg on room air. A bronchoalveolar lavage is positive for methenamine silver staining material. Which of the following statements is correct concerning the current clinical situation?

    (A) Transbronchial biopsy should be carried out to confirm the diagnosis
    (B) Corticosteroids are contraindicated given the risk of other opportunistic infections in Kaposi's sarcoma
    (C) Pentamidine therapy by the aerosolized route would be appropriate if the patient has a known allergy to sulfa drugs
    (D) Trimethoprim-sulfamethoxazole and pentamidine should be administered in combination
    (E) Trimethoprim-sulfamethoxazole alone should be administered

13. A 50-year-old woman emigrated from El Salvador approximately 10 years ago and currently resides in Washington, DC. She complains of shortness of breath. Chest x-ray reveals biventricular cardiac enlargement. Echocardiographic study shows biventricular enlargement, thin ventricular walls, and an apical aneurysm. The patient has no history of alcohol abuse, thyroid disease, risk factors for atherosclerotic heart disease, or family history of hemochromatosis. In considering a potential etiology for the patient's current problem, which of the following statements is correct?

   (A) The etiologic agent can be demonstrated on Giemsa stain of the peripheral blood
   (B) Other manifestations of infection could include involvement of the gastrointestinal tract
   (C) The vector for the transmission of this disease is the tsetse fly
   (D) Corticosteroids may be beneficial
   (E) Given the progressive and ultimately fatal course, cardiac transplantation should be considered

14. Production of all the following factors contributes to the pathogenicity of staphylococci EXCEPT

   (A) penicillinase production
   (B) coagulase production
   (C) enterotoxin production
   (D) exotoxin production
   (E) catalase production

15. Which of the following organisms is most likely to cause infection of a shunt implanted for treatment of hydrocephalus?

   (A) *Staphylococcus epidermidis*
   (B) *Staphylococcus aureus*
   (C) *Corynebacterium diphtheriae*
   (D) *Escherichia coli*
   (E) *Bacteroides fragilis*

16. A 14-year-old girl has fever, headache, pain on swallowing, and loss of voice. Her cervical lymph nodes are tender to palpation. Of these signs and symptoms, which is LEAST suggestive of a diagnosis of streptococcal pharyngitis?

   (A) Fever
   (B) Headache
   (C) Pain on swallowing
   (D) Loss of voice
   (E) Tender cervical lymph nodes

17. Meningococcal meningitis can be prevented by the administration of all the following preparations EXCEPT

   (A) group A vaccine
   (B) group B vaccine
   (C) group C vaccine
   (D) sulfonamides
   (E) rifampin

18. A 25-year-old man who was recently admitted to a psychiatric hospital with the diagnosis of severe depression complicated by psychosis is brought to the emergency room because of worsening mental status and fever. The patient is unable to give a history because he is profoundly confused and claims to be on Mars. The psychiatrist informs you that the patient has recently been started on haloperidol and amitriptyline. Physical findings include a rectal temperature of 40.6°C (105°F), muscle rigidity, and dry skin.

   A cooling blanket is ordered and you administer acetaminophen. Which of the following agents would be most appropriately ordered at this time?

   (A) Bromocriptine
   (B) Atropine
   (C) Levarterenol
   (D) Chlorpheniramine
   (E) Methylprednisolone

19. A 60-year-old insulin-dependent man with diabetes mellitus has had purulent drainage from his left ear for 1 week. Suddenly, fever, increased pain, and vertigo develop. The most likely causative agent is

    (A) *Aspergillus*
    (B) *Mucor*
    (C) *Pseudomonas*
    (D) *Staphylococcus aureus*
    (E) *Haemophilus influenzae*

20. Typhoid fever can be characterized by all the following statements EXCEPT

    (A) the illness usually is acquired from ingestion of contaminated food, water, or milk
    (B) leukopenia is more common than leukocytosis in acutely ill persons
    (C) rose spots are usually present at the time the fever begins
    (D) chloramphenicol is not effective in preventing relapse
    (E) fluoroquinolone antibiotics eradicate the organism even in the presence of gallstones

21. Active vaccination against which of the following is contraindicated in a person infected with the human immunodeficiency virus (HIV)?

    (A) Hepatitis B
    (B) Pneumococcal infection
    (C) Influenza
    (D) Polio
    (E) Rubella

22. Exposure to which of the following mandates passive immunization with standard immune serum globulin?

    (A) Rabies
    (B) Hepatitis A
    (C) Hepatitis B
    (D) Tetanus
    (E) Cytomegalovirus

23. *Haemophilus influenzae* infections occur with increased severity in association with all the following conditions EXCEPT

    (A) alcoholism
    (B) sickle cell disease
    (C) splenectomy
    (D) agammaglobulinemia
    (E) chronic granulomatous disease

24. To determine whether a child with paroxysmal coughing and gasping has whooping cough, a physician should order

    (A) white blood cell count and differential
    (B) Gram stain of the sputum
    (C) blood cultures
    (D) chest x-ray
    (E) lateral x-ray of the neck

25. A previously healthy 65-year-old man who underwent colonic resection for colon carcinoma 4 days ago complains of a left-sided frontal headache. Notable physical findings include a temperature of 39.4°C (103°F), an indwelling nasogastric tube, and redness and swelling around the left orbit. Which of the following is the most appropriate therapeutic strategy?

    (A) Drainage of the left ethmoidal sinus
    (B) Administration of intravenous diphenhydramine and amoxicillin-clavulanic acid
    (C) Administration of amoxicillin-clavulanic acid
    (D) Administration of oxacillin plus ceftazidime
    (E) Removal of the nasogastric tube and administration of oxacillin plus ceftazidime

26. A 25-year-old previously healthy woman presents with a 2-day history of fever, sore throat, and pain on swallowing. Speech is difficult. During the examination she leans forward; oral secretions are drooling out of her mouth. The posterior pharynx is not well seen. The most appropriate therapeutic strategy at this point would be

    (A) referral to an otolaryngologist for fiberoptic examination of the upper airway
    (B) administration of a loading dose of intravenous penicillin followed by a 10-day course of oral penicillin
    (C) administration of intravenous steroid, a loading dose of intravenous penicillin, and outpatient treatment with 10 days of penicillin
    (D) admission to the hospital
    (E) admission to the intensive care unit

27. Hypersensitivity reactions—such as erythema nodosum, erythema multiforme, arthritis, and arthralgias—are most frequently associated with which of the following infections?

    (A) Histoplasmosis
    (B) Cryptococcosis
    (C) Aspergillosis
    (D) Blastomycosis
    (E) Coccidioidomycosis

28. Imipenem, a newer antibiotic with a broad antibacterial spectrum, is coadministered with cilastatin because

    (A) the combination of these antibiotics is synergistic against *Pseudomonas* species
    (B) cilastatin aids the gastrointestinal absorption of the active moiety, imipenem
    (C) cilastatin inhibits a β-lactamase that destroys imipenem
    (D) cilastatin inhibits an enzyme in the kidney that destroys imipenem
    (E) cilastatin prevents the hypoprothrombinemic effect of imipenem

29. A 35-year-old man is seen 6 months after a cadaveric renal allograft. The patient has been on azathioprine and prednisone since that procedure. He has felt poorly for the past week with fever to 38.6°C (101.5°F), anorexia, and a cough productive of thick sputum. Chest x-ray reveals a left lower lobe (5 cm) nodule with central cavitation. Examination of the sputum reveals long, crooked, branching, beaded gram-positive filaments.

    The most appropriate initial therapy would include administration of which of the following antibiotics?

    (A) Penicillin
    (B) Erythromycin
    (C) Sulfisoxazole
    (D) Ceftazidime
    (E) Tobramycin

30. A previously healthy 28-year-old man describes several episodes of fever, myalgia, and headache that have been followed by abdominal pain and diarrhea. He has experienced up to 10 bowel movements per day. Physical examination is unremarkable. Laboratory findings are only notable for a slightly elevated leukocyte count and an elevated erythrocyte sedimentation rate. Wright stain of a fecal sample reveals the presence of neutrophils. Colonoscopy reveals inflamed mucosa. Biopsy of an affected area discloses mucosal infiltration with neutrophils, monocytes, and eosinophils; epithelial damage including loss of mucus; glandular degeneration; and crypt abscesses. The patient notes that several months ago he was at a church barbecue where several people had contracted a diarrheal illness. While this patient could have inflammatory bowel disease, which of the following pathogens is most likely to be responsible for his illness?

    (A) *Campylobacter*
    (B) *S. aureus*
    (C) *E. coli*
    (D) *Salmonella*
    (E) Norwalk agent

31. All the following are characteristic clinical features of chancroid EXCEPT

    (A) initial presentation as a tender papule
    (B) development of painful genital ulcers
    (C) tender, enlarged inguinal lymph nodes
    (D) *Haemophilus ducreyi* isolated from bacteriologic cultures
    (E) response to ampicillin therapy

32. A 62-year-old gardener who has chronic lymphocytic leukemia develops lymphangitis and a painless, nodular lesion on his wrist. Subsequently, he becomes severely ill with cavitary right-upper-lobe pneumonia; *Sporothrix schenckii* is isolated. He should be treated with

    (A) chloramphenicol
    (B) potassium iodide
    (C) penicillin
    (D) amphotericin B
    (E) flucytosine

33. An 86-year-old woman with a known history of rheumatic mitral valvular disease presents with a 2-week history of fevers and anorexia. She gives a history of dental work without prophylaxis approximately 3 weeks ago. Her laboratory examination is remarkable for an elevated erythrocyte sedimentation rate and microscopic hematuria. The patient is admitted to the hospital and treated with intravenous broad-spectrum antibiotics. Five days later blood cultures obtained prior to the start of antibiotics remain negative.

    Infection with all the following microorganisms could account for the patient's clinical endocarditis EXCEPT

    (A) *Streptococcus viridans*
    (B) *Haemophilus influenzae*
    (C) *H. parainfluenzae*
    (D) *H. aphrophilus*
    (E) *Eikenella corrodens*

34. A 19-year-old woman visits the emergency room because of a swollen left knee. She has no past medical problems. She gives a history of several days of feeling feverish and having muscle and joint aches. Specifically, her hands and wrists were painful for a few days, but at this point she is bothered only by her knee. Physical examination is remarkable only for vesiculopustular skin lesions and a mildly swollen left knee.

    The procedure most likely to yield a diagnosis at this point would be

    (A) cervical culture
    (B) blood culture
    (C) sinovial culture
    (D) serum complement assay
    (E) skin biopsy

35. Four days after he and his friends were killing muskrats along a rural creek, a boy becomes ill with headache, fever, and a macular rash. On examination, axillary adenopathy is noted, but otherwise the examination is normal. Which of the following tests would be most helpful in proving that this boy has tularemia?

    (A) Blood culture
    (B) Aspiration and culture of an axillary lymph node
    (C) Determination of serum agglutinins for *Francisella tularensis*
    (D) Bone-marrow culture
    (E) Examination of his friends

36. A 10-year-old boy is seen in a rural Arizona clinic because of prostration, fever of 40°C (104°F), and severe headache. Examination is negative for rash, stiff neck, joint tenderness, and chest and abdominal abnormalities. However, several tender, enlarged lymph nodes are palpated in the left axilla, which is very edematous. The test most likely to be of greatest help in the immediate management of this boy would be

    (A) blood culture
    (B) examination of a blood smear
    (C) biopsy of an axillary lymph node
    (D) aspiration and Gram stains of an axillary lymph node
    (E) surgical excision of an axillary node

37. A 45-year-old man with acute myeloid leukemia in second remission presents with cough, shortness of breath, and fever 3 months after an allogeneic bone marrow transplant. The patient was well prior to his transplant. At that time, serology revealed antibodies to cytomegalovirus (CMV). The graft was successful, but the patient has required the use of intermittent courses of corticosteroids to treat moderately severe graft-vs-host disease characterized by a diffusely erythematous skin rash and diarrhea.

On examination the patient appears mildly ill, has a temperature of 38.6°C (101.5°F), blood pressure of 130/80 mmHg, pulse of 110 beats per minute, and respiratory rate of 30 breaths per minute. Skin examination reveals a diffuse erythematous maculopapular rash, particularly on the arms and legs. Diffuse crackles are heard in both lungs. Chest x-ray demonstrates bilateral interstitial infiltrates, worse in the lower lobes. Examination of sputum fails to reveal a causative agent. Bronchoscopy is carried out, but the toludine blue stain, routine culture, and fungal stains are negative. Because the patient continues to have respiratory deterioration, he undergoes an open-lung biopsy. Examination of the lung tissue reveals the presence of cells that are several times larger than surrounding cells and contain a 10-μm inclusion placed centrally in the nucleus. There is also a plasmacytic and lymphocytic infiltrate in the lung. At this point, the best course of therapy would be to administer

(A) trimethroprim-sulfamethaxole
(B) acyclovir plus CMV immune globulin
(C) ganciclovir
(D) ganciclovir plus CMV immune globulin
(E) foscarnet

38. Intravenous acyclovir is indicated in each of the following situations EXCEPT

(A) clinically severe initial episode of genital herpes simplex virus infection
(B) clinically severe recurrent episode of herpes simplex virus infection
(C) oral herpes simplex 3 months after an allogeneic bone marrow transplant
(D) chickenpox in an adolescent female who is receiving steroids for lupus nephritis
(E) dermatomal herpes zoster infection in a middle-aged male being treated for large cell lymphoma

39. Which of the following organisms often causes diarrhea, confusion, and delirium in conjunction with pneumonia?

(A) *Legionella pneumophila*
(B) *Francisella tularensis*
(C) *Mycoplasma pneumoniae*
(D) *Haemophilus pneumoniae*
(E) *Klebsiella pneumoniae*

40. *Listeria monocytogenes* most frequently causes which of the following infections?

(A) Endocarditis
(B) Peritonitis
(C) Hepatitis
(D) Meningitis
(E) Conjunctivitis

41. A routine stool culture is obtained from a patient with diarrhea. Which one of the following organisms could be detected by this approach?

(A) *Campylobacter*
(B) *Yersinia*
(C) *Vibrio*
(D) *Salmonella*
(E) *Clostridium difficile*

42. Which of the following statements concerning infections with intestinal nematodes is correct?

    (A) A relatively small number of organisms typically produce severe clinical symptoms
    (B) *Ascaris* larvae enter the body via migration through dermal capillaries
    (C) Hookworm infections result from swallowing of hookworm eggs
    (D) *Strongyloides* infection is associated with recurrent urticaria
    (E) Pinworm infection is associated with iron deficiency anemia

43. Which of the following drugs would be LEAST likely to benefit a patient experiencing an acute attack of malaria?

    (A) Quinine
    (B) Chloroquine
    (C) Primaquine
    (D) Hydroxychloroquine
    (E) Mefloquine

44. Which of the following food- or waterborne bacteria responsible for diarrheal illness has the LONGEST incubation period (time from ingestion to illness)?

    (A) *Clostridium perfringens*
    (B) *Staphylococcus aureus*
    (C) *Bacillus cereus*
    (D) *Campylobacter jejuni*
    (E) *Vibrio parahaemolyticus*

45. A 22-year-old gay man from New Orleans presents with a 2-week history of fever, anorexia, and progressive diffuse lymphadenopathy. Physical findings reveal an emaciated young man who has several tongue ulcers. Hepatomegaly is noted. Laboratory examination reveals pancytopenia, an elevated alkaline phosphatase, and hyperkalemia. Chest radiograph reveals a miliary pattern of diffuse infiltration. A tongue biopsy reveals the presence of hyphae that bear both large and small spores. The correct diagnosis is

    (A) histoplasmosis
    (B) coccidioidomycosis
    (C) cryptococcosis
    (D) blastomycosis
    (E) aspergillosis

46. A 10-year-old boy presents with an abnormal appearing face. The boy lives in Rhode Island and has been playing outside a good deal this summer. He has been feeling poorly for a week with complaints of muscle aches and headache. His mother has noticed that her son had a low-grade fever and an oval rash on the back measuring about 10 cm in diameter. Physical examination reveals evidence of the oval erythema on the posterior thorax and also evidence of right facial droop. Routine laboratory studies are unremarkable. A lumbar puncture reveals an opening pressure of 80 mmHg, total protein of 46 mg/dL, and glucose of 90 mg/dL with 10 white cells, all of which are lymphocytes. The most specific diagnostic study would be

    (A) polymerase chain reaction–based DNA detection
    (B) *Borrelia* serology
    (C) blood culture for *Borrelia*
    (D) cerebrospinal fluid culture for *Borrelia*
    (E) western blot detection of *Borrelia* antigen in the cerebrospinal fluid

47. Which of the following samples of pleural fluid is most suggestive of tuberculous pleuritis?

Fluid sample	Color	pH	Protein, g/L	Glucose, mmol/L	LDH, U/mL	WBC Total (per mm³)	% Lymphocytes
(A)	Clear yellow	7.15	35	1.1	600	2,000	95
(B)	Thick green	7.00	40	1.1	600	10,000	50
(C)	Clear yellow	7.30	15	4.4	150	200	50
(D)	Pink-tinged	7.40	30	4.4	600	3,000	50
(E)	Clear yellow	7.30	35	3.3	150	2,000	95

(LDH, lactate dehydrogenase; WBC, white blood cell count)

48. A 10-year-old child has malaise, a low-grade fever, and submental lymphadenopathy. Biopsy of a cervical lymph node reveals granulomatous inflammation; the culture grows *Mycobacterium scrofulaceum.* The best treatment for this child would be

(A) excision of the infected nodes
(B) isoniazid and ethambutol
(C) streptomycin, isoniazid, and ethambutol
(D) rifampin, isoniazid, and ethambutol
(E) observation until the results of sensitivity studies are available

49. Which of the following statements concerning the use of fluoroquinolone antibiotics (e.g., ciprofloxacin, norfloxacin) is correct?

(A) Resistance can develop by bacterial plasmid-mediated expression of beta-lactamase enzyme
(B) They are bacteriostatic rather than bactericidal
(C) They have activity against all known bacterial enteric pathogens
(D) They are primarily excreted by biliary clearance
(E) They are contraindicated in patients with fever and neutropenia because of their inability to eradicate *Pseudomonas* species

50. Which of the following statements concerning syphilis in HIV-infected persons is correct?

(A) Syphilis is as common in HIV-infected persons as it is in non-HIV-infected persons, though the course of the disease is more aggressive in the HIV-infected group
(B) Serologic testing cannot be used to confirm the diagnosis of syphilis in most patients with HIV infection
(C) Failure to respond to single-dose penicillin G therapy is more likely in patients infected with both HIV and syphilis than in those infected with syphilis alone
(D) Central nervous system syphilis is rare in HIV-infected patients
(E) Syphilis is not an independent risk factor for HIV infection

51. A 40-year-old Canadian who operates a tropical fish store sees his physician because of a nonhealing ulcer on his left arm. He is afebrile and gives no history of night sweats, weight loss, or other constitutional symptoms. Biopsy of the lesion shows granulomatous inflammation and rare acid-fast organisms. A tuberculin test is negative. This man most likely has an infection caused by

(A) *Mycobacterium tuberculosis*
(B) *Mycobacterium ulcerans*
(C) *Mycobacterium kansasii*
(D) *Mycobacterium marinum*
(E) *Mycobacterium fortuitum*

52. Legionnaire's disease is characterized by all the following statements EXCEPT

   (A) the disease is not spread from person to person
   (B) diarrhea, nausea, and vomiting often are prominent early symptoms
   (C) chest x-ray usually shows few abnormalities, while chest examination usually is markedly abnormal
   (D) fever is usually prolonged
   (E) therapy with erythromycin is recommended

53. A 35-year-old HIV-infected homosexual man presents with fever, pain of the right upper quadrant, and a CT scan of the liver that shows a 10-cm, oval, hypoechoic cyst in the right lobe. An ELISA assay detects the presence of antibodies to *Entamoeba histolytica;* cysts from the same organism are found in a stool specimen. Which of the following is the most appropriate next step in management?

   (A) Administration of metronidazole
   (B) Administration of chloroquine
   (C) Drainage of the hepatic lesion for therapeutic purposes
   (D) Aspiration of the hepatic lesion for diagnosis
   (E) Hepatic resection

54. Which of the following statements concerning antifungal therapy is correct?

   (A) Dose-related hepatotoxicity is a complication of ketoconazole treatment
   (B) Clotrimazole is the preferred imidazole for the treatment of vaginal candidiasis
   (C) Oral fluconazole may be used as primary therapy in patients with hepatitis
   (D) Flucytosine may replace amphotericin B in cases of refractory hepatic candidiasis
   (E) The treatment of candidal hepatitis frequently requires 2 weeks of daily intravenous administration of amphotericin B

55. Which of the following tests is most useful for recognizing infections caused by the "newly discovered" *Legionella* species (e.g., the Pittsburgh pneumonia agent)?

   (A) Direct fluorescent antibody staining
   (B) DNA probe
   (C) Paired serologic testing
   (D) Culture of sputum
   (E) Culture of a lung biopsy specimen

56. Each of the following diagnostic tests may be indicated in the evaluation of an ulcerative genital lesion EXCEPT

   (A) Gram stain
   (B) serologic test for syphilis
   (C) biopsy
   (D) dark-field examination
   (E) viral culture

57. Which of the following statements concerning viral upper respiratory infections is correct?

   (A) Risk factors for infection with rhinovirus include exposure to cold temperatures, fatigue, and sleep deprivation
   (B) The incubation period for rhinoviral illness is approximately 1 week
   (C) Infection with respiratory syncytial virus (RSV) is unusual in older children and adults
   (D) Ribavirin given by aerosol is effective in treating infants with RSV
   (E) Pentamidine is a useful prophylactic therapy against adenovirus infections

58. A 55-year-old homeless man presents with fever and stiff neck several days after an upper respiratory infection. He also notes painful hands and hair loss. Physical examination reveals a disheveled male with a temperature of 40°C (104°F), blood pressure of 120/70, a heart rate of 70, and respiratory rate of 20. The remainder of the physical examination is remarkable for an erythematous posterior pharynx, areas of alopecia on the head and body, swollen metacarpophalangeal joints, and a stiff neck. Laboratory evaluation is remarkable for a white blood cell count of 2300/μL with 25 percent neutrophils, 65 percent lymphocytes, and 10 percent monocytes; hematocrit is 42 percent and platelet count is 55,000/μL. Other laboratory studies are unremarkable. Examination of the cerebrospinal fluid reveals normal opening pressure, total protein of 100 mg/dL, glucose of 20 mg/dL, and white count of 400/μL (80 percent lymphocytes and 20 percent neutrophils). Gram stain, acid-fast stain, and India ink stain are all negative. Which of the following statements about this patient is correct?

(A) Intravenous penicillin G is the treatment of choice
(B) The low CSF glucose is pathognomonic for bacterial meningitis
(C) A routine blood culture will likely establish the diagnosis
(D) The patient has probably come in contact with an infected rodent
(E) Alopecia is unrelated to the current infection

59. The diagnosis of relapsing fever (*Borrelia* infection) usually is made by

(A) serologic testing
(B) blood culture
(C) examination of blood smears
(D) lymph-node aspiration
(E) lumbar puncture

60. The characteristic "sulfur grains" of actinomycosis are composed chiefly of

(A) organisms
(B) neutrophils and monocytes
(C) monocytes and lymphocytes
(D) eosinophils
(E) calcified cellular debris

61. The best available therapy for disseminated *Mycobacterium avium-intracellulare* (MAI) infection in patients with AIDS is administration of

(A) isoniazid, rifampin, and ethambutol
(B) ciprofloxacin
(C) streptomycin and pyrazinamide
(D) clarithromycin
(E) clarithromycin and ethambutol

62. Three drugs that inhibit HIV reverse transcriptase are available to treat patients with HIV infection. These drugs are zidovudine (azidothymidine, or AZT), didanosine (dideoxyinosine, or ddI), and zalcitabine (dideoxycytidine, or ddC). Which of the following statements regarding these three drugs is correct?

(A) They have similar side effects
(B) The most frequent problem associated with long-term use of AZT is intolerance due to side effects
(C) The use of AZT in HIV-infected patients who have not yet developed AIDS is contraindicated
(D) ddI is indicated for HIV-infected patients who are intolerant of AZT
(E) ddC is indicated for patients who have failed therapy with AZT and with ddI

63. Antigen testing of blood and cerebrospinal fluid is most useful in the diagnosis of

(A) histoplasmosis
(B) blastomycosis
(C) cryptococcosis
(D) coccidioidomycosis
(E) sporotrichosis

64. What is the best therapy for a 23-year-old man with a purulent urethral discharge that contains intracellular gram-negative diplococci?

   (A) Benzathine penicillin
   (B) Tetracycline (or doxycycline)
   (C) Spectinomycin plus tetracycline (or doxycycline)
   (D) Ampicillin plus tetracycline (or doxycycline)
   (E) Ceftriaxone plus tetracycline (or doxycycline)

65. A 45-year-old man with acute myelogenous leukemia (AML) is seen 45 days after initial treatment with daunorubicin and cytosine arabinoside. After this therapy he sustained 22 days of neutropenia, during which time he became febrile and received broad-spectrum antibiotics. He was discharged feeling relatively well after a 28-day hospital course with a normal CBC and a normal bone marrow. Within several days after hospital discharge, he developed a fever of 38.5°C (101.3°F) and mild abdominal pain, particularly in the right upper quadrant. Physical examination is unrevealing. His CBC is normal as is the rest of his laboratory examination except for an elevated alkaline phosphatase. A CT scan of the liver is nonspecifically abnormal. The most appropriate action at this point would be

   (A) admission of the patient for administration of broad-spectrum antibacterial antibiotics
   (B) magnetic resonance imaging (MRI) of the right upper quadrant
   (C) abdominal ultrasonography
   (D) bone marrow aspirate and biopsy
   (E) liver biopsy

66. All the following antimicrobial agents inhibit synthesis of bacterial cell walls EXCEPT

   (A) bacitracin
   (B) imipenem
   (C) vancomycin
   (D) clarithromycin
   (E) ceftriaxone

67. Impaired immune competence is the predisposing factor in about half of all persons who develop

   (A) histoplasmosis
   (B) coccidioidomycosis
   (C) blastomycosis
   (D) cryptococcosis
   (E) sporotrichosis

68. A 50-year-old woman presents with fever, abdominal cramps, and watery diarrhea 1 week after finishing an oral course of ampicillin for cystitis. The best way to document pseudomembranous colitis caused by *Clostridium difficile* is

   (A) stool culture
   (B) a rise in serologic titers to *C. difficile*
   (C) the presence of characteristic pseudomembranes on endoscopy
   (D) cytopathic effect of stool filtrate on tissue culture monolayers
   (E) Gram stain of the stool showing sheets of neutrophils and gram-positive rods

69. Which of the following agents, when administered to an intubated patient in an intensive care unit, is most likely to decrease the incidence of hospital-acquired pneumonia?

   (A) Ranitidine
   (B) Cimetidine
   (C) Sucralfate
   (D) Penicillin G
   (E) Ciprofloxacin

70. The type of endocarditis most commonly found in patients who are intravenous drug abusers is

   (A) *Staphylococcus aureus* infection of the tricuspid valve
   (B) *S. aureus* infection of the mitral valve
   (C) α-hemolytic streptococcal infection of the tricuspid valve
   (D) α-hemolytic streptococcal infection of the mitral valve
   (E) *Pseudomonas aeruginosa* infection of the pulmonic valve

71. Recommended therapy for persons who have dermatophytosis, otherwise known as ringworm, includes all the following agents EXCEPT

    (A) clotrimazole
    (B) griseofulvin
    (C) miconazole
    (D) amphotericin
    (E) ketoconazole

72. Factors that contribute to blindness in persons who have trachoma include all the following EXCEPT

    (A) superficial corneal vascularization
    (B) corneal abrasion by eyelashes
    (C) bacterial superinfection
    (D) inflammatory destruction of the lacrimal glands
    (E) glaucoma due to limbic obstruction

73. A 28-year-old woman who works in a poultry processing factory develops an acute febrile illness. Which of the following signs and symptoms is LEAST suggestive of the diagnosis of psittacosis?

    (A) Shaking chills with fever to 40.6°C (105°F)
    (B) Severe headache
    (C) Nonproductive cough
    (D) Stiff back and neck
    (E) Diarrhea

74. Which of the following characteristics would be most useful in distinguishing between mumps and acute bacterial parotitis?

    (A) Age of patient
    (B) Presence or absence of fever
    (C) Presence or absence of warmth and tenderness over the parotid glands
    (D) Gram stain of parotid secretions
    (E) Serum amylase concentration

75. Which of the following is LEAST suggestive of infection with poliovirus?

    (A) Low-grade fever and malaise with complete resolution in 2 to 3 days
    (B) Biphasic illness with several days of fever, then meningeal symptoms and asymmetric flaccid paralysis 5 to 10 days later
    (C) Descending motor paralysis with preservation of tendon reflexes and sensation
    (D) Failure to isolate a virus from the cerebrospinal fluid in the presence of marked meningismus
    (E) Recovery of function up to 6 months after initial paralysis

76. A 58-year-old schoolteacher is hospitalized after 10 days of a respiratory illness. For 2 days he has had a dramatically worsening cough and shortness of breath. He also has had severe malaise, myalgias, arthralgias, rhinorrhea, and pharyngitis and has lost 2.7 kg (6 lb). No sputum or respiratory secretions can be collected. Chest x-ray shows a diffuse bronchopneumonia.

    All the following antibiotics would be acceptable for the initial treatment of this man's illness EXCEPT

    (A) penicillin G
    (B) nafcillin
    (C) vancomycin
    (D) cephalothin
    (E) clindamycin

77. Which of the following is LEAST likely to be a manifestation of late syphilis?

    (A) Lymphadenopathy
    (B) Aortitis
    (C) Papulosquamous skin rash
    (D) Hemiparesis
    (E) Ataxic gait

78. Infection with *Mycobacterium tuberculosis* is common in HIV-infected patients. Which of the following statements concerning this problem is correct?

    (A) Tuberculosis is a relatively rare presenting infection in a patient with AIDS
    (B) Extrapulmonary tuberculosis is more common than pulmonary tuberculosis in HIV-infected patients
    (C) HIV-infected patients with pulmonary tuberculosis need not be considered infectious
    (D) Initial therapy for HIV-infected patients with tuberculosis should be the same as that for non-HIV-infected patients with tuberculosis (isoniazid, rifampin, and pyrazinamide)
    (E) Isoniazid should not be administered to those with HIV infection and a positive tuberculin skin test until active infection is documented

79. Urinary tract infections would be LEAST likely to develop in association with

    (A) diabetes mellitus
    (B) sickle cell anemia
    (C) hyperparathyroidism
    (D) gout
    (E) Wilson's disease

80. A 35-year-old Jamaican emigrant develops diffuse lymphadenopathy, fever, lymphocytosis, hypercalcemia, and nodular skin infiltrates. Biopsy of a skin lesion reveals a monotonous population of lymphocytes that stain with antibody directed at CD4 (T4).

    Which infectious agent is associated with this disease?

    (A) Human immunodeficiency virus 1 (HIV-1)
    (B) HIV-2
    (C) Human T-lymphotropic virus I (HTLV-I)
    (D) HTLV-II
    (E) Feline leukemia virus (FeLV)

81. Which of the following agents is the most frequent cause of nonepidemic, sporadic encephalitis in the United States?

    (A) Togavirus
    (B) Picornavirus
    (C) Rubella virus
    (D) Epstein-Barr virus
    (E) Herpes simplex virus

82. A 29-year-old patient with acquired immunodeficiency syndrome (AIDS) has abdominal cramps and profuse watery diarrhea. The best way to establish the diagnosis of cryptosporidiosis is

    (A) acute and convalescent serologic studies
    (B) Gram stain of stool
    (C) stool culture
    (D) wet mount of stool
    (E) acid-fast staining of concentrated stool

83. There has been an outbreak of infections caused by methicillin-resistant *Staphylococcus aureus* in the surgical intensive care unit. The most effective means of limiting the spread is

    (A) treatment with cephalosporins to which most strains are sensitive
    (B) treatment with nafcillin and gentamicin, which have a synergistic effect
    (C) use of high-dose nafcillin alone, and isolation
    (D) treatment with vancomycin
    (E) minimization of use of any antibiotics in the affected patients because resistance will rapidly develop in other bacteria

84. A 40-year-old Filipino man has hypopigmented macular lesions and a palpably enlarged ulnar nerve. The diagnosis of leprosy can best be established by

   (A) positive lepromin skin test
   (B) culture of material obtained on skin biopsy
   (C) development of erythema and swelling of the lesions after a trial of dapsone therapy
   (D) demonstration of acid-fast organisms in skin or nerves
   (E) none of the above; leprosy is a clinical diagnosis

85. All the following groups have an increased risk of infection with *Giardia lamblia* EXCEPT

   (A) campers in mountainous areas
   (B) patients receiving chemotherapy
   (C) toddlers in day-care centers
   (D) patients with IgA deficiency
   (E) male homosexuals

86. A 35-year-old Samoan presents with recurrent fever, headache, photophobia, and painful lymphangitis in his left leg. The best way to diagnose filariasis caused by *Wuchereria bancrofti* is

   (A) biopsy of any inflamed lymph nodes to demonstrate the adult worm
   (B) serologic studies
   (C) observance of intense itching after a single dose of diethylcarbamazine
   (D) demonstration of microfilariae after injection of blood into mice
   (E) demonstration of microfilariae in blood taken between 9 P.M. and 2 A.M.

Questions 87–88

An 18-year-old, sexually active woman presents with fever, pleuritic pain of the right upper quadrant, and lower abdominal pain. Pelvic examination reveals mucopurulent cervicitis and tenderness upon the production of cervical motion. The right upper quadrant, uterine fundus, and adnexa are slightly tender. The white blood cell count and erythrocyte sedimentation rate are elevated, but the results of the remainder of the laboratory examination, including liver function tests, are normal.

87. Which of the following agents is the most likely cause of this clinical syndrome?

   (A) Herpes simplex virus
   (B) *Treponema pallidum*
   (C) *Neisseria gonorrhoeae*
   (D) *Chlamydia trachomatis*
   (E) *Mycoplasma hominis*

88. Because the patient appears ill, she is hospitalized. Assuming that pregnancy and appendicitis are excluded, which of the following antibiotic regimens is the best choice?

   (A) Doxycycline plus cefoxitin
   (B) Doxycycline alone
   (C) Acyclovir plus penicillin
   (D) Penicillin alone
   (E) Metronidazole plus gentamicin

89. A 65-year-old retired banker who spends summers on Nantucket Island off the Massachusetts coast returned to his home in Boston early in September. He noted the gradual onset of a febrile illness with chills, sweats, myalgias, and yellow eyes. His doctor could palpate the spleen and noted a macrocytic anemia, hyperbilirubinemia, and a high serum level of lactic dehydrogenase on laboratory examination.

    Which of the following would be the most helpful diagnostic procedure at this point?

    (A) Blood culture
    (B) Examination of leukocytes on blood film
    (C) Examination of erythrocytes on blood film
    (D) Splenic biopsy
    (E) Liver biopsy

90. All the following represent clinical syndromes produced by *Leishmania* EXCEPT

    (A) fever, pancytopenia, and splenomegaly
    (B) disfiguring facial ulcer
    (C) diffuse skin lesions
    (D) dysphagia, chest pain, and regurgitation
    (E) nasal obstruction and epistaxis

DIRECTIONS: Each question below contains five suggested responses. For **each** of the five responses listed with every question, you are to respond either YES (Y) or NO (N). In a given item **all, some, or none of the alternatives may be correct.**

91. In persons who have endocarditis, which of the following factors would *adversely* affect the prognosis?

    (A) The presence of congestive heart failure
    (B) Abscess formation
    (C) The isolation of organisms resistant to multiple antimicrobial agents
    (D) The isolation of *Staphylococcus epidermidis* shortly after cardiac surgery
    (E) A delay in instituting therapy

92. Which of the following conditions would warrant antibiotic prophylaxis against infective endocarditis in a patient experiencing invasive dental work?

    (A) Atrial septal defect
    (B) Ventricular septal defect
    (C) Coronary artery bypass grafts
    (D) Permanent transvenous pacemaker
    (E) Mitral regurgitation associated with mitral valve prolapse

93. Correct statements concerning the pathogenesis of fever include

    (A) aspirin inhibits the production of endogenous pyrogens
    (B) the major endogenous pyrogens in humans include interleukin 1 (IL-1) and tumor necrosis factor (TNF)
    (C) endogenous pyrogens are produced by bacteria, protozoa, and fungi
    (D) endogenous pyrogens raise body temperature by their effect on skeletal muscle beds
    (E) endogenous pyrogens play a role in the cachexia of chronic infections

94. True statements concerning genitourinary infections include which of the following?

    (A) A man who has dysuria, no urethral discharge, and only 1 or 2 leukocytes per high-power field on microscopic examination of material obtained by a urethral swab probably has chlamydial urethritis
    (B) A man who has a urethral discharge containing many leukocytes but only extracellular gram-negative diplococci should be treated with tetracycline, pending the results of cultures
    (C) A woman who has a watery, malodorous vaginal discharge that does not contain *Candida* or *Trichomonas* on microscopic examination should be treated with a sulfonamide vaginal cream for presumed bacterial vaginosis
    (D) A pregnant woman who has mucopurulent cervicitis without gram-negative diplococci on Gram stain or *Neisseria gonorrhoeae* isolated on culture should be treated with tetracycline for 1 to 3 weeks
    (E) In the United States, the most common cause of ulcerative genital lesions is herpes simplex virus

95. Correct statements concerning pneumo-coccal infection include which of the following?

   (A) Infections with type 3 pneumococci are associated with a higher mortality rate than infections with any other type of pneumococci
   (B) Patients who have had a splenectomy for any reason should receive pneumococcal vaccine
   (C) Pneumococcal pharyngitis is the most common precipitating event of pneumococcal meningitis in adults
   (D) The occurrence of the "crisis" in pneumococcal pneumonia generally corresponds to the time of maximum leukocytosis
   (E) Hypogammaglobulinemia is an important factor contributing to the unfavorable prognosis for pneumococcal pneumonia in alcoholic persons

96. True statements about the pathogenesis of streptococcal infections include which of the following?

   (A) Streptococcal strains without M protein in the cell wall are nonpathogenic
   (B) Manifestations of infection with group A streptococci are primarily due to direct invasion
   (C) Penicillin significantly shortens the clinical course of pharyngitis produced by group A streptococci
   (D) Nonenterococcal group D strepto-cocci cause endocarditis
   (E) Streptococcal pyoderma does not lead to acute rheumatic fever

97. Leptospirosis may be characterized by which of the following statements?

   (A) Fleas are the most important vector for transmission of *Leptospira* to humans
   (B) Leptospirosis usually begins with fever, headache, and myalgias
   (C) Leptospiral hepatitis often causes marked hyperbilirubinemia with only moderate transaminasemia
   (D) A normal glucose concentration and a moderately elevated white blood cell count (100 to 1000 cells/mm^3) are characteristic cerebrospinal fluid findings in leptospiral meningitis
   (E) The best way to diagnose acute leptospirosis is by dark-field microscopic examination of blood smears

98. *Neisseria gonorrhoeae* infections can be described by which of the following statements?

   (A) Gonococci with pili tend to be avirulent
   (B) Strains of *N. gonorrhoeae* that produce β-lactamase are resistant to penicillin but usually are sensitive to "third-generation" cephalosporins, such as ceftriaxone
   (C) Gonococcemia frequently occurs during menstruation
   (D) The skin lesions of gonococcemia usually appear first on the distal portions of the extremities
   (E) Gonococcal arthritis is usually symmetrical in distribution

99. True statements concerning *Acinetobacter* include which of the following?

 (A) This organism often is confused with *Neisseria* on Gram stain
 (B) This organism often is mistakenly identified as a diphtheroid on Gram stain
 (C) This organism can be easily mislabeled as a member of the Enterobacteriaceae family when first isolated on routine laboratory culture media
 (D) This organism usually is sensitive to penicillin and ampicillin
 (E) Organisms of the genus *Acinetobacter* are rarely isolated from normal patients

100. Correct statements concerning melioidosis include which of the following?

 (A) Infection usually is caused by person-to-person transmission
 (B) Patients with pneumonia usually have relatively few organisms in the sputum
 (C) Diagnosis usually depends on serologic testing
 (D) Cavitary lung lesions do not occur
 (E) Therapy with a combination of two or three antibiotics is recommended for acutely ill patients

101. Brucellosis can be described by which of the following statements?

 (A) Cattle are the most important source of human *Brucella* infections in the United States
 (B) Brucellosis is an important cause of abortion in cattle and pigs, but not in humans
 (C) Brucellosis should be considered in the differential diagnosis of fever of unknown origin in the United States
 (D) *Brucella* cannot be grown in usual blood culture media
 (E) A combination of tetracycline and streptomycin is the treatment of choice

102. Cholera can be characterized by which of the following statements?

 (A) In endemic areas, it is predominantly a disease of children
 (B) The most definitive means of diagnosis is by dark-field microscopy
 (C) Oral treatment must include replacement fluids containing glucose and sodium bicarbonate
 (D) Treatment with oral tetracycline shortens the duration of diarrhea
 (E) Vaccination affords good protection from infection

103. True statements about mucormycosis include which of the following?

 (A) The organism is grown easily from most clinical specimens once an adequate tissue sample is obtained
 (B) A characteristic feature of *Mucor* is its tendency to invade blood vessels
 (C) In persons with hematologic malignancies, the sinuses and lungs are the most frequent sites of infection
 (D) Diagnosis by serologic testing is not yet clinically practical
 (E) The treatment of choice is amphotericin B and surgical debridement

104. True statements about Rocky Mountain spotted fever include which of the following?

 (A) Fleas are the characteristic vector of disease spread
 (B) The disease is caused by the obligate intracellular organism *Rickettsia rickettsii*
 (C) Frank arthritis is a common early manifestation of infection
 (D) The initial skin lesions usually appear on the extremities
 (E) Treatment of choice consists of early administration of chloramphenicol or tetracycline

105. *Mycoplasma* pneumonia has which of the following characteristics?

(A) The causal organism, *Mycoplasma pneumoniae,* is gram-positive
(B) Persons older than 40 years of age rarely are affected
(C) A fourfold rise in the cold-agglutinin titer within 10 days of the onset of symptoms is specific evidence of this disease
(D) Treatment with tetracycline is effective
(E) Treatment with erythromycin is effective

106. Correct statements concerning toxic shock syndrome include which of the following?

(A) It is associated with a staphylococcal exotoxin
(B) Blood cultures are positive for *S. aureus* in approximately 50 percent of patients
(C) At least 40 percent of cases are non-menstrual
(D) Involvement of multiple organ systems often occurs
(E) Patients with postoperative staphylococcal wound infections usually have an obvious tissue focus that presents at least 1 week postoperatively

107. True statements concerning infectious mononucleosis include which of the following?

(A) The most common symptom of infectious mononucleosis is sore throat
(B) In young adults, the incubation period for infectious mononucleosis is 30 to 50 days
(C) The atypical lymphocytes associated with infectious mononucleosis are T cells
(D) Heterophil antibody titers usually decline within 3 to 6 months from the onset of symptoms
(E) Antibodies to Epstein-Barr virus (EBV) generally persist longer in the circulation than do heterophil antibodies

108. Cat-scratch disease can be described by which of the following statements?

(A) Only about half of all cases are associated with cat scratches
(B) Lymph node histopathology usually is pathognomonic
(C) Lymph node swelling usually lasts no more than 2 weeks
(D) It is caused by a bacterial pathogen
(E) Treatment with tetracycline is usually effective

109. Diphtherial infections are correctly characterized by which of the following statements?

(A) Human infection occurs only with strains that produce diphtheria toxin
(B) Serious disease can be prevented by mass immunization with diphtherial cell-wall polysaccharide
(C) A pseudomembrane can be observed in both cutaneous and respiratory forms of infection
(D) A portion of the diphtheria toxin molecule is responsible for specificity; another part inflicts cellular damage by directly inhibiting DNA repair
(E) Cardiac disease is common in those with diphtherial pharyngitis

110. Correct statements concerning non-group A streptococcal disease include which of the following?

(A) Most group B streptococcal infections occur in older, debilitated patients
(B) The terms *group D streptococci* and *enterococci* are synonymous
(C) Some species of viridans streptococci can cause serious pyogenic infections
(D) Ampicillin plus streptomycin is the regimen of choice in the treatment of enterococcal endocarditis
(E) Non-group A streptococci represent the second most common agents responsible for neonatal sepsis

111. True statements concerning *Klebsiella* infections include which of the following?

(A) Most clinical isolates are obtained from the respiratory tract

(B) Predisposing factors for *Klebsiella* pneumonia include alcoholism, diabetes mellitus, and chronic bronchopulmonary disease

(C) *Klebsiella* is closely related to *Enterobacter* and *Serratia*

(D) Finding *Klebsiella* growth from a sputum culture obtained from an intubated patient mandates treatment with an aminoglycoside or a third-generation cephalosporin

(E) At least 2 weeks is often required to successfully treat an established *Klebsiella* infection

112. True statements concerning malaria include

(A) malaria caused by each of the four plasmodial species can relapse after initial illness

(B) red cells negative for the Duffy blood group antigen are resistant to *Plasmodium vivax*

(C) renal impairment is a grave prognostic sign in falciparum malaria

(D) *Plasmodium malariae* can cause immune-mediated nephropathy

(E) massive splenomegaly can result from repeated bouts of infection

113. Well-recognized complications of infection with Epstein-Barr virus include

(A) airway obstruction
(B) lymphoma
(C) thrombocytopenia
(D) hemolytic anemia
(E) hepatitis

114. True statements describing amebiasis include which of the following?

(A) Humans are the principal reservoir

(B) Even in the presence of multiple liver abscesses, abatement of fever usually occurs promptly with medical therapy

(C) In persons who have received metronidazole for liver abscess, the amebic serology usually reverts from positive to negative within 4 to 6 weeks

(D) If the fluid aspirated from a liver cyst identified by liver-spleen scan contains no polymorphonuclear leukocytes or amebas, then amebic abscess is an unlikely diagnosis

(E) The mortality rate for intestinal amebiasis in the United States is less than 5 percent

115. Correct statements regarding liver abscess include which of the following?

(A) The prognosis for patients with multiple small liver abscesses is worse than for those with a single large abscess

(B) Serology is helpful in distinguishing between a pyogenic and an amebic liver abscess

(C) Blood cultures are rarely positive

(D) Multiple abscesses tend to present more acutely than does a single lesion

(E) The combination of clindamycin and gentamicin is reasonable empiric therapy for a suspected pyogenic liver abscess

116. Toxoplasmosis can be described by which of the following statements?

(A) A pregnant woman who has acquired *Toxoplasma* any time before pregnancy is unlikely to deliver an infected infant

(B) A woman who develops acute toxoplasmosis during one pregnancy is more likely than other women to give birth to an infected child in a subsequent pregnancy

(C) A woman who acquires toxoplasmosis during the last trimester of pregnancy is more likely to deliver an infected infant than if she acquired the infection during the first trimester

(D) Toxoplasmosis in a person with Hodgkin's disease probably is due to reactivation of a latent infection

(E) Antibody response is not a reliable diagnostic indicator of toxoplasmosis in immunocompromised patients

117. A person with liver disease caused by *Schistosoma mansoni* would be likely to have

(A) gynecomastia
(B) jaundice
(C) esophageal varices
(D) ascites
(E) spider nevi

118. True statements regarding *Shigella* and shigellosis include which of the following?

(A) *S. sonnei* is the isolate most frequently found in the United States

(B) Patients who have had gastric surgery or who are taking antacids have an increased susceptibility to infection

(C) There is increased transmission at day-care centers and among male homosexuals

(D) *Shigella* organisms are locally invasive in the bowel, but positive blood cultures are very unusual

(E) Antibiotic therapy should be avoided since it will increase the carrier rate

119. Extrapulmonary tuberculosis can be characterized by which of the following statements?

(A) Pleural effusions associated with tuberculosis usually occur in older patients with reactivation disease developing after an insidious onset

(B) Patients with laryngitis or bronchitis caused by tuberculosis are highly infectious

(C) Pott's disease, with extensive bony involvement of the midthoracic spine and paravertebral cold abscesses, will usually respond well to chemotherapy alone

(D) Cranial nerve findings are frequently associated with tuberculous meningitis because of basilar involvement by infection

(E) The stomach is most likely to be involved in patients with gastrointestinal tuberculosis

120. True statements about Lyme disease include which of the following?

(A) Transmission occurs almost exclusively in the northeastern United States

(B) A typical skin lesion, erythema chronicum migrans, usually occurs within a month of the infected tick bite

(C) Constitutional symptoms are very rare at the time of skin involvement

(D) Meningitis is the only form of neurologic involvement

(E) In patients with frank meningitis or significant cardiac conduction defects, parenteral therapy with 20 million units per day of penicillin G for at least 10 days is indicated

121. Correct statements about clostridial infections include which of the following?

    (A) Early antibiotic therapy is important after the isolation of clostridia from any wound to prevent more serious disease

    (B) Alpha toxin, a lecithinase, is one of the major clostridial toxins

    (C) *C. perfringens* is one of the most common causes of food poisoning in the United States

    (D) The diagnosis of clostridial myonecrosis can be difficult to make because few organisms are present in the skin lesions

    (E) Septicemia with *C. septicum* has been associated with gastrointestinal malignancies

122. Anaerobic organisms should be considered as potential etiologic agents in which of the following patients?

    (A) A previously healthy 18-year-old boy with sudden fever, cough, and right lower lobe infiltrate

    (B) A 50-year-old man with alcoholism who has marked cellulitis, swelling, and pain of his left lower mandible

    (C) A 40-year-old woman with a seizure disorder, low-grade fever, malaise, and a right lower lobe infiltrate

    (D) A 50-year-old woman with fever, hypoxia, and pulmonary infiltrates 4 h after having general anesthesia for a cholecystectomy

    (E) A 38-year-old man with a history of rheumatic fever and severe periodontitis in whom a low-grade fever, malaise, and a new heart murmur develop

123. True statements about varicella-zoster infection include which of the following?

    (A) Once dermatomal herpes zoster develops in a patient, repeated recurrences are the rule

    (B) Cerebellar ataxia is a serious complication of varicella in children

    (C) Chickenpox is very contagious with attack rates estimated at between 70 and 90 percent

    (D) Varicella pneumonitis, the most serious complication of chickenpox, occurs more frequently in adults than in children

    (E) If available within 72 h of exposure, varicella-zoster immune globulin should be given to all patients to prevent development of clinical disease

124. Cytomegalovirus (CMV) is accurately described by which of the following statements?

    (A) Approximately 60 percent of infants who are breast-fed by seropositive mothers become infected; this represents the majority of the cases of cytomegalic inclusion disease in newborn infants

    (B) Although 1 percent of newborn infants may be infected with CMV in the United States, less than .05 percent have symptomatic disease

    (C) CMV mononucleosis is the most common cause of heterophil-negative mononucleosis

    (D) CMV pneumonia, a major cause of morbidity and mortality in bone marrow transplant patients, can be diagnosed only by viral cultures of sputum

    (E) Cultures of CMV from urine, saliva, or buffy coat specimens confirm the presence of the virus but do not necessarily imply acute infection

125. Correct statements about viral gastroenteritis caused by rotavirus and Norwalk virus include which of the following?

   (A) Both alter cyclic nucleotide levels and cause a secretory diarrhea
   (B) Rotaviruses are the most important causes of severe diarrhea in infants
   (C) Rotavirus infection can be diagnosed only retrospectively by serologic methods since isolation from stool is very difficult
   (D) Norwalk virus has been associated with both food-borne and water-borne epidemics
   (E) Both viruses cause a self-limited disease with vomiting and diarrhea

126. True statements about influenza infection include which of the following?

   (A) Pandemics are caused by several simultaneous point mutations
   (B) Immunity is established by the development of antibodies to the neuraminidase, which prevents release of replicated viral particles
   (C) Outbreaks of influenza B tend to be smaller than those of influenza A because the virus does not undergo extensive antigenic shift as it does in influenza A
   (D) In a minority of patients, prolonged weakness and fatigue develop, associated with persistent viral shedding
   (E) Amantadine or rimantadine may be useful in prophylaxis or therapy of influenza A if started within 48 h of infection

127. Tetanus is correctly characterized by which of the following statements?

   (A) Neonatal tetanus develops after passage through a contaminated birth canal
   (B) If given early enough after exposure, human tetanus immune globulin can significantly modify the course of disease
   (C) Tetanus does not recur because lasting immunity develops
   (D) Trismus is a common manifestation
   (E) In a patient who is uncertain about his or her immunization status, both tetanus toxoid and immune globulin should be given for serious wounds

Infectious Diseases

Answers

1. **The answer is D.** *(Chap 81. Malech, N Engl J Med 317:687, 1987.)* This child most likely has chronic granulomatous disease (CGD), a group of inherited disorders that have in common defective oxidative metabolism of neutrophils. This defect results in a heightened susceptibility to infection with catalase-positive organisms such as staphylococci and *Aspergillus*. The diagnosis can be made by demonstrating abnormal neutrophil reduction of nitroblue tetrazolium. Recent studies have suggested that interferon-gamma may be useful in correcting the neutrophil dysfunction characteristic of CGD. Most patients with isolated deficiency of myeloperoxidase are not at increased risk for infection unless another defect is present, in which case infection with *Candida albicans* may be a problem. Decreased serum levels of immunoglobulins predispose to infection with encapsulated organisms such as *Haemophilus* and streptococci, while defects in T-lymphocyte function are manifested as infection with viruses and protozoal pathogens such as *Pneumocystis carinii*.

2. **The answer is D.** *(Chap 158. Bear, N Engl J Med 316:1270, 1987.)* The patient in question has been bitten by a member of a species known to carry rabies in an area in which rabies is endemic. Based on the animal vector and the fact that the skin was broken and saliva that possibly contains the rabies virus was present, postexposure rabies prophylaxis should be administered. If an animal involved in an unprovoked bite can be captured, it should be humanely killed and the head sent immediately to an appropriate laboratory for rabies examination by the technique of fluorescent antibody staining for viral antigen. If a healthy dog or cat bites a person in an endemic area, the animal should be captured, confined, and observed for 10 days. If the animal remains healthy for this period of time, the bite is highly unlikely to have transmitted rabies. Postexposure prophylactic therapy includes vigorous cleaning of the wound with a 20% soap solution to remove any virus particles that might be present. Tetanus toxoid and antibiotics should also be administered. Passive immunization with antirabies antiserum in the form of human rabies immune globulin (rather than the corresponding equine antiserum because of the risk of serum sickness) is indicated at a dose of 10 units/kg into the wound and 10 units/kg intramuscularly into the gluteal region. Secondly, one should administer active immunization with an antirabies vaccine (either human diploid cell vaccine or rabies vaccine absorbed [RVA]) in five 1-mL doses given intramuscularly, preferably in the deltoid or anterior lateral thigh area. The five doses are given over a 28-day period. The administration of either passive or active immunization without the other modality results in a higher failure rate than does the combination therapy.

3. **The answer is A.** *(Chap 159.)* The presence of IgM antibodies, either in the serum or CSF, reactive with the LaCrosse (California) arbovirus is highly suggestive of acute infection with this

agent. Moreover, the patient resides in an endemic area (the North Central states, New York, wooded areas of eastern Texas and Louisiana, and along the eastern seaboard). The virus is present in the woodland mosquito, *Aedes triseratus;* chipmunks and squirrels serve as amplifier hosts. Human infections occur most often during the summer months when the mosquito is active and usually involve 5- to 10-year-old boys who live in rural areas. The clinical presentation may be the abrupt epileptic type, as in this patient, or the more lethargic form. While EEGs are typically abnormal and imaging studies of the brain might also reveal abnormalities in the temporal lobe, the presence of the specific antibody obviates the need for brain biopsy to exclude herpes encephalitis, which is also typically localized in the temporal lobes. Despite the abrupt clinical onset and severity, there is progressive improvement beginning about the fourth day with almost all patients becoming afebrile, seizure-free, and able to leave the hospital within several weeks. The mortality is under 2 percent; however, about 15 percent of affected persons may develop short- or long-term sequelae including personality and behavioral changes.

4. **The answer is A.** *(Chap 166.)* The physical signs and symptoms listed in the question suggest infection with *Candida albicans.* These infections occur in several clinical settings: diabetes in poor control; broad-spectrum antibiotic therapy; chronic mucocutaneous candidiasis syndrome; hematologic malignancy; and administration of high doses of corticosteroids. Although some of these conditions may be associated with elevated serum levels of immunoglobulins A and E, these are nonspecific findings. On the other hand, a significantly elevated blood glucose concentration would make the diagnosis of diabetes almost certain. In complement deficiency or uremia, the defects in host defense are not characteristically manifested by vaginal candidiasis.

5. **The answer is C.** *(Chap 97.)* Infection of cannulas occurs most commonly by contamination during insertion or manipulation. Although the daily application of an antibacterial ointment is recommended by some authorities, the best way to prevent these infections is to change the cannula periodically, no less often than every 2 or 3 days. An exception is the use of cuffed catheters, which are inserted surgically into the subclavian vein and can be used for many weeks. Infections of such devices with relatively nonpathogenic organisms, such as coagulase-negative staphylococci, may be treated with intravenous antibiotics; however, gram-negative rod and candidal infections usually mandate removal of the indwelling catheter. Infections of cannulas occur much less frequently as a result of the other factors listed in the question.

6. **The answer is B.** *(Chap 83. Wolff, N Engl J Med 324:486, 1991.)* In the case presented, the history and physical examination strongly suggest gram-negative sepsis stemming from a urinary-tract infection. In older men, obstruction due to prostatic hypertrophy is usually the cause. Prompt initiation of appropriate antibiotic therapy is most important. The choice of antibiotics can be guided by the history and microscopic examination of a Gram-stained urine specimen. In the absence of definitive laboratory information, initial treatment with maximal doses of broad-spectrum antibiotics, such as gentamicin or tobramycin plus ampicillin or a cephalosporin, is indicated. Bladder catheterization may be necessary to relieve the obstruction or monitor urine flow. Intravenous infusion of bicarbonate solutions and Ringer's lactate or dextrose-in-saline solutions is needed acutely to correct acidosis, restore vascular volume, and maintain renal perfusion. Corticosteroids may protect against the lethal effects of endotoxin in experimental animals, but recent placebo-controlled trials have failed to support their use in most clinical situations. Agents that interfere with the action of cytokines (e.g., TNFα and IL-1β) that mediate the manifestations of septic shock are currently under investigation.

7. The answer is D. *(Chap 16.)* Primary *Pseudomonas* osteomyelitis is very unusual except in intravenous drug addicts, but it should be considered in a nail puncture wound that does not respond to local or oral antibiotic therapy. Ecthyma gangrenosum, an indurated black area approximately 1 cm in diameter with an ulcerated center and surrounding erythema, is highly suggestive of *Pseudomonas* bacteremia. *Pseudomonas* is the most common cause of chronic otitis externa, which usually responds to local measures. In diabetics, however, a rapidly invasive form may develop and require aggressive debridement and antibiotic therapy. *Escherichia coli* is the most frequent cause of gram-negative meningitis in neonatal infants. Development of *Pseudomonas* meningitis usually occurs only after introduction by surgery, trauma, or foreign objects such as shunts. *Pseudomonas* endocarditis may affect intravenous drug users or patients undergoing open-heart surgery.

8. The answer is D. *(Chap 184.)* This patient hails from an area where echinococcal infection is endemic. It is prevalent in areas where livestock is raised in association with dogs. Dogs, which are the definitive hosts, harbor the adult *E. granulosus* worm and pass eggs in their feces, which can then be ingested by the intermediate hosts, including sheep, cattle, and humans. After ingestion of the eggs, the hatched embryos enter the portal circulation and frequently travel to the liver or lungs. The larvae develop into fluid-filled hydatid cysts from which secondary cysts develop. A slowly enlarging mass ultimately develops. After 5 to 20 years the mass may enlarge to the point where it may cause symptoms, such as those due to compression of the bile duct. Leakage of cyst fluid into the biliary tree could also mimic recurrent cholelithiasis; episodic leakage from the cyst could produce a syndrome of fever, pruritus, and urticaria, or possibly even fatal anaphylaxis. The presence of daughter cysts within larger cysts and eggshell calcification in the wall of the cyst is essentially pathognomonic for *E. granulosus* infection and suggests that carcinoma, bacterial or amebic liver abscess, and hemangioma are less likely. Aspiration of the cyst may be conducted carefully for diagnostic purposes. Serology is not specific. Albendazole is not sufficiently effective to be used as a monotherapy. Surgery is indicated for such a space-occupying lesion, although the risks of anaphylaxis and dissemination of infectious scolices may be minimized by instilling ethanol into the cyst cavity.

9. The answer is B. *(Chap 80. Tompkins, N Engl J Med 327:1290–1297, 1992.)* Recombinant DNA technology has made it possible to identify specific microbial DNA sequences in clinical material. Although specific, this technique may be too sensitive in some cases and blur the distinction between infection and colonization. Probes have been developed for a wide variety of microorganisms, including CMV, EBV, hepatitis B virus, and HIV, as well as mycoplasma, chlamydia, legionella, and gonococci. These probes become even more sensitive with the use of the polymerase chain reaction to amplify specific sequences.

10. The answer is C. *(Chap 87. Black, Rev Infect Dis 12:S73, 1990.)* Toxigenic *Escherichia coli* is the major cause of diarrhea ("turista") for Americans abroad. *Staphylococcus aureus, Clostridium perfringens,* and *Bacillus cereus* cause various types of acute food poisoning owing to bacterial proliferation and elaboration of toxins in improperly stored food. Children throughout the developing world suffer acute diarrhea, similar to traveler's diarrhea, caused by rotavirus infection. All five of these agents cause watery diarrhea that generally is without blood, mucus, or fecal leukocytes, as opposed to illness caused by *Shigella, Salmonella,* or *Campylobacter,* which produces a more invasive, dysenteric type of disease.

11. The answer is A. *(Chap 82.)* Since BCG is a live attenuated organism and has been reported to cause disseminated infection in immunocompromised patients, it should not be administered to those with HIV infection or others with suspected immunodeficiency. Though patients with immune dysfunction often do not mount a good response to an administered vaccine, they should still receive certain preparations. Patients about to undergo splenectomy or cancer chemotherapy should, when possible, be vaccinated prior to therapy. Influenza vaccine should be given in autumn to those with any chronic medical illness in addition to those with obvious immune deficiency. The chronically ill, the immunosuppressed, and those at risk for infection with encapsulated microorganisms (e.g., anatomic or functional asplenia, multiple myeloma) should receive pneumococcal vaccine. The last group plus those with terminal complement component deficiencies should receive the quadrivalent meningococcal vaccine. Patients with HIV infection, especially those who are potential household contacts of children who are receiving the oral polio vaccine (attenuated live virus), should receive three doses of the inactivated polio vaccine.

12. **The answer is E.** *(Chap 178. NIH-University of California Expert Panel, N Engl J Med 323:1500, 1990.)* Patients with AIDS, premature malnourished infants, children with primary immunodeficiency diseases, and patients receiving immunosuppressive therapy (particularly corticosteroids for cancer or organ transplantation) are at risk for developing *Pneumocystis carinii* pneumonia. Usually confined to the lungs, disseminated infection can occur in up to 3 percent of patients. In this particular case, sputum obtained at bronchoalveolar lavage has yielded diagnostic material. Toludine blue, which also selectively stains the wall of the pneumocystis cyst, would have been appropriate as would immunofluorescent or immunoperoxidase staining. Further diagnostic studies are not required in this setting and treatment should be undertaken. For patients with severe hypoxemia, corticosteroids may be effective in mitigating immune-mediated lung damage. Steroids should be administered in conjunction with appropriate antimicrobial therapy, which includes either intravenous trimethoprim-sulfamethoxazole or intravenous pentamidine. Therapy should continue for 21 days in patients with AIDS. Aerosolized pentamidine is effective as prophylaxis but is not indicated in primary infections. Combination therapy with trimethoprim-sulfamethoxazole and pentamidine has not been shown to be more effective than either agent alone.

13. **The answer is B.** *(Chap 176. Kirchoff, N Engl J Med 329:639–644, 1993.)* This patient formerly resided in an area endemic for the protozoan parasite *Trypanosoma cruzi.* So-called American trypanosomiasis, or Chagas' disease, is found in almost all Latin American countries. Given the increased number of immigrants from these countries to the United States, the domestic prevalence of the infection is increasing. Transmission occurs by the bite of blood-sucking insects known as ruduviid bugs, in contrast to African trypanosomiasis (sleeping sickness), which is transmitted to humans by tsetse flies. The acute infection is self-limited and characterized by a mild febrile illness often associated with lymphadenopathy. Years or even decades later an estimated 10 to 30 percent of infected patients will be afflicted with symptomatic Chagas' disease. The heart is most commonly affected; manifestations include dilated biventricular cardiomyopathy, conduction disturbances, arrhythmias, and the development of mural thrombi complicated by thromboembolic phenomena. Dilation of the esophagus or colon can also be seen. The diagnosis is made by serology; active parasitic forms cannot be found in the peripheral blood. Treatment is supportive. Corticosteroids or the immunosuppression required for heart transplantation is contraindicated because of the possibility of reactivation and subsequent development of acute Chagas' disease. Prophylactic treatment with antitrypanosomal drugs such as benznidazole or nifurtimox is not effective enough to provide protection against acute infections.

14. **The answer is A.** *(Chap 102.)* The pathogenicity of staphylococci is related to a number of biologic properties, including the production of coagulase, catalase, exotoxin, and enterotoxin. Coagulase and catalase are thought to protect staphylococci within a host from being destroyed by phagocytes. Some staphylococcal strains produce exotoxins that can cause intraepidermal cleavage and bullae formation, as well as toxic shock syndrome. Other strains elaborate an enterotoxin that produces gastrointestinal disease. The production of penicillinase, though rendering a pathogenic organism harder to destroy pharmacologically, does not contribute to pathogenicity.

15. **The answer is A.** *(Chaps 102, 374.)* Probably because of its ubiquity and ability to stick to foreign surfaces, *Staphylococcus epidermidis* is the most frequent cause of infections of central nervous system shunts, as well as an important cause of infection on artificial heart valves and orthopedic prostheses. *Corynebacterium* species (diphtheroids), just like *S. epidermidis,* colonize the skin. When these organisms are isolated from cultures of shunts, it is often difficult to be sure if they are the cause of disease or simply contaminants. Leukocytosis in cerebrospinal fluid, consistent isolation of the same organism, and the character of a patient's symptoms all are helpful in deciding whether treatment for infection is indicated.

16. **The answer is D.** *(Chap 103.)* Streptococcal pharyngitis, usually caused by group A streptococci, is an exceedingly common bacterial infection, especially in school-age and adolescent children. Symptoms commonly include sudden sore throat and pain on swallowing, fever, headache, malaise, anorexia, nausea, and abdominal pain; aside from edema, erythema, and lymphoid hyperplasia of the posterior pharynx, physical signs also include tender, enlarged cervical lymph nodes. Because involvement of the larynx does not occur, loss of voice would not be expected. Eradication of pharyngeal streptococcal infection is important in the prevention of acute rheumatic fever.

17. **The answer is B.** *(Chap 109.)* Vaccines prepared from high-molecular-weight antigens of *Neisseria meningitidis,* serotypes A and C, have proved effective, but an effective group B vaccine is not available. Although sulfonamide resistance is an important problem in meningococcal epidemics with sulfonamide-sensitive organisms, sulfonamides remain a good choice for prophylaxis. When sulfonamide-resistant strains are isolated but the sensitivity of the organism is not known, rifampin therapy is generally recommended.

18. **The answer is A.** *(Chaps 16, 398. Caroff, Med Clin North Am 77:185, 1993.)* This patient is suffering from the neuroleptic malignant syndrome, which is characterized by muscle rigidity, autonomic dysregulation, and hyperthermia. The patient has probably been exposed to phenothiazines for the first time given his relatively recent admission to the psychiatric facility. This syndrome represents an idiosyncratic reaction to inhibition of central dopamine receptors, which results in increased heat production and a failure of heat dissipation. In addition to rapid physical cooling and administration of an antipyretic or acetaminophen (but not aspirin), the use of the dopamine agonist bromocriptine or dantrolene should be strongly considered. Dantrolene reverses the hypothalamic dysfunction caused by major tranquilizers.

19. **The answer is C.** *(Chap 116.)* *Pseudomonas* organisms can cause a rapidly invasive infection of the external ear that results in extensive bony erosion in diabetics. Aggressive surgical debridement and parenteral administration of antibiotics are required. *Aspergillus* organisms can be isolated frequently from external ear swabs but do not cause invasive disease. Mucormycosis must be considered in any seriously ill diabetic patient with sinus or ocular involvement. Infection usually spreads from the nasal cavity and does not involve the ears. Insulin-dependent diabetics are likely to have their skin colonized by *S. aureus,* but this is not associated with external otitis. *H. influenzae* is a frequent cause of otitis media, especially in children, but not of otitis externa.

20. **The answer is C.** *(Chap 117. Cherubin, Rev Infect Dis 13:343–344, 1991.)* *Salmonella typhi* survives well in food and water and generally causes infection by penetrating the intestinal mucosa and entering the bloodstream. Usually at the time that affected persons present with fever and

other signs of an acute illness, the white blood cell count is depressed. In contrast, rose spots usually do not occur until the second week of illness. Therapy with chloramphenicol does not prevent relapses but does alter the course of the acute illness. A chronic carrier state can develop in large part because of the propensity of *S. typhi* to seed and inhabit the gallbladder, especially in adults with gallstones. The fluoroquinolones are becoming the treatment of choice to eradicate the chronic carrier state.

21. The answer is D. *(Chap 82.)* HIV-infected persons in general have not demonstrated an increased risk of adverse events from inactivated vaccines; however, the immune response in such patients may not be sufficient for complete protection. Furthermore, most live vaccines are safe, except for the oral polio vaccine, for which an increased risk of virus proliferation and paralytic polio has been shown. The inactivated polio virus–enhanced (IPV-e) vaccine can be used for household contacts. The pneumococcal vaccine is a bacterial polysaccharide, the influenza vaccine is usually inactivated virus or a viral component, and the hepatitis B vaccine is a viral antigen; as such, these are quite safe in people who are immunocompromised. While the measles, mumps, and rubella vaccine contains live virus for each disease, no change in the usual immunization schedule is recommended for children who are HIV-infected. Nonetheless, if there is a documented exposure to measles, measles immunoglobulin should be administered.

22. The answer is B. *(Chap 82.)* Passive immunization can be used to provide temporary immunity in a person who is exposed to an infectious disease and has not been previously actively immunized. Standard human immune serum globulin does not contain known antibody content for a specific agent, unlike special immune serum globulins that exist for treatment of susceptible patients exposed to hepatitis B, varicella (which is indicated for postexposure prophylaxis of susceptible immunocompromised persons, susceptible pregnant women, and exposed newborn infants), rabies, tetanus, and cytomegalovirus (used in bone marrow and kidney transplant recipients). Intramuscular immune globulin can be used for hepatitis A pre- and postexposure prophylaxis as well as hepatitis non-A, non-B (C) postexposure prophylaxis; it is of questionable efficacy in postexposure prophylaxis for hepatitis B and rubella, but may have a role in postexposure prophylaxis for immunocompromised persons exposed to measles.

23. The answer is E. *(Chap 112. Farley, Ann Intern Med 116:806–812, 1992.)* Persons who have sickle-cell disease or agammaglobulinemia and those who have been splenectomized have immune systems that poorly opsonize encapsulated bacteria such as *Haemophilus influenzae*. *Haemophilus influenzae* infections also are more common in alcoholic persons, in part because of abnormal cellular defense mechanisms. Persons who have chronic granulomatous disease have problems combating infection with *Staphylococcus aureus*, *Salmonella*, and *Serratia*, but not *Haemophilus influenzae*. Other important risk factors for *Haemophilus influenzae* include pregnancy, steroid therapy, diabetes, and malignancy (with or without chemotherapy).

24. The answer is A. *(Chap 114.)* Because a marked lymphocytosis characteristically is observed in children (less commonly in older persons) who have *Haemophilus pertussis* infection (whooping cough) and is rare in other respiratory illnesses, white blood cell count with differential would be useful in making the diagnosis. Blood cultures would be negative, and Gram stain of the sputum and chest and neck x-rays would show nonspecific changes. The diagnosis of pertussis is confirmed in most cases by nasopharyngeal culture, though ELISA and DNA-based detection methods are alternative diagnostic procedures.

25. **The answer is E.** *(Chap 84.)*   Patients in the intensive care unit whose treatment includes prolonged intubation with a nasotracheal or nasogastric tube are at risk for the development of nosocomial sinusitis. Sinusitis in this setting may be due to obstruction of the ostia of the ethmoidal sinus by the tube. While the bacteriology of acute sinusitis generally includes *S. pneumoniae, H. influenzae,* and streptococci, gram-negative organisms must also be considered when an antibiotic therapy is planned for nosocomial sinusitis. Complications of sinusitis include osteomyelitis, cerebral abscess, subdural empyema, and cortical thrombophlebitis. In the case of cavernous sinus thrombosis, cranial nerve palsies (nerves III, IV, V, and VI) may be seen. Finally, as is the case with this patient, the infection may spread to the orbit from an infected ethmoidal sinus. This patient displays the characteristic findings of orbital sinusitis: pain, lid edema, and conjunctival chemosis (erythema and swelling). Coverage is required for all potential pathogens, including organisms that would routinely cause sinusitis, *S. aureus* and gram-negative enteric organisms. An important additional step is the removal of the obstructing tube.

26. **The answer is E.** *(Chap 84.)*   This young adult is presenting with acute bacterial epiglottitis with symptoms highly suggestive of impending severe upper airway obstruction. Because the airway is larger in an adult than a child with a similar clinical scenario, tracheotomy is usually not necessary, but the possibility of complete airway obstruction still exists. Fiberoptic examination, contraindicated in children, may confirm the diagnosis in adults. The findings include an edematous, cherry-red epiglottis with surrounding edematous pharyngeal mucosa. In children a lateral radiograph of the neck will reveal an enlarged epiglottis, the so-called thumb sign. In adults, fiberoptic examination should be performed only after preparations have been made for endotracheal intubation or tracheotomy. The patient should be admitted to an intensive care unit where adequate monitoring is available. In addition to confirmation of the diagnosis, administration of intravenous antibiotics (i.e., cefuroxime or cefotaxime), oxygen, humidified air by face tent, and possibly (but not definitively) glucocorticoids should be performed. Discharge from the intensive care unit should not occur until the acute cellulitis has resolved.

27. **The answer is E.** *(Chap 163.)*   Coccidioidomycosis, caused by the inhalation of *Coccidioides immitis,* may present clinically with manifestations of hypersensitivity reactions. Arthralgias and frank arthritis (so-called desert rheumatism) as well as such skin reactions as erythema nodosum and erythema multiforme are associated far more frequently with coccidioidomycosis than with the other mycoses listed in the question. Delayed hypersensitivity to *C. immitis* antigens tends to be a good prognostic sign.

28. **The answer is D.** *(Chap 100.)*   Imipenem is a novel β-lactam antibiotic in the carbapenem class with activity against most gram-positive organisms, including those that produce β-lactamase. In addition to most strains of *Pseudomonas,* imipenem inhibits the growth of *B. fragilis.* This drug must be given intravenously because of its instability in gastric acid. Since imipenem is hydrolyzed in the renal tubule by dihydropeptidase I, the coadministration of cilastatin, an inhibitor of this enzyme, serves to markedly boost levels of this broad-spectrum antibiotic. Clavulanate is a β-lactamase inhibitor used with partial success when combined with amoxicillin (Augmentin) for treatment of resistant otitis and urinary tract infections.

29. **The answer is C.** *(Chap 126.)*   This patient is chronically immunosuppressed from his antirejection prophylactic regimen, which includes both corticosteroids and azathioprine. However, the finding of a cavitary lesion on chest x-ray considerably narrows the possibilities and increases the likelihood of nocardial infection. The other clinical findings including production of profuse, thick sputum, fever, and constitutional symptoms, are also quite common in patients who have pulmonary nocardiosis. The Gram stain, which demonstrates filamentous gram-positive organisms, is characteristic. Most species of *Nocardia* are acid-fast if a weak acid is used for decolorization (e.g., modified Kinyoun method). These organisms can also be visualized by silver staining. They

grow slowly in culture and the laboratory must be alerted to the possibility of their presence on submitted specimens. Once the diagnosis, which may require an invasive approach, is made, sulfonamides are the drugs of choice. Sulfadiazine or sulfisoxazole from 6 to 8 g/d in four divided doses is generally administered, but doses up to 12 g/d have been given. The combination of sulfamethoxazole and trimethoprim has also been used as have the oral alternatives minocycline and ampicillin and intravenous amikacin. There is little experience with the newer β-lactam antibiotics including the third-generation cephalosporins or imipenem. Erythromycin alone is not effective, though it has been given successfully along with ampicillin. In addition to appropriate antibiotic therapy, the possibility of disseminated nocardiosis must also be considered; sites include brain, skin, kidneys, bone, and muscle.

30. **The answer is A.** *(Chap 119.)* Campylobacters are motile, curved gram-negative rods. The principal diarrheal pathogen is *C. jejuni*. This organism is found within the gastrointestinal tract of many animals used for food production and is usually transmitted to humans in raw or undercooked food products or through direct contact with infected animals. Over half the cases are due to insufficiently cooked, contaminated poultry. *Campylobacter* is a common cause of diarrheal disease in the United States. The illness usually occurs within 2 to 4 days after exposure to the organism in food or water. Biopsy of an affected patient's jejunum, ileum, or colon reveals findings indistinguishable from those of Crohn's disease or ulcerative colitis. While the diarrheal illness is usually self-limited, it may be associated with constitutional symptoms, last more than 1 week, and recur in 5 to 10 percent of untreated patients. Complications include pancreatitis, cystitis, arthritis, meningitis, and Guillain-Barré syndrome. The symptoms of *Campylobacter* enteritis are similar to those due to infection with *Salmonella, Shigella,* and *Yersinia;* all these agents cause fever and the presence of fecal leukocytes. The diagnosis is made by isolating *Campylobacter* from the stool, which requires selective media. *E. coli* (enterotoxogenic) is not generally associated with the finding of fecal leukocytes, nor is the Norwalk agent. *Campylobacter* is a far more common cause of a recurrent relapsing diarrheal illness that could be pathologically confused with inflammatory bowel disease than are *Yersinia, Salmonella, Shigella,* and enteropathogenic *E. coli.*

31. **The answer is E.** *(Chap 112.)* *Haemophilus ducreyi* causes painful genital ulcers, which begin as small tender papules. In contrast, syphilitic ulcers are usually painless, and the initial lesions of genital herpes simplex infections are usually vesicular. The organism causing the chancroid can be isolated from both the ulcers and affected lymph nodes; in fact, culturing the lymph nodes may produce a pure culture of this organism. Unlike infection with other members of the genus *Haemophilus,* chancroid is not effectively treated with ampicillin. Trimethoprim-sulfamethoxazole and erythromycin are the antibiotic agents of choice.

32. **The answer is D.** *(Chap 169.)* Patients who have localized sporotrichosis can be treated successfully with potassium iodide. However, systemic infections, particularly pneumonia in immunocompromised persons, should be treated with amphotericin B. Untreated persons can develop chronic sporotrichosis. Itraconazole may also be effective in this condition.

33. **The answer is B.** *(Chap 112.)* The classic organisms responsible for subacute bacterial endocarditis following a dental procedure are viridans streptococci. However, certain *Haemophilus* species as well as other members of the so-called HACEK group, fastidious organisms that require incubation in an atmosphere containing carbon dioxide, may also account for infective endocarditis in patients with underlying valvular disease or prosthetic valves or those who have used intravenous drugs. Vegetations may be large and embolization is not infrequent. Therapy should be based on antibiotic sensitivity, though initial treatment with ampicillin and an immunoglycoside in combination is recommended. Blood cultures must be observed for at least 7 days because of the slow growth of these organisms. The HACEK group includes *Haemophilus aphrophilus, H. paraphrophilus, H. parainfluenzae, Actinobacillus actinomycetemcomitans, Cardiobacterium hominis, Eikenella corrodens,* and *Kingella kingae.*

34. The answer is A. *(Chaps 91, 110.)*   One of the most common causes of infectious arthritis in young adults, particularly in urban medical centers, is gonococcal infection. Entry occurs via sites of sexual contact, either the genitourinary tract, oropharynx, or rectum. Infection at one of these sites, particularly in menstruating females, pregnant women, or those with complement deficiencies, may lead to dissemination. Such an occurrence produces a biphasic illness first manifested by constitutional symptoms, migratory arthritis (particularly in the knee, shoulder, wrists, and interphalangeal joints of the hand), tenosynovitis, and vesiculopustular skin lesions. While these symptoms may abate, joint involvement may progress to a purulent mono- or polyarticular arthritis. Synovial culture and Gram stain are usually negative early in the course of the illness, but may be positive at later stages. Blood cultures may be positive, but only in the early stage of the illness. Complement deficiencies are present only in those patients who have congenital hypocomplementemia. Gonococci are demonstrable by Gram stain in the skin lesions in about two-thirds of cases. However, diagnosis is best made by observing the intracellular gram-negative diplococci in leukocytes from Gram-stained smears of urethral or endocervical exudates. Because of the presence of other gram-negative diplococci in normal oral flora, Gram stains of pharyngeal smears are not specific. Selective media, such as Thayer-Martin, should be used to culture gonococcus from the urethra, endocervix, pharynx, or rectum. The endocervical culture is positive in 80 to 90 percent of women with gonorrhea. Treatment for disseminated gonococcal infection includes hospitalization and administration of either ceftriaxone, ceftizoxime, or cefotaxime. If the patient is proved to have gonorrhea, a serologic test for syphilis and confidential testing for HIV infection should also be undertaken.

35. The answer is B. *(Chap 122.)*   Aspiration and culture of an enlarged axillary lymph node would be most helpful in yielding a diagnosis of tularemia in the case described. Blood and bone-marrow cultures rarely are positive for *Francisella (Pasteurella) tularensis.* Agglutinin reactions ordinarily are not positive for a least 1 week after infection. A wide variety of animals and insects can transmit tularemia to humans.

36. The answer is D. *(Chap 123.)*   In the case presented, the diagnosis of plague (*Yersinia pestis* infection) must be considered. To make this diagnosis, affected lymph nodes should be aspirated and the contents Gram-stained. In most cases of bubonic plague, lymph-node aspirates teem with pleomorphic gram-negative bacilli, which can be definitively identified by immunofluorescent staining of the specimen. Blood culture, bone-marrow examination, and lymph-node biopsy might be used to diagnose plague, but with undue delay. In this situation, great care should be exercised in handling the infected materials—there is a significant risk of infection for the laboratory workers.

37. The answer is D. *(Chap 146. Emmanuel, Ann Intern Med 109:777, 1988.)*   Cytomegalovirus (CMV), a double-stranded herpes virus, is transmitted by intimate contact. Once infected, a patient carries the virus for life with actual disease only occurring in the setting of immunosuppression. However, congenital CMV infections may result in significant psychomotor, hearing, ocular, or developmental abnormalities. Secondly, the most common clinical manifestation of CMV infection, CMV mononucleosis, occurs in normal hosts and resembles the mononucleosis syndrome caused by Epstein-Barr virus, although pharyngitis and lymphadenopathy are much less common with CMV infection. The bone marrow transplant recipient described in the question is clearly at increased risk for CMV-associated syndromes, which may include fever and leukopenia, hepatitis, pneumonitis, esophagitis, gastritis, colitis, and retinitis. Risk factors for infection in transplant patients include the presence of graft-vs-host disease, older age, and known CMV seropositivity in the recipient. Pneumonitis is often manifested by tachypnea, hypoxia, and nonproductive cough. Chest x-ray may reveal bilateral interstitial or reticulonodular infiltrates, particularly beginning in the lower lobes. Since the number of organisms that cause such diffuse pulmonary changes in the posttransplant setting is large, it is important to determine the specific diagnosis. Virus isolation from the specimen obtained at bronchoscopy would be the ideal way to make the diagnosis, but cultures may be falsely negative and results take several days to return. Cytomegalic cells, demonstrated at open-lung biopsy, are the pathologic hallmark of CMV infection. Cytomegalic cells are characterized by large size and the presence of an 8- to 10-μm intranuclear inclusion that is centrally placed and sometimes surrounded by a clear halo ("owl's eye" appearance). Cytoplasmic inclusions may also be found. The use of blood from seronegative donors, deglycerolized packed red blood cells, and leukoreduced transfusions may all reduce the risk of transfusion-associated CMV in the posttransplant period. Other prophylactic measures include the use of acyclovir (in high doses) or the use of immunoglobulin. The best results for an active infection have been obtained with the use of ganciclovir, a drug similar in structure to acyclovir, but with more activity against CMV than the parent compound. While ganciclovir alone has been most effective for the treatment of CMV retinitis or colitis, in bone marrow transplant patients who develop CMV pneumonia, ganciclovir is more effective when combined with CMV immunoglobulin. Prolonged therapy may be required. Foscarnet inhibits viral DNA polymerase and may be effective in ganciclovir-resistant CMV infections. Foscarnet is considerably more toxic than is ganciclovir; side effects include renal failure, electrolyte wasting, seizures, and fever.

38.   The answer is B.   *(Chap 142. Whitley, N Engl J Med 327:782–789, 1992.)*   Acyclovir is one of the most important antiviral agents currently available. It is converted by herpes virus–encoded thymidine kinase to acyclovir monophosphate and then subsequently to the triphosphate form. This process does not occur in uninfected mammalian cells. Acyclovir triphosphate inhibits viral DNA synthesis much more specifically than it does cellular DNA polymerase. The drug is active against herpes simplex virus type I, herpes simplex virus type II, and varicella-zoster virus. Intravenous acyclovir is highly effective for the first episode of genital herpes and will result in a significant reduction in the duration of viral shedding and in the length of time to complete healing. However, because of the requirement for hospitalization, such therapy should be reserved for patients who are severely affected. On the other hand, recurrent genital herpes, even when severe, is only slightly improved after the administration of oral acyclovir and there is no known role for intravenous acyclovir. Most patients with allogeneic bone marrow transplants currently receive acyclovir prophylaxis. However, in those patients who develop mucocutaneous herpes in the peritransplant period, intravenous acyclovir should be administered. Oral acyclovir will reduce the duration of new lesions in patients with chickenpox and does improve constitutional symptoms. Intravenous use is certainly not appropriate for the average youngster who develops chickenpox, but intravenous acyclovir has been shown to improve the outcome in immunocompromised children with chickenpox. The increased frequency of morbidity in immunocompromised adults who develop herpes zoster, even dermatomal, suggests that intravenous acyclovir therapy is indicated. Severely immunocompromised patients, such as those receiving combination chemotherapy, including steroids, for large cell lymphoma, or marrow transplant recipients should be treated with intravenous acyclovir even in cases when dissemination is not apparent.

39.   The answer is A.   *(Chap 113.)*   Legionnaire's disease is caused by *Legionella pneumophila*. It occurs sporadically or in outbreaks and often begins with myalgias, headache, and fever. Diarrhea and delirium also are early features in many cases. Gastrointestinal symptoms should suggest the possibility of this diagnosis, particularly in persons who have severe pneumonia, scant production of sputum, and other extrapulmonary abnormalities. Of the other organisms listed in the question, all can cause pneumonia; *Mycoplasma pneumoniae* infection is most likely to be confused with Legionnaire's disease.

40. The answer is D. *(Chap 105.)* *Listeria monocytogenes* is a gram-positive motile bacillus that tends to infect infants as well as persons over the age of 55 years. Major illnesses in both groups are meningitis and other forms of central nervous system infection. Many of the older patients are immunosuppressed because of disease (e.g., cancer), immunosuppressive drug therapy, or both. Endocarditis, peritonitis, hepatitis, and conjunctivitis also can be caused by *Listeria* infection.

41. The answer is D. *(Chap 80.)* It is important to alert the microbiology laboratory to the clinical suspicions of the ordering physician. Stool for routine culture, which includes incubation on MacConkey's medium, will detect *Salmonella, Shigella,* and other Enterobacteriaceae. If *Campylobacter, Yersinia,* or *Vibrio* species are suspected, appropriate enrichment techniques and, in the case of *Vibrio* species, appropriate collection and transport methods must be employed.

42. The answer is D. *(Chap 181.)* Infection with intestinal nematodes is extraordinarily common worldwide, particularly in tropical developing countries. Usually, large worm burdens are required to elicit clinical manifestations of disease. However, in the case of *Ascaris lumbricoides,* single worms (reaching up to 40 cm in length) can cause biliary obstruction or cholecystitis. *Ascaris* is transmitted by the hand-to-mouth fecal carriage route with subsequent larval development followed by hematogenous migration to the lungs (possibly resulting in eosinophilic pneumonitis [Loeffler's syndrome]). On the other hand, hookworm larvae are hatched in the soil, where, after a 1-week development period, the infectious filariform larvae penetrate the skin and reach the lungs by way of the bloodstream. They are then swallowed and may reach the small intestine, where they produce epigastric pain, diarrhea, and iron deficiency if the worm burden is high enough. Unlike other nematodes, *Strongyloides* replicates in humans, which permits many cycles of autoinfection with intestinal production of larvae. These infections can persist for decades. As is the case for hookworms, *Strongyloides* larvae hatch in the soil, penetrate the skin or mucous membranes, and ultimately reach the small intestine. Migrating larvae may elicit a pathognomonic serpiginous eruption, which can cause intense pruritus and may be recurrent over a period of many years. Nausea, diarrhea, bleeding, colitis, and weight loss may also be seen with high-burden *Strongyloides* infection. Many American schoolchildren are infected with pinworm (*Enterobius vermicularis*). Eggs are released only in the perianal region and may be transmitted by hand to mouth to complete the life cycle. Perianal pruritus is the most typical clinical symptom. The diagnosis may be made by applying clear cellulose tape to the perianal region in the morning and transferring the tape to a microscopic slide where the characteristic pinworm eggs may be demonstrated.

43. The answer is C. *(Chap 172.)* Most antimalarial drugs—including quinine, 4-aminoquinolines (e.g., chloroquine, hydroxychloroquine), and 4-quinoline-methanols (e.g., mefloquine)—concentrate in erythrocytes and thereby destroy the intracellular schizonts responsible for the acute manifestations of malarial illness. However, these drugs do not readily concentrate in the liver, and they therefore allow survival of hepatic schizonts and reinfection at a later date. In contrast, primaquine, an 8-aminoquinoline, can eradicate hepatic parasites but is not effective in acute illness.

44. The answer is D. *(Chap 87.)* Bacteria that cause diarrhea via elaboration of toxins are generally associated with a shorter time from ingestion to illness than are invasive strains. For example, enterotoxigenic *E. coli* (the most common cause of traveler's diarrhea), *C. perfringens* (associated with poorly cooked meat or poultry), *S. aureus* (associated with improperly refrigerated dairy foods), and *B. cereus* (associated with grossly contaminated uncooked rice) all have incubation periods of 24 h or less. Even though the pathogenesis may depend on direct mucosal damage, *V. parahaemolyticus,* which is present in inadequately cooked seafood, can cause a diarrheal illness within 6 to 48 h after consumption of a contaminated food. Ingestion of water contaminated with the intestinal flora of wild or domestic animals may cause infection with *C. jejuni*, a frequent cause of acute, sometimes bloody diarrhea. The incubation period for this invasive bacterium is 2 to 6 days, longer than that associated with other pathogens. Therapy is usually supportive, though erythromycin will shorten the duration of illness.

45. **The answer is A.** *(Chap 162. Wheat, Medicine 69:361, 1990.)* The patient in question is presumably an HIV-infected man with acute disseminated histoplasmosis, often mistaken for miliary tuberculosis because of its similar pattern of constitutional findings and diffuse chest x-ray abnormalities. Indurated ulcers of the mouth, tongue, nose, or larynx also occur in about 25 percent of patients with acute disseminated histoplasmosis. Addison's disease, granulomatous hepatitis, gastrointestinal ulcerations, endocarditis, or chronic meningitis may also be seen. Since patients with HIV infection may present with febrile syndromes on the basis of multiple organisms and since serologic tests for histoplasmosis are plagued by frequent false negative and false positive results, definitive diagnosis requires demonstration of the organism by culture or histology. The classic morphology of hyphae that bear large and small spores in this clinical setting is diagnostic. Treatment requires prolonged administration of amphotericin B.

46. **The answer is C.** *(Chap 137. Spach, N Engl J Med 329:936–947, 1993.)* Ninety percent of cases of Lyme disease (Lyme borreliosis) have occurred in northeastern coastal states. The principal vectors for the causative agent of this disease, *Borrelia burgdorferi*, are the *Ixodes* ticks. Less than half the patients with Lyme disease recall receiving a tick bite. Most infections occur during the months of May to August when human outdoor activities are maximal and coincide with the time when nymphal *Ixodes* ticks are most active. Like syphilis, another spirochete-mediated disease, the affliction occurs in stages. The initial localized stage is frequently characterized by a macular dermatitis, erythema migrans, which develops at the site of the tick bite. The incubation period is 7 to 10 days and is frequently accompanied by constitutional symptoms. Erythema migrans is typically oval, well demarcated, and more than 5 cm in diameter. Within a few days to weeks after initial infection, dissemination occurs. The most frequent neurologic manifestation of early disseminated Lyme disease is cranial neuritis, especially facial palsy. Peripheral neuropathy or lymphocytic meningitis may also occur. Nonneurologic manifestations of Lyme disease include atrioventricular block, myopericarditis, and chronic arthritis. The diagnosis is generally made on clinical grounds; however, the most specific diagnostic test for Lyme disease is isolation of the causative organism from blood or erythematous lesions. An ELISA-based antibody test is frequently plagued by false positive and false negative results. Detection of the presence of the organism by a DNA-based method (polymerase chain reaction) remains experimental.

47. **The answer is A.** *(Chap 130.)* The diagnosis of a tuberculous pleural effusion is suggested by the following set of pleural-fluid findings: color, clear yellow; pH, < 7.20; protein, > 30 g/L; glucose, < 1.2 mmol/L (25 mg/dL); lactate dehydrogenase (LDH), > 450 U/mL; and a lymphocytosis. Tubercle bacilli rarely are identified on a smear of infected pleural fluid, and cultures are positive in no more than one-quarter of cases. Antituberculous treatment should commence as soon as the diagnosis is suspected.

48. **The answer is A.** *(Chap 132.)* Two of the lesser-known species of *Mycobacterium, M. scrofulaceum* and *M. avium-intracellulare,* cause lymphadenitis in children. Lymph nodes that drain the buccal mucosa are usually affected. Both *M. scrofulaceum* and *M. avium-intracellulare* respond poorly to chemotherapy. Treatment of choice, therefore, is prompt lymph-node excision before rupture has occurred.

49. The answer is C. *(Chap 100. Hoper, N Engl J Med 324:384–394, 1991.)* The fluoroquinolones are an important new class of antimicrobial agents with excellent bioavailability. They are renally excreted and their concentrations do increase in chronic renal failure, but generally not to toxic levels. Adverse effects are rare; gastrointestinal symptoms, headache, sleep disturbances, and allergic reactions occur in less than 4 percent of patients. Theophylline clearance is inhibited by these agents and care must be taken if coadministration is necessary. Their mechanism of action is novel: they appear to inhibit bacterial topoisomerase II (also known as DNA gyrase), an enzyme involved in the uncoiling of DNA. Their spectrum of activity includes most Enterobacteriaceae, *H. influenzae, Neisseria* species, *Pseudomonas aeruginosa,* and *Staphylococcus aureus* (including the penicillin-resistant variety). In addition, activity against *Chlamydia, Mycoplasma,* and *Legionella* species has been demonstrated. They are bactericidal and have a wide range of potential roles, but they may be preferred in complicated urinary tract infections (because of their excellent concentration in the urine with activity against many otherwise difficult-to-treat species), chronic *Salmonella* carriage, exacerbation of cystic fibrosis (because of excellent activity against *Pseudomonas aeruginosa*), gram-negative osteomyelitis, and malignant otitis externa. Finally, fluoroquinolone antibiotics may be the treatment of choice for patients with bacterial gastroenteritis who are ill enough to require treatment. These agents are effective against enterotoxigenic *E. coli,* which often causes traveler's diarrhea, as well as *Shigella.*

50. The answer is C. *(Chap 133. Hook, N Engl J Med 326:1060–1069, 1992.)* Syphilis, like other diseases associated with genital ulcers, is more common in HIV-infected patients probably because of the increased efficiency of HIV inoculation via the ulcer itself. It is unclear, however, if syphilis in patients coinfected with HIV actually follows an accelerated clinical course. Though the serologic analysis of syphilis in patients with HIV infection is altered, accurate information is still provided for most patients with HIV infection. Significantly higher serum antitreponemal titers have been reported in patients with HIV compared with those not infected with the virus. Patients with documented secondary syphilis may fail to exhibit positive serology. False positive serologic studies are also possible in HIV-infected patients who may exhibit polyclonal B-cell activation early in the course of their infection. It has been consistently shown that single-dose penicillin therapy of early syphilis is more prone to failure in HIV-infected patients than in those who are not infected with the virus. It is particularly troubling that the central nervous system may be a sanctuary from penicillin.

51. The answer is D. *(Chap 132.)* *Mycobacterium marinum* is known as the "swimming pool" or "fishtank" bacillus because ulcerative cutaneous infections can be acquired from contact with contaminated swimming pools and aquariums. *M. ulcerans* also causes ulcerative skin lesions but characteristically is confined to tropical regions. Other "atypical" mycobacteria that cause cutaneous infections in humans include *M. avium-intracellulare, M. scrofulaceum, M. kansasii,* and *M. fortuitum.*

52. The answer is C. *(Chap 113.)* Person-to-person spread of *Legionella pneumophila* has not been documented. Gastrointestinal symptoms that precede pneumonia are sometimes a clue to the diagnosis. In many cases, chest x-ray shows dense infiltrates despite a paucity of physical signs, such as rales or rhonchi; in this regard, the disease resembles *Mycoplasma* pneumonia. Although *L. pneumophila* has been found in vitro to be sensitive to several drugs, erythromycin is the treatment of choice.

53. The answer is A. *(Chap 173. Reed, Am J Med 90:269, 1991.)* AIDS patients, particularly homosexual men, have a significant incidence of infection with *Entamoeba* species, though they are frequently asymptomatic. The most common amebic-related syndrome is that of colitis. Extraintestinal infection by the organism *E. histolytica* usually involves the liver. While the symptoms (fever, pain in the right upper quadrant, and pleural effusion) and the radiologic findings (hypoechoic hepatic cysts) are nonspecific and could also be seen in bacterial abscesses or cancer, such symptoms in a patient with positive serology are quite helpful in making the diagnosis of invasive amebiasis. For that reason, no further diagnostic studies are indicated in the patient. Except in patients with threatened imminent rupture of the cyst, drainage or aggressive aspiration is not necessary. The drug of choice is metronidazole, though the less effective agent chloroquine might also be considered.

54. The answer is A. *(Chap 161.)* Successful treatment of antifungal infections is not as straightforward as that for bacterial infections. The topical imidazoles that are available for treatment of vaginal candidiasis include miconazole, clotrimazole, and butoconazole; the triazole terconazole is also available. No substantial difference in efficacy or toxicity among these agents has been noted. Ketoconazole therapy is useful in the treatment of several fungal infections, including esophageal candidiasis, but is associated with several dose-related toxicities including inhibition of steroidogenesis in the adrenal cortex or gonads and hepatotoxicity. Fluconazole is an orally administered triazole that may have activity in candidal infection. Amphotericin B itself is a difficult drug to administer because of frequent toxicities including azotemia, anemia, hypokalemia, nausea, anorexia, weight loss, phlebitis, and hypomagnesemia. Nonetheless, amphotericin B is indicated for treatment of invasive infections such as candidal hepatitis. Given a daily dose of about 0.5 mg/kg and the requirement that at least 2 g of the drug should be given in this situation, prolonged therapy is required. Flucytosine, a synthetic oral drug converted to the antimetabolite 5-FU in the fungal cell, may aid in the treatment of refractory invasive candidal disease not responsive to amphotericin B alone. Flucytosine is not substituted for, but is rather added to amphotericin B. Patients on flucytosine should be monitored carefully, since this drug may be myelosuppressive.

55. The answer is E. *(Chap 113.)* Since the recognition of *Legionella pneumophila,* many other species of *Legionella* have been discovered. These organisms can be detected by silver staining, immunofluorescent staining, and culture of infected materials. It is much better to culture lung tissue or pleural fluid than sputum because sputum contains a mixture of other organisms that tend to overgrow *Legionella.* Aside from direct methods of diagnosis, serologic tests run on paired serum specimens also are useful. Detecting genomic DNA common to all *Legionella* species can be accomplished with a radiolabeled nucleic acid hybridization kit; false positives have been reported. Direct fluorescent antibody staining is specific but relatively insensitive.

56. The answer is A. *(Chap 88. Krockta, Infect Dis Clin North Am 1:217, 1987.)* The presence of vesicles in addition to ulcerative lesions strongly suggests herpes simplex infection. If no vesicles are present, dark-field examination should be performed in order to diagnose syphilis. In all other patients a serologic test for syphilis should be performed. Without a documented etiology after the preceding evaluation, especially with the association of painful lymphadenopathy, additional diagnostic tests are required. Such tests may include a viral culture to define occult herpetic infection, a bacterial culture on special media to isolate *Haemophilus ducreyi* (chancroid), or biopsy to rule out malignancy, lymphogranuloma venereum, and donovanosis (granuloma inguinale).

57. The answer is D. *(Chap 150.)* While the clinical syndromes induced by viruses that cause upper respiratory illness are not sufficiently distinct to delineate which virus is the cause of a given clinical syndrome, knowledge of the epidemiologic setting does aid in diagnosis. Rhinoviruses are a frequent cause of the common cold. They are spread by direct contact with infected secretions and efficiently transmitted by hand-to-hand contact. Rhinoviral infections are generally uncomplicated; the incubation period is about 2 days. Respiratory syncytial virus (RSV) infections are a major cause of lower respiratory disease in infants, but the virus may also infect older children and adults. Reinfection with this agent is frequent. Though most patients recover in a week or two, occasionally more severe illness may develop and require admission to an intensive care unit. The diagnosis of RSV infection can be made by culturing the agent from nasal swabs or respiratory secretions or by demonstrating the preserved anti-RSV antibodies. While therapy for RSV infection is mainly symptomatic, aerosolized ribavirin will speed resolution in affected infants. Adenoviruses are also a common cause of upper respiratory infection in infants, children, and adults, especially in military personnel. There is no active therapy available for this infection; however, live viral vaccines, which have been administered to military recruits, may be useful.

58. The answer is D. *(Chap 160.)* Lymphocytic choriomeningitis (LCM) virus is an RNA virus associated with both an influenza-like illness manifested by rash, arthritis, or orchitis and aseptic meningitis. These two syndromes may occur simultaneously or consecutively. Mice and other rodents are the major natural hosts for LCM infection. Human infections generally are due to residence in a rodent-infested house, but laboratory animals and pets may also be vectors. The mode of entry is the respiratory tract with subsequent penetration of the blood-brain barrier. An influenza-like illness may resolve but be followed by arthralgias (particularly in the hands), hair loss, testicular pain or orchitis, bradycardia, pharyngeal injection, and occasionally axillary adenopathy. Most patients recover within 1 to 4 weeks, though those who develop encephalitis have a significant risk of long-term neurologic sequelae. Laboratory findings include leukopenia and thrombocytopenia (during the first week of the illness). In those with meningeal signs examination of the CSF reveals lymphocytosis (up to 1000 lymphocytes/μL), as well as elevated CSF protein and a normal or low glucose, a finding unusual in nonbacterial infections. Culturing the virus from blood or the spinal fluid requires a biosafety level 3 facility; antibody detection methods are available. Since there is no specific treatment available, supportive care is the optimum approach.

59. The answer is C. *(Chap 136.)* Relapsing fever can be diagnosed by finding spirochetal borreliae in a peripheral blood smear with Wright's stain. Sometimes it is necessary to examine thick smears or to use phase microscopy to see the organisms. In the western United States, especially in areas where tick bites are likely to occur, relapsing fever should be suspected in persons with acute febrile illnesses characterized by headache, photophobia, and muscle pains.

60. The answer is A. *(Chap 127.)* In the examination of purulent material from persons suspected of having actinomyosis, it is important to search the material for the characteristic "sulfur grains" and then to examine the grains for organisms. Actinomycetes are gram-positive, branching organisms. If they are detected in a patient presenting with a suggestive clinical picture, such as a chronic draining sinus in the oropharyngeal area, the gastrointestinal tract, or the pelvic area, then the diagnosis of actinomycosis is confirmed.

61. The answer is E. *(Chap 129.)* MAI infections are often considered to be rapidly fatal in patients with AIDS. Until recently there was no effective treatment. However, the new macrolide antibiotic clarithromycin (6-O-methylerythromycin) appears to be the best available drug for disseminated MAI infections in those with AIDS. It is similar to erythromycin in its mechanism of action but does not cause the gastrointestinal distress seen after exposure to the parent compound. Because the MAI organism may acquire resistance to clarithromycin, it should be combined with other antimycobacterial agents such as ethambutol or rifampin or both. The standard dose of clarithromycin is 500 mg twice daily. Standard triple-drug therapy with isoniazid, rifampin, and ethambutol may be useful for the treatment of MAI lung disease in HIV-negative patients.

62. The answer is D. *(Chap 142. Hirsch, N Engl J Med 328:1686-1695, 1993.)* The three available antiretroviral drugs are nonnucleoside inhibitors of viral reverse transcriptase. AZT has been shown to be effective in patients with advanced AIDS; several studies have suggested that its use in patients with low CD4 cell counts (prior to the development of frank AIDS) is beneficial. Nonetheless, because of some recently negative results in patients with early HIV infection, the optimum time to begin therapy is unclear. The current recommendations in the U.S. are to begin therapy with AZT in all HIV-infected patients whose CD4 counts drop below 500/μL. The major side effects of treatment with AZT include anemia and leukopenia, which may respond to therapy with erythropoietin or granulocyte colony stimulating factor (G-CSF). However, the most important problem associated with long-term use of this drug is its lack of continued efficacy, probably due to the acquisition of viral resistance. ddI, like AZT, is a pro-drug that requires phosphorylation for activation, and it is useful in patients who are intolerant of AZT. Its side-effect profile differs from that of AZT in that neuropathy is much more common than with AZT. ddC is currently not approved for use as a single agent for the treatment of HIV infection, but rather it should be used in conjunction with AZT in patients with low CD4 counts who are clinically deteriorating.

63. The answer is C. *(Chap 165.)* Initial diagnosis of cryptococcal meningitis usually is based on finding encapsulated yeast on an India ink preparation. This test, however, is positive in only about half of cases in which the diagnosis is eventually made. Testing of serum and cerebrospinal fluid for cryptococcal antigen is a very helpful adjunctive test because antigen is found in about 90 percent of cases. In pulmonary cryptococcosis, only about one-third of affected persons are antigen-positive.

64. The answer is E. *(Chaps 88, 110.)* Because of the emergence of antibiotic-resistant strains of *Neisseria gonorrhoeae,* the Centers for Disease Control (CDC) published new guidelines for treatment of gonorrhea in 1989. The antibiotic resistance could be on the basis of penicillinase production, plasmid-encoded tetracycline resistance, or chromosomally mediated resistance to both drugs. Also prompting the new guidelines were requirements for effective single-dose therapy and the frequent coexistence of chlamydial infection. Therefore, a single intramuscular dose of ceftriaxone plus a 7-day course of doxycycline (or tetracycline) represents the currently recommended therapy for uncomplicated infection. Erythromycin should be substituted for tetracycline in the pregnant female. Intravenous therapy is probably required in most cases of disseminated gonococcal infection.

65. The answer is E. *(Chaps 96, 166. Thaler, Ann Intern Med 198:88, 1988.)* This patient represents a classic case of hepatic candidiasis, which might be better termed *disseminated candidiasis* because in addition to hepatic involvement the disease also often involves other tissues such as the kidneys. Prolonged neutropenia with concomitant administration of broad-spectrum antibacterial antibiotics, especially during induction therapy for acute myeloid leukemia, is an important risk factor for the development of invasive candidiasis. A fever that develops around the time of neutrophil recovery, especially if associated with pain of the right upper quadrant or elevated alkaline phosphatase (which should be proved to be of hepatic origin), is strongly suggestive of hepatic candidiasis. Definitive diagnosis depends upon documentation of yeast or pseudohyphae in a granulomatous lesion obtained from infected tissue. Empiric amphotericin B may be indicated. While a CT or MRI scan may reveal "bull's eye" lesions, a tissue diagnosis is required. If the liver biopsy was nonspecific and failed to reveal organisms and the patient was persistently febrile, especially if his alkaline phosphatase value continued to rise, a more aggressive attempt at diagnosis, possibly even including an open biopsy, would be required. Prolonged administration of amphotericin B is often needed (up to 2 to 4 g) to effect an improvement in the clinical and laboratory findings.

66. **The answer is D.** *(Chap 100.)* Since mammalian cells do not possess a cell wall, antibiotics that target synthesis of bacterial cell walls have intrinsic selectivity. Both gram-positive and gram-negative bacteria possess a peptidoglycan cell wall; gram-negative bacteria also possess another membrane external to the aforementioned layer. The classic cell wall–specific antibiotics include β-lactam-ring agents such as the penicillins, cephalosporins, carbapenems, and monobactams. These drugs prevent the cross-linking reaction that forms peptide cross-bridges (due to the cleavage of a terminal D-alanine residue) in the cell wall. The target enzyme, a transpeptidase, actively binds β-lactam antibiotics. Preventing cell wall synthesis in this fashion not only results in loss of cell wall integrity, but also induces the bacteria's own cell wall–remodeling enzymes (autolysins) that may actually cause the microorganisms' "self-destruction." The glycopeptide vancomycin binds to the terminal D-alanine component of the bacterial cell wall peptide and thereby inhibits the addition of subunits to the peptidoglycan backbone. Bacitracin prevents the generation of an active lipid carrier that moves the peptidoglycan subunits through the cell membrane to the cell wall. The macrolide antibiotics erythromycin and clarithromycin bind specifically to a 50S portion of the bacterial ribosome and thereby inhibit peptide chain elongation. Bacteria frequently develop resistance to β-lactam antibiotics, often by elaborating antibiotic-destroying enzymes known as β-lactamases, which hydrolyze the antibiotic's critical ring. One strategy to deal with this problem is to combine the antibiotic with a molecule, such as clavulanic acid or sulbactam, that inhibits β-lactamases.

67. **The answer is D.** *(Chap 165.)* Fungal and yeast infections, predominantly candidiasis, aspergillosis, and mucormycosis, occur frequently in severely immunosuppressed patients, particularly those who have received broad-spectrum antibiotics for a prolonged period. A number of other types of fungal infection occur in these patients. About 75 percent of all cases of *Cryptococcus neoformans* infection occur in persons who have lymphoma, are taking glucocorticosteroids, or are otherwise immunocompromised. The association of cryptococcal meningitis and Hodgkin's disease is important clinically.

68. **The answer is D.** *(Chap 108.)* *Clostridium difficile* can be isolated on selective agar media, but this method is not dependable for diagnosis. Pseudomembranous colitis (PMC) is caused by the local action of at least two enterotoxins, toxins A and B. Serologic tests are not helpful. The punctate plaques on a hyperemic mucosa are characteristic of PMC, but similar pathologic changes can be seen with ischemic colitis. The best diagnostic test is the demonstration of *C. difficile* cytotoxin, an assay that can be positive in 24 h. Clostridia are part of normal fecal flora, so a Gram stain of the stool would not be helpful.

69. **The answer is C.** *(Chaps 97, 98.)* Nosocomial (hospital-acquired) pneumonias are common in intubated patients. Other patients at risk include those with altered levels of consciousness, those with nasogastric tubes, elderly persons, patients with chronic obstructive lung disease, and postoperative patients. It has been recently noted that oropharyngeal and subsequent gastric colonization with potentially pathogenic organisms is quite common in such patients. Aspiration of these colonized gastrointestinal contents occurs frequently in patients with nasogastric tubes or decreased gag reflexes. Bacterial colonization of the stomach is increased in the presence of decreased acidity due to H_2 blockers or antacids. Sucralfate heals ulcers but does not alter gastric pH; it is an ideal medicine for ICU use if the goal of preventing nosocomial pneumonias is paramount. Neither of the two antibiotics listed in the question would be appropriate prophylactic agents since penicillin G would not cover the gram-negative rod organisms that are frequent pathogens in this setting and ciprofloxacin would be relatively ineffective for *Staphylococcus aureus*, which is also a frequent cause of nosocomial pneumonia.

70. **The answer is A.** *(Chaps 85, 94.)* *S. aureus* accounts for well over half of all endocarditis infections in intravenous drug users. Unfortunately, a substantial proportion of such infections are due

to methicillin-resistant strains, which are now frequently isolated from skin sites of such persons. *S. aureus* is frequently found in association with right-sided lesions, particularly those on the tricuspid valve, which could be a function of its bombardment with injected particulate matter. Tricuspid valve endocarditis is associated with a high fever and frequent pulmonary involvement. There have been epidemics of *Pseudomonas* endocarditis in drug users, but such infections are much less frequent than those due to staphylococci. The least pathogenic organisms such as viridans streptococci and enterococci are much less common and tend to infect previously damaged or diseased left-sided valves. Diagnosis involves obtaining a positive blood culture. Treatment consists of the administration of the appropriate antibiotic for 4 weeks.

71. **The answer is D.** *(Chap 169.)* As primary therapy for dermatophytosis (ringworm), miconazole, clotrimazole, and tolnaftate usually are recommended. In severe cases, griseofulvin generally is used, with ketoconazole recommended for griseofulvin-resistant cases. Amphotericin is recommended for invasive fungal infections, not dermatophytosis.

72. **The answer is E.** *(Chap 140.)* Trachoma remains the most important cause of preventable blindness in the world. Blindness occurs primarily because of damage to the cornea and eyelids. Corneal abrasion, scarring of the lids, secondary infections, and loss of lacrimal function are the principal problems.

73. **The answer is E.** *(Chap 140.)* Fever, chills, headache, cough, and myalgias are the typical presenting signs and symptoms of psittacosis. Gastrointestinal symptoms also may occur but are much less frequent. The diagnosis of psittacosis usually depends on serologic tests or cultures of respiratory secretions. Even a low-titer positive complement fixation antibody test, in conjunction with the clinical setting described, would strongly suggest the diagnosis of psittacosis and warrant the use of tetracycline.

74. **The answer is D.** *(Chap 157.)* Both mumps and bacterial parotitis produce fever, and both may be associated with elevated serum amylase levels because of the release of salivary amylase into the blood. In persons who have mumps, the parotid glands are usually not as warm and tender as in persons who have bacterial parotitis. Mumps tends to be a disease of children and young adults, whereas bacterial parotitis tends to affect the elderly. The most useful distinguishing feature, however, is probably the nature of the parotid secretions. In bacterial parotitis, significant numbers of leukocytes and bacteria, usually staphylococci, are found in parotid secretions; in mumps, only a small amount of parotid fluid, and no pus, is observed.

75. **The answer is C.** *(Chap 154.)* As many as 90 percent of the patients with poliovirus are asymptomatic or have only a self-limited febrile illness. Paralytic polio is characterized by an initial febrile illness that resolves and is followed by development of aseptic meningitis and asymmetric paralysis. In contrast to polio, the Guillain-Barré syndrome is characterized by symmetric muscle weakness with frequent paresthesias but normal reflexes. Motor neurons are primarily affected by poliovirus infection with resultant loss of reflexes and flaccid paralysis. Return of neuronal function may be possible for up to 6 months after infection.

76. **The answer is A.** *(Chap 152.)* The man described in the question has symptoms that suggest influenza complicated by bacterial pneumonia. Pneumococci and staphylococci are the leading pathogens that cause secondary bacterial infection in this situation, and effective therapy would include drugs that act against penicillinase-producing staphylococci. The agent of choice is nafcillin or another semisynthetic penicillinase-resistant penicillin; penicillin G would be an ill-advised choice. Other acceptable alternative therapies include vancomycin, clindamycin, and cephalothin.

77. The answer is A. *(Chap 133.)* Lymphadenopathy and a papulosquamous rash that includes the palms and soles characteristically accompany secondary syphilis, which appears about 8 weeks after healing of the primary chancre. Lymphadenopathy is not a well-recognized manifestation of late syphilis. The inflammatory lesions of late syphilis are diverse and range from asymptomatic neurosyphilis, characterized only by pleocytosis or elevated protein on CSF examination, to the complex intellectual and functional disturbances caused by parenchymal damage of brain tissue (general paresis). Meningovascular syphilis can lead to middle cerebral artery strokes, which produce hemiparesis and dysphasia. Demyelinization of the posterior columns will lead to the ataxic gait and destroyed joints from loss of position sense characteristic of tabes dorsalis. About 10 percent of patients with late untreated syphilis will experience cardiovascular complications, usually in the form of aneurysms of the ascending aorta. Gummas are nodules of granulomatous inflammation that involve the skin and skeleton. Gummas of the skin may take the form of nodules, a papulosquamous eruption, or ulcers.

78. The answer is D. *(Chap 130. Barnes, N Engl J Med 324:1644–1650, 1991.)* The resurgence of tuberculosis in the United States may well be due to the increase in the number of HIV-infected patients and the frequency of tuberculosis in this risk group. Tuberculosis usually occurs in HIV-infected patients without preexisting AIDS, probably because *M. tuberculosis* is more virulent than other HIV-associated pathogens that occur at a stage of disease when the T4 count is more profoundly affected. Extrapulmonary tuberculosis is quite common in patients with HIV infection, but pulmonary involvement occurs in 74 to 100 percent of such patients. Therefore, tuberculosis remains a critical diagnostic consideration in those with abnormal chest roentgenograms. Hilar adenopathy, pleural effusions, and cavitation are most useful diagnostically, since they are rarely seen in other common causes of pneumonia in HIV-infected patients. Though more prolonged treatment is recommended in those with HIV infection compared with non-HIV-infected patients, the initial drug treatment strategy is identical and appears to be effective. This treatment involves the use of three drugs: isoniazid, rifampin, and pyrazinamide. Those with pulmonary tuberculosis are highly infective because of the generally high titers of organisms present in these immunocompromised patients. Though false negative skin tests are not uncommon, the newly positive intradermal reaction against tuberculosis bacilli should mandate a prophylactic year of antituberculosis therapy, just as it would in a non-HIV-infected patient.

79. The answer is E. *(Chap 90.)* Precisely how diabetes mellitus and sickle cell disease predispose to urinary tract infection is unclear. In persons with diabetes, glycosuria and neuropathic changes in bladder function are probably contributory. In association with both diabetes and sickle cell disease, avascular areas in the kidney probably provide sites for bacterial multiplication remote from phagocytic cells. In hyperparathyroidism and gout, stone formation leads to obstruction and infection. Although in Wilson's disease copper is deposited in the kidney and tubular dysfunction occurs, urinary infections generally are not a major problem.

80. The answer is C. *(Chap 151.)* Retroviruses contain an RNA genome that requires reverse transcription into DNA after entrance to the host cell. The DNA copy of the viral genome may then integrate into the host genome, which enables viral gene transcription and ultimately leads to complete viral replication. AIDS, the best known human retroviral disease, is caused by human immunodeficiency virus 1 (HIV-1), which attaches to CD4 molecules on lymphocytes and monocytes and produces lymphopenic immunodeficiency. HIV-2, isolated in Africa, appears to be an infrequent cause of AIDS. The two retroviruses associated with transformation of human cells are human T-lymphotropic viruses I and II (HTLV-I and HTLV-II). The role of HTLV-II in human disease is unclear, although the virus was originally isolated from a patient with a T-cell variant of hairy cell leukemia. One to three percent of those infected with HTLV-I develop a fulminant and refractory malignancy of CD4-positive lymphocytes called *adult T-cell leukemia/lymphoma*, characterized by lymphocytosis, leukemic skin infiltrates, bone lesions, and hypercalcemia. Increased numbers of interleukin 2 (IL-2) receptors can be found on the surface of the malignant cells. A demyelinating disorder termed *tropical spastic paraparesis* and a chronic T-cell leukemia represent other diseases associated with HTLV-I infection. Feline leukemia virus (FeLV), responsible for tumors in cats, does not cause human disease.

81. **The answer is E.** *(Chaps 143, 375.)* Among the many viruses that can cause acute encephalitis, the most frequent cause in the United States is herpes simplex. A few years ago, this fact would have been of academic interest only, but with the availability of antiviral chemotherapy, establishment of the specific diagnosis can be fruitful. Brain biopsy and CT scanning are the most helpful procedures for establishing this diagnosis, but empiric therapy with acyclovir is frequently employed.

82. **The answer is E.** *(Chap 179.)* Cryptosporidia, which are protozoa, cannot be cultured from the stool. They stain with iodine but not Gram stain. Investigational serologic tests appear promising but are not readily available. Because of their small size (5 μm) and lack of motility, detection of cysts by wet mounts is very difficult. By using acid-fast stains or rhodamine fluorescence, even a few cysts can be detected easily and the diagnosis of cryptosporidiosis made. No effective antimicrobial therapy has been defined.

83. **The answer is D.** *(Chap 102.)* Methicillin-resistant *Staphylococcus aureus* has become a major source of morbidity and mortality. In vitro sensitivity testing may demonstrate sensitivity to cephalosporins, but these tests are unreliable and all strains are resistant in vivo. These strains have an altered penicillin-binding protein and are resistant to all penicillinase-resistant penicillins, alone or in combination with an aminoglycoside. Resistance is not plasmid-mediated, and there is no risk of spread to other bacteria. Administration of vancomycin is the most effective treatment.

84. **The answer is D.** *(Chap 131.)* A papular reaction usually develops in patients with tuberculoid leprosy a month after injection of killed suspensions of *Mycobacterium leprae,* but it is not diagnostic since positive reactions occur in nearly all adults. Culture of *M. leprae* is exceedingly difficult and can only be accomplished in mice or armadillos. A minimum of 6 months is usually required before the results are available; therefore cultures are not practical for diagnosis. Erythema of existing skin lesions with dapsone therapy is not diagnostic. Demonstration of the organism on microscopic examination of a biopsy specimen is the only definitive way to make the diagnosis of leprosy. A sensitive serologic assay effective in diagnosing lepromatous disease has recently been developed.

85. **The answer is B.** *(Chap 179.)* The infective cysts of *G. lamblia* can survive for several months in cold water and have been responsible for large epidemics in communities such as Vail, Colorado. Immunity to *Giardia* is not well understood, but there is no increased incidence in granulocytopenic patients. Intestinal IgA may be important, as deficient patients appear to be at increased risk of infection. Transmission is primarily by the fecal-oral route, which results in higher incidence in male homosexuals, retarded patients in institutions, and children in day-care centers.

86. **The answer is E.**   *(Chap 182.)*   Adult worms do reside in lymph nodes, but biopsy is relatively contraindicated because of the potential to exacerbate problems with lymphatic drainage. Serologic testing is available at specialized centers with indirect hemagglutination, but cross-reactions with other filariae are common. Intense pruritus and a rash after administration of diethylcarbamazine (Mazzotti test) suggest dermal microfilariae; this reaction typically occurs in patients with onchocerciasis. Maintenance of filariae in cultures or animals is extremely difficult. The best animal model is in cats, but this technique plays no role in clinical diagnosis. Diagnosis is best made by demonstrating microfilariae on a Giemsa stain of blood. *W. bancrofti* microfilariae usually maintain a nocturnal periodicity and are found in the bloodstream in greatest numbers at night. The exact reason for the periodicity is not known, but it may be related to oxygen tension in the pulmonary vessels.

87. **The answer is C.**   *(Chap 89.)*   The findings on pelvic examination coupled with the elevated sedimentation rate in this setting strongly suggest acute pelvic inflammatory disease (PID). About 5 percent of women with PID will have associated perihepatitis, termed the Fitz-Hugh–Curtis syndrome, manifested by pleuritic pain of the right upper quadrant and tenderness on palpation, along with normal liver function tests and ultrasound of the right upper quadrant. *N. gonorrhoeae* is the primary pathogen in this condition, but chlamydial salpingitis is increasing in incidence, particularly in higher socioeconomic groups.

88. **The answer is A.**   *(Chap 89. CDC, MMWR 40RR-5:1, 1992.)*   It is important to pick a well-tolerated regimen with good activity against both *N. gonorrhoeae* (including penicillinase-producing strains) and *C. trachomatis* for the treatment of patients with severe pelvic inflammatory disease (PID). Activity against vaginal anaerobes and members of the Enterobacteriaceae family, which may also play a role in the pathogenesis of this disorder, would also be desirable. A combination of doxycycline and cefoxitin offers the broad-spectrum coverage required for optimal treatment. Clindamycin plus gentamicin acutely, plus a 2-week course of doxycycline to definitively treat *C. trachomatis,* is an acceptable alternative regimen. The combination of metronidazole and gentamicin lacks adequate coverage against both *Chlamydia* and *N. gonorrhoeae* and is therefore not appropriate in this setting.

89. **The answer is C.**   *(Chap 174.)*   This patient was in the right location and has the typical clinical features of a patient infected with *Babesia,* tick-borne protozoa that multiply in red blood cells. Clinical manifestations can be more severe in splenectomized persons. The best way to make the diagnosis is to demonstrate the parasite's presence in erythrocytes in Giemsa-stained peripheral blood smears. Serologic confirmation can also be helpful. The combination of quinine and clindamycin is the most effective treatment.

90. **The answer is D.**   *(Chap 175.)*   The four major clinical syndromes of leishmaniasis—visceral (kala azar), cutaneous, diffuse cutaneous, and mucocutaneous—represent sandfly-borne disease caused by members of the protozoal genus *Leishmania*. Kala azar is manifested by fever, cough, diarrhea, splenomegaly, and pancytopenia and may be diagnosed by buffy coat examination. A number of species in each hemisphere account for the various cutaneous syndromes. In the Middle East and in the Republic of Georgia, *L. tropica* causes ulcerating facial lesions. Mucocutaneous leishmaniasis, or espundia, is caused by *L. braziliensis,* which can produce (after a long initial quiescent period) excessive destruction of facial soft tissue, including nasal obstruction and epistaxis, as well as systemic signs and symptoms. Massive dissemination of skin lesions without visceral involvement can also occur. This form is refractory to therapy, which usually consists of antimony. Esophageal dysfunction is seen in Chagas' disease, a trypanosomal-mediated infestation.

91. The answer is A-Y, B-Y, C-Y, D-Y, E-Y. *(Chap 85.)* Subacute bacterial endocarditis can be treated quite successfully. However, for persons in whom the offending organisms are highly resistant to β-lactam antibiotics, such as fungi and gram-negative bacteria, the prognosis is less favorable. Delay in therapy also compromises the prognosis. The development of congestive heart failure is a most ominous sign. Endocarditis due to *Staphylococcus epidermidis* carries a poor prognosis if acquired at the time of cardiac surgery or if complicated by the adverse factors mentioned above. Valve ring or myocardial abscess also indicates a failure of medical therapy.

92. The answer is A-N, B-Y, C-N, D-N, E-Y. *(Chap 85. Kaye, Ann Intern Med 114:803-804, 1991.)* After transient bacteremia, subacute endocarditis may develop at endocardial sites at which a jet of blood flows from a high-pressure to a low-pressure area. Such lesions include ventricular septal defects and mitral regurgitation. Blood flow velocity across an isolated atrial septal defect is much lower and endocarditis is extremely uncommon in this condition. Similarly, long-standing permanent pacemakers and coronary bypass grafts very rarely result in the degree of turbulent blood flow necessary to incite endocardial infection. The degree of mitral insufficiency associated with mitral valve prolapse that requires prophylaxis is not clear. A reasonable approach is mandatory prophylaxis only in the setting of holosystolic murmur and prolapse.

93. The answer is A-N, B-Y, C-N, D-N, E-Y. *(Chap 16. Dinarello, Rev Infect Dis 10:168, 1988.)* A host of stimuli, including infection with virtually any microorganism, cause macrophages, lymphocytes, fibroblasts, and other cells to elaborate the key mediators of fever production such as TNFα, TNFβ (lymphotoxin), interferon α, and the interleukins, which are 17-kilodalton (kDa) glycoproteins that promote the synthesis of E series prostaglandins in the hypothalamus and thereby reset the central thermostat at a higher level. Aspirin and nonsteroidal anti-inflammatory agents act by inhibiting cyclooxygenase activity so that prostaglandin E_2 (PGE_2) cannot be synthesized; they do not act by reducing TNF and IL-1 production. Glucocorticoids suppress fever both by interfering with arachidonic acid metabolism and down-regulating the production of endogenous pyrogens. TNF and IL-1 also possess diverse effects, including the induction of cachexia by TNF.

94. The answer is A-N, B-Y, C-N, D-N, E-Y. *(Chap 88.)* A man who has dysuria but no urethral exudate or leukocytes in a urethral swab specimen, especially if confirmed one week later, probably does not have a chlamydial infection. On the other hand, if he has an exudate in which intracellular gram-negative diplococci are not seen, he should be considered to have chlamydial urethritis and treated presumptively with tetracycline, an antibiotic also effective against gonococci. A pregnant woman with presumed chlamydial cervicitis should be treated with erythromycin because tetracycline can produce fetal complications. Sulfa creams are ineffective in the treatment of bacterial vaginosis; metronidazole is the preferred form of therapy. Intravaginal clindamycin cream is useful in treating the pregnant female. Organisms cultured in women with this condition include *Gardnerella vaginalis, Mycoplasma hominis,* and various anaerobic bacteria. Genital ulcers in U.S. residents are due most frequently to herpes simplex virus; elsewhere in the world, syphilis and chancroid are more common.

95. The answer is A-Y, B-Y, C-N, D-N, E-N. *(Chap 101. Shapiro, N Engl J Med 325:1453, 1991.)* Type 3 pneumococci cause the most severe of all pneumococcal pneumonias, possibly because such infections occur in debilitated persons. All splenectomized patients, even those without underlying disease, should receive pneumococcal vaccine. The "crisis" in pneumococcal pneumonia ordinarily corresponds to the appearance of type-specific antibodies, not maximum leukocytosis. Alcoholic persons who develop pneumococcal pneumonia have a poor prognosis for several reasons: their tendency to aspirate pharyngeal flora, poor functioning of bronchial clearance mechanisms, and impaired leukocyte response (hypogammaglobulinemia generally is not a contributing factor). Pneumococcal pneumonia frequently precedes pneumococcal meningitis. Pneumococci cause pharyngitis extremely rarely.

96. The answer is A-Y, B-N, C-N, D-Y, E-Y. *(Chap 103.)* Streptococcal M protein is the factor most strongly associated with virulence—strains rich in M protein resist phagocytosis. Streptococcal pyoderma may lead to acute glomerulonephritis but not to acute rheumatic fever. The reason for this phenomenon remains unexplained. Group A streptococci elaborate a host of toxins important in infections: membrane-damaging streptolysins, DNAses, proteases, and pyrogenic exotoxins A, B, and C. Penicillin therapy for streptococcal pharyngitis decreases the incidence of suppurative and nonsuppurative complications but does not alter the duration of the sore throat. Nonenterococcal group D streptococci, such as *S. bovis,* are quite pathogenic and tend to cause endocarditis in patients with colonic neoplasms.

97. The answer is A-N, B-Y, C-Y, D-Y, E-N. *(Chap 135.)* Leptospirosis can be transferred from infected animals directly to humans who contact contaminated tissue or urine. Leptospirosis often is confused with influenza because of its initial manifestations: fever, headache, and myalgias. It causes hepatitis often associated with very elevated serum bilirubin levels, probably a result of both intravascular hemolysis and impaired bilirubin excretion. Leptospiral meningitis resembles a viral, or aseptic, meningitis; cerebrospinal fluid has a normal glucose concentration, and although a few neutrophils may be present, lymphocytes are the predominant cell type observed. The diagnosis of acute leptospirosis is made best by blood cultures; dark-field microscopy too often gives false positive or false negative results.

98. The answer is A-N, B-Y, C-Y, D-Y, E-N. *(Chap 110.)* Gonococcemia tends to be a problem of menstruating women, although men also are affected. The characteristic skin lesions are small pustules that usually occur first on the fingers and feet. The arthritis associated with gonococcemia is rarely symmetrical, a clinical finding that is often helpful in making the diagnosis. Gonococci that produce β-lactamase are resistant to penicillin and ampicillin but are sensitive to the newer cephalosporins, such as ceftriaxone. Treatment with spectinomycin is also effective; this agent usually is recommended as the first choice for treatment failures attributed to penicillinase production by the organism. Gonococci with pili are more virulent than gonococci without pili (pili may help the organism stick to epithelial cells to initiate infection), but the latter type may facilitate spread.

99. The answer is A-Y, B-N, C-Y, D-N, E-N. *(Chap 115.)* *Acinetobacter,* previously called *Mimae herellae* and *Bacterium anitratum,* is a ubiquitous commensal organism that is an important cause of bacteremia, pneumonia, and other serious infections. It is a gram-negative rod that can be confused with *Neisseria* on Gram stain because of its pleomorphic appearance. It is also confused with Enterobacteriaceae species in cultures because of its simple growth requirements. Unlike *Neisseria,* it is resistant to penicillin and ampicillin but sensitive to gentamicin and tobramycin; this difference in antibiotic sensitivity makes it very important to distinguish this organism from *Neisseria* in clinical isolates from patients with serious illnesses.

100. The answer is A-N, B-N, C-N, D-Y, E-Y. *(Chap 116.)* Melioidosis is caused by *Pseudomonas pseudomallei,* a gram-negative bacillus ubiquitous in many tropical areas of Asia and Africa. Infection occurs from contact with contaminated soil. Pulmonary infections are most frequent; in patients acutely ill with pneumonia, many organisms can be detected in sputum. The organisms can be grown on routine culture media. Serologic tests are used largely for epidemiologic studies. Melioidosis, particularly the chronic form, may be mistaken for tuberculosis; granulomas may develop, but calcification of cavitary lung lesions does not occur. In acute melioidosis, therapy with tetracycline and chloramphenicol or ceftazidime plus trimethoprim-sulfamethoxazole is recommended. Although the organism is usually sensitive to each of these agents, the high fatality rate of this disease (greater than 50 percent) has led to the use of a multiple antibiotic regimen.

101. **The answer is A-Y, B-Y, C-Y, D-N, E-Y.** *(Chap 121.)* Brucellosis is an important veterinary disease in those parts of the world from which it has not yet been eradicated. It is still a problem in cattle-raising areas of the United States. The disease usually presents with low-grade fever and constitutional symptoms; affected persons have lymphadenopathy, splenomegaly, and, sometimes, hepatomegaly. During the early bacteremic phase of the illness, *Brucella* can be isolated using routine cultures, provided they are kept long enough (i.e., up to 4 weeks). The diagnosis also is made using agglutination tests. Therapy with streptomycin and tetracycline still is best.

102. **The answer is A-Y, B-N, C-Y, D-Y, E-N.** *(Chap 120.)* *Vibrio cholerae* enterotoxin causes a diffuse, noninflammatory secretion of isotonic intestinal fluid without injury to the absorptive surface. Early diagnosis is aided by dark-field microscopy or immobilization of organisms with type-specific antisera; definitive diagnosis, however, depends on culturing the organisms. Oral therapy with solutions that contain sodium bicarbonate and either glucose or sucrose is recommended. This therapy usually is begun on the basis of a presumptive diagnosis in endemic areas. Oral tetracycline also is useful because it can shorten the symptomatic period, but it is not recommended for children under age 8. Infection confers some immunity, so that in endemic areas children are usually the ones affected. Cholera vaccine is not particularly effective and is now not ordinarily recommended for travelers to endemic areas.

103. **The answer is A-N, B-Y, C-N, D-Y, E-Y.** *(Chap 168.)* The molds *Mucor* and *Rhizopus,* the main causes of mucormycosis, are more often seen in than grown from pathologic specimens. The reasons they are so hard to grow have not been identified. Fungal hyphae tend to invade blood vessels, which leads to hemorrhagic necrosis. Sinusitis is the predominant illness in infected persons who have diabetes mellitus; in persons with hematologic malignancies, pulmonary disease is more common. Diagnosis is best accomplished by biopsy and histologic examination (serology is still in the investigative stages). Amphotericin is the only known nonsurgical treatment of mucormycosis.

104. **The answer is A-N, B-Y, C-N, D-Y, E-Y.** *(Chap 138.)* Rocky Mountain spotted fever is a tick-borne disease caused by *Rickettsia rickettsii,* an obligate intracellular organism. The disease is associated with severe headache, myalgias, and arthralgias, but not frank arthritis. The characteristic rash is at first macular and confined to the extremities; after several days, the rash spreads to involve the buttocks, trunk, axilla, neck, and face and becomes maculopapular, then hemorrhagic, and finally ulcerative. Treatment with chloramphenicol or tetracycline, which are rickettsiostatic agents, is most effective if begun before the rash has become hemorrhagic. Ticks found on household pets should be removed carefully with tweezers, and not by hand, in order to prevent infection through minor skin abrasions.

105. **The answer is A-N, B-Y, C-N, D-Y, E-Y.** *(Chap 139.)* *Mycoplasma pneumoniae* is an important cause of pneumonia, particularly in young adults. The organism cannot be seen by Gram stain because it does not retain the dye-iodine complex. The cold-agglutinin test is nonspecific; firm serologic evidence of mycoplasma infection may be derived from a complement-fixation test (other specific serologic tests also are available). Treatment with either tetracycline or erythromycin is effective. In nonepidemic situations in which it is often difficult to know whether a person has a pneumococcal or *Mycoplasma* infection, erythromycin is the drug of choice.

106. The answer is A-Y, B-N, C-Y, D-Y, E-N. *(Chap 102. Arbuthnot, Rev Infect Dis 11 [suppl 1]:51, 1989.)* Toxic shock syndrome (TSS) is a toxin-mediated disorder that has been linked to the ability of hyperabsorbent tampons to provide the surface area required to promote *S. aureus* growth and toxin (TSST-1) production. Though the patients may appear to be in shock with refractory hypotension, blood cultures are almost uniformly negative. With the increased recognition and prevention of menstruation-associated TSS, the relative frequency in nonmenstruating women and in men is increasing. In the severe form of the syndrome, gastrointestinal, hepatic, renal, muscular, and CNS involvement occurs not infrequently. The diagnosis of TSS in a postsurgical patient may be a clinical challenge since the signs of infection are usually minimal and occur as soon as 2 days after the operation. Treatment includes antistaphylococcal antibiotics, drainage of focal collections, and supportive care.

107. The answer is A-Y, B-Y, C-Y, D-Y, E-Y. *(Chap 145.)* The most common features of infectious mononucleosis are fever, sore throat, and lymphadenopathy. Sore throat, the most commonly described symptom, is observed in about 80 percent of young adults with this infection. Atypical lymphocytes, identified as T cells with suppressor-cytotoxic action responding to EBV-infected B lymphocytes, appear in the peripheral blood during the first week of illness. Heterophil antibodies, which are sheep red-cell agglutinins associated with the immunoglobulin M serum fraction, usually persist in the serum for a few months. On the other hand, antibodies to Epstein-Barr virus, especially to EBV nuclear antigens, often can be detected for years in the serum of persons who have had infectious mononucleosis. The incubation period in young adults is thought to be 30 to 50 days; in children, the incubation period is much shorter.

108. The answer is A-N, B-N, C-N, D-Y, E-N. *(Chap 98. Hainer, J Fam Pract 25:497, 1987.)* Cat-scratch disease, as the name implies, is transmitted to humans chiefly by cat scratches. Other animal vectors have not been definitively recognized. Lymphadenopathy often persists for weeks; examination of a lymph-node biopsy specimen may show the granulomatous inflammation also noted in lymphogranuloma venereum, tularemia, brucellosis, tuberculosis, and some lymphomas. Splenomegaly generally does not develop. Antibiotics are ineffective in treating persons with cat-scratch disease, although it is now recognized that the etiologic agent is a bacterium with a defective cell wall.

109. The answer is A-N, B-N, C-Y, D-N, E-Y. *(Chap 104.)* The gram-positive rod *Corynebacterium diphtheriae* may produce human disease upon infection of skin or mucous membranes. Specific viruses, termed *corynephages,* must infect *C. diphtheriae* to convert the bacterium to a toxin-producing strain. Disease can occur as a result of infection with toxin-producing or toxin-negative strains, but the serious manifestations of carditis and neuritis occur as a result of toxins. The toxin, elaborated as a single polypeptide chain by the lysogenized bacteria, is proteolytically cleaved into an A portion, which binds to cell membranes, and a B portion, which catalyzes the adenosine diphosphate ribosylation and inactivation of elongation factor 2, a vital element in ribosome-mediated protein synthesis. Most unimmunized patients with diphtherial pharyngitis experience myocardial abnormalities with manifestations ranging from an abnormal electrocardiogram to congestive heart failure and ventricular fibrillation. Formaldehyde-treated diphtheria toxin creates toxoid, a vaccine component that can provide 10 years of protection against serious disease. Pharyngeal and cutaneous infections with toxigenic strains produce edema, hyperemia, and a dense, fibrinopurulent exudate (termed a *pseudomembrane*) teeming with *C. diphtheriae*. Formation of the pseudomembrane can lead to obstruction of the upper airway. Administration of antitoxin is the primary specific modality of treatment for those with suspected infections.

110. The answer is A-N, B-N, C-Y, D-N, E-Y. *(Chap 103.)* Differences in cell-wall carbohydrates account for the alphabetized classification system used to describe streptococcal strains. Group A streptococcal infection is usually associated with pharyngitis or pyoderma and is notable for the incidence of poststreptococcal nonsuppurative complications (acute rheumatic fever and acute glomerulonephritis). The beta-hemolytic and bacitracin-resistant group B streptococci colonize the female genital tract and are the second most common cause, after *E. coli,* of neonatal sepsis and meningitis. Systemic disease, including urinary tract infections and endocarditis, in debilitated adults may also be caused by group B streptococci. Group D streptococci include both enterococcal and nonenterococcal forms. Unlike most streptococci, which are exquisitely penicillin-sensitive, enterococci are relatively resistant. Enterococcal endocarditis should be treated with the synergistic combination of ampicillin plus an aminoglycoside. The aminoglycoside of choice is gentamicin, since many strains are now highly resistant to the formerly administered streptomycin. Nonenterococcal group D strains, typified by *Streptococcus bovis,* which tends to cause bacteremia in patients with colonic neoplasia, can be identified by their ability to grow in 6.5% NaCl. Viridans streptococci inhabit the mouth and are the organisms most frequently associated with subacute bacterial endocarditis. Certain subtypes of viridans streptococci, including *Streptococcus milleri,* can cause major suppurative disease, such as liver abscesses and empyema.

111. **The answer is A-N, B-Y, C-Y, D-N, E-Y.** *(Chap 115.)* *Klebsiella* and the related *Serratia* and *Enterobacter* are the most important enteric organisms other than *E. coli* to infect humans. Although respiratory disease is important (*Klebsiella* accounts for 1 percent or less of community-acquired pneumonia), most clinical isolates now come from the urinary tract. All three genera are important pulmonary nosocomial pathogens. However, merely finding these organisms growing in the sputum of a very ill hospitalized patient does not necessarily implicate the bacteria as pathogenic in that particular circumstance and may indicate colonization rather than infection. Clinical context and procurement of the sample in a sterile fashion (transtracheal aspiration, bronchoscopy) will aid in diagnosis. Chronic alcoholics, diabetics, and those with chronic lung disease are at increased risk for *Klebsiella* pneumonia, a difficult disease to treat because of the frequency of suppurative complications (empyema and abscess) with the associated requirement for prolonged (>2 weeks) therapy.

112. **The answer is A-N, B-Y, C-N, D-Y, E-Y.** *(Chap 174.)* Only in *P. vivax* and *P. ovale* infections may relapses occur because a portion of the intrahepatic forms remain dormant. *P. vivax* depends upon the Duffy antigen to enter red cells; patients who lack this antigen are resistant. *P. falciparum* produces a form of disease that can lead to coma and death. Seizures and hypoglycemia, grave prognostic signs, may also be present. Renal failure in falciparum malaria seems to occur on the basis of tubular sequestration of parasitized erythrocytes and tends to abate. Renal failure with *P. malariae* infection may be due to deposition of soluble immune complexes in glomeruli. Repeated malarial infections can result in massive splenomegaly.

113. **The answer is A-Y, B-Y, C-Y, D-Y, E-Y.** *(Chap 145.)* Serious complications of infectious mononucleosis (IM) due to infection with Epstein-Barr virus (EBV) are uncommon. Mild hepatitis occurs in 90 percent of patients. Airway obstruction, which is sensitive to glucocorticoid therapy, is sometimes a result of the massive pharyngeal adenopathy accompanying IM. IgM antibodies elicited by EBV may be directed against the i antigen on red blood cell membranes, which thereby causes a transient autoimmune hemolytic anemia. Mild antibody-mediated thrombocytopenia is common, but a serious drop in the platelet count is unusual. Some patients develop cranial nerve palsies and encephalitis as the result of EBV infection. There is growing recognition of the association between EBV infection and B-cell lymphoproliferative disorders in immunocompromised patients.

114. **The answer is A-Y, B-Y, C-N, D-N, E-Y.** *(Chap 173.)*   Although *Entamoeba histolytica* can infect some animals, the principal hosts are humans. Even in the presence of large or multiple amebic liver abscesses, defervescence usually occurs in 1 to 3 days with appropriate medical therapy. The abscess cavity in an amebic liver abscess usually contains no neutrophils or amebas; the infection does not evoke a typical acute inflammatory response, and amebas are found only at the edge of the advancing infection. Amebic serologic tests stay positive for up to 1 year despite therapy. Deaths from amebiasis are uncommon; however, failure to make the diagnosis in a timely fashion is among the most important causes of mortality.

115. **The answer is A-Y, B-Y, C-N, D-Y, E-Y.** *(Chap 86. Barnes, Medicine 66:472, 1987.)*   Unlike liver abscesses caused by bacteria, amebic abscesses rarely need to be drained. A positive serology for *Entamoeba histolytica,* which indicates prior exposure to this organism, is a most helpful differential point in deciding between the two causes. Bacterial hepatic abscesses may be caused by ascending cholangitis, bacteremia, direct extension (including peritoneal infection), or trauma. In the former two cases, especially in the instance of complete biliary obstruction, the presentation is more likely to be acute and the abscesses are more likely to be multiple; multiple abscesses carry a poorer prognosis than does a solitary abscess. Blood cultures enable noninvasive, specific diagnosis (although not all organisms in the abscess may grow in the blood) about one-third of the time. Given the preponderance of anaerobic (including the penicillin-resistant *B. fragilis*) and gram-negative bacterial forms in the biliary and GI tracts, empiric therapy, if required, should include an aminoglycoside and clindamycin.

116. **The answer is A-Y, B-N, C-Y, D-Y, E-Y.** *(Chap 177.)*   Toxoplasmosis is a relatively common infection; serologic data indicate that possibly as many as two-thirds of the U.S. adult population have had some form of the infection. The most serious manifestations appear to arise when the disease is acquired during pregnancy. Infection during the first trimester can result in spontaneous abortion, stillbirth, prematurity, or severe disease in any of several organ systems; infection during the third trimester more commonly leads to neonatal disease, which, however, tends to be asymptomatic. Infections acquired before pregnancy generally are of little consequence to the offspring. Immunocompromised persons usually have recrudescent disease. Diagnosis in these patients is often difficult to make, in part because the serologic responses are blunted by the underlying disease process. Serologic screening of asymptomatic immunocompromised patients may be helpful for recognizing toxoplasmosis at a later date.

117. **The answer is A-N, B-N, C-Y, D-N, E-N.** *(Chap 183.)*   *Schistosoma mansoni* infection of the liver causes cirrhosis from vascular obstruction due to periportal fibrosis but relatively little hepatocellular injury. Hepatosplenomegaly, hypersplenism, and esophageal varices develop quite commonly, and schistosomiasis usually is associated with eosinophilia. Spider nevi, gynecomastia, jaundice, and ascites are uncommon.

118. **The answer is A-Y, B-N, C-Y, D-Y, E-N.** *(Chap 118.)*   *Shigella sonnei* is the most common isolate in developed countries, while *S. dysenteriae* and *S. flexneri* predominate in tropical areas. Fewer than 100 organisms can cause disease irrespective of gastric acidity. Transmission by the fecal-oral route is the most important and occurs most frequently in areas of crowding and poor sanitation. Bacteremia with *Shigella* organisms is distinctly unusual, probably because the organism is sensitive to complement-mediated lysis. Unlike such therapy for infection with *Salmonella* organisms, antibiotic therapy of shigellosis can shorten both symptoms and fecal shedding.

119. The answer is A-N, B-Y, C-Y, D-Y, E-N. *(Chap 130.)* Pleural effusions occur most frequently in young patients with primary infection associated with an abrupt onset of symptoms. Effusions are being noted more frequently in older patients with reactivation disease, but they still account for less than one-third of patients in North America with pleurisy. Laryngeal and bronchitic tuberculosis are very infectious because the bacilli are readily aerosolized. Response to therapy is usually good. In the absence of neurologic abnormalities, extensive bony involvement by tuberculosis usually requires chemotherapy alone. Involvement of the basilar meninges is very common in meningeal tuberculosis and results in cranial nerve abnormalities. Gastrointestinal infection usually occurs in association with cavitary disease with large numbers of organisms. The terminal ileum and cecum are the most common sites, which results in disease that can be difficult to differentiate from Crohn's disease. The stomach is very resistant to infection.

120. The answer is A-N, B-Y, C-N, D-N, E-Y. *(Chap 137.)* The complete clinical spectrum of Lyme disease was first identified in the northeastern United States, but it is now recognized to have a worldwide distribution. Erythema chronicum migrans usually starts as an erythematous macule at the site of the tick bite and eventually forms a characteristic annular lesion with central clearing, which is present in approximately 90 percent of patients within a month. Constitutional symptoms including headache, fever, chills, and fatigue are common at the time of onset of skin lesions. Approximately 10 to 15 percent of patients have neurologic involvement with Lyme disease, which can be manifested as meningitis (with a lymphocytic pleocytosis), cranial neuritis, chorea, mononeuritis multiplex, or motor and sensory radiculoneuritis. Parenteral therapy with penicillin or ceftriaxone is recommended for patients with significant neurologic or cardiac involvement.

121. The answer is A-N, B-Y, C-Y, D-N, E-Y. *(Chap 108.)* *Clostridium* species are present in high numbers in normal intestinal flora and soil, and it is not surprising that they are frequent isolates from wound cultures. The presence of necrotic tissue and a low oxidation reduction potential are necessary to establish severe disease. Treatment is based on the clinical setting, and a culture positive for clostridia alone does not warrant therapy. *Clostridium perfringens* produces at least 12 toxins, one of the most important of which is the alpha toxin. It has been associated with hemolysis and capillary and platelet damage. *C. perfringens* is a common cause of food poisoning associated with contaminated meats and poultry. The serous discharge from the overlying skin in a patient with gas gangrene has many gram-positive rods but few inflammatory cells, which emphasizes the importance of an early Gram stain when the diagnosis is suspected. More than 70 percent of cases of *C. septicum* septicemia reported in the literature are associated with malignant neoplasms, especially of the gastrointestinal tract.

122. The answer is A-N, B-Y, C-Y, D-N, E-N. *(Chap 128.)* Anaerobic pulmonary infections most often develop in the setting of aspiration. The sudden development of a bacterial pneumonia in a healthy teenager would most likely be caused by *Streptococcus pneumoniae*. Both anaerobic and aerobic organisms are implicated in Ludwig's angina, an infection that originates in the third molar and can rapidly spread through soft tissues of the mandible and pharynx. Pharyngeal anaerobic bacteria, including *Bacteroides melaninogenicus, Fusobacterium* sp., and anaerobic cocci, cause bacterial aspiration pneumonia in a patient who has a diminished gag reflex, such as with a seizure disorder. It is important to differentiate bacterial aspiration, which requires antibiotic therapy, from aspiration of stomach contents, which usually occurs after general anesthesia and resolves with symptomatic therapy. Anaerobic bacteria are a very unusual cause of endocarditis, which—as is the case with aerobic gram-negative organisms—may in part be explained by a failure to adhere to damaged valves.

123.   The answer is A-N, B-Y, C-Y, D-Y, E-N.   *(Chap 144.)*   Less than 5 percent of patients will have a second recurrence of herpes zoster unless they are immunosuppressed. Acute cerebellar ataxia is the most common form of neurologic involvement in children. This benign condition usually develops 3 weeks after the rash and resolves spontaneously. Chickenpox is one of the most contagious diseases; it infects up to 90 percent of seronegative persons, presumably via the respiratory route. Varicella pneumonia can cause fever and severe hypoxia and thus complicate the course of chickenpox infection in up to 20 percent of adults. Varicella-zoster immune globulin is recommended only for immunodeficient patients under the age of 15 years who have been exposed to varicella.

124.   The answer is A-N, B-Y, C-Y, D-N, E-Y.   *(Chap 146. Drew, Rev Infect Dis 10:S468, 1988.)*   Perinatal transmission of CMV occurs by passage through an infected birth canal or through the breast milk of a seropositive mother. Though such transmission is very common, symptomatic infection is distinctly unusual except in premature infants in whom interstitial pneumonitis may develop. Congenital infection with CMV occurs in approximately 1 percent of births in the United States, but detectable disease develops in less than 0.05 percent of births, almost exclusively in association with primary maternal infections. CMV produces a syndrome very similar to mononucleosis associated with EBV. Cervical lymphadenopathy and exudative pharyngitis are usually not present, however, and heterophil antibodies are absent. CMV pneumonia can prove fatal in greater than 80 percent of bone marrow transplant patients. Salivary excretion of the virus or positive sputum cultures do not implicate CMV as the cause of pulmonary infiltrates. Definitive diagnosis rests on the demonstration of the characteristic pathologic finding—intranuclear inclusions in enlarged, epithelial cells—on lung biopsy. Diagnosis of CMV infection rests on characteristic pathologic findings, a fourfold rise in serology titer, or culture of CMV, usually from urine, saliva, or buffy coat. Because viral excretion can continue for weeks to months, isolation of CMV does not always implicate acute infection.

125.   The answer is A-N, B-Y, C-N, D-Y, E-Y.   *(Chap 153.)*   Both Norwalk virus and rotavirus infect the small intestinal epithelium and cause malabsorption and osmotic diarrhea. Worldwide, rotavirus is the most important cause of dehydrating diarrhea in infants. Rotavirus is shed in large quantities in the stool allowing for easy diagnosis by culture or immunoassays to detect viral antigens. Norwalk virus is presumably spread by the fecal-oral route and has also been implicated in food-borne and water-borne epidemics. The clinical manifestations of infection by both viruses are characterized by vomiting, diarrhea, and, occasionally, low-grade fever. Rotavirus is a major cause of diarrhea in children under 3 years of age, while Norwalk virus causes disease more often in older children and adults.

126.   The answer is A-N, B-N, C-Y, D-N, E-Y.   *(Chap 152. CDC, MMWR 40:1, 1991.)*   Major epidemics are associated only with influenza A and have been attributed to "antigenic shifts" or reassortment of genomic segments possibly with animal strains. Between pandemics, minor antigenic variations ("drifts") occur through point mutations. Antibodies against the hemagglutinin are most important presumably because they prevent viral attachment. Influenza B tends to cause smaller outbreaks, with less severe disease, because there is no animal reservoir and major antigenic shifts do not occur. Prolonged fatigue or "postinfluenzal asthenia" may occur, but the etiology is not known. Viral shedding usually stops 2 to 5 days after symptoms in uncomplicated influenza. Both amantadine and rimantadine can either prevent or attenuate infection with influenza A. In major outbreaks, therapy may be useful until immunity can be established by immunization.

127. **The answer is A-N, B-Y, C-N, D-Y, E-Y.** *(Chap 106.)* Neonatal tetanus is associated with a more than 60 percent mortality rate. It is caused by infections of the umbilical stump. In third-world countries the infection is often associated with practices of applying dirt or feces to the umbilical stump to speed sloughing. Human immune globulin cannot affect tetanus toxin that is already bound in the central nervous system, but it can be helpful if given early to bind any free toxin. Such small amounts of tetanospasmin are present that no immunity develops and active immunization must be initiated. Trismus, or lockjaw, is the most common manifestation of tetanus; it is caused by neuromuscular blockade and central disinhibition of motor neurons. Immune globulin provides protective antibody levels for up to 4 weeks and should be given along with toxoid for serious wounds if fewer than two previous doses of toxoid have been given.

Disorders of the Heart and Vascular System

DIRECTIONS: Each question below contains five suggested responses. Choose the **one best** response to each question.

128. A 48-year-old man is admitted to the coronary care unit with an acute inferior myocardial infarction. Two hours after admission, his blood pressure is 86/52 mmHg; his heart rate is 40 beats per minute with sinus rhythm. Which of the following would be the most appropriate initial therapy?

(A) Immediate insertion of a temporary transvenous pacemaker
(B) Intravenous administration of atropine sulfate, 0.6 mg
(C) Administration of normal saline, 300 mL over 15 min
(D) Intravenous administration of dobutamine, 0.35 mg/min
(E) Intravenous administration of isoproterenol, 5.0 µg/min

129. A 68-year-old man with a history of hypertension, diabetes, and urinary retention awoke feeling nauseated and light-headed. He did not respond to questions from his wife. When the emergency medical technicians arrived his blood pressure was 60 by palpation. IV fluids and oxygen were administered. Vital signs obtained in the ER were blood pressure 60, heart rate 120 and regular, temperature 38.9°C (102°F), and respiratory rate 30. A brief physical examination revealed coarse rales approximately halfway up in the chest bilaterally and inaudible heart sounds. An indwelling urinary catheter was placed with drainage of 10 to 20 mL of dark urine. Chest x-ray revealed bilateral interstitial infiltrates; the ECG was unremarkable except for sinus tachycardia. Antibiotics were administered and the patient was transferred to the ICU, where a right heart catheterization was performed. Pulmonary capillary wedge pressure was 28 mmHg. The cardiac output was 1.9 L/min. Right atrial mean pressure was 10 mmHg. The most likely cause of this man's hypotension was

(A) left ventricular dysfunction
(B) right ventricular infarction
(C) gram-negative sepsis
(D) gastrointestinal bleeding
(E) pulmonary emboli

130. A middle-aged man who suddenly collapsed on the golf course is brought to the emergency department. The emergency medical technicians had diagnosed cardiorespiratory arrest, performed CPR, applied a 200-joule shock to the patient's chest, and inserted an endotracheal tube and an intravenous line. At the time of arrival in the emergency room, the patient has no spontaneous pulse or respiration. After viewing the rhythm strip shown below, you order additional defibrillatory shocks: first 200 joules, then 300 joules, and finally 360 joules. CPR is continued. Which of the following is the most appropriate drug to administer at this time?

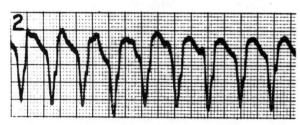

From Schlant, et al: *Hurst's The Heart*, 8/e. New York, McGraw-Hill, 1994, with permission.

(A) Procainamide
(B) Bretylium tosylate
(C) Epinephrine
(D) Lidocaine
(E) Sodium bicarbonate

131. All the following are features of captropril EXCEPT that it

(A) decreases plasma renin activity
(B) retards the degradation of circulating bradykinin
(C) inhibits formation of angiotensin II
(D) can be used safely in combination with a beta blocking agent
(E) is contraindicated in patients with bilateral renal artery stenosis

132. Which of the following physical findings is associated with the chest x-ray shown below?

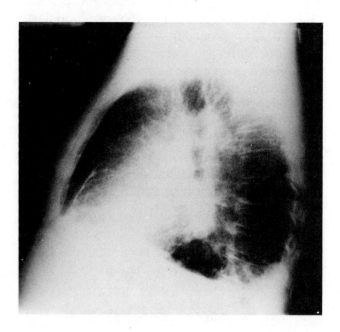

(A) Wide splitting of the second heart sound
(B) Opening snap and diastolic rumble
(C) Pericardial knock
(D) Late-peaking systolic ejection murmur
(E) Central cyanosis

133. Which of the following statements concerning the therapeutic role of isoproterenol is correct?

(A) Its alpha-adrenergic effects make it useful in cardiogenic shock
(B) It increases cardiac contractility but not cardiac rate
(C) It is useful in asthma because it is a beta$_2$-adrenergic agonist
(D) Severe vasoconstriction may occur due to stimulation of alpha-adrenergic receptors
(E) It functions as a dopaminergic agonist at low doses

134. A 55-year-old man with known coronary heart disease develops recurrent anginal symptoms 2 months after having undergone an apparently successful percutaneous transluminal coronary angioplasty (PTCA) procedure. The original PTCA procedure was performed because of angina unresponsive to medical therapy in the setting of two proximal 90 percent occlusions (one in the right coronary artery and the other in the left circumflex). Cardiac catheterization now reveals that the left circumflex lesion has reoccluded. Which of the following statements concerning the patient's current condition is correct?

(A) The patient will likely require coronary artery bypass surgery
(B) Had the patient been treated with aspirin daily from the time of his initial PTCA, this problem would have been less likely
(C) A cholesterol-lowering agent would have been useful in preventing this problem
(D) The administration of warfarin therapy for 6 months after PTCA is indicated to prevent this problem
(E) Coronary artery smooth muscle hyperplasia probably played a role in the current problem

135. Combined echocardiographic and Doppler echocardiographic studies are useful in the evaluation of all the following disorders EXCEPT

(A) aortic stenosis
(B) atrial septal defect
(C) tricuspid regurgitation
(D) mitral stenosis
(E) calcification of the left coronary artery

136. A 73-year-old man recently began having frequent syncopal episodes upon rising from recumbency. Associated complaints include constipation, difficulty voiding, and dry skin. Evaluation reveals orthostatic hypotension in the absence of compensatory tachycardia while the man is standing, but no evidence of degeneration of the central nervous system, including the extrapyramidal tracts and basal ganglia. Glucocorticoid and mineralocorticoid secretion is normal; plasma norepinephrine concentration, measured while the man is supine, is low. The treatment LEAST likely to benefit this man is

(A) high salt intake
(B) elastic supportive hose
(C) fludrocortisone acetate (Florinef)
(D) ephedrine sulfate
(E) tyramine

137. A 67-year-old man who has experienced recurrent episodes of dizziness over the last several months is admitted to the hospital because of a fainting episode. No evidence of acute myocardial infarction is documented. On the evening of the admission the patient tells his nurse that approximately 10 min ago he experienced several minutes of dizziness. His current rhythm appears to be normal sinus; however, a monitoring strip obtained at the time of this episode reveals absent QRS complexes every third beat. The PR interval, while slightly prolonged, is constant from beat to beat. P waves are present at regular intervals. Which of the following is the most appropriate therapeutic action?

(A) Insertion of permanent cardiac pacemaker
(B) Insertion of temporary cardiac pacemaker followed by insertion of permanent cardiac pacemaker
(C) Administration of atropine, 2 mg IV
(D) Administration of isoproterenol, 2 mg/min IV
(E) No specific therapy is required for this benign arrhythmia

138. Each of the following events is known to be a consequence of ligand binding to an alpha-adrenergic receptor EXCEPT

(A) increases in intracellular cyclic adenosine monophosphate (AMP)
(B) conformational change of guanosine-binding protein
(C) activation of phospholipase C
(D) activation of the calcium-sensitive protein kinase C
(E) synthesis of inositol triphosphate

139. A 42-year-old woman has bilateral ankle edema of recent onset. On examination, her jugular venous pulse is 5 cmH$_2$O and the hepatojugular reflux is negative. All the following should be considered in the differential diagnosis of the woman's ankle edema EXCEPT

(A) pelvic thrombophlebitis
(B) venous varicosities
(C) cyclic edema
(D) hypoalbuminemia
(E) right heart failure

140. All the following causes of congestive heart failure are associated with a widened arterial–mixed venous oxygen difference EXCEPT

(A) tricuspid stenosis
(B) alcoholic cardiomyopathy
(C) Paget's disease
(D) constrictive pericarditis
(E) right ventricular infarction

141. Examination of the carotid pulse reveals two impulses or peaks during ventricular systole. Which of the following physical findings would likely be associated with this finding?

(A) Diastolic murmur beginning after an opening snap
(B) Decrease in systolic arterial pressure during inspiration
(C) Systolic murmur increasing during the Valsalva maneuver
(D) Right-sided third heart sound
(E) Left-sided third heart sound

142. The electrocardiogram shown below is consistent with which of the following clinical situations?

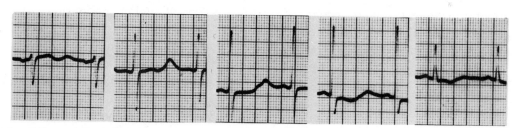

From Schlant, et al: *Hurst's The Heart*, 8/e. New York, McGraw-Hill, 1994, with permission.

(A) A 55-year-old man complaining of crushing substernal chest pain
(B) A 25-year-old woman with acute renal failure due to lupus nephritis
(C) A 27-year-old man with prolonged neutropenia after induction therapy for acute myeloid leukemia who is receiving amphotericin B
(D) A 57-year-old woman with metastatic breast cancer receiving etidronate
(E) A 72-year-old woman receiving digitalis therapy for chronic congestive heart failure

143. Digitalis glycosides enhance myocardial contractility primarily by which of the following mechanisms?

(A) Opening of calcium channels
(B) Release of calcium from the sarcoplasmic reticulum
(C) Stimulation of myosin ATPase
(D) Stimulation of membrane phospholipase C
(E) Inhibition of membrane Na^+-K^+-ATPase

144. An elderly person who has been taking digitalis for heart failure is brought to the hospital because of anorexia and nausea. On examination, ventricular bigeminy is noted. Digoxin level is 1.5 pg/L. All the following factors would be expected to contribute to digitalis intoxication EXCEPT

(A) chronic obstructive lung disease with hypoxemia
(B) addition of quinidine to the therapeutic regimen
(C) diuretic therapy with loop diuretics
(D) hyperthyroidism
(E) hyperparathyroidism

145. Which of the following is likely to be the clinical consequence of an irregularly shaped mass in the right atrium noted on two-dimensional echocardiography?

(A) Pleuritic chest pain
(B) Right-sided weakness
(C) Substernal chest pain
(D) Pedal edema
(E) Orthopnea

146. A 65-year-old man with a long history of untreated hypertension complains of recurrent shortness of breath on minimal exertion. Examination of the cardiovascular system is normal except for a prominent precordial impulse. Chest x-ray is normal except for a prominent left ventricular shadow. An exercise tolerance test with thallium scanning reveals no evidence of myocardial ischemia. Two-dimensional echocardiography reveals left ventricular hypertrophy. Radionuclide ventriculography reveals a normal right and left ventricular ejection fraction. What is the most likely explanation for the patient's symptoms?

(A) Chronic obstructive pulmonary disease
(B) Reactive airways disease
(C) Systolic congestive heart failure
(D) Diastolic congestive heart failure
(E) Myocardial ischemia

147. Clues to the presence of atrioventricular nodal block (as opposed to trifascicular block) would include all the following EXCEPT

(A) clinical evidence of inferior myocardial infarction
(B) Wenckebach periodicity to conduction
(C) escape-focus rate faster than 50 beats per minute
(D) a narrow QRS complex at the escape focus
(E) unresponsiveness of the escape focus to atropine

148. A 79-year-old woman has daily episodes of lightheadedness. A rhythm strip shows sinus bradycardia at 52 beats per minute and 2.5-s sinus pause that produces no symptoms. The next step in this woman's management should be

(A) implantation of a permanent demand ventricular pacemaker
(B) trial of a temporary transvenous pacemaker
(C) institution of sublingual isoproterenol therapy
(D) continuous 24-h Holter monitoring
(E) exercise tolerance testing

149. Which of the following agents has been shown to reduce mortality in patients with congestive heart failure?

(A) Digitalis
(B) Furosemide
(C) Enalapril
(D) Procainamide
(E) Aspirin

150. A 68-year-old Haitian man presents with a chronic nonproductive cough, dyspnea on exertion, and chronic nonexertional chest pain. The patient notes a loss of 10 pounds over the past 6 months, decreased appetite, and swelling of the ankles. Physical findings reveal an ill-appearing man with decreased skeletal mass. Blood pressure is 100/70 without a significant inspiratory decrease in systolic pressure. Heart rate is 110; respiratory rate is 25; temperature is 37.2°C (99.0°F) orally. Significant physical findings include the absence of rales on chest examination and the presence of jugular venous distention with a decline during inspiration. The apical cardiac pulse is reduced. The heart sounds are distant; an early third heart sound occurs very shortly after aortic valve closure; there are no murmurs. Both the liver and spleen are enlarged and there is a fluid wave on abdominal examination. Electrocardiography displays low QRS voltage but is otherwise unremarkable. Chest x-ray reveals clear lungs and an enlarged cardiac silhouette. Which of the following findings is most likely to be found on echocardiographic examination?

(A) Enlarged right ventricular size
(B) Pericardial effusion
(C) Thickened myocardium
(D) Thickened pericardium
(E) Right ventricular diastolic collapse

151. A 60-year-old man is admitted to a hospital because of respiratory failure and tachycardia. His rectal temperature is 38.3°C (101°F), respiratory rate 32 breaths per minute, and blood pressure 100/60 mmHg. His admission electrocardiogram is shown below. Which of the following measures would constitute the most appropriate management for this man?

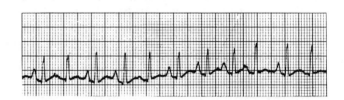

(A) Electrical cardioversion after the blood pressure is raised
(B) Supplemental oxygenation or mechanical ventilation
(C) Administration of digitalis
(D) Administration of quinidine
(E) Administration of verapamil

152. A 57-year-old previously healthy woman develops atrial flutter, 2:1 atrioventricular conduction, and a ventricular rate of 150 beats per minute. Her ventricular rate could be decreased safely with the use of all the following EXCEPT

(A) digoxin
(B) verapamil
(C) propranolol
(D) quinidine
(E) carotid sinus massage

153. Each of the following patients was noted to have an abnormally high serum cholesterol and was placed on a reduced calorie, cholesterol, and fat diet for the past 3 months. None has any history of ischemic heart disease. In which of the following patients would it be most appropriate to recommend lipid-lowering drug therapy at this time?

(A) A 52-year-old smoker and diabetic with an LDL cholesterol value of 3.2 mmol/L (120 mg/dL)

(B) A 60-year-old hypertensive woman with an LDL cholesterol value of 3.5 mmol/L (140 mg/dL)

(C) A 50-year-old man with cholesterol of 6 mmol/L (230 mg/dL)

(D) A 45-year-old man with LDL cholesterol of 5 mmol/L (200 mg/dL)

(E) A 58-year-old male smoker with cholesterol of 5.5 mmol/L (220 mg/dL) and LDL cholesterol of 4 mmol/L (150 mg/dL)

154. Which of the following statements regarding lipid-lowering agents is correct?

(A) Cholestyramine decreases LDL and VLDL lipoprotein levels

(B) Nicotinic acid lowers both LDL and VLDL levels and raises HDL cholesterol

(C) Lovastatin promotes gastrointestinal lipid clearance

(D) Gemfibrozil lowers LDL levels but increases VLDL

(E) Estrogens increase both VLDL and LDL levels

155. All the following statements regarding secundum atrial septal defect are true EXCEPT

(A) surgical correction is advisable when the pulmonary-to-systemic flow ratio has reached 2.0

(B) affected persons are usually asymptomatic in childhood

(C) electrocardiography shows a leftward axis

(D) echocardiography shows abnormal ventricular septal motion

(E) atrial arrhythmias are common

156. The chest x-rays below would likely have been taken of which of the following persons?

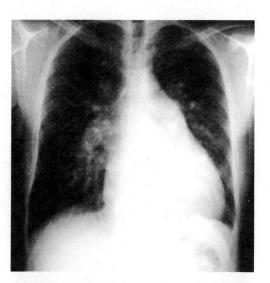

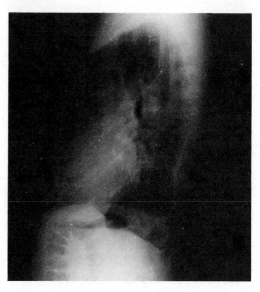

(A) A 38-year-old woman who has hemoptysis, dyspnea on exertion, and fatigability

(B) A 36-year-old woman who has a heart murmur but is asymptomatic

(C) A 32-year-old woman who has a continuous murmur, widened systemic pulse pressure, and dyspnea on exertion

(D) A 40-year-old woman who has a loud first heart sound, a diastolic rumble, a large *v* wave in her jugular pulse, and ascites

(E) None of the above

157. A 75-year-old man presents with recurrent episodes of shortness of breath on minimal exertion. He has no prior significant past medical history. Physical examination reveals blood pressure of 110/70 without pulsus paradoxus, heart rate of 110, respiratory rate of 25; and temperature of 37°C (98.6°F) orally. Jugular veins are distended and the heart sounds are distant but there are third and fourth extra heart sounds. The liver is enlarged and pedal edema is present. The electrocardiogram shows nonspecific ST-T wave changes and occasional premature ventricular contractions. The chest x-ray reveals clear lung fields and a mildly dilated cardiac silhouette. Echocardiography reveals normal systolic function and thickened ventricular walls with a "speckled" appearance. Which of the following conditions is most consistent with the patient's clinical presentation?

(A) Alcoholic cardiomyopathy
(B) Hemochromatosis
(C) Amyloidosis
(D) Viral myocarditis
(E) Tuberculosis

158. A 20-year-old woman has mild pulmonic stenosis (transvalvular gradient is 20 mmHg). All the following statements regarding this situation are true EXCEPT

(A) heart size on chest x-ray is likely to be normal
(B) electrocardiogram is likely to be normal
(C) her jugular *a* wave is likely to be prominent
(D) compared to other valvular defects, the risk of endocarditis is relatively low
(E) frequent monitoring for progression of the stenosis is indicated

159. A 23-year-old female medical student undergoes a routine physical examination. An echocardiogram, ordered because of the finding of a systolic murmur, reveals a ventricular septal defect. The patient is totally asymptomatic at this time. Which of the following statements concerning the patient's condition is correct?

(A) No further intervention is required
(B) If the patient becomes symptomatic, then further evaluation would be required
(C) Cardiac catheterization is required to clarify the anatomic and hemodynamic details
(D) Catheterization is unnecessary; the patient should be taken to surgery at this time
(E) The patient requires surgery at this time, but catheterization should be performed to clarify anatomic details for the surgeon

160. All the following findings would be expected in a person with coarctation of the aorta EXCEPT

(A) a systolic murmur across the anterior chest and back and a high-pitched diastolic murmur along the left sternal border
(B) a higher blood pressure in the right arm than in the left arm
(C) inability to augment cardiac output with exercise
(D) rib notching on chest x-ray
(E) persistent hypertension despite complete surgical repair

161. A 15-year-old boy residing with his parents on a military base presents with a fever of 38.6°C (101.5°F) and complains of lower back, knee, and wrist pain. The arthritis is not localized to any one joint. He gives a history of a severe sore throat several weeks ago. Physical examination of the skin reveals pea-sized swellings over the elbows and wrists. He also has two serpiginous, erythematous, pink areas on the anterior trunk, each of about 5 cm in diameter. Laboratory investigation includes negative blood cultures, negative throat culture, normal CBC, and erythrocyte sedimentation rate (ESR) of 100. An antistreptolysin-O (ASO) titer is elevated. At this point, appropriate therapy would be

(A) supportive care alone
(B) parenteral penicillin
(C) parenteral penicillin and glucocorticoids
(D) parenteral penicillin and aspirin
(E) parenteral penicillin, aspirin, and diazepam

162. Each patient below is alert and oriented and has a blood pressure of 110/60. In which patient would adenosine be appropriate initial therapy?

(A) A 65-year-old man with no ischemic heart disease and wide complex tachycardia
(B) A 65-year-old woman with known ischemic disease and narrow complex tachycardia
(C) A 25-year-old woman with known preexcitation syndrome and narrow complex tachycardia
(D) A 28-year-old man with known preexcitation syndrome and wide complex tachycardia
(E) A 44-year-old man with atrial fibrillation without prior history of heart disease

163. Factors accounting for the pedal edema associated with congestive heart failure include all the following EXCEPT

(A) increased secretion of aldosterone
(B) increased effective arterial blood volume
(C) increased level of plasma renin
(D) renal vasoconstriction
(E) sympathetic nervous system–mediated renal vasoconstriction

164. Which of the following statements best describes long-acting nitrate preparations?

(A) Tolerance often develops
(B) Their effect can be blocked by high doses of beta$_2$ selective inhibitors
(C) Transdermal patches are more likely to be associated with headaches than are sublingual nitrates
(D) Oral preparations are more effective than sublingual ones
(E) Oral administration of isosorbide should not exceed 15 mg every 3 to 4 h

165. A 70-year-old retired banker with no past medical history presents to the emergency department 4 h after the onset of severe substernal crushing chest pain with radiation to the left arm and neck. Electrocardiogram reveals significant ST-segment elevation in leads I, L, V$_5$, and V$_6$. The patient has no clear-cut medical contraindications to anticoagulation. Which of the following would be the optimal management strategy at this time?

(A) Intravenous tissue plasminogen activator alone
(B) Intravenous tissue plasminogen activator and aspirin
(C) Intravenous tissue plasminogen activator and heparin
(D) Intravenous tissue plasminogen activator, heparin, and aspirin
(E) Thrombolytic therapy is contraindicated because of the patient's age

166. Aspirin has been shown to reduce the risk of myocardial infarction in all the following groups EXCEPT

    (A) patients with chronic stable angina
    (B) patients who have survived unstable angina
    (C) patients who have survived myocardial infarction
    (D) patients experiencing unstable angina
    (E) patients with ischemic cardiomyopathy

167. A 62-year-old woman was started on a regimen of quinidine sulfate because of asymptomatic ventricular couplets. One week later, she was admitted to the hospital after a syncopal episode. Serum electrolyte concentrations were normal. The arrhythmia shown below appeared transiently on her cardiac monitor. The recommended course at this time is to

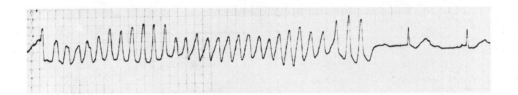

    (A) increase the quinidine dose
    (B) discontinue administration of quinidine and observe
    (C) begin intravenous administration of procainamide 2 mg/min
    (D) administer sodium bicarbonate, 70 meq, intravenously
    (E) administer potassium chloride, 10 meq, intravenously over 1 h

168. A 45-year-old man with essential hypertension was treated with enalapril 5 mg daily. After 6 months of therapy, the arterial pressure was measured at 150/100 mmHg. His physician advised sodium restriction and doubled the dose of enalapril to 10 mg daily. His blood pressure was unchanged after 3 additional months. At this point, the next recommended intervention would be

    (A) double the dose of enalapril
    (B) add 25 mg of hydrochlorothiazide daily
    (C) double the dose of enalapril and add 25 mg of hydrochlorothiazide
    (D) switch to captopril 50 mg three times per day
    (E) add diltiazem 360 mg per day

169. This two-dimensional echocardiogram was most likely recorded in which of the following patients?

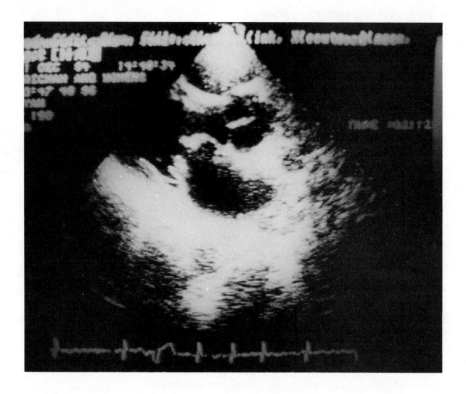

(A) A 54-year-old man with syncopal episodes when bending forward
(B) A previously healthy 68-year-old man with sudden onset of pulmonary edema and a new holosystolic murmur
(C) A 17-year-old girl with atypical chest pain and a midsystolic click
(D) A 42-year-old woman with palpitations, exertional dyspnea, and episodes of hemoptysis
(E) An asymptomatic 32-year-old cardiologist

170. A 63-year-old black woman with a long history of hypertension and diabetes is brought to the emergency department by relatives because she has become incoherent over the past 24 h. Physical examination reveals a disoriented woman whose blood pressure is 230/160, respiratory rate 25, and pulse 110. The patient is afebrile. The chest reveals bibasilar rales. Cardiac examination is remarkable only for the presence of an S_4. There is no organomegaly or focal neurologic findings. The patient is oriented to person only.

The family revealed that the patient has not been taking her antihypertensive medicines in the past several weeks. The patient is placed on a cardiac monitor and both intravenous and intraarterial lines are placed. An emergent CT scan reveals no evidence for hemorrhage or mass lesion. The next most appropriate step in management would be to

(A) observe the patient in a quiet room for 1 h prior to administering therapy
(B) wait for laboratory values to return before deciding on specific therapy
(C) administer sodium nitroprusside
(D) administer diazoxide
(E) administer intravenous nicardipine

171. A previously healthy 58-year-old man is admitted to the hospital because of an acute inferior myocardial infarction. Within several hours, he becomes oliguric and hypotensive (blood pressure is 90/60 mmHg). Insertion of a pulmonary artery (Swan-Ganz) catheter reveals the following pressures: pulmonary capillary wedge, 4 mmHg; pulmonary artery, 22/4 mmHg; and mean right atrial, 11 mmHg. This man would best be treated with

(A) fluids
(B) digoxin
(C) norepinephrine
(D) dopamine
(E) intraaortic balloon counterpulsation

172. All the following statements regarding myocardial hypertrophy are true EXCEPT

(A) norepinephrine induces the synthesis of fetal myosin forms
(B) the proto-oncogenes c-*sis*, c-*myc*, c-*ras*, and c-*fos* are all induced in myocardial tissue during hypertrophy
(C) a gene responsible for familial hypertrophic cardiomyopathy has been mapped to chromosome 14
(D) angiotensin II can stimulate hypertrophy by direct effects on smooth muscle
(E) hypertrophy due to hemodynamic overload is accompanied by a similar synthetic induction of fetal myosin forms to that observed in the hypertrophy associated with hyperthyroidism

173. Which of the following patients should undergo operative excision of an abdominal aortic aneurysm and replacement with a vascular graft?

(A) A 58-year-old man with an 8-cm abdominal aneurysm who sustained a myocardial infarction 3 months ago
(B) A 65-year-old man with a 7-cm aneurysm who sustained a myocardial infarction 1 year ago
(C) A 65-year-old woman with a 4-cm aneurysm and no prior history of heart or lung disease
(D) A 58-year-old man with a 7-cm aneurysm and FEV_1 of 0.8 L
(E) A 67-year-old man with an 8-cm aneurysm and creatinine 3.2 mg/dL

174. A 72-year-old man with a history of diabetes, mild chronic renal insufficiency, hypertension, and chronically severe angina develops a rash several hours after undergoing cardiac catheterization. The patient complains of diffuse pain and tenderness. Skin is notable for localized areas of tenderness and pallor in a mottled appearance (livedo reticularis). His right great toe is cold and blue. Which of the following procedures would be the best way to establish the diagnosis?

(A) Femoral angiography
(B) Abdominal CT scan
(C) Blood culture
(D) Urinalysis
(E) Skin biopsy

175. All the following statements regarding physiologic maneuvers used to distinguish one cardiac condition from another are true EXCEPT

(A) the Valsalva maneuver results in a decreased length and intensity for most systolic murmurs, except those due to mitral valve prolapse and hypertrophic cardiomyopathy
(B) in the case of mitral valve prolapse, squatting results in increased intensity of the systolic murmur
(C) handgrip exercise increases the intensity of the murmurs of mitral stenosis and mitral regurgitation
(D) murmurs of tricuspid regurgitation and tricuspid stenosis increase during inspiration
(E) the murmur of aortic stenosis increases following a ventricular premature beat

176. A 68-year-old man who has had a recent syncopal episode is hospitalized with congestive heart failure. His blood pressure is 160/80 mmHg, his pulse rate is 80 beats per minute, and there is a grade III/VI harsh systolic murmur. An echocardiogram shows a disproportionately thickened ventricular septum and systolic anterior motion of the mitral valve. Which of the following findings would most likely be present in this man?

(A) Radiation of the murmur to the carotid arteries
(B) Decrease of the murmur with hand grip
(C) Delayed carotid upstroke
(D) Reduced left ventricular ejection fraction
(E) Signs of mitral stenosis

177. Which factor accounts for the prolonged QRS complex depicted in this figure?

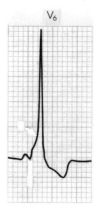

(A) Left ventricular hypertrophy
(B) Accessory conducting fibers parallel to the AV junction
(C) Right ventricular infarction
(D) Left bundle branch block
(E) Right bundle branch block

178. Each of the following techniques can detect nonviable myocardium EXCEPT

   (A) positron emission tomography (PET)
   (B) thallium 210 scintigraphy
   (C) technetium 99m stannous pyrophosphate scintigraphy
   (D) standard computed tomography (CT)
   (E) echocardiography

179. For the last 6 h, a 33-year-old man has had sharp, pleuritic, substernal chest pain that is relieved when he sits upright. His electrocardiogram shows diffuse ST-segment elevation. Which of the following observations would LEAST support a diagnosis of acute pericarditis?

   (A) Frequent atrial premature beats
   (B) PR-segment depression
   (C) Diffuse T-wave inversion with ST-segment elevation
   (D) Twice-normal serum creatine phosphokinase concentration
   (E) No rub

180. All the following electrocardiographic findings may represent manifestations of digitalis intoxication EXCEPT

   (A) bigeminy
   (B) junctional tachycardia
   (C) atrial flutter
   (D) atrial tachycardia with variable block
   (E) sinus arrest

181. All the following are indications for surgical intervention in the treatment of dissection of the aorta EXCEPT

   (A) compromised femoral pulse
   (B) new murmur of aortic regurgitation
   (C) persistent chest pain
   (D) involvement of the ascending aorta
   (E) involvement of the descending aorta

182. All the following congenital cardiac disorders will lead to a left-to-right shunt, generally without cyanosis, EXCEPT

   (A) anomalous origin of the left coronary artery from the pulmonary trunk
   (B) patent ductus arteriosus without pulmonary hypertension
   (C) total anomalous pulmonary venous connection
   (D) ventricular septal defect
   (E) sinus venosus atrial septal defect

183. Clear contraindications to the use of thrombolytic agents in the setting of an acute anterior myocardial infarction include all the following EXCEPT

   (A) left carotid artery occlusion with hemiparesis 1 month ago
   (B) transurethral resection of the prostate 1 week ago
   (C) diastolic blood pressure of 110 mmHg during chest pain
   (D) patient age greater than 70
   (E) epigastric pain and melena 1 week ago treated with histamine receptor antagonists

184. True statements describing dissection of the aorta include all the following EXCEPT

   (A) nearly all cases involve medial necrosis
   (B) coexisting hypertension is present in more than two-thirds of the patients
   (C) all false aneurysms begin with rupture of the aorta
   (D) dissection associated with Marfan's syndrome (type II dissection) stops before the great vessels arising from the aortic arch
   (E) appropriate medical management could consist of labetolol or a combination of nitroprusside and a beta blocker

185. Which of the following situations in the periinfarction period would suggest the presence of ventricular septal perforation?

  (A) Systolic murmur, large v waves in pulmonary capillary wedge tracing; P_{O_2} in right atrium equals that in right ventricle

  (B) Systolic murmur, large v waves in pulmonary capillary wedge tracing; P_{O_2} in right atrium is greater than that in the right ventricle

  (C) Systolic murmur, large v waves in pulmonary capillary wedge tracing; P_{O_2} in right atrium is less than that in the right ventricle

  (D) Diastolic murmur, large v waves in the pulmonary capillary wedge tracing; P_{O_2} in the right atrium is less than that in the right ventricle

  (E) Diastolic murmur, large v waves in the pulmonary capillary wedge tracing; P_{O_2} in the right atrium is greater than that in the right ventricle

186. A 50-year-old man with a history of smoking, hypertension, and chronic exertional angina develops several daily episodes of chest pain at rest compatible with cardiac ischemia. The patient is hospitalized. All the following would be part of an appropriate management plan EXCEPT

  (A) intravenous heparin
  (B) aspirin
  (C) intravenous nitroglycerin
  (D) lidocaine by bolus infusion
  (E) diltiazem

187. Cardiac catheterization disclosing decreased cardiac output, elevation of right and left end-diastolic pressures, and a dip and plateau configuration during the diastolic portion of the ventricular pressure tracing could be seen in all the following conditions EXCEPT

  (A) Duchenne's muscular dystrophy
  (B) amyloidosis
  (C) hemochromatosis
  (D) hypereosinophilic syndrome
  (E) endomyocardial fibrosis

188. All the following patients are at increased risk for the development of deep venous thrombosis EXCEPT

  (A) a 35-year-old woman with systemic lupus erythematosus and a prolonged partial thromboplastin time

  (B) a 75-year-old woman with a Colles fracture of the wrist

  (C) a normotensive 18-year-old woman taking an oral contraceptive

  (D) a 55-year-old man 3 days after an uncomplicated inferior myocardial infarction

  (E) a 55-year-old man 5 days after complete resection of a squamous cell carcinoma of 2 cm in diameter in the periphery of the right lung

189. This figure most likely represents the pulmonary capillary wedge and left ventricular pressure tracing from which of the following patients?

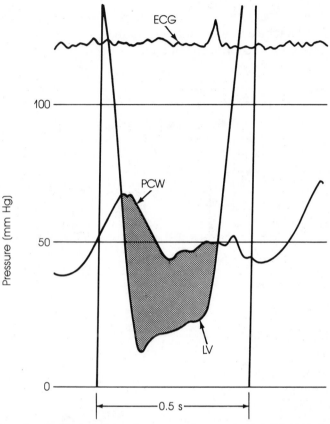

From Grossman W (ed): *Cardiac Catheterization and Angiography*, 3d ed. Philadelphia, Lea & Febiger, 1986, with permission.

(A) A 40-year-old woman with a history of rheumatic fever, orthopnea, and hemoptysis

(B) A 24-year-old intravenous drug abuser with fever, holosystolic murmur, and large mitral valve vegetation

(C) A 26-year-old man with long arms, abnormal lenses, and a diastolic murmur

(D) A 72-year-old man with left ventricular hypertrophy, syncope, and a systolic murmur

(E) A 35-year-old woman with elevated neck veins and a large mediastinal mass due to non-Hodgkin's lymphoma

DIRECTIONS: Each question below contains five suggested responses. For **each** of the five responses listed with every question, you are to respond either YES (Y) or NO (N). In a given item **all, some, or none** of the responses may be correct.

190. A 62-year-old man loses consciousness in the street, and resuscitative efforts are undertaken. In the emergency room an electrocardiogram is obtained, part of which is shown below. Which of the following disorders could account for this man's presentation?

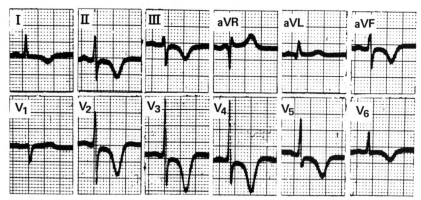

From Marriott HJL: *Practical Electrocardiography*, 7th ed. Baltimore, Williams & Wilkins, 1983, p 400, with permission.

    (A)   Subendocardial infarction
    (B)   Hyperkalemia
    (C)   Intracerebral hemorrhage
    (D)   Myocardial ischemia
    (E)   Hypocalcemic tetany

---

191. A loud first heart sound is associated frequently with

    (A)   hypothyroidism
    (B)   Lown-Ganong-Levine syndrome
    (C)   mitral stenosis
    (D)   mitral regurgitation
    (E)   fever

192. Acute hyperkalemia is associated with which of the following electrocardiographic changes?

    (A)   QRS widening
    (B)   Prolongation of the ST segment
    (C)   Decrease in the P wave
    (D)   Prominent U waves
    (E)   Peaked T waves

193. True statements regarding exercise tolerance tests include which of the following?

(A) Requiring $\geq$ 2.0 mm of ST depression to define a test as positive enhances the sensitivity of the test compared with a situation in which only 0.5 mm of ST depression is required to count as positive

(B) Given a specificity of 90 percent and a sensitivity of 80 percent, a positive test in a patient whose prior probability of having coronary artery disease (based on clinical factors) is 10 percent suggests a greater than 80 percent likelihood that the patient actually has coronary artery disease

(C) Thallium 201 exercise scanning increases both the sensitivity and specificity for detecting ischemic heart disease

(D) A thallium 201 scan done at peak exercise that reveals a nonperfused area of myocardium indicates that the patient has suffered a prior myocardial infarction

(E) A marked increase in blood pressure during the test suggests poor conditioning and will likely cause the test to be nondiagnostic

194. The rhythm shown on the electrocardiogram below can be associated with

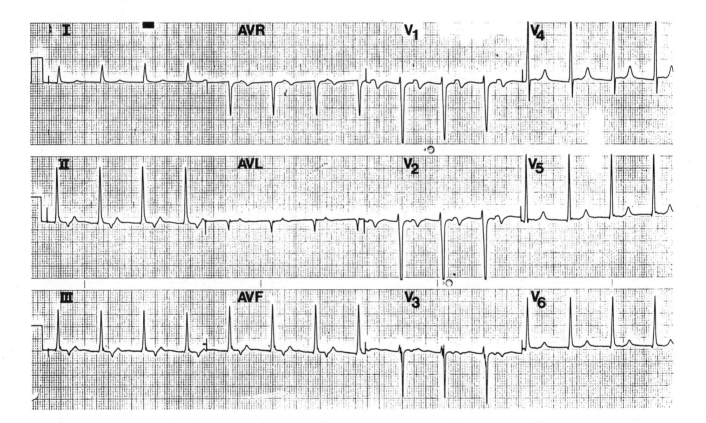

(A) digitalis toxicity
(B) acute myocarditis
(C) anterior myocardial infarction
(D) mitral valve surgery
(E) hypercalcemia

195. Features of chest pain that increase the probability that the patient has myocardial ischemia include which of the following?

(A) Radiation of pain to the forehead
(B) Abrupt, sharp pain in the substernal area radiating to the back
(C) Relief of pain 2 min after the administration of sublingual nitroglycerin
(D) Relief of pain seconds after recumbency
(E) Radiation of pain to the teeth

196. Mild heart failure due to left ventricular dysfunction is accurately described by which of the following statements?

(A) Cardiac output would be depressed at rest
(B) Plasma norepinephrine levels would be higher than in normal controls during exercise
(C) Myocardial norepinephrine content would be high
(D) Left ventricular end-diastolic pressure would rise more during exercise than in normal controls
(E) Cardiac output would fail to rise appropriately when oxygen consumption is increased during exercise

197. Drugs that would *antagonize* the interaction of catecholamines with adrenergic receptors include

(A) prazosin
(B) clonidine
(C) phenylephrine
(D) yohimbine
(E) isoproterenol

198. Sudden cardiac death is accurately described by which of the following statements?

(A) Ventricular tachycardia or ventricular fibrillation during the convalescent phase (3 days to 8 weeks) after a myocardial infarction is a risk factor for subsequent sudden cardiac death
(B) A patient convalescing from a myocardial infarction displaying a salvo of three ventricular premature beats is at greater risk than a similar patient who has 35 unifocal premature beats per hour
(C) If only one person is present to provide basic life support, chest compressions should be performed at a rate of 80 per minute and breaths twice in succession every 15 s
(D) Assuming there is no spontaneous pulse, a 400-joule shock should be delivered immediately upon recognition of ventricular tachycardia or ventricular fibrillation
(E) Intravenous sodium bicarbonate should be given approximately every 5 min during cardiac arrest

199. A 37-year-old man with Wolff-Parkinson-White syndrome develops a broad-complex irregular tachycardia at a rate of 200 beats per minute. He appears comfortable and has little hemodynamic impairment. Useful treatment at this point might include

(A) digoxin
(B) quinidine
(C) propranolol
(D) verapamil
(E) direct-current cardioversion

200. A 17-year-old girl has an atrial septal defect of the sinus venosus type, with a 3:1 pulmonary-to-systemic blood flow ratio. True statements concerning her condition include which of the following?

(A) She is probably asymptomatic
(B) She probably has partial anomalous connection of the pulmonary veins
(C) The magnitude of the shunt is a function of the amount of total blood flow
(D) A systolic murmur would likely be due to flow across the defect
(E) A diastolic rumble would strongly suggest coexistence of mitral stenosis (Lutembacher's syndrome)

201. For which of the following patients would cardiac surgery be appropriately recommended?

(A) An asymptomatic 18-year-old woman who has an atrial septal defect with a 2:1 pulmonary-to-systemic flow ratio
(B) An asymptomatic 19-year-old man who has a loud murmur and ventricular septal defect with a 1.5:1 pulmonary-to-systemic flow ratio
(C) A 33-year-old man who has chest pain, fatigue, cyanosis, a large ventricular septal defect, a 2:1 right-to-left shunt, and a normal pulmonary outflow tract and pulmonic valve
(D) A 52-year-old man who has chronic mitral regurgitation and has recently developed pulmonary edema associated with the onset of rapid atrial fibrillation
(E) A 54-year-old man who has aortic stenosis and has chest pain on moderate-to-strenuous exertion

202. The initial positive deflection in the jugular venous pulse (*a* wave) can be accentuated in which of the following conditions?

(A) Junctional rhythm
(B) Tricuspid stenosis
(C) Atrial fibrillation
(D) Multiple pulmonary emboli
(E) Complete heart block

203. A 64-year-old man with aortic stenosis is admitted to the hospital because of the recent onset of congestive heart failure. True statements characterizing his condition include which of the following?

(A) The development of atrial fibrillation (ventricular response of 70 beats per minute) could explain the deterioration of his condition
(B) The absence of left ventricular hypertrophy on the electrocardiogram excludes severe obstruction
(C) Absence of aortic valve calcification on echocardiography rules out severe aortic stenosis
(D) Once his congestive heart failure is treated, he may do well for several more years
(E) If an echocardiogram shows cusp calcification, then his aortic stenosis is likely to be severe

204. True statements regarding balloon valvuloplasty include

(A) balloon dilation of a stenotic pulmonary valve is not feasible because of the danger of rupture of the thin-walled pulmonary artery
(B) mitral valvuloplasty increases the effective diastolic valve area to normal size
(C) balloon aortic valvuloplasty is contraindicated in calcific aortic stenosis because the fracture of calcium deposits on the leaflets leads to cerebral emboli
(D) restenosis after aortic valvuloplasty is a significant problem
(E) aortic valvuloplasty results in symptomatic improvement for most patients

205. True statements regarding hemodynamic changes occurring during exercise include which of the following?

   (A) Venous return is augmented by the pumping action of skeletal muscles
   (B) The increased adrenergic nerve impulses to the heart as well as an increased concentration of circulating catecholamines help to augment the contractile state of the myocardium
   (C) Venoconstriction in exercising muscles as well as increased cardiac output leads to marked increases in systemic blood pressure
   (D) End-diastolic volume increases in the failing heart during exercise
   (E) Stroke volume and heart rate increase

206. A 34-year-old woman is bothered by palpitations and chest pain. On auscultation, the first heart sound is normal, but there is a midsystolic click and a late systolic murmur. Her electrocardiogram shows T-wave inversions in leads II, III, and aVF. True statements concerning her condition include which of the following?

   (A) An exercise stress test would most likely be positive
   (B) An echocardiogram may show abrupt posterior displacement of both mitral leaflets
   (C) The woman's chest pain could be due to excessive stress on the papillary muscles
   (D) The click and murmur would be expected to occur later in systole when the woman stands
   (E) Prophylactic measures should be taken to prevent subacute bacterial endocarditis

207. A permanent atrioventricular sequential pacemaker (DDD) would be preferred to a standard ventricular pacemaker (VVI) in which of the following patients?

   (A) A 64-year-old woman with atrial fibrillation and a ventricular rate of 40 beats per minute
   (B) A 56-year-old man with complete heart block and a global left ventricular ejection fraction of 36 percent
   (C) An active 46-year-old man with high-grade atrioventricular block
   (D) An 80-year-old woman with symptomatic bradyarrhythmias and normal left ventricular function
   (E) A 50-year-old man with hypertrophic cardiomyopathy and infranodal second-degree atrioventricular block

208. A 58-year-old man with a history of severe hypertension, three prior myocardial infarctions, and a left ventricular ejection fraction of 15 percent presents with a 30-pound weight loss. Workup for malignancy is negative. Which of the following factors could explain the patient's cachexia and weight loss?

   (A) Digitalis intoxication
   (B) Protein loss in the gastrointestinal tract due to high right-sided pressures
   (C) Elevation of the metabolic rate
   (D) Malabsorption of nutrients
   (E) Incomplete gastric filling

209. Correct statements regarding cardiac transplantation include

   (A) the 5-year survival is 25 to 50 percent
   (B) two P waves are typically evident on the electrocardiogram of patients with a transplanted heart
   (C) risk factors for accelerated coronary vascular disease include the number of rejection episodes and hyperlipidemia
   (D) coronary disease accounts for the majority of late (> 1 year after transplant) deaths
   (E) immunosuppressive drugs can be discontinued after 5 years since the risk of rejection after that point is extremely low

210. A 70-year-old man with a history of the "bradytachy syndrome" treated by insertion of a ventricular demand pacemaker (VVI) develops fatigue, dizziness, and syncope. Assuming no deterioration in his intrinsic cardiac function, which of the following factors could account for his symptoms?

(A) Pacemaker-mediated triggering of tachyarrhythmias due to ventriculoatrial conduction

(B) Loss of atrial contribution to ventricular systole

(C) Large *a* waves on the jugular venous pulse

(D) Systemic and pulmonary venous regurgitation due to atrial contraction against a closed AV valve

(E) Intermittent ventricular tachycardia induced by chronic irritation of the right ventricular wall by the pacemaker lead

211. A 50-year-old woman with a history of hypertension (but who is taking no medication currently) presents to the emergency ward with a complaint of sudden palpitations and faintness. Her pulse is 120 and the 12-lead ECG discloses a wide-complex tachycardia. Which of the following characteristics would suggest a ventricular origin for her tachycardia rather than supraventricular tachycardia with aberrant conduction?

(A) A QRS complex of 0.12 s

(B) A QRS complex of 0.22 s

(C) Very irregular rhythm

(D) Atrioventricular dissociation

(E) A Q wave in lead V_6 and a broad R wave in V_1

212. True statements about the side effects of antiarrhythmic drugs include which of the following?

(A) Verapamil can cause hemodynamic collapse if administered to patients with sustained ventricular tachycardia

(B) Blue-gray skin pigmentation, thyroid abnormalities, and corneal deposits are seen with prolonged use of flecainide

(C) Thrombocytopenia is a well-recognized, occasional consequence of procainamide

(D) Glaucoma can develop after the institution of disopyramide for ventricular tachycardia

(E) Quinidine can precipitate digitalis toxicity

213. A 23-year-old man has had recent onset of exertional dyspnea. A grade III/VI systolic murmur is heard at the left sternal border. Electrocardiography shows apical and lateral Q waves and left ventricular hypertrophy. Echocardiography reveals asymmetric septal hypertrophy without evidence of obstruction. Correct statements regarding this clinical situation include which of the following?

(A) The man's dyspnea is best explained by lateral wall infarction

(B) First-degree relatives should be evaluated

(C) The risk of sudden death is low

(D) Calcium-channel blockers may relieve symptoms

(E) The man's heart is normal histologically, aside from changes of infarction

214. Aortic regurgitation is accurately characterized by which of the following statements?

(A) Most cases of aortic regurgitation (with or without associated lesions) are due to congenital (including Marfan's syndrome), syphilitic, or spondylitic causes

(B) *Quincke's pulse* refers to the pistol-shot sound audible over the femoral arteries

(C) The Graham Steell murmur of pulmonary regurgitation is frequently associated

(D) The echocardiogram frequently reveals fluttering of the anterior leaflet of the mitral valve

(E) Surgical correction can be delayed if the patient is asymptomatic and retains normal left ventricular function

215. Correct statements regarding the laboratory evaluation of suspected myocardial infarction include which of the following?

(A) Creatine phosphokinase usually rises 4 h after a myocardial infarction

(B) A rise in lactic dehydrogenase (LDH) following the death of myocardium may persist for 14 days

(C) Increased LDH isoenzyme 1 (LDH$_1$) is a more sensitive indicator of myocardial infarction than is total LDH

(D) In hypothyroid patients, serum creatine phosphokinase levels will not rise even after a myocardial infarction

(E) The opening of a coronary occlusion after an infarction will lead to a delayed and blunted elevation of creatine phosphokinase

216. Which of the following findings would likely be present in a patient who sustained recurrent pulmonary emboli?

(A) Decreased lung volumes on spirometric testing

(B) Enlarged P waves on electrocardiographic examination

(C) Tricuspid regurgitant flow on Doppler echocardiography

(D) Positive right ventricular uptake on thallium 201 scintigraphy

(E) Prominent *a* waves on physical examination of jugular venous pulsation

217. True statements regarding the effect of alcohol on the heart include which of the following?

(A) Chronic ingestion of alcohol will lead to a restrictive cardiomyopathy

(B) Once heart failure develops, discontinuing consumption of alcohol will not appreciably affect the natural history of the disease

(C) If thiamine deficiency is present in the alcoholic, high output failure is noted

(D) If the patient with heart failure due to ethanol continues to drink, he or she is unlikely to be alive in 3 years

(E) The most common arrhythmia associated with a drinking binge is ventricular tachycardia

218. A 45-year-old woman with a history of metastatic breast cancer develops shortness of breath, cardiomegaly, and elevated neck veins. Findings consistent with pericardial involvement by tumor include

(A) a right ventricular free-wall collapse during left ventricular systole on the echocardiogram

(B) a 15 mmHg decrease in systolic arterial pressure during inspiration

(C) a prominent *x* descent on jugular venous pressure tracing

(D) pericardial pressure equal to right atrial pressure

(E) left ventricular systolic pressure equal to right ventricular end-systolic pressure

219. True statements regarding cardiac neoplasms include

    (A) lymphoma is the most common malignant neoplasm to primarily involve the heart

    (B) the most common site for a myxoma is the left atrium

    (C) myxomas may arise as part of a familial syndrome that also includes pigmented skin lesions and endocrine abnormalities

    (D) a midsystolic "plop" typically indicates the presence of a cardiac myxoma

    (E) weight loss and fever are frequent presenting manifestations of cardiac myxoma

220. True statements regarding risk factors for accelerating atherosclerosis include which of the following?

    (A) Increasing risk for the development of premature heart disease can be detected at serum cholesterol levels higher than 5.2 mmol/L (200 mg/dL)

    (B) Hypertriglyceridemia without a concomitant increase in cholesterol level is an independent risk factor for premature ischemic heart disease

    (C) All adults should have at least one lipoprotein electrophoresis as part of routine health care screening

    (D) Hyperlipidemia may be exacerbated by any of the following conditions: hypothyroidism, uremia, diabetes mellitus, and multiple myeloma

    (E) Reduction of serum glucose levels in a patient with diabetes mellitus will lower the risk of development of premature atherosclerosis

221. For the purpose of diagnosing secondary causes of high blood pressure, which of the following patients with hypertension should have workup beyond routine laboratory studies (blood urea nitrogen, glucose, creatinine, calcium, uric acid, potassium, cholesterol, triglycerides, electrocardiogram, and chest x-ray)?

    (A) A 35-year-old man with a prior history of normotension who presents with a blood pressure of 160/105 but an otherwise normal physical examination

    (B) A 35-year-old woman with a prior history of normotension who presents with a blood pressure of 160/105 and an abdominal bruit

    (C) A 60-year-old man with a prior history of normotension who presents with a blood pressure of 160/100

    (D) A 40-year-old woman with a prior history of normotension who presents with a blood pressure of 160/105 unresponsive to enalapril and hydrochlorothiazide

    (E) A 45-year-old man with an unknown prior history who presents with a blood pressure of 160/100 and left ventricular heave on physical examination

222. Peripheral arterial insufficiency is correctly characterized by which of the following statements?

    (A) Pentoxifylline is useful in the treatment of patients with claudication

    (B) At least 70 percent of femoral occlusions treated with a saphenous vein bypass graft remain open at 3 years

    (C) Patients with claudication should be advised to stay off their feet until a definitive treatment plan is outlined

    (D) A ratio of ankle to brachial artery pressures of 1.2:1 indicates arterial occlusive disease

    (E) Pain at rest due to arterial insufficiency mandates either angioplasty or arterial reconstruction

DIRECTIONS: The group of questions below consists of lettered headings followed by a set of numbered items. For each numbered item select the **one** lettered heading with which it is **most** closely associated. Each lettered heading may be used **once, more than once, or not at all.**

Questions 223–226

Match each of the causes of right heart failure below with the most characteristic set of hemodynamic measurements.

	Right Atrial Pressure, mmHg	Pulmonary Arterial Pressure, mmHg	Pulmonary Capillary Wedge Pressure, mmHg
(A)	16	75/30	11
(B)	16	35/17	16
(C)	16	100/30	28
(D)	16	45/22	20
(E)	16	22/12	10
Normal values	0–5	12–28/3–13	3–11

223. Right ventricular infarction

224. Cor pulmonale from bronchitis

225. Mitral stenosis

226. Constrictive pericarditis

Disorders of the Heart and Vascular System

Answers

128. The answer is B. *(Chap 202.)* The combination of hypotension and bradycardia suggests a vagal response in the setting of an acute myocardial infarction. Administration of the anticholinergic agent atropine is the treatment of choice. If the bradyarrhythmia and hypotension persist after 2.0 mg of atropine has been administered in divided doses, insertion of a temporary pacemaker is indicated. Isoproterenol should be avoided in patients with acute myocardial infarction since it may greatly increase myocardial oxygen consumption and thereby intensify ischemia. Volume replacement or inotropic support may be required if hypotension persists after correction of the bradyarrhythmia, but they are not indicated as initial therapies.

129. The answer is A. *(Chaps 34, 202.)* A patient presenting with hypotension and oliguria is critically ill and demands urgent definition of the etiology of this condition. The clinical presentation with shock, fever, and pulmonary infiltrates is consistent either with noncardiogenic or cardiogenic pulmonary edema. The elevated pulmonary capillary wedge pressure strongly suggests failure of left ventricular output, either due to primary myocardial dysfunction or obstruction caused by pericardial tamponade. Pulmonary emboli, septic shock, and hypovolemia from gastrointestinal blood loss would all cause the pulmonary capillary wedge pressure to be decreased. Though pericardial tamponade could produce an elevated pulmonary capillary wedge pressure, the obstruction to right ventricular inflow should be associated with equally abnormal right atrial mean, right ventricular end-diastolic, and pulmonary artery end-diastolic pressure. Therefore, this patient is suffering from cardiogenic shock due to left ventricular myocardial dysfunction on the basis of either myocardial infarction, severe cardiomyopathy, or myocarditis. Given the relatively normal electrocardiogram and a fever, the last condition is a distinct possibility.

130. The answer is D. *(Chap 35. Standards and guidelines for cardiopulmonary resuscitation [CPR] in emergency cardiac care [ECC]. JAMA 255:2905, 1986.)* The successful resuscitation of a patient suffering cardiac arrest depends on the rapidity of the initiation of resuscitative efforts, the clinical status of the patient prior to the arrest, and the mechanism of the event. In this case the patient has a reasonable chance of recovery based on his good initial performance status (the event occurred while he was golfing), rapid institution of CPR by trained personnel, and sustained ventricular tachycardia (VT) as the mechanism for the event. The most appropriate management of cardiac arrest induced by VT is an initial 200-joule defibrillation. Additional shocks at higher energies, up to a maximum of 360 joules, should be attempted in the event of the initial failure to abolish the VT. Whether the initial defibrillation attempt is successful or not, lidocaine should be given intravenously as a 1 mg/kg bolus to be followed in 2 min by the same dose if the arrhythmia is persistent.

Second-line drugs that can be used in the event of lidocaine failure include intravenous procain-amide and bretylium. If persistent ventricular fibrillation (VF) is the cause of the event, epineph-rine may be administered every 5 min. Intravenous sodium bicarbonate and calcium are no longer considered safe or necessary for routine administration. Intravenous calcium gluconate would be indicated in the setting of hyperkalemia as the triggering event for resistant VF, in the presence of known hypocalcemia, or in those who have received high doses of calcium channel antagonists.

131. The answer is A. *(Chap 209. Williams, N Engl J Med 319:1517, 1989.)* Captopril is an inhibitor of angiotensin-converting enzyme, and thus it impairs the production of angiotensin II, a potent vasoconstrictor. Through removal of feedback inhibition, renin secretion is *increased*. Additional antihypertensive effects of captopril result from a reduction of bradykinin degradation and stimu-lation of vasodilating prostaglandin production. Converting-enzyme inhibitors can be added to a regimen of beta blockade for an additional antihypertensive effect. Captopril is contraindicated in patients with bilateral renal artery stenosis since reduction in systemic arterial pressure may lead to progressive renal hypoperfusion.

132. The answer is C. *(Chap 206.)* The lateral-view chest film demonstrates calcification of the an-terior pericardium, consistent with constrictive pericarditis. This pattern is seen in approximately one-half of patients with long-standing constriction, and pericardial thickening can often be con-firmed by echocardiography. In patients with this disease, a pericardial knock is often heard 0.06 to 0.12 s after aortic valve closure, corresponding to the sudden cessation of ventricular filling. Murmurs are typically absent.

133. The answer is C. *(Chap 68.)* Basic knowledge of adrenergic, dopaminergic, and cholinergic phys-iology is necessary for understanding the treatment of a multitude of cardiovascular and respiratory disorders. Catecholamines influence a wide variety of cells by interacting with one of two popu-lations of adrenergic receptors, alpha or beta. Each of these categories is further divided into type 1 and type 2 subgroups. The alpha$_1$ receptor mediates what have come to be known as classic alpha effects, mainly vasoconstriction. Phenylephrine, used in refractory hypotension, is a selective alpha$_1$ agonist; prazosin is a fairly selective alpha$_1$ blocker used in the treatment of hypertension. Activation of the alpha$_2$ receptor causes presynaptic inhibition of epinephrine release from adren-ergic nerves and also inhibits acetylcholine release from cholinergic nerves. Other effects include the inhibition of lipolysis and insulin secretion as well as stimulation of platelet aggregation and vasoconstriction in some vascular beds. For example, clonidine is a specific alpha$_2$ agonist that exerts an antihypertensive effect by stimulating alpha$_2$ receptors in the brainstem. The beta$_1$ recep-tor mediates cardiac stimulation, both contractility and increased heart rate. The beta$_2$ receptor, more responsive to epinephrine than to norepinephrine, mediates vasodilation and bronchodila-tion. Isoproterenol stimulates both beta$_1$ and beta$_2$ receptors; as such, it is useful both in the situ-ation of cardiogenic shock and, as an inhaled agent, in the treatment of asthma. Selective beta$_2$ agonists, such as albuterol, are useful in asthma where bronchodilation is desired but not cardio-stimulatory effects. Since isoproterenol has relatively few alpha effects, vasoconstriction is not a major problem.

134. The answer is E. *(Chap 193.)* PTCA to reduce one or more coronary stenoses in the treatment of chronic angina unresponsive to medical therapy, unstable angina, or acute myocardial infarction has been employed with increasing frequency. The risks and benefits of PTCA compare favorably with those of conventional surgery. Given the decreased cost and recovery and hospitalization time, PTCA is preferred whenever possible. While the current PTCA success rate exceeds 90 percent, a return of cardiac ischemia within 6 months strongly suggests restenosis of the dilated segment. Such restenosis appears to result from excessive local smooth muscle cell hyperplasia, triggered by platelet adhesion on the balloon-damaged surface. While the use of nitrates, calcium channel antagonists, heparin, and aspirin just before and up to 6 months after the procedure helps to prevent an acute closure due to spasm and thrombus formation, no anatomic or pharmacologic strategy has substantially reduced the restenosis rate. When recurrent ischemia develops more than 6 months after a PTCA, progression of disease at another site is more likely than restenosis. However, repeat PTCA is quite successful in treating patients with restenosis; bypass surgery will be required in 10 percent or fewer of such patients.

135. **The answer is E.** *(Chap 190.)* Two-dimensional and M-mode echocardiograms directly image the intracardiac valves and are extremely useful in the detection of valvular stenosis. Doppler echocardiography permits the calculation of the pressure gradient across the intracardiac valves. Regurgitant lesions, such as those of the tricuspid valve, can be detected and the severity estimated by this technique. Although the echocardiographic findings of atrial septal defect are nonspecific (right ventricular volume overload pattern), Doppler studies can determine the presence of the transatrial shunt. Coronary calcification cannot at present be imaged with a high degree of sensitivity.

136. **The answer is E.** *(Chap 17.)* Chronic idiopathic orthostatic hypotension, most common among elderly men, is characterized by orthostatic hypotension in the absence of reflex tachycardia. Other autonomic disturbances typically are present, including anhidrosis, difficulty with urination, and constipation. In this condition, peripheral norepinephrine synthesis is deficient and plasma norepinephrine levels are low. Treatment consists of increasing intravascular volume and venous return as well as administering directly acting sympathomimetic agents. Tyramine and other indirectly acting sympathomimetic agents are not helpful. In central preganglionic autonomic insufficiency, a condition related to chronic idiopathic orthostatic hypotension, peripheral norepinephrine stores and plasma levels are normal but release of norepinephrine is deficient; this condition, which is associated with a variety of central nervous system manifestations, may respond to tyramine.

137. **The answer is A.** *(Chap 197.)* The electrocardiogram discloses sudden failure of atrial ventricular conduction without a preceding change in the PR interval, termed Mobitz type II second-degree AV block, which usually reflects significant disease of the conduction system. It may occur after a significant anterior myocardial infarction or in Lev's disease, which involves calcification and sclerosis of the fibrous cardiac skeleton (frequently involving the aortic and mitral valves), or in Lenegre's disease, which involves only the conducting system. Mobitz type II block is inherently unstable and tends to progress to complete heart block with a slow, lower escape pacemaker. Therefore, pacemaker implantation is necessary in this condition, particularly if the patient is symptomatic, as in this case.

138. **The answer is A.** *(Chaps 69, 187.)* Understanding the molecular mechanisms involved in the signaling cascade engendered by catecholamine adrenergic receptor binding may allow rational drug design. It is now known that the type of G protein (guanosine-binding regulatory proteins) will explain the results of such an interaction. For example, binding of dobutamine to the beta-adrenergic receptor–G protein complex results in a conformational change of the G-stimulatory protein (G_s). G_s activates adenylate cyclase, which in turn increases the level of cyclic AMP. Cyclic AMP stimulates myocardial contractility. On the other hand, G proteins coupled to alpha$_1$-adrenergic receptors activate an enzyme called phospholipase C, which hydrolyzes membrane phospholipids, into inositol triphosphate, which liberates calcium inositol from intracellular stores, and diacylgylcerol, the endogenous activator for the important enzyme calcium-sensitive protein kinase C. Activation of protein kinase C, a serine/threonine kinase, regulates myocyte ion channels and leads to myocardial hypertrophy by causing changes in gene expression.

139. The answer is E. *(Chaps 33, 195.)* Many persons who have ankle edema are inappropriately diagnosed as having heart failure. In particular, the diagnosis of right heart failure should not be made in the absence of jugular venous distention. Venous varicosities, cyclic edema, thrombophlebitis, and hypoalbuminemia all cause ankle edema and should be considered in the differential diagnosis.

140. The answer is C. *(Chap 195.)* Congestive heart failure associated with pulmonary and systemic venous congestion may occur either with low cardiac output and widened arterial–mixed venous oxygen difference or with high output and normal or narrowed arterial–mixed venous oxygen difference. High-output states are associated with usually low systemic vascular resistance and peripheral shunting. If Paget's disease is widespread, increased bony vascularity and overlying cutaneous vasodilation can lead to shunting and a high-output state. Venous congestion occurs when the ventricles are unable to handle the increased venous return.

141. The answer is C. *(Chaps 188, 205.)* Assessment of the central aortic pulse wave is best carried out by examination of the carotid pulsations. Normally, the carotid pulse is characterized by a fairly rapid rise to a somewhat rounded peak. If two such peaks are found, diagnostic considerations include aortic regurgitation and hypertrophic cardiomyopathy. In the latter condition, obstruction to outflow usually occurs in midsystole. Moreover, obstruction is more manifest during reduced left ventricular size, such as after a Valsalva maneuver with subsequent decreased venous return. A brief decline in pressure follows the sudden decrease in the rate of left ventricular ejection during midsystole because of the development of obstruction. The second peak is caused by a smaller positive pulse wave produced by the remainder of ventricular ejection and by reflected waves from peripheral sources. The so-called bisferiens pulse should be distinguished from pulsus alternans in which there is a regular alteration of the pressure pulse amplitude from beat to beat, usually associated with severe impairment of left ventricular function and therefore occurring in the setting of a third heart sound. Pulsus paradoxus, found in pericardial tamponade, severe airway disease, or superior vena cava obstruction, reflects an exaggerated decrease in systolic arterial pressure during inspiration.

142. The answer is C. *(Chap 189.)* This ECG reveals an abnormal increase in the amplitude of the U wave, a small deflection following the T wave usually having the same polarity as the T wave. Recognition of a pronounced U wave is important, for it may represent an increased susceptibility to a torsades de pointes type of ventricular tachycardia. Prominent U waves are most commonly seen subsequent to use of antiarrhythmic drugs such as quinidine, procainamide, and disopyramide or to hypokalemia. The latter condition would be typical of a patient receiving amphotericin B, which typically produces severe renal potassium wasting due to renal tubular damage. The patient with acute renal failure and hyperkalemia would display peaked T waves or an increased QRS duration on the ECG. Hypercalcemia, such as in patients with metastatic breast cancer, and digitalis intoxication tend to produce short QT intervals. Inverted U waves are sometimes a subtle sign of myocardial ischemia.

143. The answer is E. *(Chap 195.)* Digitalis glycosides augment contractility of the heart and slow atrioventricular condition and heart rate. The primary mechanism of action is inhibition of Na^+-K^+-ATPase, which is located in the sarcolemmal membrane. This action leads to intracellular accumulation of sodium and, subsequently, calcium by way of a sodium-calcium exchange mechanism.

144. The answer is D. *(Chap 195.)* Elderly persons are particularly prone to develop digitalis intoxication at relatively low doses and apparently normal serum levels (<2.0 pg/L). Exacerbating factors in the development of toxicity are hypoxemia and hypercalcemia. Potassium wasting and, perhaps, hypomagnesemia from potent loop diuretics also can foster toxicity. By reducing both its renal and nonrenal elimination, quinidine can increase the serum levels of digoxin, thereby inducing toxicity. Hyperthyroidism tends to decrease the efficacy of digitalis, while hypothyroidism enhances the likelihood of toxicity.

145. The answer is A. *(Chap 190. Popp, N Engl J Med 323:101–108, 165–172, 1990.)* Not only is it possible to diagnose right and left atrial enlargement with a two-dimensional echocardiogram, this technique is also the procedure of choice for documenting abnormal masses, such as myxomas or thrombi. An echocardiogram of an irregularly shaped mass in the right atrium that is able to move to and through the tricuspid valve could explain a patient's complaint of pleuritic chest pain. Such a mass, or part of the mass, could easily embolize through the right ventricular outflow tract and cause symptoms of pulmonary emboli. Echocardiographic documentation of such benign cardiac tumors is so convenient and specific that angiography is probably not required before surgery.

146. The answer is D. *(Chap 195. Grossman, N Engl J Med 325:1557–1564, 1991.)* Despite the fact that this patient's ejection fraction is normal, the presence of left ventricular hypertrophy, suggested by physical examination and confirmed by noninvasive testing, implicates the heart as the source of the problem. The patient has no evidence of either ischemic heart disease or lung disease, yet his ejection fraction is normal. However, it is now increasingly recognized that increased resistance to filling of one or more cardiac ventricles, so-called diastolic heart failure, can produce increased pulmonary capillary wedge pressures with resultant respiratory complaints. In conditions such as advanced myocardial hypertrophy, impaired diastolic relaxation occurs. While hypertrophic heart disease is probably the best recognized cause of diastolic dysfunction, resistance to filling can also be seen in a diverse spectrum of conditions including aortic valve stenosis, constrictive pericarditis, dilated cardiomyopathy, and even the "stunned" myocardium seen in ischemic heart disease. Treatment with beta blockers and calcium channel blockers may provide some degree of relief for symptoms related to diastolic dysfunction.

147. The answer is E. *(Chap 197.)* The escape focus in atrioventricular nodal block is relatively high in the conduction system in an area of vagal innervation. Thus, a beneficial response to vagolytic drugs, such as atropine, is usually apparent. The rate at the escape focus is relatively rapid, and the QRS complex is narrow. Unless complete heart block persists, some Wenckebach periodicity can be observed. Inferior myocardial infarction, mitral valve surgery, and digitalis toxicity can lead to atrioventricular nodal block.

148. The answer is D. *(Chap 197.)* Sinus bradycardia and a long sinus pause raise the possibility of sick sinus syndrome, which frequently causes lightheadedness among the elderly. It is important that the relationship between symptoms and the arrhythmias documented by Holter monitoring be clarified before implantation of a permanent pacemaker is considered. An exercise tolerance test, though it may strengthen the suspicion of sick sinus syndrome by showing an inadequate heart rate response, cannot prove that the condition is responsible for the patient's symptoms. Sublingual isoproterenol has little usefulness in the management of chronic bradyarrhythmias.

149. The answer is C. *(Chap 195. SOLVD Investigators, N Engl J Med 325:293–302, 1991.)* The agents most typically used in the treatment of congestive heart failure, diuretics and cardiac glycosides, have never been formally shown to prolong survival. However, there have now been at least four trials that have demonstrated benefit in the use of afterload reduction in the treatment of heart failure. Vasodilators including angiotensin-converting enzyme inhibitors and hydralazine reduce left ventricular afterload; in the case of angiotensin inhibitors such as enalapril, anti-ischemic properties may also play a role via inhibiting the formation of angiotensin II in the coronary artery wall. There is no role for procainamide or other antiarrhythmics in treating patients with congestive heart failure unless the presence of ventricular tachycardia has been documented. Aspirin is indicated only for those with known coronary artery disease and a history of myocardial infarction or angina.

150. The answer is D. *(Chap 206. Fowler, JAMA 266:99–103, 1991.)* Obstruction to cardiac filling and concomitant elevated right-sided pressures that produce elevated neck veins, congestive organomegaly, and pedal edema may be found in several conditions. It is often difficult to distinguish between pericardial tamponade, constrictive pericarditis, restrictive cardiomyopathy, and right ventricular myocardial infarction. In cardiac tamponade, accumulation of fluid in the pericardium is sufficient to cause significant obstruction to the inflow of blood to the ventricles. There is an elevation of intracardiac pressures, limitation to diastolic filling, and florid cardiac failure. An important physical finding in tamponade is a paradoxical pulse, which is an exaggeration of the normal inspiratory augmentation of right ventricular volume and a reciprocal reduction in left ventricular volume manifested by a significant inspiratory decrease in systolic arterial pressure. Paradoxical pulse is rare in constrictive pericarditis, restrictive cardiomyopathy, and right ventricular infarction. Right ventricular infarction is usually distinguishable by the absence of low electrocardiographic voltage and frequently by the presence of an injury current on the acute electrocardiogram. The distinction between constrictive pericarditis and restrictive cardiomyopathy is more difficult. In constrictive pericarditis, resulting from healing of a former acute pericarditis or a chronic pericardial effusion with obliteration of the pericardial cavity, filling is reduced abruptly when the elastic limit of the pericardium is reached, unlike tamponade when filling is impeded throughout diastole. Patients with constrictive pericarditis often appear to have a chronic illness. Venous pressures decline during inspiration (Kussmaul's) and congestive organomegaly is common as is ascites. The apical pulse is reduced and heart sounds are typically distant. An early heart sound, or pericardial knock, may occur 0.06 to 0.12 s after aortic valve closure, which is earlier than the third heart sound associated with ventricular failure. The electrocardiogram frequently displays low QRS voltage. Restrictive cardiomyopathy (e.g., due to amyloidosis, hemochromatosis, sarcoidosis, or scleroderma) can be distinguished from chronic constrictive pericarditis by the presence of a well-defined apical beat, frequent attacks of acute left ventricular failure, left ventricular hypertrophy, true S_3, bundle branch block, and occasional Q waves on the electrocardiogram in the latter condition. In acute pericardial tamponade, diastolic right ventricular collapse is characteristic. In restrictive cardiomyopathy, myocardial thickness is frequently increased and abnormalities of the pericardium are absent. Right ventricular size is typically enlarged in right ventricular myocardial infarction. Echocardiographic findings consistent with constrictive pericarditis include the presence of a thickened pericardium (which is often calcified) in the absence of other findings. The patient in question might well have tuberculous pericarditis that has progressed from the original acute stage to a chronic condition with obliteration of the pericardial space and loss of pericardial elasticity.

151. The answer is B. *(Chap 198.)* The rhythm demonstrated in the electrocardiogram presented is multifocal atrial tachycardia, which is characterized by variable P-wave morphology and PR and RR intervals. Control of multifocal atrial tachycardia, usually associated with severe pulmonary disease, comes with improved ventilation and oxygenation. Carotid sinus massage, electrical cardioversion, and administration of digitalis, verapamil, or quinidine are of little benefit, although verapamil may temporarily slow the ventricular rate.

152. The answer is D. *(Chap 198.)* The ventricular rate in atrial flutter can be decreased by interfering with atrioventricular conduction and slowing the atrial rate. Quinidine slows the rate but enhances conduction; the net result is 1:1 conduction at a somewhat slower atrial rate and a more rapid ventricular rate. Quinidine thus should not be used to treat atrial flutter without the addition of digoxin, verapamil, or propranolol to block atrioventricular conduction.

153. The answer is D. *(Chap 208.)* Given the clearly defined benefits of lipid lowering in patients at risk for ischemic heart disease, screening measurement of blood cholesterol levels (nonfasting) is recommended for all adult patients, especially those young patients with a family history of premature heart disease. If hyperlipidemia is detected, secondary causes such as hypothyroidism, nephrotic syndrome, and uremia should be considered as well as stopping drugs that can aggravate the condition, including oral contraceptives, estrogens, thiazides, and beta blockers. Once these effects are considered, the primary step is attention to diet. Attempts should be made to bring the patient to normal weight and to encourage the patient to undergo dietary therapy with reduced intake of calories, cholesterol, and saturated fat. However, patients who remain at high risk after 3 months of an intensive regimen of dietary therapy should be strongly considered for lipid-lowering drug therapy. Such therapy is recommended for any adult patient whose LDL cholesterol remains greater than 4.9 mmol/L (190 mg/dL) or greater than 4.1 mmol/L (160 mg/dL) in the presence of two or more risk factors. A more aggressive approach is recommended for patients with a prior history of ischemic heart disease. Other risk factors for early atherosclerosis include diabetes mellitus, hypertension, familial hyperlipidemias, hypothyroidism, systemic lupus, and homocysteinemia. Drugs that act to lower LDL cholesterol include bile acid–binding resins such as cholestyramine, nicotinic acid, and hydroxymethylglutaryl coenzyme A (HMG-CoA) reductase inhibitors.

154. The answer is B. *(Chap 208.)* Drugs that act by lowering LDL cholesterol, the major risk factor for ischemic heart disease, are the lipid-lowering drugs of choice. These drugs include the bile acid–binding resins such as cholestyramine, nicotinic acid, and HMG-CoA reductase inhibitors, such as lovastatin. These last agents block the initial step in cholesterol biosynthesis and increase LDL receptor–mediated removal of LDL lipoproteins. Their long-term tolerability is being evaluated, but side effects appear few. Nicotinic acid is one of the few drugs that lowers both LDL and VLDL levels as well as increases "good" HDL cholesterol. Nicotinic acid has been shown to reduce the risk of ischemic heart disease in randomized controlled trials, but its use is accompanied by side effects including gastrointestinal symptoms, flushing, hypoglycemia, and hepatic dysfunction. These side effects can be mitigated by lowering the dose of the agent. Estrogens clearly lower risk of heart disease and may be the first choice for postmenopausal women with high serum cholesterol levels. Cholestyramine can raise VLDL levels while lowering LDL levels. Gemfibrozil is more effective in lowering triglyceride levels; its major effect is to decrease VLDL lipoprotein.

155. The answer is C. *(Chap 199.)* Atrial septal defect (ASD) is usually asymptomatic in childhood. Clinical presentation occurs in the third or fourth decade of life and results from atrial arrhythmias and pulmonary hypertension. A frequent cause of symptoms and of right heart failure is coexistent left ventricular dysfunction—even mild left atrial pressure is not tolerated well when transmitted into the systemic venous circulation. Secundum atrial septal defect is associated with a rightward axis on electrocardiography; the axis is leftward in primum defects. Echocardiography also reveals evidence of right ventricular volume overload, including abnormal motion of the ventricular septum (i.e., right-to-left movement) during diastole. Though small shunts are well tolerated, operative repair is usually indicated when the pulmonary flow is at least 1.5 times the systemic flow.

156. The answer is B. *(Chaps 199, 201.)* The chest x-rays presented in the question show enlargement of the right ventricle and main pulmonary artery and pulmonary vascular plethora, or "shunt" vasculature—classic findings for an atrial septal defect, which could well be asymptomatic in a 36-year-old woman. The chest x-ray of a patient with mitral stenosis and hemoptysis and dyspnea would show left atrial enlargement, and in the presence of primary or secondary tricuspid regurgitation, ascites and a large jugular venous *v* wave. Continuous murmur, widened systemic pulse pressure, and dyspnea on exertion in combination to suggest patent ductus arteriosus, which would produce x-ray evidence of left ventricular and perhaps left atrial enlargement and shunt vasculature without right ventricular enlargement.

157. The answer is C. *(Chaps 205, 206.)*   The restrictive cardiomyopathies are characterized patho-physiologically by an impairment to ventricular filling. The cardiac silhouette is usually mildly, if at all, enlarged. Electrocardiography typically displays low-voltage QRS complexes, atrioventricular conduction defects, and a host of nonspecific arrhythmias. Echocardiography frequently reveals normal systolic and increased left ventricular wall thickness. In amyloidosis, the left ventricular wall appears to be "speckled." While primary cardiac amyloidosis typically produces diastolic dysfunction or restrictive cardiomyopathy as in this question, systolic dysfunction, arrhythmias, or orthostatic hypotension may be alternative presentations. Hemochromatosis may also cause a restrictive picture, but the speckled appearance noted in the echocardiogram would be absent. Alcoholism and viral infections typically cause dilated cardiomyopathies. Chronic tuberculous pericarditis can manifest clinical symptoms similar to those seen in restrictive cardiomyopathy. Patients with constrictive pericarditis have similar clinical presentations to those with restrictive cardiomyopathy, but tend to have normal ventricular wall thickness on echocardiography, pericardial calcification, and the absence of third or fourth heart sounds on chest auscultation.

158. The answer is E. *(Chap 199.)*   Adults with mild pulmonic stenosis are generally asymptomatic. Unlike congenital aortic stenosis, this condition usually does not progress; thus, follow-up need not be frequent. The risk of endocarditis is somewhat lower for pulmonic valves than for the other heart valves, whether normal or stenotic. Clinical signs of mild pulmonic stenosis include prominent *a* wave on jugular venous pulse, normal electrocardiogram, and normal cardiac size on chest x-ray.

159. The answer is C. *(Chap 199.)*   Patients with large ventricular septal defects (VSDs) may develop severe pulmonary vascular obstruction (Eisenmenger syndrome) and a right-to-left shunt, which can lead to cyanosis, clubbing, erythrocytosis, dyspnea, chest pain, syncope, and hemoptysis. Patients should be operated on prior to an increase in pulmonary vascular resistance, if possible. Other than pulmonary vascular obstruction or hypertension, right ventricular outflow tract obstruction, aortic regurgitation, and infective endocarditis may also occur. Since the spectrum of VSDs may range from spontaneous closure to severe congestive heart failure and death in infancy, it is important to define this situation by angiography and hemodynamic studies. Surgery is not recommended for patients with small shunts (pulmonary to systemic flow ratios of less than 1.5 to 2) and normal arterial pressures. However, if there is a moderate to large left-to-right shunt, in the absence of prohibitively high levels of pulmonary resistance, surgery should be undertaken to prevent the development of right-sided failure.

160. The answer is C. *(Chap 199.)*   Coarctation of the aorta usually occurs just distal to the origin of the left subclavian artery; if it arises above the left subclavian, blood pressure elevation may only be evident in the right arm. The associated murmur is continuous only if obstruction is severe; otherwise, a systolic ejection murmur is heard anteriorly and over the back. Coarctation of the aorta commonly is accompanied by a bicuspid aortic valve, which can produce the diastolic murmur of aortic regurgitation. X-ray findings include the "3" sign, caused by aortic dilation just proximal and distal to the area of stenosis, and rib notching, caused by increased collateral circulation through dilated intercostal arteries. Hypertension is the major clinical problem and may persist even after complete surgical correction. Unless hypertension is very severe, or left ventricular failure has ensued, cardiac output responds normally to exercise.

161. The answer is D. *(Chap 200.)*   Acute rheumatic fever is a nonsuppurative complication of infection with group A streptococci. While the incidence of rheumatic fever has been declining, there have been recent domestic outbreaks in military bases. In such outbreaks the attack rate of rheumatic fever following streptococcal pharyngitis may be as high as 3 percent. The diagnosis of rheumatic fever requires two of the following major manifestations of the illness: carditis, migratory polyarthritis, chorea, erythema marginatum, and subcutaneous nodules. The patient in question has three such features. In addition to fever, he also has evidence for recent history of streptococcal infection by virtue of an elevated ASO titer. Even if streptococci cannot be isolated, it is preferable to administer a therapeutic course of parenteral penicillin (a single injection of 1.2 million units of benzathine penicillin IM for 10 days). Prophylactic therapy with penicillin should be administered indefinitely to prevent recurrent attacks. Glucocorticoid therapy is probably unnecessary especially in patients without carditis. Arthritis can be managed entirely with salicylates. Prophylactic therapy for the associated movement disorder is unnecessary.

162. **The answer is B.** *(Chap 198. Oates, N Engl J Med 325:1621–1629, 1991.)* Adenosine is currently approved for the termination of paroxysmal supraventricular tachycardias at doses of 6 mg and, if 6 mg fails, 12 mg. The primary mechanism of adenosine is to decrease conduction velocity through the AV node. As such it is an ideal drug for acute termination of regular reentrant supraventricular tachycardia involving the AV node. Side effects may include chest discomfort and transient hypotension. The half-life is extremely short and the side effects tend to be brief. Patients with wide complex tachycardia suggestive of ventricular tachycardia or known preexcitation syndrome should be treated with agents that decrease automaticity such as quinidine or procainamide. However, in patients with apparent ventricular tachycardia who have neither a history of ischemic heart disease nor preexcitation syndrome, adenosine may be a useful diagnostic agent to determine whether the patient has a reentrant tachycardia, in which case the drug may terminate it; an atrial tachycardia, in which case the atrial activity may be unmasked; or a true, preexcited tachycardia, in which case adenosine will have no effect. While adenosine is not the recommended primary therapy for patients with wide complex tachyarrhythmia, patients with junctional tachycardia who have evidence of poor ventricular function or concomitant beta-adrenergic blockade may be reasonable candidates for its use.

163. **The answer is B.** *(Chap 33.)* A fall in cardiac output from any cause leads to a decrease in effective arterial blood volume. Increased release of renin from juxtaglomerular cells in the kidney leads to the release of angiotensin I from its hepatically synthesized substrate, angiotensinogen. The decapeptide angiotensin I is proteolytically cleaved to angiotensin II, a vasoconstrictor and secretagogue for aldosterone. After release from the adrenal gland, aldosterone leads to renal proximal tubular salt and water retention. Renal vasoconstriction, which also causes proximal sodium absorption by increasing the filtration fraction, is also caused by the augmented sympathetic nervous system activity associated with a diminished cardiac output. A fall in the glomerular filtration rate and the associated renal vasoconstriction furthers the edematous state.

164. **The answer is A.** *(Chap 203.)* Nitrates are generalized smooth-muscle dilators whose direct effect on the vasculature cannot be blocked by any agents presently available. Long-acting preparations of nitroglycerin may be completely degraded by the liver in some patients and thus are generally less effective than sublingual forms. Because individual variability in metabolism is considerable, dosages should be titrated against side effects and should not conform to a rigidly standardized regimen. Tolerance is common and must be considered if a patient fails to respond to a previously efficacious dose. The long-acting preparations such as transdermal patches are less likely to produce the nitrate-associated side effects of headaches and dizziness than are the more rapidly acting sublingual forms.

165. The answer is D.   *(Chap 200. Anderson, N Engl J Med 329:703–709, 1993.)*   It is now recognized that most cases of acute myocardial infarction occur because of thrombus formation at the site of an atherosclerotic plaque, with resultant sudden coronary artery obstruction. The ability to lyse such clots by means of intravenous administration of plasminogen activating agents has resulted in the reduction of early postmyocardial infarction mortality. A problem with use of thrombolytic therapy has been reocclusion of the reperfused arteries. Administration of adjunctive agents may reduce this risk. Aspirin has such an activity based on an interference with platelet aggregation. Heparin forms a complex with antithrombin 3, thereby blocking the action of several protease procoagulants, including thrombin. When given in association with tissue plasminogen activator, heparin reduces mortality to a greater degree than when tissue plasminogen activator is given alone. Thrombolytic therapy including adjunctive heparin and aspirin is beneficial in patients at least up to 75 years of age. Absolute contraindications to the use of such thrombolytic therapy include major surgery or trauma within the prior 6 weeks, gastrointestinal or genitourinary bleeding within 6 months, known history of bleeding diathesis, or the presence of aortic dissection or pericarditis. Additional risks include the presence of a known intracranial tumor, neurosurgery, stroke, or head trauma within the prior 6 months. The patient meets the required electrocardiographic criteria for an acute Q-wave infarction in evolution and is seen early enough in the event to be expected to have significant benefit from thrombolytic therapy. Even patients who are seen between 6 and 12 h after the onset of symptoms may experience some improvement from the initiation of thrombolytic therapy.

166. The answer is E.   *(Chap 203. Willard, N Engl J Med 327:175–181, 1992.)*   Management of patients with angina pectoris involves improving the ratio of oxygen delivery to oxygen utilization. As such, some degree of altered lifestyle may be necessary. Standard antianginal drugs include nitrates, beta-adrenergic blockers, and calcium-channel antagonists. Aspirin, an irreversible inhibitor of platelet cyclooxygenase, interferes with platelet activation and therefore may reduce the risk of coronary thrombosis at sites of atherosclerotic plaques. Administration of aspirin should be considered in all patients who have coronary artery disease but who do not have aspirin allergy or risk factors for bleeding. Low-dose chronic aspirin therapy (100 to 325 mg orally every day or every other day) has been shown to decrease the likelihood of myocardial infarction in asymptomatic adult men, patients with asymptomatic ischemia after myocardial infarction, patients with chronic stable angina, and patients who have survived unstable angina and myocardial infarction. Aspirin is an important part of the therapeutic strategy for patients in the midst of a myocardial infarction who require thrombolytic therapy as well as for those with unstable angina.

167. The answer is B.   *(Chap 198.)*   The rhythm strip shows polymorphic ventricular tachycardia characteristic of torsades de pointes ("twisting of the points"). This life-threatening rhythm is associated with prolongation of the QT interval, resulting, in this case, from the administration of quinidine. The appropriate therapy is to discontinue the offending agent and to withhold other agents that prolong the QT interval, such as procainamide. Hypokalemia can also prolong the QT interval and result in this rhythm; however, this patient had normal serum electrolyte concentrations.

168. The answer is B.   *(Chap 209.)*   The aim of antihypertensive drug therapy is to reduce the blood pressure to normal values with minimal side effects so as to reduce the risk of stroke, kidney failure, and heart disease. Therapy with a diuretic or beta blocker has traditionally been the initial approach, since these are the only agents shown to reduce mortality. However, angiotensin-converting enzyme inhibitors, such as captopril, and calcium-channel antagonists, such as diltiazem, are effective first-line therapy and may be better tolerated. The widespread use of diuretics as initial therapy has been tempered by the known poor compliance rates, adverse metabolic effects (hypokalemia, hypomagnesemia, hypoglycemia, and hypercholesterolemia), and the potentially increased frequency of fatal cardiac arrhythmias. Moreover, the need to coadminister potassium supplementation is another relative problem with the use of diuretics as initial therapy. Current recommendations include doubling the dose of the primary agent as the initial response to failure to lower the blood pressure to less than 140/90 mmHg. If this maneuver fails to control the blood pressure, 25 mg of hydrochlorothiazide per day should be added. Diuretics potentiate the action of angiotensin-converting enzyme inhibitors. Secondly, the adverse metabolic effects of thiazide will be partially countered by the angiotensin-converting enzyme inhibitor. Only after failure of two drugs should the primary agent be increased to full dose, which in the case of enalapril would be 20 mg per day. Additional reasons for a poor therapeutic response must be considered, including excessive sodium intake, inadequate compliance, excessive weight gain, and concomitant use of antagonistic drugs such as cold remedies and oral contraceptives. Additionally, failure to respond to adequate oral therapy would increase the prior probability that the patient might actually have secondary rather than essential hypertension.

169.   The answer is D.   *(Chaps 190, 201.)*   The echocardiogram shows that the left atrium is enlarged, and there is calcification and thickening of the mitral valve and chordal apparatus. The mitral leaflets show diastolic doming, resulting from fusion of the valve commissures. These are the typical findings of rheumatic mitral stenosis, exemplified by this 42-year-old woman. The aortic leaflets are also mildly thickened, consistent with rheumatic disease. The symptoms of the patient described in Option A are suggestive of a left atrial myxoma. The patient in Option B has acute mitral regurgitation. The patient in Option C has mitral valve prolapse.

170.   The answer is C.   *(Chap 209. Calhoun, N Engl J Med 323:1177–1183, 1991.)*   A hypertensive emergency is defined by the presence of end-organ damage in the setting of a severe elevation in blood pressure, usually with a diastolic pressure above 130 mmHg. Syndromes qualifying as a hypertensive emergency include hypertensive encephalopathy as in this patient, cerebral infarction, intracerebral hemorrhage, myocardial ischemia or infarction, pulmonary edema, aortic dissection, eclampsia, acute renal insufficiency, severe ophthalmoscopic changes, or severe microangiopathic hemolytic anemia. Those with a severe elevation of blood pressure yet without evidence of end-organ injury can be managed in a more gradual fashion with attempts to lower the blood pressure over a period of 24 to 48 h. However, for those with true hypertensive emergencies, immediate therapy, even before the results of all laboratory tests are available, should be undertaken. Hypertensive emergencies require immediate but not precipitous lowering of the mean arterial pressure by approximately 25 percent with an attempt to reduce the diastolic blood pressure to 100 to 110 mmHg over a period of minutes to hours. Sodium nitroprusside is the drug of choice because it allows for titratable blood pressure reduction. On the other hand, the administration of this agent by continuous intravenous infusion requires continuous monitoring of the arterial blood pressure, which has been provided for in this patient. Diazoxide can be used in situations where arterial monitoring is not immediately available. However, use of diazoxide may be complicated by hypotension and tachycardia (thereby exacerbating myocardial ischemia). Intravenous labetolol, a titratable beta blocker, or intravenous nicardipine, a calcium-channel antagonist, may prove to be acceptable alternatives. The symptoms of hypertensive encephalopathy may include headache, nausea, vomiting, visual disturbances, confusion, or generalized weakness. Focal neurologic signs, such as asymptomatic reflexes, may also be seen.

171.   The answer is A.   *(Chap 202.)*   The man described in the question probably has a right ventricular infarction complicating his inferior myocardial infarction because right atrial pressure is elevated out of proportion to the left atrial (pulmonary capillary wedge) pressure. Cardiac output is depressed on the basis of an insufficient left-heart filling pressure. The best treatment consists of administration of fluids.

172. The answer is E.   *(Chap 187. Jarcho, N Engl J Med 321:1372, 1989.)*   Thyroid hormone acts directly via nuclear receptors to regulate myosin heavy chain gene transcription, thus increasing the level of myosin enzyme V_1 (fast myosin), whereas in response to pressure load on the heart, fetal forms of myosin such as V_3 (slow myosin) are induced. The c-*sis* proto-oncogene, which encodes for the B chain of platelet-derived growth factor; c-*myc* and c-*fos,* which encode for nuclear proteins involved in regulation of the cell cycle; and c-*ras,* which encodes for guanosine-binding proteins are all induced in myocardial tissue undergoing hypertrophy. Lineage analysis through the use of restriction fragment length polymorphisms has allowed mapping of a gene (now known to be the adult myosin heavy chain gene) associated with familial hypertrophic cardiomyopathy to chromosome 14. Angiotensin II and beta agonists augment proto-oncogene expression, stimulate protein synthesis and induce the synthesis of fetal forms of actin and myosin, thereby leading to hypertrophy of smooth muscle.

173. The answer is B.   *(Chap 210. Ernst, N Engl J Med 328:1167–1172, 1993.)*   The vast majority of aortic aneurysms are due to atherosclerosis; 75 percent of such aneurysms are located in the distal aorta below the renal arteries. Though these aneurysms are typically asymptomatic, rupture may occur with devastating consequences. Prognosis is related to the size of the aneurysm as well as to the presence of coexistent vascular diseases. Patients with aneurysms exceeding 6 cm who are not treated surgically have a 50 percent mortality in 1 year, while those with lesions between 4 and 6 cm have a 25 percent mortality during the first year. Surgical excision and replacement with a prosthetic graft is indicated for patients with aneurysms greater than 6 cm in diameter, as well as in symptomatic patients or those with rapidly enlarging aneurysms regardless of the absolute diameter. Depending on the degree of operative risk, surgery may also be recommended in those with aneurysms whose diameters are between 5 and 6 cm. Contraindications to elective reconstruction include myocardial infarction within the past 6 months, intractable congestive heart failure, ongoing severe angina pectoris, severe obstructive lung disease, severe chronic renal failure, history of stroke with residual neurologic deficits, and life expectancy of less than 2 years. An extensive preoperative evaluation including assessment of coronary disease, renal failure, and pulmonary function studies should be carried out, and if abnormalities are found, they should be ameliorated when possible. For patients in whom the diameter of the aneurysm is less than 6 cm or in whom there is significant operative risk, serial ultrasounds may be helpful to define a group that more urgently requires surgical intervention based on expansion of 0.5 cm or more over time.

174. The answer is E.   *(Chap 211.)*   This patient has evidence of atherosclerotic vascular disease in multiple arterial beds. Such patients are at risk after procedures in which catheters may dislodge atherosclerotic plaques and thereby cause the embolization of small deposits of fibrin, platelet, and cholesterol debris. The emboli tend to lodge in small vessels of muscle and skin, and distal pulses may remain palpable since large vessels are not affected. The characteristic rash is livedo reticularis, which presents a mottled appearance. Tenderness, pallor, pain, and localized areas of necrosis and gangrene may also occur. Skin or muscle biopsy may demonstrate cholesterol crystals and confirm the diagnosis. Surgical revascularization is rarely helpful; platelet inhibitors could be used to try to prevent further atheroembolism.

175. The answer is B.   *(Chaps 188, 201.)*   Inspiration, which augments systemic venous return because of negative intrathoracic pressure, will cause accentuation of right-sided murmurs. Prolonged expiratory pressure against a closed glottis (Valsalva maneuver) reduces the intensity of most murmurs by diminishing both right and left ventricular filling. By reducing filling, and thereby reducing chamber size, the murmurs of hypertrophic cardiomyopathy and mitral valve prolapse will increase. The cycle following a premature ventricular beat will have a larger stroke volume so the gradient across an obstructed semilunar valve (aortic or pulmonary) will increase, thereby leading to a louder murmur. Squatting, which increases both venous return and chamber size as well as systemic arterial resistance, increases most murmurs except those due to hypertrophic cardiomyopathy and mitral valve prolapse. Sustained handgrip, which increases heart rate and systemic arterial pressure, often accentuates the murmurs of mitral stenosis and mitral regurgitation by impeding outflow and by decreasing diastolic filling.

176. **The answer is B.** *(Chap 205.)* Echocardiographic evidence of a disproportionately thickened ventricular septum and systolic anterior motion of the mitral valve strongly suggests idiopathic hypertrophic subaortic stenosis (IHSS). The typical harsh systolic murmur does not usually radiate to the carotid arteries and decreases when ventricular volume enlarges with isometric exercise (e.g., handgrip). The carotid upstroke is brisk, often bifid. Congestive failure often occurs because of reduced ventricular compliance despite normal ventricular systolic function. Malposition of the mitral apparatus, a result of the distorted septum, often leads to some degree of mitral regurgitation.

177. **The answer is B.** *(Chap 189.)* A delta wave or slowed QRS upstroke is depicted. This finding occurs in the Wolff-Parkinson-White syndrome in which accessory Kent bundles result in an apparently short PR interval caused by the bypassed AV node and early onset of the QRS complex. Left bundle branch block could result in marked initial delay, whereas right bundle branch block results in late delay. Left ventricular hypertrophy causes minor uniform QRS prolongation. Right ventricular infarction has little effect on QRS duration in the absence of right bundle branch block.

178. **The answer is D.** *(Chaps 190, 191.)* Lack of motion (akinesis) in a segment of myocardium visualized by echo indicates tissue death, as does an area of reduced thallium accumulation during exercise that fails to "fill in" at rest. Since pyrophosphate appears to bind calcium and macromolecules in irreversibly damaged myocardial cells, an area of increased uptake indicates myocardial infarction if the injection is performed between 48 and 72 h after suspected transmural infarction. Using a combination of $[^{13}N]H_3$ (blood flow marker) and $[^{18}F]$deoxyglucose (glucose uptake), PET can identify nonviable myocardium if there is a defect in the uptake of both isotopes. Standard CT cannot detect global or regional left ventricular function, although fast, or cine, CT may be able to detect infarction by monitoring changes in ventricular volume and wall thickness.

179. **The answer is C.** *(Chap 206.)* Acute pericarditis is associated with ST-segment elevation and, frequently, PR-segment depression. Usually, reciprocal ST-segment depression is not present. T waves begin to invert only *after* the ST segment becomes isoelectric. Elevations in serum creatine phosphokinase levels to twice normal may be associated with uncomplicated pericarditis.

180. **The answer is C.** *(Chap 195.)* Digitalis glycosides are effective in increasing myocardial contractility and in treatment of certain atrial tachyarrhythmias. However, digoxin actually increases myocardial automaticity (increase in premature beats) and facilitates reentry (atrial tachycardias). Digoxin also slows conduction through AV nodal tissue and has central effects that can mimic vagal influence on the heart and may thus produce sinus arrest. Paroxysmal atrial tachycardia with variable block represents the classic rhythm of digitalis intoxication. Digoxin is profibrillatory, but its administration should not lead to atrial flutter.

181. **The answer is E.** *(Chap 210.)* Complications of dissection of the aorta include loss of a major pulse, dissection into the pericardial or pleural space, and acute aortic regurgitation. When these events occur, surgical intervention is required. Because the risk of these complications is higher in persons with dissection of the ascending aorta, these persons usually are treated surgically. In contrast, persons with dissection of the descending aorta often can be treated medically. Persistence of pain, which suggests that dissection is continuing, is another indication for surgery.

182. The answer is C. *(Chap 199.)*   Left-to-right shunts occur in all types of atrial and ventricular septal defects, but generally do not result in cyanosis, whereas large right-to-left shunts frequently do. The magnitude of the shunt depends on the size of the defect, the diastolic properties of both ventricles, and the relative impedance of the pulmonary and systemic circulations. Defects of the sinus venosus type occur high in the atrial septum near the entry of the superior vena cava or lower near the orifice of the inferior vena cava and may be associated with anomalous connection of the right inferior pulmonary vein to the right atrium. In the case of anomalous origin of the left coronary artery from the pulmonary artery, as pulmonary vascular resistance declines immediately after birth, perfusion of the left coronary artery from the pulmonary trunk ceases and the direction of flow in the anomalous vessel reverses. Twenty percent of patients with this defect can survive to adulthood owing to myocardial blood supply totally through the right coronary artery. In the absence of pulmonary hypertension, blood will flow from the aorta to the pulmonary artery throughout the cardiac cycle, which results in a "continuous" murmur at the left sternal border. In total anomalous pulmonary venous connection, all the venous blood returns to the right atrium; therefore, an interatrial communication is required and right-to-left shunts with cyanosis are common.

183. The answer is D. *(Chap 202.)*   While prompt initiation of thrombolytic therapy during an acute myocardial infarction is associated with improvement in mortality and limitation of the size of infarct, all thrombolytic agents, including tissue plasminogen activator, are associated with an increased risk of major bleeding. These agents should not be given if there is a history of a cerebrovascular accident, a surgical procedure within 2 weeks, active peptic ulcer disease, or marked hypertension during acute presentation (systolic pressure greater than 180 or diastolic pressure greater than 100 mmHg). Other situations in which the risk of bleeding might be higher (such as advanced age) are not absolute contraindications, but the potential benefit of administration of thrombolytic therapy should be carefully considered in each case.

184. The answer is D. *(Chap 210.)*   Factors predisposing to aortic dissection include hypertension (present in at least 70 percent of cases), cystic medial necrosis, Marfan's syndrome, coarctation, bicuspid aortic valve, and third trimester of pregnancy. Dissection of the aorta is a disease of the media, either from arteriosclerosis or cystic medial necrosis. The associated intimal tear that initiates the dissection almost always begins in the ascending aorta (2 to 5 cm above the valve) or just distal to the left subclavian artery; at these two points the aorta is relatively fixed, so that shear forces are increased. Type I dissections extend around the aortic arch and can affect the abdominal aorta; most type II (ascending aorta only) dissections proceed variably into the arch or reach the left subclavian artery. Type III dissections begin in the descending aorta and propagate distally. Dissection can result in aortic rupture, which can result in a false aneurysm (an "aneurysm" contained within the adventitia or a clot) or, if the dissection is of the ascending aorta, in hemopericardium. Medical therapy should be aimed at reducing both cardiac contractility and systemic arterial pressure in order to reduce shear stress on the aortic wall. This can be accomplished either by labetolol, a combined alpha and beta blocker, or by simultaneous administration of nitroprusside and a beta blocker.

185. The answer is C. *(Chap 202.)*   Apical systolic murmurs associated with a myocardial infarction may represent either mitral regurgitation (on the basis of papillary muscle rupture or newly dilated heart size) or ventricular septal defect. In both conditions large *v* waves may be recorded in the pulmonary capillary wedge position. In the case of ventricular septal defect, but not mitral regurgitation, there will be an increase in the partial pressure of oxygen as a catheter is advanced from the right atrium to the right ventricle.

186. The answer is D. *(Chap 203. Fuster, N Engl J Med 326:242, 310, 1992.)* Any patient with recent onset of severe and frequent angina, accelerating angina, or angina at rest is considered to have unstable angina. Such patients are likely to have one or more stenoses in major coronary arteries and require emergent management. Hospitalization with identification and treatment of predisposing conditions (e.g., heart failure, fever, thyrotoxicosis) is indicated. Since thrombus formation frequently complicates this condition, intravenous heparin followed by oral aspirin should be given. Beta blockers and calcium channel blocking drugs should be administered if possible. Antiarrhythmics are only required in the presence of specific arrhythmias. Intravenous nitroglycerin is effective, but requires continuous blood pressure monitoring. If evidence of ischemia, based on clinical symptoms or electrocardiographic findings, does not abate within 24 to 48 h of aggressive medical management, then diagnostic cardiac catheterization should be performed.

187. The answer is A. *(Chaps 205, 206.)* The cardiac catheterization findings described are consistent with increased impedance to ventricular filling as may be seen in either restrictive cardiomyopathies or constrictive pericarditis. Restrictive cardiomyopathies often are due to myocardial infiltration with neoplastic cells, eosinophils, iron, amyloid, or fibrous tissue. The transmural necrosis noted in patients with Duchenne's muscular dystrophy can lead to a dilated cardiomyopathy.

188. The answer is B. *(Chap 211.)* Conditions associated with stasis, vascular damage, or hypercoagulability lead to an increased risk for deep venous thrombosis. Risk is increased by any condition leading to immobility, such as recuperation after a myocardial infarction (of any severity), a major thoracic resection (even if the cancer was completely resected), and trauma or operation involving the hip or leg. A wrist fracture in an elderly woman would probably not lead to any increased risk if her baseline mobility was present. Hypercoagulable states include systemic cancers; pregnancy; exogenous or endogenous estrogens; deficiencies of antithrombin III, protein C, and protein S; circulating lupus anticoagulant (manifested by elevated partial thromboplastin time); or myeloproliferative disease.

189. The answer is A. *(Chap 192.)* A gradient between the left atrium (as measured by the pulmonary capillary wedge tracing) and the left ventricle in diastole indicates mitral stenosis as exemplified by the woman with a history of rheumatic fever and hemoptysis. The intravenous drug abuser with mitral regurgitation caused by a mitral valve vegetation would exhibit large *v* waves on the pulmonary capillary wedge tracing. The aortic regurgitation associated with Marfan's syndrome would cause an equilibration between left ventricular and peripheral pressures. A feature of severe aortic regurgitation that occurs when left ventricular pressure exceeds pulmonary capillary wedge (i.e., left atrial) pressure during early diastole may result in premature mitral valve closure. In aortic stenosis, as exemplified by the elderly man with left ventricular hypertrophy, the left ventricular pressure is higher than aortic pressure during systole. In pericardial tamponade, as might be seen in the patient with lymphoma, there is equalization of right and left diastolic pressures.

190. The answer is A-Y, B-N, C-Y, D-Y, E-N. *(Chap 189.)* The electrocardiographic T wave represents myocardial repolarization, and its configuration can be altered nonspecifically by metabolic abnormalities, drugs, neural activity, and ischemia by a dispersion effect on the activation or repolarization of action potentials. Although myocardial ischemia and subendocardial infarction can produce deep, symmetric T-wave inversions, which would result in tachyarrhythmias and syncope, such noncardiac phenomena as intracerebral hemorrhage can similarly affect ventricular repolarization. Hyperkalemia is manifested by tall, peaked T waves, not inverted ones. Hypocalcemia is manifested by prolonged QT intervals.

191. **The answer is A-N, B-Y, C-Y, D-N, E-Y.** *(Chap 188.)* The intensity of S_1 is determined by the contractility of the left ventricle ("slamming the door shut"), the degree of separation of mitral leaflets at the onset of contraction, and the thickness and pliability of the mitral leaflets. Contractility increases with fever but is diminished in hypothyroidism. Lown-Ganong-Levine syndrome is associated with a short PR interval, so that atrial contraction just precedes ventricular contraction; S_1 tends to be loud. Mitral regurgitation may lead to poor leaflet apposition and a soft S_1; on the other hand, mitral stenosis is associated with a loud S_1, unless the thickened valve leaflets are restricted in motion by heavy calcification.

192. **The answer is A-Y, B-N, C-Y, D-N, E-Y.** *(Chap 189.)* Hyperkalemia leads to partial depolarization of cardiac cells. As a result, there is slowing of the upstroke of the action potential as well as reduced duration of repolarization. The T wave becomes peaked, the RS complex widens and may merge with the T wave (giving a sine-wave appearance), and the P wave becomes shallow or disappears. Prominent U waves are associated with hypokalemia; ST-segment prolongation is associated with hypocalcemia.

193. **The answer is A-N, B-N, C-Y, D-N, E-N.** *(Chaps 2, 190, 203.)* Making a test's cutoff point for positivity more stringent (i.e., > 2.0 mm of ST depression rather than 0.5 mm) will enhance specificity (there will be fewer false positives) at the expense of sensitivity (there will be more false negatives). Bayesian analysis dictates that low prior probability (e.g., 10 percent—odds 1:9) can only be enhanced to a 50 percent posttest (or posterior) probability for a test with the given operating characteristics [1:9 × sensitivity/(1 − specificity)], where sensitivity is defined as the probability of a positive test in a patient with the disease and specificity is defined as the probability of a negative test result in a patient without the disease. Thallium scans can increase the sensitivity for detecting coronary artery disease by about 20 percent and increase specificity by 10 percent. Such scans are most useful in patients with an uninterpretable or nondiagnostic electrocardiogram due to failure to achieve 85 percent of predicted maximal heart rate, left ventricular hypertrophy, left bundle branch block, or drug effects. A prior myocardial infarction can be inferred if a defect on thallium scintigraphy noted during exercise also fails to be perfused at rest. Blood pressure and heart rate should rise during a normal exercise tolerance test. Failure of the blood pressure to rise or an actual decrease may suggest global left ventricular dysfunction.

194. **The answer is A-Y, B-Y, C-N, D-Y, E-N.** *(Chaps 189, 198.)* The electrocardiogram presented in the question demonstrates nonparoxysmal junctional tachycardia. The junctional rhythm is at a rate of 82 beats per minute, which is faster than the usual escape nodal rhythm. Retrograde P waves can be seen. This rhythm can occur following mitral valve surgery and in association with digitalis toxicity, acute myocarditis, and inferior myocardial infarction. These processes all can irritate the atrioventricular node and accelerate its action.

195. **The answer is A-N, B-N, C-Y, D-N, E-Y.** *(Chap 12.)* Angina is usually described as a vague substernal pain that is precipitated by exercise or emotion and may radiate into the left arm or jaw. The discomfort may radiate into the teeth, but rarely above the maxilla. A sharp pain radiating to the back, particularly if long-lasting, suggests aortic dissection. Relief of pain at rest (but not by change of position) or within 5 min of sublingual nitroglycerin is highly suggestive of pain due to coronary ischemia.

196. **The answer is A-N, B-Y, C-N, D-Y, E-Y.** *(Chap 194. Cohn, N Engl J Med 311:819, 1984.)* Stroke volume and cardiac output at rest are not sensitive indexes of myocardial dysfunction. Stroke volume is often normal, though at the expense of higher end-diastolic volume (Frank-Starling mechanism). Even when stroke volume begins to diminish, cardiac output can be maintained by

increases in heart rate. However, when the heart is stressed by exercise, cardiac output does not rise proportionately to oxygen consumption, and left ventricular end-diastolic pressure rises more than in normal controls. Although plasma norepinephrine levels are elevated in persons with left ventricular dysfunction, myocardial levels are typically low.

197. **The answer is A-Y, B-N, C-N, D-Y, E-N.** *(Chap 68.)*   The antihypertensive agent prazosin blocks alpha$_1$ receptors that mediate vasoconstriction. Clonidine is also an antihypertensive agent but works by stimulating alpha$_2$ receptors in the brainstem, thereby reducing sympathetic outflow. Phenylephrine, an alpha$_1$ agonist with pressor effects, is frequently employed in over-the-counter nasal decongestants. By antagonizing presynaptic alpha$_2$ receptors, yohimbine increases parasympathetic activity that may augment penile blood flow and may be useful in the treatment of erectile impotence. Isoproterenol stimulates beta$_1$ and beta$_2$ receptors and can increase chronotropy in the setting of heart block.

198. **The answer is A-Y, B-Y, C-Y, D-N, E-N.** *(Chap 35.)*   Frequent premature ventricular complexes (defined as >30 per minute), salvos or nonsustained ventricular tachycardia, and a low ejection fraction (<20 percent) are associated with an increased risk of sudden cardiac death. Advanced forms (triplets or longer) are more predictive of risk than even a high density of unifocal premature beats. It is unclear whether suppressing ectopic activity can reduce risk. Conventional techniques of cardiopulmonary resuscitation require lung inflation every 15 s and chest compressions 80 times per minute if only one provider is present. In the case of ventricular fibrillation or ventricular tachycardia in a pulseless patient, the first shock should be delivered at 200 joules, followed by additional higher energy shocks (up to 360 joules in the absence of response). Intravenous sodium bicarbonate, formerly recommended, is no longer considered routinely necessary and may be dangerous (unless pH monitoring indicates profound acidosis).

199. **The answer is A-N, B-Y, C-N, D-N, E-Y.** *(Chap 198.)*   Persons who have Wolff-Parkinson-White syndrome are predisposed to developing two major types of atrial tachyarrhythmias. The first, which resembles paroxysmal supraventricular tachycardia (SVT) with reentry, involves the atrioventricular node in anterograde conduction and the bypass tract in retrograde conduction. This tachycardia typically has a narrow QRS complex and can be treated similarly to other forms of SVT. The other, more dangerous tachyarrhythmia (present in the man described in the question) is atrial fibrillation, which usually is conducted anterograde down the bypass tract and has a wide QRS configuration. The ventricular rate in such a situation is quite rapid, and cardiovascular collapse or ventricular fibrillation may result. Usual treatment is direct-current cardioversion, though quinidine may slow conduction through the bypass tract. Verapamil and propranolol have little effect on the bypass tract and may further depress ventricular function, which already is compromised by the rapid rate. Digoxin may accelerate conduction down the bypass tract and lead to ventricular fibrillation.

200. **The answer is A-Y, B-Y, C-N, D-N, E-N.** *(Chap 199.)*   Atrial septal defects (ASD) of the sinus venous type are located high in the atrial septum and commonly are associated with anomalous pulmonary venous return. The magnitude of the shunt depends upon defect size, relative ventricular compliance, and the relative resistances in the pulmonary and systemic circuits, but *not* upon total blood flow. The systolic ejection murmur associated with ASD arises from increased flow across the pulmonic valve; a diastolic rumble due to increased flow across the tricuspid valve is common and should not necessarily be attributed to mitral stenosis, which is associated with ASD in a disorder known as Lutembacher's syndrome. Most persons even with a large ASD are asymptomatic until late in adult life.

201. **The answer is A-Y, B-N, C-N, D-N, E-Y.** *(Chaps 199, 201.)* The risks of cardiac surgery always must be weighed against the potential benefits. The risk is extremely low in the correction of atrial septal defects, and surgery may prevent the development of atrial arrhythmia and pulmonary hypertension, complications that can arise later in life. Small ventricular septal defects, on the other hand, almost never cause hemodynamic problems later in life. The presence of Eisenmenger's reaction—cyanosis and a right-to-left shunt from pulmonary hypertension—is a contraindication to surgery, regardless of the underlying lesion. Persons with symptomatic aortic stenosis warrant consideration for surgery because hemodynamic deterioration can ensue quickly. Chronic mitral regurgitation, however, is far more indolent, and mild symptoms or acute decompensation from a correctable cause does not necessarily require surgical intervention.

202. **The answer is A-Y, B-Y, C-N, D-Y, E-Y.** *(Chap 188.)* Large *a* waves indicate contraction of the right atrium against increased resistance, such as might occur with obstruction at the tricuspid valve (tricuspid stenosis) or more commonly with increased resistance to right ventricular filling. Right ventricular filling could be impaired in pulmonary stenosis or any condition that causes pulmonary hypertension, such as multiple pulmonary emboli. The *a* wave will also be pronounced if the right atrium contracts while the tricuspid valve is closed by right ventricular systole, as would be the case in atrioventricular dissociation, complete heart block, or junctional rhythm. The *a* wave is absent in patients with atrial fibrillation, since no organized atrial contraction occurs.

203. **The answer is A-Y, B-N, C-Y, D-N, E-N.** *(Chap 201.)* Although aortic stenosis may be present in affected persons for several decades, survival for more than 2 years is unlikely once symptoms of heart failure occur. Atrial fibrillation with the loss of synchronized atrial systole can precipitate clinical deterioration. Stenosis of the aortic valve becomes of critical importance when the effective orifice is reduced to less than 0.7 cm^2/m^2 body surface area. Absence of calcification in aortic valve cusps studied by fluoroscopy or echocardiography essentially rules out severe aortic stenosis in adults; this relationship, however, does not apply to plain chest x-ray. Normal boxlike separation of the aortic cusps on echocardiography excludes the presence of severe aortic stenosis; however, cusp calcification and poor mobility may not necessarily indicate significant valvular stenosis. While in advanced cases a strain pattern on the electrocardiogram is present, there is no close correlation between the electrocardiogram and the hemodynamic severity of the lesion.

204. **The answer is A-N, B-N, C-N, D-Y, E-Y.** *(Chap 193. Kuntz, N Engl J Med 325:17, 1991.)* Safe and effective (it reduces gradients from 75 to 15 mmHg), balloon valvuloplasty is the preferred treatment for pulmonary stenosis. Rheumatic mitral stenosis secondary to commissural fusion with associated leaflet thickening is the mitral lesion most amenable to treatment with balloon dilation. Such dilation can increase valve size to 2.0 cm^2 or more, but usually not to the normal 3.5 to 5.0 cm^2 area. The indications for balloon aortic valvuloplasty in patients who are poor operative risks include congenital, rheumatic, or acquired calcific aortic stenosis. In the last group, valvuloplasty fractures leaflet calcium and provides new hinge points along which leaflets may open. Surprisingly, stroke is an uncommon complication of this procedure and most patients experience a reduction in symptoms. The best results are obtained in patients with preserved left ventricular function before the procedure. Restenosis is common, but can be treated with repeat aortic valvuloplasty.

205. **The answer is A-Y, B-Y, C-N, D-Y, E-Y.** *(Chap 194.)* The cardiac output must increase during exercise since oxygen demand is greater. This increase is accomplished by a physiologic augmentation in stroke volume and heart rate. The pumping action of hyperventilation increases ventricular filling and thereby stroke volume rises. Catecholamine synthesis and secretion increase, which leads to faster heart rate and greater stroke volume through augmented myocardial contractility. Since blood pressure is determined by cardiac output and resistance, once cardiac output increases, blood pressure would also tend to rise. However, vasodilation in muscle beds counteracts this tendency somewhat. In the normal heart, catecholamine-mediated changes in the force-volume curve lead to decreased or similar end-diastolic volumes (filling pressure) during exercise; heart failure is characterized by marked and sometimes dangerous rises in end-diastolic volume, possibly even to the point of pulmonary edema.

206. **The answer is A-N, B-Y, C-Y, D-N, E-Y.** *(Chap 201. Marks, N Engl J Med 320:1031, 1989.)* The systolic click-murmur syndrome is associated with mitral valve prolapse, which can place excessive stress on the papillary muscles and lead to ischemia and chest pain. Although often associated with inferior T-wave changes, the systolic click-murmur syndrome only occasionally results in an ischemic response to exercise. On standing or during Valsalva's maneuver, as ventricular volume gets smaller the click and murmur move earlier in systole. Echocardiography reveals midsystolic prolapse of the posterior mitral leaflet, or on occasion both mitral leaflets, into the left atrium. Persons with mitral regurgitation from prolapse are at risk for developing subacute bacterial endocarditis and should be treated accordingly.

207. **The answer is A-N, B-Y, C-Y, D-N, E-Y.** *(Chap 197.)* The choice of a permanent pacemaker type depends on the underlying conduction disease and the patient's clinical profile. DDD pacing preserves the normal relationship between atrial and ventricular contraction, and physiologic atrial sensing with ventricular pacing improves exercise tolerance in young, active persons. As this form of pacing preserves the normal atrial contribution to cardiac output, it is desired in patients with decreased left ventricular function or hypertrophied ("stiff") left ventricular chambers. DDD pacing is contraindicated in atrial fibrillation or flutter since the ventricular rate response is unpredictable.

208. **The answer is A-Y, B-Y, C-Y, D-Y, E-Y.** *(Chap 195.)* With severe chronic heart failure from any cause there may be severe weight loss due to (1) elevation of the metabolic rate, which results from extra respiratory muscle work; (2) anorexia, nausea, and vomiting due to central causes, digitalis intoxication, or congestive hepatomegaly and abdominal fullness (including ascites with impairment of gastric filling and early satiety); (3) impaired intestinal absorption due to intestinal venular congestion; and (4) a protein-losing enteropathy.

209. **The answer is A-N, B-Y, C-Y, D-Y, E-N.** *(Chap 196.)* A 5-year survival rate of 70 percent suggests that cardiac transplantation is the therapy of choice for patients with end-stage heart disease. Because the posterior walls of the host's atria are left in place at the time of transplantation, the recipient's sinus node remains innervated and under the influence of the autonomic nervous system, but the donor sinus node controls the rate of the transplanted heart (and has a regular PR interval in contrast to the dissociated P waves generated by the residual host atria). Accelerated coronary vascular disease (chronic rejection) is the major factor limiting long-term survival. The vascular disease, which may be ameliorated somewhat by early posttransplant use of diltiazem, is a consequence of fibrointimal hyperplasia brought on by injury during rejection episodes and high serum lipids. The high serum lipids are a side effect of the immunosuppressive medicines that must be administered. Immunosuppression must continue for a lifetime. Neoplasia, particularly Epstein-Barr virus–associated lymphomas, represent another class of late complications.

210. **The answer is A-N, B-Y, C-Y, D-Y, E-N.** *(Chap 197.)* The standard VVI pacemaker paces the ventricle, senses the ventricle, and is inhibited by spontaneous ventricular activity. Thus it will only fire in backup situations when the ventricular rate is lower than its set point. The right ventricular wire is rarely if ever irritating itself and does not cause ventricular tachycardia. Since the patient has a single-chamber, nontriggered pacer, triggering after ventriculoatrial conduction is not possible. On the other hand, since the VVI only paces the ventricle, the normal physiologic augmentation of cardiac output by atrial contraction is lost. Moreover, atrial contraction will occur at the wrong time if the AV valve is closed, thereby leading to large *a* waves (and a vasodepressor reflex) as well as systemic and pulmonary venous regurgitation.

211. **The answer is A-N, B-N, C-N, D-Y, E-Y.** *(Chap 198.)* Ventricular tachycardia (VT) generally accompanies some form of structural heart disease, most commonly chronic ischemic heart disease associated with a prior myocardial infarction. The ECG diagnosis of VT is suggested by a wide-complex tachycardia at a rate exceeding 100 beats per minute. It is important, however, to differentiate supraventricular tachycardia with aberration of intraventricular conduction from VT since the clinical implications and managements of these two entities are so different. A very irregular rhythm suggests atrial fibrillation (AF) with conduction via a bypass tract (WPW syndrome). If a tracing previously obtained during sinus rhythm demonstrates a bundle branch block pattern with the same morphologic features as those during the tachycardia, then supraventricular origin is favored. Characteristics of the 12-lead ECG during the arrhythmia that suggest a ventricular origin are (1) a QRS complex >0.14 s in the absence of antiarrhythmic therapy (although a QRS complex >0.20 s suggests a preexcitation syndrome); (2) AV dissociation or variable retrograde conduction; (3) a superior QRS axis in the presence of a right bundle block pattern; (4) concordance of the QRS pattern in all precordial leads; and (5) other QRS patterns that are inconsistent with typical bundle branch block patterns. Intracardiac electrical recordings would be required to confirm this important distinction.

212. **The answer is A-Y, B-N, C-N, D-Y, E-Y.** *(Chap 198.)* The calcium channel blocker verapamil is a very effective agent in the treatment of atrial and AV nodal reentrant tachycardias, but can cause hemodynamic collapse if given to a patient with sustained VT or atrial fibrillation/flutter and preexcitation and can raise serum levels of digoxin. Therefore it should be used with extreme caution in any patient with a wide-complex tachycardia. Amiodarone is useful in the treatment of refractory atrial and ventricular tachyarrhythmias, but is associated with a host of side effects including prolonged QT interval, peripheral neuropathy, abnormalities of thyroid function, pulmonary fibrosis, and various ocular and cutaneous problems, including corneal deposits and skin pigmentation. Flecainide may result in AV block, polymorphic VT, or heart failure if given in the face of severe left ventricular dysfunction. Reversible agranulocytosis occurs rarely after institution of procainamide therapy, while thrombocytopenia may be associated with quinidine use. Quinidine can also cause elevation of serum digoxin levels. Disopyramide may cause blurred vision and narrow-angle glaucoma.

213. **The answer is A-N, B-Y, C-N, D-Y, E-N.** *(Chap 205.)* The symptoms of dyspnea in persons with asymmetric septal hypertrophy are related as much to decreased left ventricular (diastolic) compliance as to the degree of obstruction. Use of calcium-channel blockers often relieves dyspnea by decreasing left ventricular stiffness. Sudden death in affected persons does not correlate with the degree of obstruction and is thought to be due to arrhythmias. On electrocardiography, Q waves commonly are seen and do not imply a coexistent infarction. Histologic abnormalities consist of disorganized arrangements of myocytes in the ventricular septum. As many as 50 percent of the cases have familial predisposition, often due to one of several mutations in the beta cardiac myosin heavy chain gene on chromosome 14.

214. **The answer is A-N, B-N, C-N, D-Y, E-Y.** *(Chap 201.)* In approximately two-thirds of patients with aortic regurgitation (AR), the disease is rheumatic in origin, although such an etiology is less common in those with isolated AR. Manifestations of the rapidly falling arterial pressure during late systole and diastole include Corrigan's "water-hammer" pulse, capillary pulsations visible at the root of nails (Quincke's pulse), a pistol-shot (Traube's) sound over the femoral arteries, and a to-and-fro murmur (Duroziez's sign) audible over a lightly compressed femoral artery. In addition to a midsystolic ejection murmur, a second associated murmur may be the Austin Flint murmur, a low-pitched, rumbling diastolic bruit. Such a murmur is produced by the anterior displacement of the anterior leaflet of the mitral valve by the aortic regurgitant stream (characteristically seen at echocardiography). Close follow-up by means of echocardiography is necessary to ensure that an operation is undertaken before irreversible left ventricular dysfunction occurs.

215. **The answer is A-N, B-Y, C-Y, D-N, E-N.** *(Chap 202.)* Creatine phosphokinase (CK) rises within 8 to 24 h of infarction and returns to normal in 2 or 3 days, while the lactic dehydrogenase (LDH) level rises at 2 to 3 days, but may remain elevated for 2 weeks. LDH isoenzyme 1 (LDH$_1$) predominates in the heart and is a relatively specific indicator of myocardial damage. Coronary reperfusion leads to a rapid washout (early sharp rise and quick fall) of serum CK levels. Hypothyroidism can actually account for misleadingly elevated CK levels.

216. **The answer is A-N, B-Y, C-Y, D-Y, E-Y.** *(Chap 204.)* Pulmonary hypertension due to chronic pulmonary vascular disease such as that produced by multiple pulmonary emboli produces characteristic findings on physical examination, including a loud pulmonary second heart sound, a prominent *a* wave in the jugular venous pulse, and the systolic murmur of tricuspid regurgitation (the abnormal jet of blood flow is easily detectable on Doppler echocardiography). Pulmonary function testing may reveal an enlarged dead space, but there are usually no abnormalities on spirometry. Usual findings on the ECG include P pulmonale (tall, peaked P waves) and right axis deviation. The hypertrophied right ventricle can be imaged on thallium 201 scintigraphy, whereas this chamber normally remains invisible because of the marked uptake of the left ventricle.

217. **The answer is A-N, B-N, C-N, D-Y, E-N.** *(Chap 205.)* Chronic alcoholics may develop a clinical picture virtually identical to that of idiopathic dilated cardiomyopathy. Ceasing consumption of alcohol may well result in halting the progression of heart disease. With continued alcohol abuse, however, 75 percent of afflicted persons will die within 3 years. While beriberi heart disease leads to high output failure, alcoholic cardiomyopathy is associated with a low cardiac output. Atrial arrhythmias, particularly fibrillation, are the most common electrical disorder seen in what is termed "holiday heart syndrome."

218. **The answer is A-N, B-Y, C-Y, D-Y, E-N.** *(Chap 206.)* The manifestations of pericardial tamponade include equalization of pressures in the pericardial space, right atrium, pulmonary artery wedge, right ventricle, and pulmonary artery during diastole. The systolic pressure in the left ventricle, unlike the diastolic, may be greater than the right-sided pressure. Right ventricular free-wall diastolic collapse is a characteristic echocardiographic feature of tamponade. The normal small decrease in left ventricular stroke volume during the negative intrathoracic pressure created by inspiration is magnified by the nondistensible sac containing the diseased pericardium; this leads to pulsus paradoxus (a greater than 10 mmHg drop in systolic blood pressure with inspiration). In tamponade there is a prominent *x* descent with a small *y* descent on the jugular venous pressure contour.

219. **The answer is A-N, B-Y, C-Y, D-N, E-Y.** *(Chap 207.)* The most common type of primary cardiac tumor is the benign myxoma, which most frequently arises in the left atrium. Auscultation may reveal a "tumor plop" in diastole as the tumor hits the ventricular wall. Although most myxomas are sporadic, some are familial with autosomal dominant inheritance. Features of the familial syndromes associated with cardiac myxomas include pigmented nevi, nodular disease of the adrenal cortex, mammary fibroadenomas, and testicular and pituitary tumors. Systemic symptoms that are typically confused with those of endocarditis, noncardiac malignancy, or collagen vascular disease may be associated with myxomas. Sarcoma is the most common primary malignant cardiac tumor.

220. The answer is A-Y, B-N, C-N, D-Y, E-N. *(Chap 208. National Cholesterol Education Program, Arch Intern Med 148:36, 1988.)*   An increasing risk of premature ischemic heart disease can be detected when the cholesterol level exceeds 5.2 mmol/L (200 mg/dL); men with levels above 6.21 mmol/L (240 mg/dL) have a threefold risk of death from myocardial infarction compared with men whose cholesterol is below 5.2 mmol/L (200 mg/dL). Pure hypertriglyceridemia does not appear to be an independent risk factor for atherosclerotic heart disease, but this condition can exacerbate the problem for those who have other risk factors such as uremia, smoking, and hypertension. Hyperlipidemia is best confirmed by measurement of total cholesterol, high-density lipoprotein cholesterol, and triglycerides in serum or plasma in a sample obtained after an overnight fast. Routine use of lipoprotein electrophoresis adds little information. Secondary causes of hyperlipidemia include uncontrolled diabetes mellitus, hypothyroidism, uremia, nephrotic syndrome, obstructive liver disease, dysproteinemias, and drugs (alcohol, estrogens, glucocorticoids, and antihypertensives). Such conditions must be considered and ruled out before an appropriate decision on treatment can be made. There is no compelling evidence that lowering blood sugar per se decreases the death rate from ischemic heart disease in those with diabetes.

221. The answer is A-N, B-Y, C-Y, D-Y, E-N. *(Chap 209.)*   The abrupt onset of severe hypertension or the onset of high blood pressure of any severity in a person under the age of 25 or after the age of 50 should lead to additional tests to exclude renovascular hypertension and pheochromocytoma. The presence of an abdominal bruit (though not a very sensitive screening test) should prompt a workup for renovascular hypertension. Any patient whose hypertension is not controlled by a two-drug regimen such as an angiotensin-converting enzyme inhibitor and a diuretic at adequate doses should undergo further workup. While evidence for left ventricular hypertrophy on physical examination or electrocardiography suggests long-standing hypertension, such a finding does not necessarily imply the presence of Cushing's syndrome, pheochromocytoma, or a renovascular disease.

222. The answer is A-Y, B-Y, C-N, D-N, E-Y. *(Chap 211.)*   Pentoxifylline may have clinical utility in the treatment of claudication by increasing blood flow to the microcirculation through the mechanism of decreasing blood viscosity and enhancing red cell flexibility. Doppler measurements can be used to assess blood pressure in the ankle, which, in the absence of occlusive disease, is greater than that in the brachial artery. In addition to control of blood pressure and cholesterol level, patients with claudication should be advised to exercise regularly to progressively higher levels. Revascularization or angioplasty should be reserved for those patients who suffer from pain at rest or from progressive and disabling symptoms. Patency rates of femoral-popliteal saphenous vein bypass grafts approach 95 percent at 1 year and 70 to 80 percent at 3 years.

223–226. The answers are 223-E, 224-A, 225-C, 226-B. *(Chaps 201, 204, 206.)*   Right heart failure, or elevated right-heart filling pressure, can develop from many causes. Right heart failure most commonly occurs as a result of pulmonary artery hypertension. Pulmonary artery hypertension, in turn, arises either from increased pulmonary vascular resistance with lung disease, in which case the pulmonary capillary wedge pressure (left atrial pressure) is not elevated, or from left-sided failure or valvular disease, in which case left atrial pressure is increased. Massive right ventricular infarction can cause the right side of the heart to fail at low systolic pressures. With primary myocardial disease, both left and right atrial pressures are elevated; however, when diastolic pressures are *equal* in the left and right cardiac chambers, external compression, such as constrictive pericarditis, must be the suspected cause.

Disorders of the Respiratory System

DIRECTIONS: Each question below contains five suggested responses. Select the **one best** response to each question.

227. The most useful and predictive tool in evaluating the condition of a patient with an acute asthmatic attack and in assessing response to therapy is

    (A) chest radiography
    (B) arterial blood gas measurement
    (C) measurement of pulsus paradoxus
    (D) observation of accessory muscle use
    (E) measurement of peak expiratory flow or FEV_1

228. A 24-year-old woman presents with a 1-year history of chronic painless hemoptysis. She has coughed up clotted blood on several occasions without significant additional sputum production. She is otherwise well. Her past medical history is unremarkable. Her only medicine is an oral contraceptive pill. Evaluation includes a chest x-ray, which is unremarkable, and a ventilation-perfusion nuclear medicine scan, which is normal. Which of the following is the most likely diagnosis?

    (A) Pulmonary thromboembolism
    (B) Primary pulmonary hypertension
    (C) Chronic bronchitis
    (D) Bronchial adenoma
    (E) Cystic fibrosis

229. A young male is brought to the emergency department after having been submerged for a prolonged period of time at a nearby pond. Cardiopulmonary resuscitation was performed at the scene. The patient is being ventilated by mask and bag upon arrival in the emergency department. A brief examination reveals that the patient has no obvious sites of trauma and is conscious but not communicative. His blood pressure is 90/60, pulse 120, temperature 36°C (96.8°F), and respiratory rate 30. Cardiac rhythm reveals sinus tachycardia. Pulse oximetry reveals oxygen saturation of 83 percent. Which of the following is the best method to reverse the patient's apparent hypoxemia?

    (A) Administration of sodium bicarbonate
    (B) Administration of acetazolamide
    (C) Administration of supplemental oxygen
    (D) Application of continuous positive airway pressure and administration of supplemental oxygen
    (E) Administration of supplemental oxygen and endotracheal suction to remove aspirated fluid

230. A patient who is being evaluated for shortness of breath is found to have an arterial P_{O_2} of 7.9 kPa (59 mmHg) while breathing room air at sea level and an arterial P_{O_2} of 8.1 kPa (61 mmHg) while breathing 40% inspired O_2. In each case the arterial P_{CO_2} is normal. Which of the following conditions would be LEAST likely to account for these findings?

(A) Idiopathic pulmonary fibrosis
(B) Atelectasis
(C) *Klebsiella* pneumonia
(D) Cardiogenic pulmonary edema
(E) Osler-Rendu-Weber syndrome

231. A 63-year-old man has pneumococcal pneumonia with extensive air-space consolidation in the left upper and left lower lobes. He complains of extreme shortness of breath when positioned with his left side down. An arterial blood sample drawn in this position shows a P_{O_2} of 6.2 kPa (46 mmHg); 10 min earlier, an arterial blood sample drawn while his right side was dependent had revealed a P_{O_2} of 8.2 kPa (66 mmHg). The most likely explanation for the drop in P_{O_2} when the man was lying on his left side is

(A) increased blood flow to the dependent lung
(B) reduced ventilation to the dependent lung
(C) increased airway resistance in the dependent lung
(D) accumulation of interstitial edema in the dependent lung
(E) increased stiffness of the chest wall on the dependent side

232. A 65-year-old man presents with progressive shortness of breath. Other than a history of heavy tobacco abuse, the patient has a benign past medical history. Breath sounds are absent two-thirds of the way up on the left side of the chest. Percussion of the left chest reveals less resonance than normal. While you place your hand on the left side of the chest and have the patient say "99," no tingling is appreciated in the hand. The trachea appears deviated toward the left. Which of the following diagnoses is most likely?

(A) Bacterial pneumonia
(B) Viral pneumonia
(C) Bronchial obstruction
(D) Pleural effusion
(E) Pneumothorax

233. The best way to make a diagnosis of cystic fibrosis in a patient suspected of having this disorder is

(A) sweat chloride test
(B) sputum culture
(C) pulmonary function testing
(D) stool for fetal fat content
(E) DNA analysis

234. Asthmatic attacks may be precipitated in susceptible persons by a wide variety of stimuli. All the following have been demonstrated to produce airway obstruction in certain asthmatic subjects EXCEPT

(A) viral respiratory infections
(B) cold air
(C) sodium salicylate
(D) exercise
(E) airborne allergens

235. A 21-year-old college student with no prior medical problems begins working as a laboratory technician. He subsequently presents because of several recent episodes of shortness of breath, cough, fever, chills, and malaise. Each episode has lasted several days. The patient is seen during the recovery phase of such an episode; findings at physical examination are normal. Chest x-ray reveals several ill-defined, diffuse, patchy infiltrates. The laboratory evaluation is positive only for an increased erythrocyte sedimentation rate. Pulmonary function studies display reduced lung volumes.

On further questioning it is learned that these episodes begin on days the patient is required to tend to experiments involving laboratory rats at the animal facility. What is the best treatment for this condition?

(A) Inhaled cromolyn sodium
(B) Prednisone
(C) Inhaled beclomethasone
(D) Discontinuation of visits to the animal facility
(E) No treatment

236. The primary pathophysiologic problem in idiopathic pulmonary fibrosis is believed to be

(A) microorganism-mediated activation of pulmonary neutrophils
(B) immune complex–mediated activation of alveolar macrophages
(C) direct immune complex–mediated pulmonary interstitial damage
(D) primary fibroblast proliferation
(E) viral-mediated pulmonary epithelial damage

237. A 59-year-old man with a long-standing smoking history presents with persistent dyspnea. His FEV_1 is 1.0 L/min, arterial blood gas reveals P_{O_2} 60 mmHg, P_{CO_2} 40 mmHg, pH 7.45, and O_2 saturation of 90 percent. He has hyperlucent lungs on chest x-ray and decreased breath sounds on physical examination. The patient's current medical regimen consists of theophylline (300 mg twice daily) and inhaled isoproterenol. The most important addition to the patient's therapy would be

(A) trimethoprim-sulfamethoxazole
(B) substitution of albuterol for isoproterenol
(C) oxygen therapy
(D) prednisone
(E) addition of inhaled beclomethasone

238. Although asthma is a heterogeneous disease, a given individual with asthma would be most likely to

(A) relate a personal or family history of allergic diseases
(B) conform to a characteristic personality type
(C) display a skin-test reaction to extracts of airborne allergens
(D) demonstrate nonspecific airway hyperirritability
(E) have supranormal serum immunoglobulin E

239. A diagnosis of allergic bronchopulmonary aspergillosis in a person who has asthma, recurrent pulmonary infiltrates, and eosinophilia would be supported by all the following findings EXCEPT

    (A) delayed, tuberculin-type skin-test reaction to *Aspergillus fumigatus*
    (B) sputum culture positive for *A. fumigatus*
    (C) immediate skin test reaction to *A. fumigatus*
    (D) marked elevation of serum immunoglobulin E level
    (E) radiographic evidence of bronchiectasis

240. A 22-year-old woman with a history of intermittent wheezing in response to exercise presents to the emergency room with shortness of breath. Her attack occurred during an aerobics class. At this point she is having obvious difficulty breathing and has diffuse wheezes on pulmonary examination. O_2 saturation is 95 percent by pulse oximetry. The most effective treatment at this point would be

    (A) intravenous aminophylline
    (B) inhaled cromolyn sodium
    (C) inhaled albuterol
    (D) intravenous hydrocortisone
    (E) inhaled beclomethasone

241. A 55-year-old woman presents with a cough. Chest x-ray reveals a right hilar mass. Computed tomography of the chest revealed a 5-cm tumor near the right mainstem bronchus within about 4 cm of the carina. Mediastinoscopy and bronchoscopy reveal that the mass is positive for small cell lung carcinoma and that lymph nodes in the right hilar subcarinal regions are also involved. The most appropriate therapy at this time is

    (A) combination chemotherapy
    (B) combination chemotherapy plus radiation therapy
    (C) surgery
    (D) surgery plus radiation therapy
    (E) radiation therapy

242. The dyskinetic ciliary syndromes, including Kartagener's syndrome, can produce all the following manifestations EXCEPT

    (A) bronchiectasis
    (B) sinusitis
    (C) recurrent bronchitis
    (D) interstitial pulmonary fibrosis
    (E) infertility

243. All the following characteristics distinguish small cell lung carcinoma from non-small cell lung carcinoma EXCEPT

    (A) neuroendocrine properties (e.g., neuron-specific enolase staining, presence of dense core granules ultrastructurally) are more common in small cell tumors
    (B) higher rate of response to chemotherapy in small cell tumors
    (C) higher rate of response to radiation therapy in small cell tumors
    (D) higher overall 5-year survival in small cell tumors
    (E) more common inactivation of retinoblastoma gene in small cell tumors

244. A patient with advanced adult respiratory distress syndrome (ARDS) has suffered a pneumothorax after being exposed to 10 cmH_2O positive end-expiratory pressure (PEEP). Which of the following modes of mechanical ventilation would be best?

    (A) Assist/control mode of ventilation
    (B) Synchronized intermittent mandatory ventilation
    (C) Pressure-control ventilation
    (D) Pressure-support ventilation
    (E) Continuous positive airway pressure

245. A 48-year-old Haitian man presents with shortness of breath. Chest x-ray reveals a right pleural effusion extending about halfway up the chest. The patient has no other known medical problems and is on no medicines. The rest of the general physical examination is unremarkable. Diagnostic thoracentesis reveals the following: lactate dehydrogenase 1.7 μkat/L (100 U/L), glucose 6.4 mmol/L (150 mg/dL), and amylase 1.6 μkat/L (90 U/L). Cell count reveals 1000 red cells per microliter and 1000 white cells per microliter (differential: 50 percent neutrophils, 25 percent lymphocytes, and 25 percent monocytes). A ventilation-perfusion lung scan is indeterminate on the right side because of the large effusion, but there are no ventilation-perfusion mismatches elsewhere. The next most appropriate step would be

(A) pulmonary arteriogram
(B) abdominal CT
(C) chest CT
(D) needle biopsy of pleura
(E) administration of isoniazid with ethambutol

246. A 45-year-old woman presents with fever and cough. She has had no past medical problems and was well until about 3 days ago. Physical examination is remarkable for a temperature of 39°C (102.2°F) and the presence of diffuse rales on chest examination. Except for an elevated white count with a left-shifted differential, her blood tests are normal. Chest radiography reveals patchy bilateral infiltrates. She is unable to produce sputum. Which is the most reasonable choice of antibiotics at this time?

(A) Penicillin G
(B) Cefotaxime
(C) Erythromycin
(D) Ampicillin plus sulbactam
(E) Ampicillin plus sulbactam plus erythromycin

Questions 247–248

A 60-year-old man with emphysema and bronchitis is brought to an emergency room by an ambulance crew that has been giving him oxygen by mask. Three days ago, he noted that his sputum had changed color and increased in amount. His wife called the ambulance when he became suddenly short of breath and confused. On arrival at the hospital he is somnolent. Mid-inspiratory crackles and diffuse expiratory wheezes are audible on examination of the chest, and he has marked peripheral edema and ascites. Hemoglobin is 180 g/L (18 g/dL). Arterial blood gases are pH 7.08, P_{O_2} 19.8 kPa (148 mmHg), and P_{CO_2} 14.2 kPa (106 mmHg).

247. The most appropriate immediate therapy for the man described above would be

(A) intravenous infusion of sodium bicarbonate
(B) endotracheal intubation and assisted ventilation
(C) administration of isoetharine by air-compressor nebulizer
(D) discontinuation of supplemental oxygen
(E) subcutaneous injection of epinephrine

248. In this patient, manifestations of right ventricular heart failure would best be treated with

(A) diazoxide
(B) digoxin
(C) hydralazine
(D) oxygen
(E) phlebotomy

249. A 45-year-old sandblaster develops shortness of breath. Chest x-ray reveals diffuse miliary infiltration and calcified hilar nodes. Which of the following statements considering the patient's current condition is correct?

   (A)   Lung damage is due to asbestos exposure
   (B)   There is an increased risk of tuberculosis
   (C)   The disease is likely to abate if the occupational exposure ends
   (D)   An obstructive pattern is likely on pulmonary function studies
   (E)   Angiotensin-converting enzyme levels will be high

250. A 34-year-old man complains of shortness of breath after minimal exertion. He has no systemic symptoms. He developed a nonproductive cough 10 months ago. A chest x-ray, which was reportedly normal, was done at that time. Examination now reveals a respiratory rate of 28 breaths per minute, and diffuse end-inspiratory crackles are heard over his lower lung fields. His chest x-ray is shown below. An arterial P_{O_2} measured while the patient is breathing room air is 55 mmHg, and arterial P_{CO_2} is 26 mmHg. Routine blood counts are normal. The next step in his evaluation should be

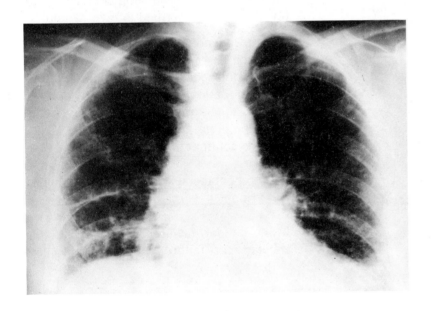 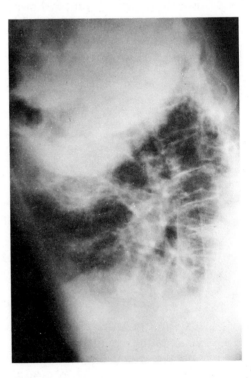

   (A)   angiotensin-converting enzyme level
   (B)   transbronchial biopsy
   (C)   bronchoalveolar lavage
   (D)   salivary gland biopsy
   (E)   serology for rheumatoid factor

251. A 23-year-old woman complains of dyspnea and substernal chest pain on exertion. Evaluation for this complaint 6 months ago included arterial blood-gas testing, which revealed pH 7.48, P_{O_2} 79 mmHg, and P_{CO_2} 31 mmHg. Electrocardiography then showed a right axis deviation. Chest x-ray now shows enlarged pulmonary arteries but no parenchymal infiltrates, and a lung perfusion scan reveals subsegmental defects that are thought to have a "low probability for pulmonary thromboembolism." Echocardiogram demonstrates right heart strain, but no evidence of primary cardiac disease. The most appropriate diagnostic test now would be

(A) open lung biopsy
(B) Holter monitoring
(C) right-heart catheterization
(D) transbronchial biopsy
(E) serum α_1-antitrypsin level

252. A 53-year-old man is noted to be tachypneic and confused 48 h after suffering multiple orthopedic and internal injuries in an automobile accident. Chest x-ray is interpreted as normal, but arterial blood-gas values are as follows: pH 7.49, P_{O_2} 52 mmHg, and P_{CO_2} 30 mmHg. The course of action most likely to confirm the diagnosis of this man's condition would be to

(A) order a ventilation-perfusion scan
(B) order pulmonary angiography
(C) order impedance plethysmography
(D) order blood testing for fibrin split products
(E) repeat the physical examination

253. A 42-year-old man who is a heavy cigarette smoker develops chills, malaise, and tenderness at the angle of the jaw a week after onset of a sore throat. He is febrile and tachypneic, and a pleural friction rub is audible over the left chest. Chest x-ray reveals several nodular densities in both lung fields. The most likely diagnosis is

(A) osteoma of the tonsil
(B) retropharyngeal abscess
(C) peritonsillar cellulitis
(D) pharyngeal tuberculosis
(E) postanginal sepsis

254. A 52-year-old woman with long-standing rheumatoid arthritis is hospitalized for total knee replacement. On her admission chest x-ray, a 2-cm nodule is noted near the right hilus. She has smoked one pack of cigarettes daily for the last 32 years. The most appropriate management of this woman's pulmonary condition would be

(A) observation with chest x-rays every 4 months
(B) therapy for 2 months with oral corticosteroids
(C) an upper gastrointestinal series
(D) scalene node biopsy
(E) exploratory thoracotomy

255. The most sensitive noninvasive test for bilateral diaphragmatic paralysis is

(A) testing of vital capacity
(B) "sniff test"
(C) chest x-ray
(D) fluoroscopy
(E) physical examination

256. All the following statements about obstructive sleep apnea syndrome are true EXCEPT

(A) men are affected more often than women
(B) systemic hypertension is a common finding
(C) alcohol can be a contributing factor
(D) estrogens are frequently useful
(E) personality changes may be the presenting complaint

257. A 54-year-old man has a nonproductive cough and exertional breathlessness. He also notes low-grade fever, malaise, and a weight loss of 7 kg (15 lb) over 6 weeks. His white blood cell count is 13,500/mm³. He has a history of mild asthma. A chest x-ray discloses peripheral lung infiltrates. The most likely diagnosis is

(A) idiopathic pulmonary fibrosis
(B) alveolar proteinosis
(C) polymyositis
(D) chronic eosinophilic pneumonia
(E) lymphangiomyomatosis

258. Owing to profound hypoxemia, tracheal intubation is performed on a drowning victim, and mechanical ventilation is begun. Inspired oxygen concentration is 80%. Initially, the man is agitated and fights the respirator. Arterial blood gases are obtained and show pH 7.21, P_{O_2} 70 mmHg, and P_{CO_2} 56 mmHg. The most appropriate management step at this time would be to

   (A) add positive end-expiratory pressure (5 cmH$_2$O)
   (B) sedate the man and control his ventilation
   (C) infuse sodium bicarbonate intravenously
   (D) raise the inspired oxygen concentration
   (E) initiate extracorporeal membrane oxygenation

259. One week following a right total hip replacement a 65-year-old woman develops the sudden onset of shortness of breath. Workup reveals normotension, a prominent second heart sound, hypoxemia, sinus tachycardia with new right axis deviation on the electrocardiogram, and a normal chest x-ray. Oxygen is administered. Impedance plethysmography is consistent with a large proximal clot in the left leg. Which of the following would be the most reasonable next step?

   (A) Performance of a pulmonary angiogram
   (B) Performance of perfusion scintigraphy
   (C) Administration of tissue plasminogen activator
   (D) Administration of heparin
   (E) Administration of warfarin

260. Which of the following is LEAST likely to be associated with cystic fibrosis?

   (A) Intestinal obstruction
   (B) Sinusitis
   (C) Steatorrhea
   (D) Dextrocardia
   (E) Clubbing

DIRECTIONS: Each question below contains five suggested responses. For **each** of the five responses listed with every question, you are to respond either YES (Y) or NO (N). In a given item **all, some, or none** of the alternatives may be correct.

Questions 261-262

A 35-year-old man seeks medical attention for breathlessness on exertion. He has never smoked cigarettes and has not been coughing. One sibling died at 40 years of age of respiratory failure. His three children are healthy. Physical examination reveals him to be tachypneic as he exhales through pursed lips. His chest is tympanitic to percussion, and breath sounds are poorly heard on auscultation. Chest x-ray shows flattened diaphragms with peripheral attenuation of bronchovascular markings most noticeable at the lung bases.

261. Expected results of the pulmonary function testing of the man described above would include

    (A) increased lung elastic recoil
    (B) increased total lung capacity
    (C) reduced functional residual capacity
    (D) reduced vital capacity
    (E) increased diffusing capacity

262. Initial laboratory assessment of the man described above should include

    (A) measurement of oxygen consumption during exercise
    (B) measurement of sweat chloride concentration
    (C) serum protein electrophoresis
    (D) complete spirometry
    (E) arterial blood-gas determination

263. Hypoxemia occurring after pulmonary thromboembolism can result from

    (A) lowered mixed venous P_{O_2} due to heart failure
    (B) perfusion of atelectatic areas
    (C) increased dead-space ventilation in the area of vascular occlusion
    (D) perfusion of areas poorly ventilated because of airway constriction
    (E) inadequate time for oxygen diffusion secondary to a reduction in the capillary bed

264. Correct statements concerning the pathogenesis of α_1-antitrypsin deficiency include which of the following?

    (A) Emphysema results from an inability to inhibit alveolar destruction by neutrophils
    (B) Clinical deficiency of α_1-antitrypsin usually results from one of several missense mutations that cause a truncated mRNA
    (C) Most α_1-antitrypsin is synthesized by alveolar macrophages
    (D) Mutations of the α_1-antitrypsin gene of the S type produce less severe emphysema than do mutations of the Z type
    (E) Treatment with purified α_1-antitrypsin can raise the serum level to that associated with lung protection

265. A middle-aged woman has a large central mass on chest x-ray. Sputum cytology is positive for squamous cell carcinoma. Which of the following conditions would be considered a contraindication for operation on this woman?

    (A) Resting P_{CO_2} above 50 mmHg
    (B) Syndrome of inappropriate antidiuretic hormone secretion
    (C) Malignant pleural effusion
    (D) Recurrent laryngeal nerve paralysis
    (E) Metastasis to lobar lymph nodes

266. Which of the following conditions would be likely to result in an increased residual volume on plethysmographic pulmonary function testing?

(A) Emphysema
(B) Sarcoidosis
(C) Cystic fibrosis
(D) Fracture of the cervical spine
(E) Kyphoscoliosis

267. In order to decrease the likelihood of drug toxicity, theophylline dosage should be reduced in a patient with asthma who is

(A) older than 70
(B) taking erythromycin for *Mycoplasma* pneumonia
(C) taking phenytoin for seizures
(D) heavily abusing marijuana
(E) taking allopurinol for gout

268. Known consequences of asbestos exposure include

(A) pulmonary fibrosis
(B) pleural effusion
(C) small cell carcinoma
(D) peritoneal mesothelioma
(E) pleural plaques

269. A 51-year-old man develops pancreatitis associated with the passage of a gallstone. His treatment includes meperidine and intravenous normal saline. Two days later, he becomes anxious, tachypneic, and short of breath. An emergency chest x-ray demonstrates diffuse, bilateral interstitial and alveolar infiltrates. A year ago, he suffered a myocardial infarction, but since then he has had no evidence of congestive heart failure. In this case, adult respiratory distress syndrome can be distinguished from cardiogenic pulmonary edema by

(A) measurement of lung water
(B) measurement of protein concentration in edema fluid
(C) measurement of pulmonary artery wedge pressure
(D) measurement of lung compliance
(E) calculation of the alveolar-arterial P_{O_2} difference

270. A 65-year-old man with chronic bronchitis presented to the emergency room 2 weeks ago with acute respiratory failure. He was intubated and treated with diuretics and antibiotics. However, after apparent improvement during a 1-week stay in the intensive care unit on mechanical ventilation, he has since failed three attempts at being weaned from the ventilator. Which of the following factors could account for the difficulty in removing this patient from the ventilator?

(A) Metabolic acidosis
(B) Benzodiazepines
(C) A P_{CO_2} too high prior to extubation
(D) Hypokalemia
(E) Hypothyroidism

271. True statements regarding idiopathic pulmonary fibrosis include

(A) the FEV_1/FVC ratio is reduced
(B) therapy with corticosteroids and cyclophosphamide may be beneficial
(C) serial chest x-rays are helpful in following response to therapy
(D) the carbon monoxide diffusing capacity is a useful indicator of response to therapy
(E) lung transplantation should be considered

Disorders of the Respiratory System

Answers

227. The answer is E. *(Chap 217.)* Several investigators have shown that the most efficient means of assessing the severity of an asthmatic attack and of following the therapeutic response is the measurement of some parameter of respiratory function such as peak flow or forced expiratory volume in 1 s (FEV_1). The chest radiograph will frequently show only hyperinflation in attacks of varying degrees of severity. Arterial blood gases will reflect hypoxemia and hypocapnia in all but the most severe episodes, when they may reflect respiratory fatigue and severe obstruction as rising P_{CO_2} levels. Accessory muscle use and the presence of pulsus paradoxus reflect changes in intrathoracic pressure and the work of breathing, and they may actually disappear if the patient's breathing worsens to the point of becoming shallow. Thus, these signs may be misleading.

228. The answer is D. *(Chap 30.)* The evaluation of hemoptysis must begin with confirmation that the blood is actually coming from the respiratory tract, rather than nasopharyngeal or gastrointestinal sites. If blood-tinged sputum is the primary symptom, the most likely diagnosis is chronic bronchitis. Chronic and recurrent hemoptysis in a young, otherwise asymptomatic female strongly suggests the diagnosis of a bronchial adenoma. Bronchiectasis is usually associated with extensive sputum production and "tram-tracking" (abnormal air bronchograms) on chest radiography. Given the absence of physical examination evidence for primary pulmonary hypertension (e.g., an accentuated second heart sound), a negative perfusion scan, a normal physical examination, and the chronic history without chest pain, thromboembolic disease is unlikely, even though the patient is on oral contraceptive pills. The patient should undergo bronchoscopy to define the location of the putative adenoma so that it can be removed surgically.

229. The answer is D. *(Chap 399. Modell, N Engl J Med 328:253–256, 1993.)* Ninety percent of drowning patients aspirate fluid; however, the vast majority aspirate less than 22 mL/kg. Though aspiration of fresh water can produce acute hypervolemia with dilutional hyponatremia and possibly even hemolysis, these are rare occurrences. Aspiration of sea water can cause hypovolemia with ensuing hypernatremia. In the absence of documentation of such an electrolyte problem, no specific therapy is required. Aspiration of water of any type leads to considerable venous admixture (i.e., ventilation-perfusion abnormalities), which can produce hypoxemia. The most important therapeutic maneuvers, after resuscitation on the scene, are to provide supplemental oxygen, intravenous access, and transportation to a hospital where the patient can be evaluated for adequacy of ventilation, cardiac function, and blood volume. The best way to reverse drowning-associated hypoxemia is the application of continuous positive airway pressure (CPAP). CPAP may be combined with mechanical inflation of the lung as needed; the latter technique may be particularly effective in those who have aspirated fresh water, which leads to a change in surface-tension characteristics of pulmonary surfactant. Correction of severe metabolic acidosis with bicarbonate is controversial. Finally, the universal need for corticosteroid therapy and antibiotics is no longer accepted.

230. The answer is A. *(Chap 214.)* General mechanisms responsible for hypoxemia include alveolar hypoventilation, impaired diffusion, ventilation/perfusion inequality, and shunting (blood bypassing ventilated areas of the lung). In each of these cases, except for shunting, the arterial P_{O_2} increases significantly when the inspired P_{O_2} is raised. Examples of shunts (which could account for the lack of response to oxygen therapy described in the question) include congenital heart disease that produces direct right-to-left intracardiac flow (usually associated with pulmonary hypertension), intrapulmonary vascular shunting (i.e., congenital telangiectatic disorders such as Osler-Rendu-Weber syndrome), or most commonly perfused alveoli that are not ventilated because of atelectasis or fluid buildup (pneumonia or pulmonary edema). Since impaired diffusion is usually not severe enough to lead to disordered gas exchange except during exercise, most cases of normocapnic hypoxemia are due to ventilation-perfusion mismatch. Many processes that affect the lungs (alveolar disease, interstitial lung disease, pulmonary vascular disease, airway disease) do so unevenly, which leads to some areas with adequate perfusion and poor ventilation and some with good ventilation and poor perfusion.

231. The answer is A. *(Chap 214.)* In a person standing erect, blood flow per unit volume increases from the apex of the lung to the base. Ventilation also increases from apex to base, but the gradient is less than that for blood flow, making the ventilation-perfusion ratio less at the bottom of the lung than at the top. Both ventilation and perfusion are affected by posture; as a general rule, the dependent regions are better perfused than ventilated and have the lowest ratio of ventilation to perfusion. Thus, a person with unilateral air-space disease may have an increase in venous admixture when the diseased lung is dependent. In that situation, blood flow increases to the diseased lung, perfusing atelectatic and poorly ventilated alveoli, and hypoxemia ensues.

232. The answer is C. *(Chap 212.)* In evaluating the patient with shortness of breath, examination of the thorax is crucial. Tracheal deviation to the left indicates either a pleural effusion on the right or loss of volume on the left. Volume loss is typically due to an obstructed bronchus producing atelectasis in the affected segment or lobe. Loss of aerated lung will be reflected in dullness to percussion, absent breath sounds on auscultation, and decrease in tactile fremitus. A consolidative process, such as bacterial pneumonia, might well produce increased fremitus as well as bronchial breath sounds and whispered pectoriloquy since sounds are well transmitted through a consolidated area. In a pneumothorax, a percussion of the chest would reveal hyperresonance, although breath sounds and fremitus would also be absent. A possible cause of obstruction and atelectasis of a large amount of left lung tissue could be obstruction of a major bronchus by carcinoma of the lung, especially in an older patient who is a heavy smoker.

233. The answer is A. *(Chap 222. Collins, Science 256:774, 1992.)* Cystic fibrosis, an autosomal recessive disease, results from a mutation in a gene located on chromosome 7. Because of the multiple potential mutations in this gene that have been described, it is currently not feasible to use DNA-based diagnosis for identification of patients with this disorder or heterozygous carriers. The gene codes for a protein called the cystic fibrosis transmembrane regulator (CFTR), which is a single-chain 1480 amino acid–containing protein that functions as a cyclic AMP-regulated chloride channel. All affected tissues, including airway and intestinal epithelium, sweat ducts, and exocrine pancreatic ducts, express an abnormal CFTR protein. The most common mutation in this protein is an absence of phenylalanine in amino acid position 508, resulting from a 3-base pair DNA deletion. A consequence of this and the other mutations in the CFTR protein is failure of normal calcium chloride transport. Therefore, secretions are dehydrated and poorly cleared. The diagnosis of cystic fibrosis now depends on a combination of clinical criteria and a demonstration that sweat chloride values are abnormally low. About half of the 1 to 2 percent of patients with cystic fibrosis who have normal sweat chloride values have a specific single G to T mutation in the CFTR gene.

234. The answer is C. *(Chap 217.)* Respiratory infections, particularly those that are viral in origin, are common precipitants of acute asthmatic attacks. Bacterial infections are relatively less common precipitants; in fact, they may be implicated wrongly in acute asthma if purulent sputum due to sputum eosinophilia is mistakenly attributed to bacterial disease. Hyperventilation with cold air is now used as a bronchoprovocation test in some pulmonary function laboratories to identify asthmatic subjects. Heat loss across the respiratory mucosa is believed to be the stimulus producing airway narrowing in asthmatic persons who breathe cold air and who have exercise-induced asthma. Although some persons with asthma develop bronchospasm after ingestion of acetylsalicylic acid or tartrazine dye, they tolerate sodium salicylate without symptoms. In allergic asthma subjects, inhalation challenge testing with appropriate antigens causes reproducible bronchospasm.

235. The answer is D. *(Chap 218.)* Given the temporal relationship of the symptoms to the work with rats, serologic evidence for inflammation, the nonspecific radiographic findings, and the restrictive pulmonary physiology suggested by spirographic examination, the most likely diagnosis is acute hypersensitivity pneumonitis with male rat urine probably the offending antigen. Without treatment, the patient could develop the subacute or chronic form of the disease with potentially serious physiologic impairment. While steroids can be helpful in severe or chronic cases, the best therapy is to remove the offending antigen or to remove the patient from an environment where exposure is inevitable. This approach is difficult when the patient's life-style or livelihood requires a radical change; in the case presented, however, simply restricting the student's laboratory efforts to those not involving direct animal care seems relatively nondisruptive.

236. The answer is B. *(Chaps 213, 224.)* Bronchoalveolar lavage in patients with idiopathic pulmonary fibrosis, a chronic inflammatory disorder of the lower respiratory tract characterized by dyspnea and reticulonodular infiltrates on chest radiography, discloses an abundance of alveolar macrophages. Probably related to locally generated immune complexes, alveolar macrophages become activated and then produce several mediators that recruit and induce fibroblast proliferation, which causes secondary damage. Macrophage-derived mediators believed to be important in this process include fibronectin, a 200-kDa dimeric glycoprotein that interacts with connective tissue matrix as well as specific receptors on fibroblasts, and platelet-derived growth factor, whose beta chain is encoded by the c-*sis* proto-oncogene. Platelet-derived growth factor is believed to play an important role in recruiting fibroblasts to the site of inflammation. Macrophages also produce chemotaxins such as leukotriene B_4 and interleukin 8, which attract neutrophils and eosinophils into the region.

237. The answer is C. *(Chap 223. Weinberger, N Engl J Med 328:1389–1397, 1993.)* The patient has evidence for obstructive lung disease based on hyperinflation, decreased breath sounds, and decreased FEV_1, and a heavy smoking history. He has chronic hypoxemia and a moderate degree of CO_2 retention. He may have an intermediate syndrome between emphysema and chronic bronchitis. Smoking cessation, yearly vaccination against influenza, and a one-time vaccination against *S. pneumoniae* infection are definitely indicated. There are no definitive data to support the use of chronic antibacterial prophylaxis or systemic glucocorticoids, though occasional patients will benefit from steroid therapy given either systemically or by inhalation. The major issue is hypoxemia, which should be treated with continuous (at least nocturnal) oxygen therapy. Several trials have documented the benefit of oxygen therapy for lowering mortality, improving neuropsychological status, and decreasing the incidence of heart failure. Albuterol, a selective beta$_2$ agonist, induces bronchodilation with few cardiac side effects; however, the benefit of oxygen therapy is likely to be much greater than that of changing the inhaled sympathomimetic.

238. The answer is D. *(Chap 217.)*   The importance of immune mechanisms in the pathogenesis of asthma is suggested by the common association between the disease and the presence of allergic diseases, skin-test sensitivity, and increased serum IgE levels. In addition, many susceptible persons develop bronchospasm after inhalation challenge with airborne allergens. A large proportion of asthmatic subjects, however, have none of these markers of immunologic activity and are classified as having idiosyncratic asthma. When tested for bronchial hyperirritability with various nonantigenic bronchoprovocational agents (e.g., histamine or cold air), asthmatic subjects are found to be more sensitive than normal; the reason for this airway hyperirritability, which is a common feature of all asthmatic persons, is unknown. Although psychologic factors certainly influence the expression of asthma, no single personality type is considered "asthmatic."

239. The answer is A.   *(Chap 218. Greenberger, Chest 91:165S, 1987.)*   Allergic bronchopulmonary aspergillosis is a hypersensitivity pneumonitis involving an allergic reaction to antigens from *Aspergillus* species, most commonly *A. fumigatus*. The diagnosis should be suspected in asthmatic persons who have recurrent pulmonary infiltrates associated with peripheral blood or sputum eosinophilia. Suggestive laboratory findings include serum immunoglobulin E levels elevated many times normal and the presence of aspergilli in the sputum. Antigenic skin testing is positive both in immediate (type I, wheal and flare) reaction and reaction evident after 4 to 6 h (type III, erythema and induration). Delayed, tuberculin-type (type IV, cell-mediated) reactions, however, do not occur. Serum precipitins to aspergilli are found in a majority of affected persons. The inflammatory response leads to dilatation of central airways and often is evident radiographically as mucoid impaction.

240. The answer is C.   *(Chap 217. McFadden, N Engl J Med 327:1928–1937, 1992.)*   Asthmatic patients who present with an acute attack and lack signs of impending ventilatory collapse should be treated with an inhaled aerosolized beta$_2$ agonist such as albuterol or isoproterenol. Such medicines can be given up to every 20 min by inhaled nebulizer for three doses with the frequency reduced thereafter. Such drugs are five times more effective than intravenous aminophylline. Intravenous or inhaled steroids will have a delayed onset of action, if they are destined to be beneficial at all. Patients should be reassured that mortality from asthma is unlikely; however, it is nonetheless advisable to respect an acute asthmatic attack, especially if accompanied by CO_2 retention.

241. The answer is B.   *(Chap 227. Ihde, N Engl J Med 327:1434–1441, 1992.)*   The treatment of patients with small cell lung cancer differs markedly from the approach to patients with non-small cell lung cancer. Chemotherapy is the treatment of choice for essentially all patients with small cell carcinoma. In contrast, non-small cell lung cancer is best treated with local therapy. As such, small tumors with minimal lymph node involvement should be surgically removed. Radiation therapy with or without surgery is appropriate if more extensive lymph node involvement is detected or if the primary tumor is large or invades the chest wall, diaphragm, or pleural surfaces. The patient in this question has stage T2N2 (IIIA) small cell lung cancer. Actually, a more useful staging system for small cell lung cancer is based on limited (confined to one hemithorax) versus extensive disease. Combination chemotherapy for patients with limited small cell cancer can be expected to result in complete or partial responses in 90 percent; recent studies have documented a benefit if thoracic radiation therapy is added to chemotherapy. While there is a demonstrable increase in survival with the use of combined modality therapy compared with chemotherapy alone, there is also a greater degree of toxicity. Chemotherapy in non-small cell lung cancer, associated with a much lower response rate than in small cell disease, may have limited benefit in those with metastatic cancer and is being studied as an adjunctive approach to locally advanced disease.

242. The answer is D. *(Chap 221.)* Cilia, responsible for the motility and mucous clearance functions of many cell types, are composed of a double tubular structure. Abnormalities in one or another of the anatomic components of cilia can lead to a lack of coordinated ciliary action. Kartagener's syndrome, the best known of the dyskinetic ciliary syndromes, is caused by an absence of the inner or outer dynein arms normally present in functional cilia. Impaired ciliary motion is most prominently reflected in the lack of sperm motility and in the impaired epithelial function of the fallopian tubes and respiratory tract. Infertility results from impaired motility of sperm and epithelial function of fallopian tubes, while chronic sinopulmonary infections result from impaired function of the respiratory tract. Recurrent bronchitis and pneumonia due to impaired removal of airway secretions can lead to diffuse bronchiectasis with abnormally dilated airways and copious sputum production, but not to interstitial pulmonary fibrosis.

243. The answer is D. *(Chap 227. Carbone, Adv Intern Med 37:145, 1991.)* The distinction between small cell (also called oat cell) and non-small cell (adenocarcinoma, large cell, squamous cell) is made on morphologic, biochemical, and biologic grounds. While these differences bear heavily on the understanding of the neoplastic process, they also have important clinical implications because major treatment decisions rest on the differentiation of small cell and non-small cell lung tumors. Most small cell tumors present at a stage beyond the limits of reasonable resectability; however, they are much more responsive to radiation therapy and sensitive to chemotherapy than are the non-small variants. Complete regression of a non-small cell lung tumor would be rare with either modality, but such regression occurs about half the time with small cell tumors. Some 10 to 20 percent of patients with small cell disease limited to one hemithorax are long-term survivors; however, because most patients present with incurable, extensive disease, the overall 5-year survival for both non-small cell and small cell variants is under 10 percent. Small cell tumors are believed to originate from neuroendocrine cells because of the frequent presence of neuron-specific enolase, chromogranin, and secretory granules, as well as neuropeptides such as vasopressin and ACTH. Perhaps also indicative of the distinctive pathogenesis of small cell tumors is the frequent finding of retinoblastoma gene abnormalities and deletions in the long arm of chromosome 3.

244. The answer is C. *(Chap 231.)* A patient with the stiff lungs characteristic of the adult respiratory distress syndrome often requires the institution of 0 to 5 cmH$_2$O of positive end-expiratory pressure to maintain adequate oxygenation. However, such high pressures may disrupt lung tissue, causing subcutaneous emphysema or pneumothorax. Patients with such complications will probably be best served by use of pressure-control ventilation, in which a given pressure is imposed at the airway opening during the inspiratory phase and will deliver whatever tidal volumes and inspiratory flow rates are possible based on the set pressure. In addition to its use in situations where barotrauma has occurred, pressure-control ventilation may also be helpful in postoperative thoracic surgical patients who have newly created suture lines. Because of the asynchronous nature of pressure-control ventilation relative to the patient's own ventilatory efforts, such ventilation usually requires heavy sedation. However, newer modifications of pressure-control ventilation allow the patient to initiate breaths to be given at a set pressure, thereby allowing its use without such sedation.

245. The answer is D. *(Chap 228. Burkmann, Postgrad Med J 69:12, 1993.)* The initial step in the evaluation of a pleural effusion is the determination of the presence of either a transudative effusion, usually due to congestive heart failure, cirrhosis, or nephrotic syndrome, or an exudative pleural effusion, which may be due to a host of causes. The working definition of an exudative effusion is one that meets any of the following criteria: (1) pleural fluid to serum protein concentration ratio of greater than 0.5; (2) pleural fluid to serum lactate dehydrogenase (LDH) concentration ratio greater than 0.6; or (3) pleural fluid LDH concentration greater than two-thirds of the upper limit of normal serum LDH. This patient's effusion is an exudate. Additional studies to be done include measurement of pleural glucose and cultures for bacterial mycobacteria and fungi. If the glucose is less than 60 mg/dL, malignancy, empyema, or rheumatoid pleuritis should be considered. Esophageal rupture, pancreatitis, or malignancy can cause an elevated pleural fluid amylase. If no diagnosis is apparent after the above studies, then occult pulmonary embolism should be considered. If there is still no diagnosis based on the aforementioned studies, it is then appropriate to perform a needle biopsy of the pleura with particular attention to histologic analysis for tuberculosis or cancer.

246. The answer is E. *(Chap 220. Fang, Medicine 69:307–316, 1992.)* Patients who require hospitalization for pneumonia acquired in the community optimally require prompt microbiologic diagnosis. Recent studies have shown that about one-third of patients with such community-acquired pneumonias are either alcohol abusers or have COPD. The potential microbiologic etiology for this spectrum of disease is *S. pneumoniae, H. influenzae, Legionella* species, *Chlamydia*, anaerobes, *S. aureus*, and *Mycoplasma*. If the likelihood of pneumococcal pneumonia is high based on the sputum Gram stain, then penicillin or ampicillin still remain the drugs of choice, given a relatively low rate of penicillin-resistant organisms. However, if the likelihood of aerobic bacterial infection is high, then second-generation cephalosporins, such as cefotaxime, are appropriate. If anaerobic infection is considered likely, then metronidazole or ampicillin plus sulbactam should be used. In the current case, given the lack of clear-cut microbiologic evidence for a specific infection, the absence of sputum, and the equivocal findings on the chest x-ray, *Chlamydia* or *Legionella* should be strongly considered. The best empiric regimen in this situation would be ampicillin plus sulbactam in addition to erythromycin. A microbiologic diagnosis should be made in the next few days to allow narrowing of the antibiotic regimen.

247. The answer is B. *(Chap 223.)* Certain persons with severe obstructive lung disease appear to respond to uncontrolled oxygen therapy by dangerously reducing their minute ventilation. Because they are relatively insensitive to changes in arterial P_{CO_2}, hypoxemia is the major ventilatory stimulus in these persons. When hypoxemia is suddenly treated with supplemental oxygen therapy given in an uncontrolled fashion, ventilation drops, arterial P_{CO_2} rises, acidosis results, and coma may develop. However, abrupt removal of supplemental oxygen may precipitate life-threatening hypoxemia. Because acidosis must nevertheless be rapidly reversed by increasing ventilation, endotracheal intubation should be performed, followed by mechanical ventilation of sufficient amount to return arterial pH to physiologic range. Inhaled bronchodilators cannot be given to comatose, unintubated persons. Epinephrine is relatively ineffective in persons with acute or chronic respiratory failure and is dangerous in elderly, acidemic patients.

248. The answer is D. *(Chap 223.)* Right ventricular failure in persons with chronic pulmonary disease is usually evident as edema and ascites—that is, signs of increased extravascular water. Evidence also suggests that increased right ventricular filling pressures contribute to increases in lung water. Treatment should be aimed at reducing the afterload of the right ventricle. This goal can be accomplished most physiologically by increasing alveolar oxygen tension with supplemental oxygen therapy. Although hydralazine and diazoxide are vasodilators with important effects on the pulmonary circulation, they would not be needed in the case described and may, in fact, worsen gas exchange. Although the usefulness of digoxin therapy in cor pulmonale is debated, the drug generally is reserved for treating persons who have coexisting left ventricular disease. Phlebotomy, although it may improve oxygen delivery in persons with right ventricular failure and elevated hemoglobin concentrations (>200 g/L [20 g/dL]), would not be a reliable remedy for the ascites and edema in the patient presented.

249. The answer is B. *(Chap 219.)* Exposure to free silica (SiO_2) remains a major occupational hazard in the U.S. despite the use of protective garb. Workers at high risk for the development of pulmonary silicosis include stone cutters, sandblasters, foundry workers, and granite quarriers. Pulmonary fibrosis tends to develop in a dose-responsive manner but can progress even after exposure ceases. Radiographic findings include a diffuse miliary or consolidative pattern as well as eggshell-type calcification of hilar nodes. Reticular densities may occur in the upper lung zones. Both restrictive and obstructive components are typically associated with advanced fibrosis secondary to silicosis. Pulmonary tuberculosis very commonly accompanies severe silicosis. Any patients with silicosis and a positive tuberculin skin test should be treated with antituberculous therapy.

250. The answer is B. *(Chap 224.)* The chest x-rays presented show diffuse, severe interstitial infiltrates without hilar adenopathy. Although sarcoidosis may produce this radiographic picture, it is also compatible with idiopathic interstitial pneumonitis, hypersensitivity pneumonitis, collagen vascular disease, inhalation of inorganic dusts, and many other processes. The degree of respiratory system dysfunction demonstrated by this patient necessitates rapid evaluation and a definitive histologic diagnosis so that appropriate therapy can be initiated. Angiotensin-converting enzyme levels, although elevated in many patients with sarcoidosis, are not sufficiently sensitive or specific to replace tissue biopsy in the workup of persons with interstitial infiltrates. Although biopsy of extrapulmonary tissue may demonstrate noncaseating granulomas in patients with sarcoidosis, such biopsies may be negative in patients with active disease. A pathologic diagnosis is absolutely required in patients presenting with interstitial lung disease of uncertain etiology. Fiberoptic bronchoscopy should be performed to rule out infection or malignancy; an accompanying transbronchial biopsy may yield a diagnosis about 25 percent of the time. Bronchoalveolar lavage to assess the degree of inflammation may be helpful in monitoring disease activity, but its precise role in interstitial lung disease remains to be defined. Despite its relatively low yield, the relatively low risk makes an attempt at transbronchial biopsy reasonable prior to definitely obtaining tissue at open lung biopsy.

251. The answer is C. *(Chap 225. Rich, Prog Cardiovasc Dis 31:205, 1988.)* Primary pulmonary hypertension is an uncommon disease that usually affects young women. Early in the illness affected persons often are diagnosed as psychoneurotic because of the vague nature of presenting complaints—for example, dyspnea, chest pain, and evidence of hyperventilation without hypoxemia on arterial blood-gas testing. However, progression of the disease leads to syncope in approximately one-half of cases and signs of right heart failure on physical examination. Chest x-ray typically shows enlarged central pulmonary arteries with or without attenuation of peripheral markings. The diagnosis of primary pulmonary hypertension is made by documentation of elevated pressures by right heart catheterization and by exclusion of other pathologic processes. Lung disease of sufficient severity to cause pulmonary hypertension would be evident by history and on examination. Major differential diagnoses include thromboemboli and heart disease; outside the United States, schistosomiasis and filariasis are common causes of pulmonary hypertension, and a careful travel history should be taken.

252. **The answer is E.** *(Chap 226.)* The clinical triad of dyspnea, confusion, and petechiae in a person who has had recent long-bone fractures establishes the diagnosis of fat embolism syndrome. This disorder, which usually occurs within 48 h of injury, may lead to respiratory failure and death. Petechiae most often are found across the neck, in the axillae, and in the conjunctivae; however, their appearance is often evanescent. No laboratory test is specific for fat embolism.

253. **The answer is E.** *(Chaps 93, 128, 220.)* Postanginal sepsis is a complication of acute bacterial pharyngitis in which a tonsillar abscess leads to infection of the ipsilateral carotid sheath and suppurative thrombophlebitis of the jugular vein. Anaerobic organisms are most commonly cultured from the blood and metastatic foci of infection. At the time of dissemination of infection the pharynx may not be painful, so the origin of the infection may be unsuspected.

254. **The answer is E.** *(Chap 227.)* A solitary lung nodule in a middle-aged person who is a cigarette smoker requires surgical resection. Although a rheumatoid nodule would be in the differential diagnosis of the lesion described in the case, such nodules are usually subpleural and are more common in men than in women. The central location and small size of the lesion described make it relatively inaccessible to nonsurgical biopsy techniques. Because 95 percent of malignant solitary nodules originate in the lung, an undirected search for a primary source is likely to be fruitless. Mediastinoscopy has largely replaced scalene node biopsy in most centers, but because the incidence of mediastinal metastases in malignant solitary nodules is less than 10 percent, surgical exploration would be indicated for the woman described in the question.

255. **The answer is E.** *(Chap 228.)* When the diaphragm is completely paralyzed, it behaves as a floppy membrane. With inspiration, the intercostal and other accessory muscles of respiration contract, causing intrathoracic pressure to become more negative. A floppy diaphragm would then be drawn upward into the chest, and the anterior abdominal wall would move inward. This "paradoxical" motion of the abdominal wall, which is best seen while an affected person is supine, is the most sensitive sign of bilateral diaphragmatic paralysis. Other disorders, such as severe obstructive lung disease, may also produce paradoxical motion of the anterior abdominal wall; however, the paradoxical motion usually improves when a person with this disorder is supine.

256. **The answer is D.** *(Chap 229. Fujita, Ear Nose Throat J 72:67, 1993.)* Obstructive sleep apnea syndrome is a complex entity that involves intermittent upper-airway obstruction during sleep. Most of the manifestations, such as hypertension, cor pulmonale, chronic fatigue, personality changes, and disordered sleep behavior, resolve when obstruction is bypassed by a tracheostomy or endotracheal tube. Although the syndrome is more common in men, the prevalence increases in women after menopause. Alcohol and sedatives can exacerbate ventilatory obstruction by decreasing upper-airway muscle tone. Treatment of severe obstructive sleep apnea includes tricyclics to improve upper-airway muscle tone, uvulopalatopharyngoplasty to create a more spacious airway, continuous nasal positive airway pressure to prevent muscular collapse, and tracheostomy to completely bypass the obstruction. Estrogens, once thought beneficial in improving respiratory drive, are not now considered a mainstay of treatment.

257. **The answer is D.** *(Chap 218. Allen, N Engl J Med 321:569, 1989.)* Chronic eosinophilic pneumonia is an interstitial lung disorder of unknown cause that produces a systemic illness characterized by fever, weight loss, and malaise. Although lung biopsy shows an eosinophilic infiltrate involving both the interstitium and the alveolar space, there may not be an associated eosinophilia in the peripheral blood. The diagnosis should be suggested by the "photonegative pulmonary edema" pattern, with central sparing and nonsegmental, patchy infiltrates in the lung periphery. This disorder often responds dramatically to corticosteroid therapy. Idiopathic pulmonary fibrosis and polymyositis produce diffuse reticular, nodular, or reticulonodular infiltrates on chest x-ray. Alveolar proteinosis is a rare disorder that most often produces a diffuse air-space filling pattern radiating from hilar regions on chest x-ray, often with air bronchograms. Alveolar proteinosis does not cause fever unless complicated by infection such as nocardiosis. Lymphangiomyomatosis is also rare. It occurs exclusively in women of childbearing age. The chest x-ray shows reticulono-dular infiltration but the lungs often appear hyperinflated. Lymphangiomyomatosis is complicated by pleural effusion and pneumothorax, but not fever.

258. The answer is B. *(Chap 231. Hinson, Annu Rev Med 43:341, 1992.)* Some persons who become agitated or anxious while on a mechanical ventilator receive inadequate ventilation because they are breathing out of phase with the machine. The man described in the question has adequate oxygenation—a P_{O_2} of 70 mmHg means his hemoglobin is more than 90 percent saturated. However, he is hypoventilating and has developed an acute respiratory acidosis. Positive end-expiratory pressure (PEEP) improves oxygenation by raising the lung volume and reducing shunting but it does not have a large effect on carbon dioxide clearance. Therefore, the appropriate first step in management would be to administer a sedative and control the man's ventilation in order to reduce arterial P_{CO_2} and raise pH.

259. The answer is D. *(Chap 226.)* Patients at high risk for thromboembolic disease include those who have had recent anesthesia, recent childbirth, heart failure, leg fracture, prolonged bed rest, obesity, estrogen use, or cancer. The clinical scenario presented is highly consistent with a pulmonary embolism arising from venous thrombosis of a proximal lower extremity in a postoperative patient. While the electrocardiogram is usually normal except for sinus tachycardia, the finding of new right heart strain is compatible with a significant pulmonary embolus. The positive impedance plethysmogram for an above-the-knee venous thrombosis obviates the need for additional diagnostic testing. The patient must receive antithrombotic therapy (heparin) in an attempt to inhibit clot growth, promote resolution, and prevent recurrence. Warfarin requires several days to achieve anticoagulation and is therefore not appropriate for the acute setting. While thrombolytic therapy can clearly hasten the resolution of thrombi and may be appropriate for large, deep venous thromboses and pulmonary embolisms large enough to cause hypotension, its role in altering the natural history of this disorder remains to be defined. Furthermore, recent surgery is a contraindication to the use of thrombolytic agents, which, even in the case of more specific newer agents such as tissue plasminogen activator, carry significant hemorrhagic risk.

260. The answer is D. *(Chap 222.)* Although the majority of patients with cystic fibrosis are diagnosed in childhood, a significant number of patients will not be identified until their late teens, twenties, or even thirties. Accurate diagnosis requires that the sweat chloride test be given to all patients with clinical features of cystic fibrosis. Airway obstruction resulting from bronchiectasis is associated with sinusitis and infertility in males with both cystic fibrosis and the immotile cilia syndrome, but only males with immotile cilia have Kartagener's syndrome (bronchiectasis, sinusitis, and dextrocardia). Patients with cystic fibrosis may have any of several gastrointestinal manifestations including obstruction, intussusception, fecal impaction, volvulus, portal hypertension, and steatorrhea. Steatorrhea is a manifestation of pancreatic insufficiency. Nearly all patients with cystic fibrosis display clubbing.

261. **The answer is A-N, B-Y, C-N, D-Y, E-N.** *(Chap 223.)* The man described in the question presents physical signs (pursed lip breathing, chest hyperexpansion) and radiographic evidence (flattened diaphragms, attenuated markings) suggestive of obstructive lung disease with loss of lung tissue. Reduced expiratory air-flow rates are produced by narrowing of airways (e.g., in asthma), by loss of airways (e.g., in bronchiolitis obliterans), or by loss of elastic tissue (e.g., in emphysema). Pathophysiologically, these conditions cause increased resistance as airways are narrowed or collapse, as well as decreased driving pressure, representing loss of elastic recoil. Air-trapping and reduced lung recoil lead to an increase in both total lung capacity (TLC) and functional residual capacity (FRC), which is the volume at which the tendency of the lung to recoil inward is just balanced by the tendency of the chest to recoil outward. Although TLC is increased, vital capacity, the maximum amount of gas that can be exhaled from the lungs with a single breath, is reduced owing to the great increase in residual volume produced by gas-trapping. Not only is vital capacity reduced, but it takes longer to empty the lungs; thus, forced expiratory volume in 1 s (FEV_1) is reduced as a percentage of vital capacity. When alveolar capillaries are destroyed by emphysema, the diffusing capacity, which reflects in part the surface area of alveolar membrane available for gas exchange, is reduced.

262. **The answer is A-N, B-N, C-Y, D-Y, E-Y.** *(Chap 223.)* To establish baseline information in persons who have emphysema, spirometry should be performed, and for those persons with significant complaints or physical findings, arterial blood gases also should be checked. Although cigarette smoking accounts for the vast majority of cases of emphysema, a small percentage of persons who develop this illness have had no exposure to tobacco products. A subset of this nonsmoking, emphysematous population is deficient in α_1-antitrypsin, which is a protease inhibitor normally found in the serum. It is currently believed that release of proteolytic enzymes from inflammatory cells accounts for the lung destruction that typifies emphysema, and α_1-antitrypsin deficiency, a familial disorder diagnosed by serum protein electrophoresis, permits this destruction to occur unimpeded. Exercise testing is not necessary as an initial screening test for emphysema but should be considered before oxygen therapy is prescribed. A male who has emphysematous respiratory failure, who gives no history of respiratory infections, and who has children would not have cystic fibrosis (affected men are sterile); therefore, a sweat chloride test would not be a useful procedure.

263. **The answer is A-Y, B-Y, C-N, D-Y, E-N.** *(Chap 226.)* Hypoxemia occurs commonly after massive pulmonary thromboembolism, although normal arterial oxygen tension does not exclude the diagnosis. The most important mechanism producing hypoxemia in this setting is an increase in venous admixture due to continued perfusion of poorly ventilated areas. Ventilation may be decreased by atelectasis or by airway constriction in response to the release of bronchoactive mediators. A fall in cardiac output producing a low mixed venous P_{O_2} can increase the effect of venous admixture. Increased dead-space ventilation would not be a cause of hypoxemia.

264. **The answer is A-Y, B-N, C-N, D-Y, E-Y.** *(Chaps 213, 223. Stockley, Lung 169:61, 1991.)* Reduced serum levels of the antiprotease α_1-antitrypsin, which is primarily synthesized in the liver, are associated with an inability to control the alveolar-damaging effects of neutrophil elastase and clinical emphysema. α_1-Antitrypsin is encoded by a 7-exon gene spanning 12.2 kilobases on chromosome 14. Common disease-producing mutations of the normal M gene are the Z type, in which a single amino-acid substitution results in a hyperaggregative, improperly processed protein, and the S type, which results in a product with a shortened half-life and is also due to a single amino-acid change. Since the S type produces less clinical antiprotease "deficiency," the pulmonary disease produced in SS homozygotes is much less than that seen in patients whose genotype is ZZ. Intravenous administration of normal human purified α_1-antitrypsin can increase serum levels to a point at which sufficient antiprotease activity is provided to protect alveoli from elastase-induced damage.

265. **The answer is A-Y, B-N, C-Y, D-Y, E-N.** *(Chap 227.)* Although persons with pulmonary lesions often require sophisticated pulmonary function testing to determine their suitability for surgery, hypercapnia at rest usually is considered a contraindication to resection. Obviously, metabolic and other causes of hypoventilation must be excluded. The presence of systemic syndromes, including syndrome of inappropriate antidiuretic hormone secretion (SIADH), does not rule out surgery; in fact, these syndromes often remit following surgical resection of the pulmonary lesion. Malignant pleural effusion or paralysis of either the recurrent laryngeal nerve or the phrenic nerve indicates that the affected person has nonoperable disease. Although metastatic invasion of mediastinal lymph nodes usually is considered an indication not to operate, metastatic spread to lobar lymph nodes that could be included in the resection does not rule out surgery.

266. **The answer is A-Y, B-N, C-Y, D-Y, E-N.** *(Chap 214.)* The volume remaining in the lungs at the conclusion of a complete forced expiration is termed the *residual volume* and can be determined either by the body plethysmography or helium dilution methods. At the residual volume there is a balance between the intrinsic outward recoil of the chest wall and the force maintained by the respiratory muscles to decrease lung volumes further. Therefore, increases in the residual volume can result from the functionally weak musculature of the chest wall that might be observed in neuromuscular disorders that affect the ability to expire forcefully (Guillain-Barré syndrome, muscular dystrophies, cervical spine injury). Furthermore, diseased airways will collapse at low lung volumes, preventing further emptying and also producing an abnormally high residual volume. Thus, any condition in which airway obstruction plays a major role (chronic bronchitis, emphysema, asthma, cystic fibrosis) may be associated with increased residual volume. On the other hand, pulmonary parenchymal disease (e.g., sarcoidosis) produces normal expiration and reduced lung volumes. If inspiratory dysfunction is the primary chest wall problem (as in kyphoscoliosis and obesity), then residual volume will be relatively unaffected or slightly decreased.

267. **The answer is A-Y, B-Y, C-N, D-N, E-Y.** *(Chap 217.)* Although inhaled sympathomimetics are now considered the first-choice treatment for acute asthmatic attacks, the methylxanthines such as theophylline are effective bronchodilators and continue to be extensively used in this disorder. The therapeutic plasma concentration is 10 to 20 μg/mL, but the dose required to achieve these levels varies widely depending on the clinical situation. Theophylline dosage should be reduced in any condition in which the clearance of this drug is significantly impaired, such as in the very young, the elderly, and in those with liver or cardiac dysfunction. Many drugs interfere with the metabolism of theophylline. Commonly used agents including allopurinol, propranolol, cimetidine, and erythromycin all interfere with theophylline clearance and thereby lead to increased levels of this methylxanthine. Drugs that activate hepatic microsomal enzymes—such as cigarettes, marijuana, phenobarbital, and phenytoin—may lower theophylline levels.

268. **The answer is A-Y, B-Y, C-N, D-Y, E-Y.** *(Chap 219.)* Inhalation of asbestos fibers for 10 years or more may lead to interstitial fibrosis that typically begins in the lower lobes and later spreads to mid and upper lung fields. This fibrosis is associated with a restrictive pattern on pulmonary function testing. The chest x-ray shows linear densities, thickening or calcification of the pleura (pleural plaques), and, in severe cases, honeycombing. Exposure to asbestos may also cause exudative pleural effusions. These effusions are often blood-stained and may be painful. The diagnosis may be elusive if a careful occupational exposure is not obtained. These effusions are benign, but affected persons may later sustain malignant mesotheliomas of the pleura or peritoneum. Unlike pulmonary fibrosis, pleural effusions and mesotheliomas may develop after brief exposures to asbestos, often of 1 to 2 years. Mesotheliomas are not associated with cigarette smoking, but the combination of exposure to asbestos and cigarette smoking has a multiplicative effect on the risk of development of lung cancer. Exposure to asbestos increases the risk for both adenocarcinoma and squamous cell (but not small cell) carcinoma of the lung, which suggests that lung cancer screening may be useful in selected individuals.

269. The answer is A-N, B-Y, C-Y, D-N, E-N. *(Chap 230. Bone, Chest 101:320, 1992.)*   The adult respiratory distress syndrome (ARDS) is a clinical triad of hypoxemia, diffuse lung infiltrates, and reduced lung compliance not attributable to congestive cardiac failure. This syndrome's many causes suggest its complex pathogenesis. However, the pathologic outcome is the same: an increase in lung water due to an increase in alveolar capillary permeability. This noncardiogenic pulmonary edema is identical to congestive cardiac pulmonary edema in its effect on the mechanical properties of the lung and on gas exchange. Just as in cardiac pulmonary edema, the increase in lung water associated with ARDS produces interstitial edema and alveolar collapse, so the affected lung becomes stiff and the alveolar-arterial oxygen tension difference widens. Unlike cardiac edema, however, the increase in lung water in ARDS occurs as a result of an increase in alveolar capillary permeability and is not due to an increase in hydrostatic forces. Edema fluid in ARDS, therefore, often contains macromolecules (such as serum proteins), and measurement of pulmonary artery wedge pressure is normal or low. In clinical practice, determination of pulmonary artery wedge pressure is the most helpful discriminant between ARDS and cardiac failure.

270. The answer is A-N, B-Y, C-N, D-Y, E-Y. *(Chap 222.)*   There are many reasons why patients fail removal from assisted ventilation. Sedatives, commonly prescribed earlier in the hospital stay for agitation or sleep, may not yet have been discontinued or metabolized and could contribute to impairment of respiratory drive. Persistent secretions that could be removed by suctioning might also contribute to the problem. A very important issue is maintenance of a continued drive to breathe. The central respiratory centers are sensitive to blood pH and will promote ventilation when sufficient acidosis (greater than that normally noted in the bronchitic patient with chronic CO_2 retention) ensues. Thus, creation of metabolic alkalosis with diuretic therapy or running the assisted minute ventilation too high (i.e., lower P_{CO_2} and higher pH than normal for the patient) could account for failed extubation. Neuromuscular weakness caused by diuretic-induced hypokalemia, malnutrition, and occult hypothyroidism are potential factors leading to difficulty in independent ventilation and trouble in weaning.

271. The answer is A-N, B-Y, C-N, D-Y, E-Y. *(Chap 224. DuBois, Annu Rev Med 44:441, 1993.)*   A nonproductive cough, dyspnea, hypoxemia with normo- or hypocapnia at rest, bibasilar reticular infiltrates on chest x-ray, and restrictive pulmonary function tests (normal or increased FEV_1/FVC ratio, reduced lung volumes) should suggest the diagnosis of idiopathic pulmonary fibrosis. This diagnosis can only be confirmed after the host of other entities causing interstitial lung disease are excluded by appropriate clinical and pathologic examination. Inasmuch as activated alveolar macrophages (possibly activated by immune complexes) are believed to be pathogenetically responsible for this disease, it is not surprising that immunosuppressive therapy with corticosteroids with or without cyclophosphamide has been beneficial. While chest x-ray correlates poorly with disease activity, the carbon monoxide diffusing capacity, usually reduced in idiopathic pulmonary fibrosis, is a useful test in assessing therapeutic response. Given the initial success with the procedure, lung transplantation (heart-lung or single-lung) should be considered in severe or unresponsive cases.

Disorders of the Kidney and Urinary Tract

DIRECTIONS: Each question below contains five suggested responses. Choose the **one best** response to each question.

272. A patient with lymphoma known to excrete 1.5 g urinary protein per day has a negative dipstick evaluation for urinary protein. The reason for the seeming inconsistency is

    (A) the size of the excreted protein is too small to be picked up by the test strip
    (B) the urine is not concentrated enough
    (C) only heavy-chain sequences are recognized by the test strip
    (D) Tamm-Horsfall protein blocks the reaction between the secreted protein and the test strip
    (E) dipsticks preferentially detect albumin compared with immunoglobulin because the former is negatively charged

273. A 75-year-old female nursing home resident is brought to the emergency department because of increasing obtundation. She is found to be poorly communicative. Brief physical examination reveals skin turgor. Blood pressure is 100/60, pulse 120, respiratory rate 20, and temperature 37°C (98.6°F). Blood tests reveal the following serum electrolytes: sodium 160 mmol/L, potassium 5.0 mmol/L, bicarbonate 30 mmol/L, chloride 110 mmol/L. The most appropriate management at this time would include administration of 5% dextrose in

    (A) normal saline, 100 mL/h
    (B) normal saline solution, 250 mL/h
    (C) half normal saline, 100 mL/h
    (D) half normal saline, 200 mL/h
    (E) water, 150 mL/h

274. Laboratory evaluation of a 19-year-old man being worked up for polyuria and polydipsia yields the following results:

Serum electrolytes (mmol/L): Na$^+$ 144; K$^+$ 4.0; Cl$^-$ 107; HCO$_3^-$ 25
BUN: 6.4 mmol/L (18 mg/dL)
Blood glucose: 5.7 mmol/L (102 mg/dL)
Urine electrolytes (mmol/L): Na$^+$ 28; K$^+$ 32
Urine osmolality: 195 mosmol/kg water

After 12 h of fluid deprivation, body weight has fallen by 5 percent. Laboratory testing now reveals the following:

Serum electrolytes (mmol/L): Na$^+$ 150; K$^+$ 4.1; Cl$^-$ 109; HCO$_3^-$ 25
BUN: 7.1 mmol/L (20 mg/dL)
Blood glucose: 5.4 mmol/L (98 mg/dL)
Urine electrolytes (mmol/L): Na$^+$ 24; K$^+$ 35
Urine osmolality: 200 mosmol/kg water

One hour after the subcutaneous administration of 5 units of arginine vasopressin, urine values are as follows:

Urine electrolytes (mmol/L): Na$^+$ 30; K$^+$ 30
Urine osmolality: 199 mosmol/kg water

The likely diagnosis in this case is

(A) nephrogenic diabetes insipidus
(B) osmotic diuresis
(C) salt-losing nephropathy
(D) psychogenic polydipsia
(E) none of the above

275. A 70-year-old man with diabetes mellitus and hypertension has the following serum chemistries:

Electrolytes (mmol/L): Na$^+$ 138; K$^+$ 5.0; Cl$^-$ 106; HCO$_3^-$ 20
Glucose: 11 mmol/L (200 mg/dL)
Creatinine: 176 μmol/L (2.0 mg/dL)

All the following may contribute to worsening hyperkalemia EXCEPT

(A) propranolol
(B) indomethacin
(C) captopril
(D) digitalis
(E) carbenicillin

276. The following laboratory serum values are obtained:

Electrolytes (mmol/L): Na$^+$ 122; K$^+$ 4.2; Cl$^-$ 88; HCO$_3^-$ 24
BUN: 2.8 mmol/L (8 mg/dL)
Creatinine: 71 μmol/L (0.8 mg/dL)
Osmolality: 245 mosm/kg

These findings are most consistent with

(A) multiple myeloma
(B) acute bacterial meningitis
(C) congestive heart failure
(D) Addison's disease
(E) diabetes mellitus

277. A normotensive patient is found to have a serum potassium level of 3 mmol/L. The urine potassium excretion is 10 mmol/L. The serum bicarbonate is 32 mmol/L. Based on the available data, what is the most likely cause for the patient's hypokalemia?

(A) Diuretic use
(B) Gastrointestinal loss
(C) Renal tubular acidosis
(D) Bartter's syndrome
(E) Malignant renin-secreting tumor

278. A 40-year-old alcoholic male presents with a 6-day history of binge drinking. Serum chemistry tests reveal the following:

Electrolytes (mmol/L): Na$^+$ 145; K$^+$ 5.0; Cl$^-$ 105; HCO$_3^-$ 15
BUN: 7.1 mmol/L (20 mg/dL)
Creatinine: 133 μg/L (1.5 mg/dL)
Glucose: 9.6 mmol/L (172 mg/dL)

The nitroprusside (Acetest) agent gives a minimally positive result. Optimal therapy to ameliorate the patient's acid-base disorder would include 5% dextrose in

(A) water
(B) normal saline
(C) normal saline, insulin, and sodium bicarbonate
(D) half normal saline and insulin
(E) half normal saline, insulin, and sodium bicarbonate

279. A 45-year-old woman who has had slowly progressive renal failure begins to complain of increasing numbness and prickling sensations in her legs. Examination reveals loss of pinprick and vibration sensation below the knees, absent ankle jerks, and impaired pinprick sensation in her hands. Serum creatinine concentration, checked during her most recent clinic visit, is 790 μmol/L (8.9 mg/dL). The woman's physician should now recommend

(A) a therapeutic trial of phenytoin
(B) a therapeutic trial of pyridoxine (vitamin B_6)
(C) a therapeutic trial of cyanocobalamin (vitamin B_{12})
(D) initiation of maintenance hemodialysis
(E) neurologic referral for nerve conduction studies

280. In patients with chronic renal failure, all the following are important contributors to bone disease EXCEPT
(A) impaired renal production of 1,25-dihydroxyvitamin D_3
(B) hyperphosphatemia
(C) aluminum-containing antacids
(D) loss of vitamin D and calcium via dialysis
(E) metabolic acidosis

281. A 50-year-old man is hospitalized for treatment of enterococcal endocarditis. He has been receiving ampicillin and gentamicin for the past 2 weeks but is persistently febrile. Laboratory results are as follows:

Serum electrolytes (mmol/L): Na^+ 145; K^+ 5.0; Cl^- 110; HCO_3^- 20
BUN: 14.2 mmol/L (40 mg/dL)
Serum creatinine: 300 μmol/L (3.5 mg/dL)
Urine sodium: 20 mmol/L
Urine creatinine: 3000 mmol/L (35 mg/dL)

Which of the following is the most likely cause of this patient's acute renal failure?

(A) Tubular necrosis
(B) Insensible skin losses
(C) Renal artery embolism
(D) Cardiac failure
(E) Nausea and vomiting

282. The mechanism of cyclosporine-induced acute renal failure is most likely due to

(A) interstitial nephritis
(B) acute tubular necrosis
(C) intrarenal vascular constriction
(D) renal artery spasm
(E) immune-mediated glomerular injury

283. A 72-year-old man becomes oliguric following surgery for repair of an abdominal aortic aneurysm. He is alert, oriented, and able to take fluids and medications by mouth. Laboratory testing done on the fourth postoperative day reveals the following:

Serum electrolytes (mmol/L): Na^+ 139; K^+ 5.1; Cl^- 104; HCO_3^- 17
Serum chemistries: BUN 32 mmol/L (90 mg/dL); creatinine 740 μmol/L (8.4 mg/dL); calcium 2.0 mmol/L (8.0 mg/dL); phosphorus 3.4 mmol/L (10.4 mg/dL); uric acid 1070 μmol/L (18.0 mg/dL); glucose 7.8 mmol/L (140 mg/dL)
Urine volume: approximately 400 mL/d (Foley catheter in place)
Urine electrolytes (mmol/L): Na^+ 50; K^+ 30; Cl^- 40

All the following orders would be appropriate in the management of this man EXCEPT

(A) discontinue drainage by Foley catheter
(B) give oral aluminum hydroxide gel (Amphogel), 60 mL four times daily
(C) give oral allopurinol, 300 mg once daily
(D) limit total fluid intake to 800 mL per day
(E) ensure daily intake of at least 100 g of carbohydrate

284. Which of the following case histories would most likely be associated with the urinary sediment depicted?

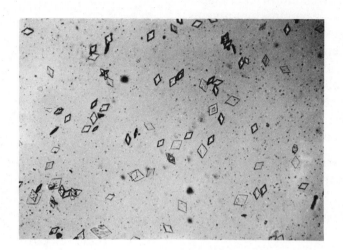

(A) A 23-year-old man with newly diagnosed lymphoblastic lymphoma who is found to have a rising creatinine level 2 days after the administration of combination chemotherapy
(B) A 23-year-old woman 1 year after surgery performed because of morbid obesity
(C) A 45-year-old woman with a history of multiple urinary tract infections with urea-splitting organisms
(D) A 40-year-old man with edema, hypoalbuminemia, and proteinuria
(E) An 18-year-old man with flank pain, hematuria, and a positive family history for renal stones in youth

285. Which of the following is the mechanism of hypocalcemia during acute renal failure?

(A) Hyperphosphatemia
(B) Failure of parathyroid hormone release
(C) Metabolic acidosis
(D) Tubular calcium losses
(E) Hypermagnesemia

286. A 55-year-old man with end-stage renal disease is undergoing his first hemodialysis treatment. Part way through the session he develops confusion, followed by a generalized seizure. The most likely reason for this complication is

(A) induction of hypotension
(B) rapid osmolality flux
(C) hypocalcemia
(D) complement activation
(E) rapid change in pH

287. The condition of a 50-year-old obese woman with a 5-year history of mild hypertension controlled with a thiazide diuretic is being evaluated because proteinuria was noted on her routine yearly medical visit. Physical examination disclosed a height of 167.6 cm (66 in); weight 91 kg (202 lb); blood pressure 130/80 mmHg; and trace pedal edema. Laboratory values are as follows:

Serum creatinine: 106 μmol/L (1.2 mg/dL)
BUN: 6.4 mmol/L (18 mg/dL)
Creatinine clearance: 87 mL/min
Urinalysis: pH 5.0; specific gravity 1.018; protein 3+ ; no glucose; occasional coarse granular cast
Urine protein excretion: 5.9 g/d

The results of a renal biopsy are shown below. Sixty percent of the glomeruli appeared as shown (by light microscopy); the remainder were unremarkable.

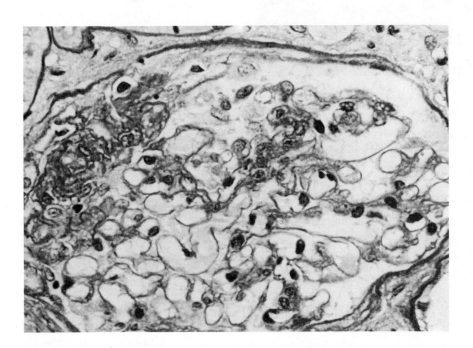

The most likely diagnosis is

(A) hypertensive nephrosclerosis
(B) focal and segmental sclerosis
(C) minimal-change (nil) disease
(D) membranous glomerulopathy
(E) crescentic glomerulonephritis

288. In a person who has carcinoma of the lung and the depicted urinalysis, renal biopsy would most likely show

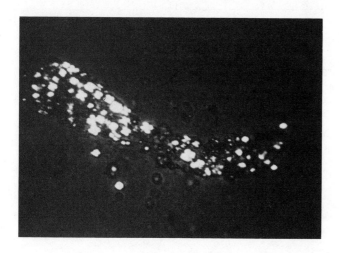

    (A) minimal-change disease
    (B) diffuse proliferative glomerulonephritis
    (C) membranoproliferative glomerulonephritis
    (D) membranous glomerulopathy
    (E) focal glomerulosclerosis

289. Management of renal allograft recipients now includes the more frequent use of cyclosporine compared with azathioprine. This change in immunosuppressant therapy has resulted in

    (A) equivalence between living related donor transplants and cadaveric donor transplants in terms of rate of long-term kidney survival
    (B) an improvement in the survival of living related donor grafts at 1 year
    (C) an equivalence in the allograft survival rates at 1 year in cadaveric donors and living related donors
    (D) a 95 percent 1-year graft survival rate with cadaveric renal allografts
    (E) a marked increase in the rate of death due to hepatic failure

290. A 23-year-old man has recurrent episodes of hematuria over the past year. Each of the episodes seems to be associated with an upper respiratory infection. Physical examination currently is normal. Urinalysis reveals a relatively bland sediment; dipstick is positive for both protein and blood. Renal biopsy would reveal

    (A) extensive extracapillary proliferation on light microscopy
    (B) diffuse mesangeal proliferation on light microscopy
    (C) diffuse capillary deposition of IgG on immunofluorescence
    (D) diffuse mesangeal deposition of IgA on immunofluorescence
    (E) deposition of C3 in capillary walls on immunofluorescence

291. A 19-year-old U.S. Marine, who has had a feeling of malaise for a few hours, begins passing coffee-colored urine. During the next 2 days pedal edema develops. Urinalysis reveals 4+ hematuria, 3+ proteinuria, and a sediment containing many red-cell and white-cell casts. Serum testing shows that the BUN level is 14 mmol/L (40 mg/dL) and creatinine concentration is 350 μmol/L (4.0 mg/dL). Renal biopsy reveals diffuse endocapillary proliferative lesions with infiltration of glomeruli by polymorphonuclear leukocytes. All the following conditions could produce this clinical picture EXCEPT

    (A) infectious mononucleosis
    (B) streptococcal infection
    (C) heroin abuse
    (D) acute viral hepatitis
    (E) falciparum malaria

292. All the following represent potential complications of chronic hemodialysis EXCEPT

    (A) autonomic neuropathy
    (B) cerebral vascular accidents
    (C) osteomalacia
    (D) gastrointestinal bleeding
    (E) dementia

293. A 19-year-old man with nephrotic syndrome on the basis of membranous glomerulonephritis is receiving corticosteroids. He now presents with flank pain and swelling of his left testicle. Which of the following would be the best study to confirm the likely diagnosis?

(A) Ultrasonography
(B) Angiography
(C) Renal biopsy
(D) Computed tomography of the abdomen
(E) Renal scan (nuclear medicine)

294. A 72-year-old woman with rheumatic heart disease is being treated with ampicillin and gentamicin for enterococcal endocarditis. One week into her course she develops a morbilliform skin rash and fever. Laboratory evaluation is remarkable for a doubling of her serum creatinine and blood urea nitrogen from their baseline values. Urinalysis dipstick is positive for blood, protein, and white cells. Ultrasonography reveals bilaterally enlarged kidneys. Based on the available data, the most likely cause of the patient's azotemia is

(A) tubular necrosis due to aminoglycoside
(B) membranous nephropathy due to endocarditis
(C) enterococcal pyelonephritis
(D) cystitis
(E) hypersensitivity reaction to ampicillin

295. A 40-year-old woman who has never had significant respiratory disease is hospitalized for evaluation of hemoptysis. Urinalysis reveals 2+ proteinuria and microscopic hematuria. BUN concentration is 7.1 mmol/L (20 mg/dL), and serum creatinine concentration is 177 µmol/L (2.0 mg/dL). Serologic findings include normal complement levels and a negative assay for fluorescent antinuclear antibodies. Renal biopsy reveals granulomatous necrotizing vasculitis with scattered immunoglobulin and complement deposits. The most likely diagnosis in this case is

(A) mesangial lupus glomerulonephritis
(B) Henoch-Schönlein purpura
(C) microscopic polyarteritis
(D) Wegener's granulomatosis
(E) Goodpasture's syndrome

296. Which of the following patients is LEAST likely to develop destruction of renal papillae with concomitant tubulointerstitial damage?

(A) A middle-aged man who has consumed "moonshine" alcohol distilled in automobile radiators
(B) An older man with repetitive episodes of acute urinary retention due to prostatic hypertrophy
(C) A young adult woman with sickle cell anemia
(D) An older woman who uses analgesics for chronic headaches
(E) A middle-aged woman with a history of multiple urinary tract infections associated with pyuria, flank pain, fever, and poor response to short courses of oral antibiotics

297. A 45-year-old woman with long-standing systemic lupus erythematosus who has had intermittent bouts of acute renal failure over the last 6 years now presents with anorexia. Physical examination is noncontributory. Laboratory evaluation includes hematocrit 29 percent, white count 5000 with a normal differential, and platelet count 27,500/μL. The following values are also found:

Serum electrolytes (mmol/L): Na$^+$ 136, K$^+$ 6, Cl$^-$ 90, HCO$_3^-$ 20
BUN: 35.5 mmol/L (100 mg/dL)
Serum creatinine: 665 μmol/L (7.5 mg/dL)

Anti-double-strand DNA and C3 levels have been stable. Renal biopsy shows obliterative sclerosing glomerular lesions. The most appropriate management strategy would be

(A) high-dose intravenous methylprednisolone
(B) high-dose intravenous methylprednisolone and azathioprine
(C) high-dose intravenous methylprednisolone and intravenous cyclophosphamide (500 mg/m^2)
(D) intravenous cyclophosphamide (500 mg/m^2) plus low-dose prednisone
(E) dialysis

298. A patient being examined for acute renal failure has a urine sodium concentration of 15 mmol/L and a urine osmolality of 510 mosmol/kg. These findings might be consistent with all the following conditions EXCEPT

(A) acute poststreptococcal glomerulonephritis
(B) acute partial urinary obstruction
(C) cholesterol embolization of the kidneys
(D) rhabdomyolysis
(E) cirrhosis of the liver with ascites

299. A 30-year-old woman with diabetic nephropathy received a cadaveric renal allograft. On the third postoperative day her serum creatinine concentration was 160 μmol/L (1.8 mg/dL). She is being treated with cyclosporine and prednisone. On the sixth postoperative day she experiences a decrease in urine output from 1500 mL/d to 1000 mL/d; the serum creatinine concentration increases to 194 μmol/L (2.2 mg/dL). Her blood pressure remains stable at 170/90 mmHg and her temperature is 37.2°C (99°F). The best initial step in management would be to

(A) decrease the dose of cyclosporine
(B) obtain ultrasonography of the renal allograft
(C) obtain a biopsy of the renal allograft
(D) administer pulsed steroid therapy
(E) administer an intravenous bolus of furosemide

300. A 55-year-old man undergoes intravenous pyelography (IVP) as part of a workup for hypertension. A solitary radiolucent mass, 3 cm in size, is noted in the left kidney; the study otherwise is normal. The man complains of no symptoms referable to the urinary tract, and examination of urinary sediment is within normal limits. Which of the following studies should be performed next?

(A) Repeat intravenous pyelography in 6 months
(B) Early-morning urine collections for cytology (three samples)
(C) Selective renal arteriography
(D) Renal ultrasonography
(E) CT scanning (with contrast enhancement) of the left kidney

301. Risk factors for carcinoma of the bladder include all the following EXCEPT

  (A)   exposure to cigarette smoke
  (B)   use of cyclophosphamide
  (C)   exposure to dyes
  (D)   positive family history
  (E)   schistosomal infestation

302. A 10-year-old girl complaining of profound weakness, occasional difficulty walking, and polyuria is brought to her pediatrician. Her mother is sure her daughter has not been vomiting frequently. The girl takes no medicines. She is normotensive and no focal neurologic abnormalities are found. Serum chemistries include sodium 142 mmol/L; potassium 2.5 mmol/L; bicarbonate 32 mmol/L; chloride 100 mmol/L. A 24-h urine collection on a normal diet reveals sodium 200 mmol/d, potassium 50 mmol/d, and chloride 30 mmol/d. A stool phenolphthalein test and urine screen for diuretics are negative. Plasma renin levels are found to be elevated. Which of the following conditions is most consistent with the above data?

  (A)   Conn's syndrome
  (B)   Chronic ingestion of licorice
  (C)   Bartter's syndrome
  (D)   Wilms's tumor
  (E)   Proximal renal tubular acidosis

303. A previously healthy 55-year-old man presents with confusion that began 2 days ago. Serum values (in mmol/L) include Na$^+$ 120, K$^+$ 4.0, Cl$^-$ 90, and HCO$_3^-$ 23. The patient is not edematous. Which of the following conditions is LEAST likely to explain the preceding information?

  (A)   Subdural hematoma
  (B)   Occult alcoholism with hepatic cirrhosis
  (C)   Lung cancer
  (D)   Addison's disease
  (E)   Hypothyroidism

304. A previously healthy 45-year-old man who developed weight gain, fatigue, and vomiting within the past week presents to his physician. He had been seen 3 months earlier for a routine check-up, at which time a physical examination, complete blood count, and serum chemistries were all normal. Relevant physical findings now include a blood pressure of 155/110 mmHg and periorbital edema. Serum studies reveal a BUN of 30 mmol/L (85 mg/dL) and a creatinine of 796 μmol/L (9 mg/dL). Urinalysis reveals 2+ proteinuria and the sediment findings depicted below. Which of the following statements is LEAST likely to be correct?

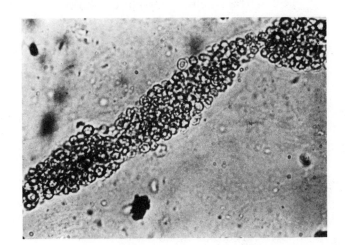

  (A)   Renal biopsy is indicated
  (B)   Poststreptococcal glomerulonephritis is an important diagnostic consideration
  (C)   Extracapillary proliferation is probable
  (D)   Spontaneous resolution of the renal disease is likely
  (E)   A trial of high-dose glucocorticoids is indicated

DIRECTIONS: Each question below contains five suggested responses. For **each** of the five responses listed with each item, you are to respond either YES (Y) or NO (N). In a given item **all, some, or none** of the alternatives may be correct.

305. A 43-year-old construction worker is noted to be anuric following a crush injury to the lower extremities. Serum electrolytes (mmol/L) obtained 8 h following admission are Na^+ 138, K^+ 8.8, Cl^- 100, and HCO_3^- 19. Electrocardiography reveals peaked T waves, prolongation of the PR interval, and widening of the QRS complex. Which of the following measures would rapidly lower serum potassium concentration in the man described?

    (A) Intravenous infusion of 10 mL of a 10% calcium gluconate solution
    (B) Intravenous infusion of 10 mL of a 10% magnesium sulfate solution
    (C) Intravenous infusion of 50 mL of a 50% glucose solution with 10 units of regular insulin
    (D) Intravenous infusion of 2 ampules of sodium bicarbonate
    (E) Administration by nasogastric tube of 60 mL of a potassium-binding resin

306. Rhabdomyolysis or acute myoglobinuric renal failure can develop as a result of

    (A) strenuous muscular exercise
    (B) cocaine overdose
    (C) ethanol ingestion
    (D) hypokalemia
    (E) volume depletion

307. Patients in whom the mechanism leading to their urinary incontinence puts them at risk for hydronephrosis include those with

    (A) Alzheimer's dementia
    (B) Guillain-Barré syndrome
    (C) normal pressure hydrocephalus
    (D) diabetes mellitus
    (E) hypothyroidism

308. Metabolic abnormalities associated with the nephrotic syndrome include

    (A) increased serum lipid levels
    (B) increased serum thyroxine levels
    (C) reduced serum calcium levels
    (D) reduced serum zinc levels
    (E) increased serum antithrombin III (heparin cofactor) levels

309. True statements about acute poststreptococcal glomerulonephritis (PSGN) include which of the following?

    (A) The latent period appears to be longer when PSGN is associated with cutaneous rather than with pharyngeal infections
    (B) Serologic evidence of a streptococcal infection may not be forthcoming if antimicrobial therapy is begun early
    (C) Antimicrobial therapy for streptococcal infection is without value once the presence of renal disease is established
    (D) Long-term antistreptococcal prophylaxis is indicated following documented cases of PSGN
    (E) Lasting and progressive deterioration in renal function is more common in adults than in children with PSGN

310. The inheritance of a tendency to develop adult polycystic kidney disease is correctly described by which of the following?

    (A) A mutation on the short arm of chromosome 16 has been linked to the disease
    (B) A polymorphic locus near the alpha-globin gene cluster has been linked to the disease
    (C) Most cases are due to new mutations
    (D) Adult polycystic kidney disease displays autosomal recessive inheritance
    (E) A person found to be homozygous at the polymorphic locus linked to the disease cannot be analyzed for predisposition to the disease

311. Which of the following patients could be appropriately matched with the urine sediment depicted?

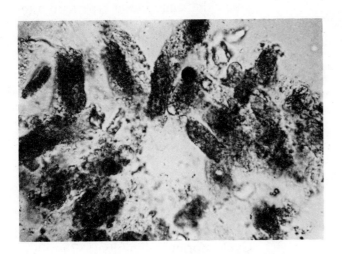

(A) A 75-year-old man 1 day after complicated surgery for the repair of an abdominal aortic aneurysm

(B) A 75-year-old man with a porcine aortic valve prosthesis, malaise, fever, and positive blood cultures

(C) A 50-year-old man with a history of chronic alcoholism who presents with stupor and a history of having been found on the street with multiple bruises

(D) A 75-year-old man with known benign prostatic hypertrophy and inability to void who presents with an enlarged bladder and a creatinine level of 220 μmol/L (2.5 mg/dL)

(E) A 35-year-old woman with idiopathic dilated cardiomyopathy and an ejection fraction of 15 percent who is awaiting cardiac transplantation

312. A 45-year-old black woman on chronic hemodialysis for renal failure due to uncontrolled hypertension has a hematocrit of 22 percent with a mean red cell volume (MCV) of 89. Correct statements about her condition include which of the following?

(A) A trial of erythropoietin is unlikely to improve her hematocrit because erythropoiesis is relatively unresponsive to this hormone in the face of chronic uremia

(B) The patient may be experiencing chronic blood loss because of the use of heparin with dialysis or the abnormal hemostasis associated with chronic renal failure

(C) Folic acid deficiency is possible, even though the anemia is normocytic

(D) Multiple blood transfusions could lead to direct heart damage

(E) If the patient requires surgery, vasopressin or cryoprecipitate could be used to ameliorate the bleeding tendency

313. A 48-year-old woman is hospitalized for elective knee surgery. Routine preoperative laboratory evaluation reveals the following:

Serum electrolytes (mmol/L): Na^+ 138; K^+ 3.5; Cl^- 110; HCO_3^- 20
Blood glucose: 5.2 mmol/L (95 mg/dL)
Serum creatinine: 160 μmol/L (1.8 mg/dL)
BUN: 7.1 mmol/L (20 mg/dL)
Urinalysis: pH 5.2; specific gravity 1.005; protein 1+; glucose 2+; 3 to 5 white blood cells per high-power field

This woman says she voids several times during the night but is unaware of any problem with her kidneys. Disorders associated with the findings in this case would include

(A) multiple myeloma
(B) diabetic nephropathy
(C) Sjögren's syndrome
(D) penicillamine-induced nephropathy
(E) analgesic abuse

314. A 45-year-old woman presents with her third episode of nephrolithiasis. Laboratory studies disclose the following:

Serum electrolytes (mmol/L): Na^+ 134; K^+ 2.5; Cl^- 106; HCO_3^- 18

Serum chemistries: creatinine 97 μmol/L (1.1 mg/dL); calcium 2.4 mmol/L (9.5 mg/dL); albumin 40 g/L (4.0 g/dL)

Arterial blood gas values: P_{CO_2} 4 kPa (30 mmHg); P_{O_2} 14 kPa (108 mmHg); pH 7.30

Urine pH: 7.2

A plain film of the abdomen is shown below. Correct statements about this clinical picture include which of the following?

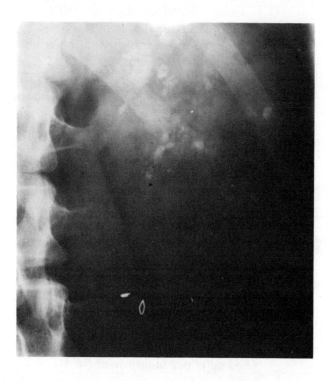

(A) The findings are consistent with the presence of multiple myeloma

(B) The findings are consistent with the presence of medullary sponge kidney

(C) There is evidence for type I distal renal tubular acidosis (RTA)

(D) Family members should be screened for electrolyte disorders

(E) Intravenous pyelography would provide further useful information

315. Correct statements regarding renal allografting include which of the following?

(A) A potential living donor that does not share the same blood type as the recipient cannot be considered even if the tissue types are HLA-identical

(B) The degree of HLA mismatch with cadaveric donor kidneys is a determinant of long-term graft survival

(C) Progressive renal failure in a transplant recipient, termed *chronic rejection,* is associated with renal vascular damage

(D) Allopurinol must be coadministered with azathioprine to prevent urate nephropathy associated with drug-induced cell turnover

(E) Cyclosporine A inhibits IL-2 production by helper T cells

316. A 42-year-old man with a history of hypertension presents to the emergency room with his third episode of severe right flank pain over the past 5 years. Correct statements include which of the following?

(A) It is likely that a scout film of the abdomen will be positive

(B) If the pain is due to a renal stone and does not remit, direct removal will be necessary

(C) The patient should be asked about a history of bowel surgery

(D) After resolution of the acute episode, urine calcium, creatinine, uric acid, citrate, and oxalate should be measured

(E) If the patient is found to have calcium stones, thiazide diuretics should be avoided

DIRECTIONS: The group of questions below consists of lettered headings followed by a set of numbered items. For each numbered item select the **one** lettered heading with which it is **most** closely associated. Each lettered heading may be used **once, more than once, or not at all.**

Questions 317–319

For each case history that follows, select the set of laboratory values with which it is most likely to be associated.

| | Na^+ | K^+ | Cl^- | HCO_3^- | Serum Creatinine | pH | |
| | | | | | (μmol/L [mg/dL]) | | |
	(Serum, mmol/L)					Arterial blood	Urine
(A)	143	4.8	100	10	265 (3.0)	7.25	5.0
(B)	135	4.5	107	21	265 (3.0)	7.37	5.0
(C)	140	2.5	114	14	265 (3.0)	7.30	6.2
(D)	139	5.1	104	21	265 (3.0)	7.37	5.0
(E)	139	6.3	108	19	265 (3.0)	7.35	5.0

317. A 28-year-old man, comatose, is believed to have been drinking ethylene glycol

318. A 48-year-old woman has been given amphotericin B for treatment of disseminated coccidioidomycosis

319. A 19-year-old man is recovering from acute poststreptococcal glomerulonephritis

Disorders of the Kidney and Urinary Tract

Answers

272. The answer is E. *(Chap 44.)* Up to 150 mg/day of protein may be excreted by normal persons. The bulk of this normal daily excretion is made up of the Tamm-Horsfall mucoprotein. Urine dipsticks may register a trace result in response to as little as 50 mg protein per liter and are definitively positive once the urine protein exceeds 300 mg/L. A false negative may occur if the proteinuria is due to immunoglobulins, which are positively charged. If proteinuria is suspected or documented, a 24-h urine collection should be undertaken to measure the absolute protein excretion. Urine immunoelectrophoresis may also identify which particular immunoglobulin is produced in excess.

273. The answer is E. *(Chap 45.)* Due to the powerful effect of ADH secretion in the setting of hypertonicity, severe persistent hypernatremia is only possible in patients who cannot respond to thirst by ingestion of water. A nursing home patient with a fever may lose significant amounts of body fluid, which could result in dangerous levels of hypernatremia. Manifestations of hypernatremia include central nervous system dysfunction such as neuromuscular irritability, seizures, obtundation, or coma. Calculation of water replacement needs is based on total body water, since water loss occurs from both intracellular and extracellular sites. In this case, a 60-kg woman has a plasma sodium of 160 mmol/L, which one would like to lower to 140 mmol/L. Total body water is 60 percent of weight (36 L). To reduce the plasma sodium, this volume must be increased to 160/140 times 36 L, or about 41 L. Thus, a positive water balance of 5 L (41 − 36) is needed. This deficit is best corrected fairly slowly with the aim to replace about half the water deficit in the first day. If correction is done in this conservative fashion, progressive central nervous system dysfunction is not likely. If the patient had signs of circulatory collapse indicating an associated sodium deficiency, then treatment would begin with normal saline to provide intracellular volume. In certain situations, such as hyperosmolar diabetic coma, the plasma osmolarity is elevated due to hyperglycemia as well as hypernatremia. Therefore, initial treatment should consist of normal saline to ensure circulatory integrity and insulin to lower plasma glucose and partially reduce intracellular osmolarity. Finally, half normal saline could be used to slowly replace the remaining water and salt deficits.

274. The answer is A. *(Chaps 44, 333.)* Failure to concentrate urine despite substantial hypertonic dehydration suggests a diagnosis of diabetes insipidus. A nephrogenic origin would be postulated if there is no increase in urine concentration after exogenous vasopressin. The only useful mode of therapy is a low-salt diet and use of a thiazide diuretic agent. The resultant volume contraction presumably enhances proximal reabsorption and thereby reduces urine flow.

275. The answer is E.   *(Chaps 44, 335.)*   This man's electrolyte pattern is consistent with the "syndrome of hyporeninemic hypoaldosteronism," or type IV renal tubular acidosis. The defect is believed to be due to an insufficiency of both angiotensin (because of impaired renin release) and adrenal mineralocorticoid secreting capacity. Inhibition of the renin-angiotensin system by nonsteroidal anti-inflammatory agents, converting enzyme inhibitors, and beta-adrenergic blockade can contribute to hyperkalemia. Beta blockade can also interfere with intracellular potassium uptake. Potassium can leak out of cells owing to the digitalis-induced poisoning of the Na, K-ATPase. Use of carbenicillin can lead to hypokalemia since this drug acts as an unresorbed anion, thereby promoting the potassium loss associated with distal tubular secretion.

276. The answer is B.   *(Chap 45.)*   The differential diagnosis of hyponatremia depends on exclusion of artifactual causes followed by an assessment of volume status. Artifactual hyponatremia can occur in the setting of hyperlipidemia (where a portion of any volume of plasma taken for analysis will be sodium-free lipid) or extreme hyperproteinemia (plasma proteins occupy more than the normal 7 percent of plasma volume) as in multiple myeloma. In these cases plasma osmolality should not be depressed. Actually, modern sodium-selective electrodes eliminate artifactual hyponatremia by measuring the sodium concentration in plasma volume only, not total plasma volume.

In diabetes with very high blood sugars, plasma osmolality may actually be increased in the face of significant hyponatremia. Plasma sodium can become diluted by the movement of water outside cells in the presence of any osmotically active solute. For every elevation of 5.5 mmol/L (100 mg/dL) of plasma glucose, plasma sodium will decrease by 1.6 mmol/L.

In congestive heart failure or any edema-forming state in which the "effective" arterial blood volume is depressed, hyponatremia may ensue. This situation is generally accompanied by alkalosis and hypokalemia because mineralocorticoid secretion is high. On the other hand, acidosis and hyperkalemia would be associated with the hyponatremia of Addison's disease (adrenal insufficiency) with insufficient aldosterone present to cause the distal tubular reabsorption of sodium bicarbonate and the concomitant extrusion of potassium chloride.

The inappropriate secretion of vasopressin, or ADH (SIADH), may occur in multiple settings including head trauma, drug use (vincristine, narcotics), pain, or bacterial meningitis. Vasopressin has little effect on the renal excretion of potassium and hydrogen ions. Patients with SIADH must be euvolemic. Thus, hyponatremia in this setting is usually not accompanied by changes in concentrations of BUN or creatinine (if anything, they are low-normal), potassium, or bicarbonate.

277. The answer is B.   *(Chap 45.)*   In the hypokalemic patient who is also hypertensive, important diagnostic considerations include high-renin states such as a renin-secreting tumor or low-renin, high-aldosterone states such as licorice ingestion or frank hyperaldosteronism. The patient in question, however, is normotensive and is excreting a relatively minimal amount of potassium. Gastrointestinal losses of potassium, such as in the case of colonic-mediated diarrhea, would be associated with low urinary potassium excretion; because of the induced alkalosis, the serum bicarbonate would be high. In diuretic excess, alkalosis also occurs but urinary potassium excretion is high. Renal tubular acidosis and Bartter's syndrome are also characterized by elevated potassium excretion.

278. **The answer is B.**   *(Chap 46. Wrenn, Am J Med 91:119, 1991.)*   A reasonable way to approach the diagnosis of metabolic acidosis is to separate patients into those with an increased anion gap and those with a normal anion gap (hyperchloremic acidosis). A calculation of these unmeasured anions is the sum of plasma bicarbonate and chloride minus the plasma sodium concentration (the normal value is 8 to 16 mmol/L). Reasons for increased acid production include diabetic ketoacidosis, alcoholic ketoacidosis (as in the patient in this question), starvation, lactic acidosis due to circulatory failure, certain drugs and toxins, and poisoning due to salicylates, ethylene glycol, or methanol. Finally, renal failure increases the anion gap because sulfate, phosphate, and organic acid ions are not excreted normally. Normal anion gap acidosis is due to renal tubular dysfunction or colonic losses. Since the ratio of beta-hydroxybutyrate to acetoacetate is high in alcoholic ketoacidosis, ketonemia can be missed by the routinely employed nitroprusside (Acetest) reagent, which detects acetoacetate but not beta-hydroxybutyrate. Patients suffering from alcoholic ketoacidosis do well with infusions of glucose and saline. Neither insulin nor alkali is required in these situations unless the acidosis is extreme (bicarbonate less than 6 to 8 mmol/L).

279. **The answer is D.**   *(Chap 237.)*   Development of advancing peripheral neuropathy is an indication for dialysis. Delaying dialysis could allow development of irreversible motor deficits, such as foot drop. Prompt institution of dialysis, on the other hand, usually prevents progression of uremic peripheral neuropathy and may ameliorate early sensory defects. No pharmacologic agent would be of significant benefit in the clinical situation described.

280. **The answer is D.**   *(Chap 237.)*   Impaired renal production of 1,25-dihydroxyvitamin D_3 leads to decreased calcium absorption from the gut. Impaired renal phosphate excretion contributes to increased calcium entry into bone. The resultant decreased serum calcium concentration leads to secondary hyperparathyroidism. Chronic metabolic acidosis leads to dissolution of bone buffers and decalcification. Aluminum administered in long-term therapy, although useful in controlling hyperphosphatemia and thereby hypocalcemia, can be taken up by bone and contribute to altered bone matrix. There is *no* significant loss of vitamin D or calcium associated with presently employed dialysis techniques.

281. **The answer is A.**   *(Chap 46.)*   In order to offer optimal management to patients with acute renal failure, it is helpful to distinguish prerenal azotemia (generally managed with volume replacement or amelioration of cardiac dysfunction) from intrinsic renal dysfunction. Sodium reabsorption, quite avid in the case of prerenal azotemia, is impaired in intrinsic renal disease. On the other hand, creatinine is reabsorbed less efficiently than sodium in both conditions. Therefore, the fractional excretion of sodium is very helpful in distinguishing between these two etiologies of renal failure. The fractional excretion of sodium is calculated by multiplying the urine sodium times the plasma creatinine, dividing this by the plasma sodium times the urine creatinine, and multiplying by 100. In this case the result is approximately 1.4, which suggests that impaired reabsorption of sodium is ongoing and that intrinsic renal failure is occurring. Only about 15 percent of patients receiving nephrotoxins such as aminoglycosides or radiocontrast agents have renal failure associated with a fractional excretion of sodium of less than 1 percent, so an elevated value in this case points in the direction of nephrotoxic injury. The other causes of acute renal failure listed will all be associated with prerenal azotemia and therefore with a more avid reabsorption of sodium than described.

282. **The answer is C.**   *(Chap 236.)*   Many drugs can produce acute renal failure. Aminoglycosides, for example, appear to disrupt membrane phospholipids in tubular cells. Cisplatin injures mitochondria and mediates free radical injury in tubular membranes. Cyclosporine and radiocontrast agents appear to provoke intrarenal vascular constriction, thereby leading to epithelial cell ischemic injury. Factors that might promote prerenal azotemia such as hypovolemia, concomitant exposure to other toxins, use of drugs such as nonsteroidal anti-inflammatory agents or angiotensin-converting enzyme inhibitors that disrupt normal renovascular dilation can promote renal injury due to cyclosporine.

283. The answer is C. *(Chap 236.)* The management of oliguric acute renal failure is largely conservative, although some clinicians believe that early dialysis and hyperalimentation lessen morbidity and speed recovery. Fluid intake should match output plus estimated insensible losses; food intake should be encouraged to lessen tissue catabolism. Continuous drainage by Foley catheter should not be routinely employed because it increases the risk of infection; however, if supervening bladder outlet obstruction is suspected, recatheterization should be considered. Reduction of high serum phosphate levels usually is recommended to reduce the risk of soft-tissue calcification. Reduction of high uric acid levels, however, is unnecessary, both because symptomatic gout is very unusual in persons with oliguric renal failure and because there is no evidence that kidneys are damaged by hyperuricemia that develops after an acute reduction in the glomerular filtration rate.

284. The answer is A. *(Chaps 242, 245.)* Cystine crystals appear as flat hexagonal plates and are found in association with cystine stones, which are caused by a hereditary deficiency in tubular cystine transport. Struvite stones result from chronic urinary tract infection with *Proteus* species. These bacteria degrade urea to carbon dioxide and ammonia, which alkalinizes the urine, thereby favoring the formation of the insoluble triple salt $MgNH_4PO_4$. Struvite crystals can appear in the urine as rectangular prisms. Patients with proteinuria due to albuminuria exhibit a sediment characteristic of the nephrotic syndrome with oval fat bodies. Patients with intestinal malabsorption with concomitant steatorrhea, such as in the case of a jejunoileal bypass done for obesity, may hyperabsorb oxalate and form calcium oxalate renal stones. Calcium oxalate crystals appear bipyramidal or as biconcave ovals. The sediment depicted here displays flat, square plates, which represent one of the several forms uric acid crystals may manifest. Hyperuricemia may accompany rapid cell turnover (as occurs in the rapid lysis of lymphomas with large tumor burdens after chemotherapy). In such settings aggressive hydration, the use of allopurinol, and urinary alkalinization may be effective prophylaxis against uric acid nephropathy.

285. The answer is A. *(Chap 236.)* High levels of serum phosphate are very common in acute renal failure. Not only is phosphate excretion impaired, the severe catabolic state that often accompanies acute renal failure, especially if due to rhabdomyolysis or tumor lysis, promotes the hyperphosphatemia. Deposition of calcium phosphate in the setting of high phosphate concentrations can lead to hypocalcemia. Tissue resistance (bone and kidney) to the actions of parathyroid hormone and reduced levels of 1,25-dihydroxyvitamin D also contribute. However, the hypocalcemia associated with acute renal failure rarely requires treatment because the effects of acidosis counterbalance the neuromuscular excitability brought on by hypocalcemia. Patients who do develop the symptoms of hypocalcemia, such as seizures, hallucinations, or prolongation of the QT interval on the electrocardiogram, can be treated with calcium carbonate or calcium gluconate infusions. The treatment of the acidosis associated with acute renal failure with bicarbonate can exacerbate the neuromuscular side effects of hypocalcemia and therefore should be used with caution.

286. The answer is B. *(Chap 238.)* Probably the most common complication of chronic hemodialysis arises from the need for access to the circulation. Arteriovenous fistulas allow such access, but infection, thrombosis, and aneurysms may complicate these connections, particularly if a prosthetic vascular channel has been used. Hypotension may occur during dialysis owing to removal of excess fluid, concomitant use of antihypertensive drugs, or infusion of acetate, which is a cardiac depressant, in the dialysate. Potassium fluxes may lead to cardiac arrhythmias. Dialysis membranes can induce complement-mediated leukopenia and hypoxemia. The rapid flux in serum osmolality can cause a dialysis disequilibrium syndrome manifested by confusion, alterations in consciousness, and seizures. Nonetheless, hemodialysis may have less of an effect on a person's life-style than peritoneal dialysis because of the relatively short treatment time and minimal interruption between treatments. Hemodialysis is also a more efficient way to remove toxins than is peritoneal dialysis.

287. The answer is B.   *(Chap 240.)*   The characteristic pattern of focal (not all glomeruli) and segmental (not the entire glomerulus) glomerular scarring is shown. The history and laboratory features are also consistent with this lesion, i.e., some associated hypertension, diminution in creatinine clearance, and a relatively inactive urine sediment. The "nephropathy of obesity" may be associated with this lesion secondary to hyperfiltration. Hypertensive nephrosclerosis exhibits more prominent vascular changes and patchy, ischemic, totally sclerosed glomeruli. In addition, nephrosclerosis seldom is associated with nephrotic-range proteinuria. Minimal-change disease is usually associated with symptomatic edema and normal-appearing glomeruli as demonstrated by light microscopy. This patient's presentation is consistent with that of membranous nephropathy but the biopsy is not. With membranous glomerular nephritis all glomeruli are uniformly involved with subepithelial dense deposits. There are no features of crescentic glomerulonephritis present.

288. The answer is D.   *(Chap 240.)*   Persons who have solid tumors and develop nephrotic syndrome usually have membranous glomerulopathy. Diagnosis of the nephrotic syndrome may precede the recognition of the primary tumor. In several cases, tumor antigens have been discovered in the glomerular deposits; the nephrotic syndrome may remit following effective tumor therapy. Patients with Hodgkin's disease may develop nephrotic syndrome on the basis of minimal-change disease (diffuse epithelial foot process effacement on ultrastructural examination).

289. The answer is C.   *(Chap 238.)*   It has been previously assumed that renal allografts from living related donors survived longer than grafts from cadaveric donors. However, in most current series in which cyclosporine is used in the immunosuppressive regimen, the 1-year graft survival rate of 80 percent is identical in transplants from cadaveric and haploidentical living related donors. Unfortunately, whether azathioprine or cyclosporine is used, the median time to graft failure is approximately 25 years with HLA-identical donors, 11 years with haploidentical donors, and 8 years with cadaveric donors. The toxic effects of cyclosporine include nephrotoxicity, hepatotoxicity, hirsutism, tremor, and gingival hyperplasia; only nephrotoxicity is commonly a difficult management problem.

290. The answer is D.   *(Chap 240.)*   One of the more common forms of asymptomatic urinary abnormalities is Berger's disease, which may be a cause of recurrent hematuria of glomerular origin. Such episodes of macroscopic hematuria may be associated with minor flulike illnesses or vigorous exercise. Skin rash, arthritis, and abdominal pain are usually absent, which tends to distinguish this entity from Henoch-Schönlein purpura. Occasionally patients develop a nephrotic or nephritic syndrome. Serum IgA levels are increased in about 50 percent of all cases, though serum complement is normal. Renal biopsy in these situations may reveal a spectrum of changes, though diffuse mesangeal proliferation or focal and segmental proliferative glomerulonephritis is most common. The essential feature of Berger's disease is the finding of diffuse mesangeal deposition of IgA on immunofluorescence microscopy. IgG, C3, and propardin, but not C1q or C4, may also be found on this study. Although the disease progresses slowly, about 50 percent of patients develop end-stage renal failure within 25 years of original presentation. There is no evidence that therapy influences the natural history, although glucocorticoids or antibiotics may reduce the frequency of episodic gross hematuria. IgA deposition in the kidney and recurrent renal failure may occur in about 35 percent of those who receive a renal allograft. Fortunately, such recurrent pathologic findings are usually not associated with loss of renal function.

291. The answer is C.   *(Chap 240.)*   The presentation and renal pathology described in the question are typical of acute glomerulonephritis. This syndrome, both when originally described and currently, occurs most often in association with streptococcal infection. Antibodies generated in response to *Streptococcus* are assumed to compose part of the immune deposits seen in damaged glomeruli. More recently, acute glomerulonephritis has been noted in association with a number of other infectious illnesses, which presumably also give rise to immune complexes capable of damaging glomerular capillaries. Heroin abuse is associated with focal and segmental glomerulo-sclerosis (focal sclerosis), not acute glomerulonephritis; proteinuria and a decline in renal function usually are the first signs.

292. The answer is A. *(Chap 238.)* Almost 100,000 Americans require chronic dialysis, with 90 percent receiving hemodialysis. Long-term complications of hemodialysis include dialysis dementia and osteomalacia, which is believed to be secondary to the aluminum to which the patient is exposed either in the dialysate or in oral preparations designed to lower serum phosphate. Immunologic derangements and need for transfusions can lead to an increased incidence of hepatitis B and C antigenemia, which in some cases can lead to liver failure or portal hypertension with resultant variceal bleeding. Moreover, the heparin required to maintain access patency also predisposes to bleeding. Fortunately the success of erythropoietin therapy has virtually eliminated anemia and has decreased the need for blood transfusions. The high incidence of heart attack and stroke in dialysis patients is probably due to the prevalence of risk factors in the uremic patients, such as hypertension and hyperlipidemia. Peripheral neuropathy, present in many with chronic renal failure, is a consequence of uremia and represents an indication for the institution of dialytic therapy.

293. The answer is B. *(Chap 240.)* The increased likelihood of thrombotic complications in patients with nephrotic syndrome is believed to be related to deficiencies of the coagulation regulatory proteins antithrombin III, protein C, or protein S, as well as hypofibrinogenemia, impaired fibrinolysis, enhanced platelet aggregation, and hyperlipidemia. Though renal vein thrombosis, suggested by unilateral or bilateral flank or groin pain, gross hematuria, left-sided varicocele, or decreased renal function, was previously thought to be a cause of nephrotic syndrome, it is now thought to be a consequence of this disorder. The most common renal lesions associated with this complication are membranous or membranoproliferative glomerulonephritis and amyloidosis. Selective renal venous angiography will provide the most specific confirmatory test. The therapeutic response to a positive angiogram is usually the administration of systemic anticoagulation, although the precise benefit of this approach has not been defined. A less aggressive approach calls for the use of systemic anticoagulation only in those patients who are found to have a pulmonary embolism. Given the low levels of antithrombin III, heparin may be less effective than in a nonnephrotic situation. The highest risk for renal vein thrombosis is in those patients who have a very low albumin level (less than 20 g/L [2 g/dL]).

294. The answer is E. *(Chap 242.)* A number of drugs may elicit an acute interstitial nephritis. The classic offender is methicillin, although ampicillin, penicillin, cephalothin, thiazides, furosemide, and nonsteroidal anti-inflammatory drugs have also been associated with this problem. Hematuria, fever, and skin rash may occur within 1 to 2 weeks of exposure to the drug. Urinalysis would reveal protein, pyuria, and eosinophiluria. Ultrasonography discloses enlarged kidneys. A biopsy (usually not necessary since withdrawal of the offending drug will lead to complete resolution) would reveal normal glomeruli but infiltration of the interstitium with polymorphonuclear leukocytes, lymphocytes, plasma cells, and eosinophils.

295. The answer is D. *(Chap 241.)* A variety of diseases involve both pulmonary and renal (and, often, also dermal) microvasculature and may present with either prominent pulmonary or renal manifestations. When a firm diagnosis cannot be made serologically or by biopsy of skin or lesions of the upper respiratory tract, renal biopsy may be necessary. In the case described in the question, the serologic findings, though not specific, are typical of Wegener's granulomatosis, a diagnosis established by the renal biopsy report. Granulomas are an uncommon microscopic finding in polyarteritis as well as in lupus nephritis and in Henoch-Schönlein purpura, though a spectrum of pathologic abnormalities may be seen in the latter two conditions. Antineutrophil antibodies in the serum would be highly suggestive of Wegener's and other systemic vasculitides. The renal biopsy in Goodpasture's syndrome usually reveals linear immunoglobulin deposits.

296. The answer is A. *(Chap 242. Bennet, N Engl J Med 320:1269, 1989.)* Patients with damage to renal papillae may be unable to excrete maximally concentrated urine owing to chronic tubular damage. Moreover, the necrosed papillae can lead to the gradual development of renal failure. Although renal papillary necrosis has been classically associated with long-term abuse of analgesics (phenacetin or acetaminophen), such a finding can also be present in those with sickle cell anemia, diabetic nephropathy, or obstructive uropathy (as in the man with prostate disease) or after many episodes of pyelonephritis due to urinary tract infections. Aspirin can potentiate the deleterious effects of chronic analgesic abuse by inhibiting the production of renal vasodilatory prostaglandins. Ingestion of lead, such as that caused by leaching out from an unusual distilling apparatus, can lead to a nephropathy manifested by tubular atrophy and fibrosis of small renal arteries.

297. The answer is E. *(Chap 241.)* The pathophysiology of nephrotoxic involvement by systemic lupus erythematosus (SLE) is thought to be immune complex deposition. Renal disease in SLE can range from mild abnormalities of the urinalysis to a fulminant inflammatory process leading to progressive renal failure. Renal biopsy findings in patients with SLE who have worsening renal function can range from minimal glomerular lesions to diffuse proliferative lupus glomerulonephritis and membranous lupus glomerulonephritis. Patients with membranous lupus glomerulonephritis may be managed conservatively with therapy directed toward extrarenal manifestations. On the other hand, those with more extensive or proliferative glomerular lesions require a more aggressive approach using corticosteroids (with or without another immunosuppressive agent such as azathioprine or cyclophosphamide). However, little is gained by using immunosuppressant therapy in patients with advanced renal failure characterized by obliterative sclerosing lesions of the glomeruli. If such patients have other indications for dialysis such as systemic symptoms or hyperkalemia, they are best managed with dialysis followed by renal transplantation. Measurement of serologic evidence of disease (e.g., double-stranded DNA autoantibodies or a decrease in serum complement components) may be helpful. Patients with end-stage lupus nephritis can actually be managed successfully with hemodialysis. Moreover, patients with SLE who have undergone renal allografting rarely experience recurrence of disease in the new kidney.

298. The answer is D. *(Chap 44.)* Cholesterol embolization of the kidneys and cirrhosis fit clearly into the "prerenal" azotemia category, with a low urine sodium concentration and high urine osmolality. Cholesterol emboli cause "plugging" of renal arterioles and cirrhosis causes hypoalbuminemia, hypovolemia, and possibly a humorally mediated reduction of renal perfusion. However, it is important to recall that other disorders associated with abrupt decline in renal function but with intact tubular integrity, such as acute partial urinary obstruction and acute glomerulonephritis, can also give urinary solute values similar to those in prerenal states if evaluated early in the process. When rhabdomyolysis causes renal damage, it typically produces the picture of acute tubular necrosis, with a urine osmolality less than 400 mosmol/kg and a urinary sodium exceeding 20 mmol/L.

299. The answer is B. *(Chap 238.)* In the first week after renal transplantation, the differential diagnosis of graft dysfunction includes early rejection, hypovolemia, cyclosporine intoxication, acute tubular necrosis, urinary obstruction, and renal artery thrombosis. Cyclosporine can mask many of the classic signs of rejection, such as fever and graft tenderness; renal biopsy is often needed to make the diagnosis. However, renal ultrasonography should precede any manipulation to rule out mechanical outflow obstruction, as it should in any patient with acute deterioration of renal function.

300. The answer is D. *(Chap 247.)* The most important differential diagnosis in the case presented is between a renal cell carcinoma and a benign cystic lesion. Urinalysis may be normal in the presence of renal cell carcinoma, and urinary cytology is unfortunately of little value in the diagnosis of this lesion. Ultrasonography will reveal whether or not the lesion is cystic. If the lesion fulfills the criteria for a simple cyst (i.e., lack of internal echoes, smooth borders, through transmission) and the patient does not have hematuria, the cyst can be considered benign with a diagnostic accuracy of 97 percent. If greater assurance is required or if there are changes on follow-up radiologic studies, then needle aspiration should be carried out. If the ultrasound appearance is not consistent with a simple cyst, then contrast-enhanced CT scanning, the optimal test for diagnosis and staging of renal cell carcinoma, should be performed.

301. The answer is D. *(Chap 247.)* Older men are the most frequent victims of carcinoma of the bladder. Transitional cell carcinoma, the most common histologic subtype of cancer of the bladder in this country, is associated with a more favorable prognosis than is adenocarcinoma or squamous carcinoma. Squamous carcinomas are more frequent in Egypt, where the prevalence of *Schistosoma haematobium* is high. The prognosis in cancer of the bladder is highly linked to the stage of the disease at presentation: muscular or perivascular fat invasion offers a much bleaker outlook (45 percent 5-year survival) than does disease confined to the mucosa. Risk factors for cancer of the bladder include exposure to the aromatic amines (cigarette smoke and products of the dye, rubber, and chemical industries), but not positive family history, as in the case of renal carcinoma. Chronic bladder irritation, such as that produced by the metabolites of cyclophosphamide as well as by recurrent stones or infections, also leads to a higher incidence of carcinoma of the bladder.

302. The answer is C. *(Chaps 45, 244. Narins, Am J Med 72:496, 1982.)* The evaluation of patients with hypokalemia should first include consideration of redistribution of body potassium into cells as occurs in alkalosis, insulin excess, vitamin B_{12} therapy, and periodic paralysis. In the last condition serum bicarbonate is normal. If urinary excretion of potassium is elevated (>20 mmol/d), then the blood pressure should be measured. If the patient is hypertensive and plasma renin is elevated, renovascular hypertension or a renin-secreting tumor (including Wilms's) must be considered and appropriate imaging studies carried out. If plasma renin levels are low, mineralocorticoid effect may be high, either due to endogenous hormone (glucocorticoid overproduction or aldosterone overproduction as in Conn's syndrome) or exogenous agents (licorice or steroids). In the normotensive patient a high serum bicarbonate excludes renal tubular acidosis. A high urine chloride excretion makes gastrointestinal losses less likely and implies primary renal potassium loss as might be seen in diuretic abuse (ruled out by the urine screen) or Bartter's syndrome. In Bartter's syndrome, hyperplasia of the granular cells of the juxtaglomerular apparatus leads to high renin levels and secondary aldosterone elevations. Such hyperplasia appears to be secondary to chronic volume depletion caused by a hereditary (autosomal recessive) defect interfering with salt reabsorption in the thick ascending loop of Henle. Chronic potassium depletion, which frequently initially presents in childhood, leads to polyuria and weakness.

303. The answer is B. *(Chap 45.)* Hepatic cirrhosis associated with hyponatremia almost always would be associated with edema, thereby defining a state of inappropriate water and sodium retention. The differential diagnosis of hypovolemic hyponatremia includes disorders associated with volume depletion in extrarenal or renal (renal failure, diuretic excess, osmotic loads, Addison's disease) losses. In almost all such cases, plasma bicarbonate and potassium tend to be elevated. The differential diagnosis of euvolemic hyponatremia includes syndromes in which vasopressin is secreted inappropriately either by the pituitary (head trauma, meningeal infection, brain disease, drugs, pulmonary disease) or directly by certain tumors (e.g., small cell carcinoma of the lung). The endocrine disorders Addison's disease and hypothyroidism should also be included in the etiology of euvolemic hyponatremia.

304. **The answer is D.** *(Chap 240.)*   The syndrome described is typical of rapidly progressive glomerulonephritis with rapid onset of acute renal failure in the setting of glomerular disease (manifested
by red blood cell casts and proteinuria). The patient's vomiting is consistent with the development
of azotemia over a short time period. Renal biopsy is highly recommended early in the course of
such a disease for the purpose of defining the nature and severity of the glomerular lesion both for
prognostic and therapeutic purposes. The hallmark pathologic lesion associated with this clinical
scenario is that of crescentic glomerulonephritis, the manifestation of extracapillary endothelial
proliferation. Such a finding on renal biopsy carries an ominous prognosis, especially if crescents
are present in more than 70 percent of glomeruli or if the GFR is <5 mL/min. Spontaneous resolution rarely occurs except in those cases associated with an infectious cause, such as endocarditis
or streptococcal disease. Though controlled trials are lacking, it appears that high-dose methylprednisolone given parenterally ("pulse steroids") can stave off the need for hemodialysis in some
patients. Plasmapheresis may also benefit some patients, especially those who have antiglomerular
basement antibodies.

305. **The answer is A-N, B-N, C-Y, D-Y, E-N.** *(Chaps 44, 236. Kupin, Contrib Nephrol 102:1, 1993.)*
Because of a beneficial effect on neuromuscular membranes intravenous calcium infusion is the
correct treatment for the cardiac disturbances caused by hyperkalemia; however, this approach
does not lower serum potassium concentration. Sodium bicarbonate infusion, on the other hand,
lowers serum potassium levels rapidly by causing potassium to move into cells. Intravenous infusion of glucose and insulin achieves the same result though slightly less rapidly. Potassium-binding
resins effectively remove potassium from the body but are slow, particularly when instilled into
the stomach. Persons who are in acute renal failure and have a large potassium load due to severe
muscle damage may require emergency dialysis. Such persons have a profound inability to excrete
magnesium, so the administration of additional magnesium would be dangerous.

306. **The answer is A-Y, B-Y, C-Y, D-Y, E-Y.** *(Chap 236.)*   Muscle cells may be sufficiently taxed
during strenuous exercise (e.g., distance running) to result in cell breakdown and myoglobin release. Muscle breakdown associated with sedative overdose is generally attributed to ischemia
caused by muscle compression in immobile, comatose patients. Muscle ischemia and breakdown
can occur from mechanical compression, vascular insufficiency, or cocaine overdose. Not only can
ethanol ingestion promote muscle breakdown in a similar manner, but also ethanol itself has a
direct toxic effect on muscle. Hypokalemia and hypophosphatemia decrease muscle-cell energy
production and thus increase the risk of rhabdomyolysis in any setting. Volume depletion can
contribute to decreased muscle perfusion and, more importantly, increase the susceptibility of the
kidneys to damage from myoglobin and other muscle breakdown products.

307. **The answer is A-N, B-Y, C-N, D-Y, E-Y.** *(Chap 44. Resnick, N Engl J Med 320:1, 1989.)*   The
force for bladder emptying is provided by the detrusor muscle, which is innervated by parasympathetic outflow from the sacral plexus. The involuntary control that prevents automatic bladder
emptying emanates from sympathetic innervation of the bladder outlet. A sacral spinal reflex arc
mediates automatic detrusor contraction when the intravesical pressure exceeds 20 cmH$_2$O (a volume of 400 mL) unless inhibited by cortical centers via the reticulospinal tracts. Diseases leading
to damage of inhibitory neural pathways in the brain or spinal cord, such as multiple strokes,
Alzheimer's disease, brain tumors, and normal pressure hydrocephalus, create detrusor instability.
In this situation the bladder will empty automatically before it is filled owing to unchecked operation of the spinal reflex arc. On the other hand, conditions leading to chronic overflow incontinence caused by obstruction at the bladder neck or a hypotonic bladder caused by autonomic
neuropathy could result in hydronephrosis and impaired renal function. The most common example
of outflow obstruction is benign prostatic hypertrophy. Examples of conditions in which autonomic

peripheral neuropathy could lead to overflow incontinence include diabetes mellitus, hypothyroidism, uremia, collagen vascular diseases, Guillain-Barré syndrome, and exposure to certain toxins (including alcohol). Cholinergic agents, such as bethanechol, can sometimes aid bladder emptying in those with overflow incontinence.

308. **The answer is A-Y, B-N, C-Y, D-Y, E-N.** *(Chap 240.)* Persons who have nephrotic syndrome may lose a variety of serum proteins other than albumin. Loss of thyroxine-binding globulin leads to reduced serum thyroxine levels, and loss of cholecalciferol-binding protein may combine with a decrease in albumin-bound calcium to reduce serum calcium levels. Loss of antithrombin III, protein C, or protein S as well as hyperfibrinogenemia have all been implicated in hypercoagulability, which affects some persons who have nephrotic syndrome. Hyperlipidemia is associated commonly with nephrotic syndrome; the cause remains uncertain, though it may be that the lowered plasma oncotic pressure stimulates hepatic lipoprotein synthesis. Loss of metal-binding proteins may lead to zinc or copper deficiency.

309. **The answer is A-Y, B-Y, C-N, D-N, E-Y.** *(Chap 240.)* Studies during epidemics of streptococcal disease have shown the latent period between symptomatic pharyngitis and the appearance of poststreptococcal glomerulonephritis (PSGN) to be between 6 and 10 days. The latent period following cutaneous infection is more difficult to establish but appears to be longer. Persons who receive early antimicrobial therapy for streptococcal infection may develop glomerulonephritis but not mount the immune response to streptococcal enzymes (e.g., streptolysin O) on which laboratory testing for antecedent streptococcal infection is based. Antimicrobial therapy is recommended for persons who have acute glomerulonephritis and continuing streptococcal infection. Long-term prophylaxis, however, is unwarranted, because affected persons are not markedly predisposed to recurrent episodes of PSGN. For unknown reasons, PSGN leads to permanent, progressive renal insufficiency more often in adults than in children.

310. **The answer is A-Y, B-Y, C-N, D-N, E-N.** *(Chap 234. Reeders, Nat Genetics 1:235–237, 1992.)* Most patients with adult polycystic kidney disease, an autosomal dominant disorder, are presumed to have a mutation at a locus on the short arm of chromosome 16. This particular locus is close to the gene coding for the alpha-globin chain. A highly polymorphic (genetic variability among individuals; less than 1 percent of the population is homozygous) locus is associated with the alpha-globin gene cluster. Thus, in an individual family with members manifesting the disease, a given polymorphic allele can be shown to be coinherited with the disease. Since such a polymorphism is inherited as a germ line sequence, DNA from any tissue in the body can be extracted, cut with the proper restriction enzyme, electrophoresed, and probed with a radioactive sequence at the polymorphic region. The presence of a fragment of the size previously established to be associated with the disease suggests a predisposition to the disease. If a person lacks the relevant fragment, even if he or she is homozygous at the polymorphism, the likelihood of disease is very low because of the proximity of this locus to the disease-specific gene. The biochemical defect has not yet been identified; patients have an increased incidence of subarachnoid hemorrhage due to berry aneurysms as well as pancreatic and hepatic cysts.

311. **The answer is A-Y, B-N, C-Y, D-N, E-Y.** *(Chap 236.)* The granular casts seen in the photograph are the hallmark of acute tubular necrosis (ATN) (ischemic or nephrotoxic acute renal failure). The most common cause of ATN is prerenal failure. Such an occurrence is not infrequent in major intravascular volume loss of a real or effective nature (burns, trauma, surgery with major blood loss or aortic compromise, severe pancreatitis, pregnancy-related catastrophe, or severe heart failure). A second important cause of ATN is that brought on by agents directly toxic to the tubules. These agents include endogenous pigments such as hemoglobin (released in hemolytic crises) or myoglobin (released in rhabdomyolysis due to any cause, including heat stroke, multiple trauma, severe exercise, or hypokalemia/hypophosphatemia). Certain antibiotics (e.g., aminoglycosides), radiographic contrast, organic solvents, and heavy metals represent examples of direct tubular toxins. The renal disease caused by endocarditis would produce red blood cell casts on urinalysis. Obstructive uropathy, as exemplified by the man with prostatism, would tend to produce few abnormalities in the urinary sediment.

312. **The answer is A-N, B-Y, C-Y, D-Y, E-Y.** *(Chap 237. Eschback, Ann Intern Med 111:992, 1989.)* Debilitating normochromic, normocytic anemia experienced by most patients with chronic renal failure (CRF) is a significant clinical problem. Fortunately, much recent evidence supports the use of recombinant human erythropoietin as a safe and effective therapy, even though bone marrow responsiveness may be somewhat decreased owing to the presence of uremic toxins. Former reliance on multiple blood transfusions was fraught with several dangers, including viral infections and hemosiderosis (chronic iron overload), which can damage many organs, including the heart and gonads. Folic acid deficiency is not uncommon in these patients, since the vitamin is lost during dialysis even though their MCV is not elevated. Clotting problems in uremia are multifactorial; however, impaired platelet function can be improved safely with the administration of cryoprecipitate, desmopressin, or erythropoietin.

313. **The answer is A-Y, B-N, C-Y, D-N, E-Y.** *(Chap 242.)* Glycosuria (with a normal blood glucose concentration), proteinuria, and hyperchloremic acidosis ("normal anion gap acidosis") are evidence of proximal renal tubular dysfunction. Frequent nocturia, presumably resulting from impaired ability to concentrate urine, also suggests renal insufficiency caused by a tubulointerstitial disease. Multiple myeloma may present in this manner, and similar renal abnormalities may be associated with analgesic abuse and Sjögren's syndrome. The findings presented in the case are not characteristic of primary glomerular diseases, such as diabetic nephropathy, or the membranous glomerulopathy induced by penicillamine.

314. **The answer is A-N, B-Y, C-Y, D-Y, E-Y.** *(Chaps 244, 245.)* This patient with recurrent renal calculi and nephrocalcinosis has a normal serum calcium concentration. The serum electrolyte pattern is typical of distal (type 1) renal tubular acidosis with evidence of renal potassium wasting, hyperchloremic metabolic acidosis, and an alkaline urine. The nephrocalcinosis and distal RTA could be consistent with hypervitaminosis D, medullary sponge kidney, hyperparathyroidism, sarcoidosis, or multiple myeloma. However, in all of these conditions except medullary sponge kidney, an increased serum calcium concentration is responsible for the nephrocalcinosis. Intravenous pyelography would better define the defect seen in medullary sponge kidney; it shows a typical "paintbrush" pattern in the renal papillae with tiny papillary cysts containing the calcium deposits. Although medullary sponge kidney is usually not inherited, type 1 distal RTA is often hereditary and relatives should be screened.

315. **The answer is A-N, B-Y, C-Y, D-N, E-Y.** *(Chap 238.)* Living volunteer donors should be healthy, have normal renal arteries, and have the same blood group as the recipient. The one exception to the last rule is in the case of a type O donor who could donate to a recipient with any blood group, since no endothelial antigens in the ABO system would be present to engender rejection. The donor and recipient should be as closely HLA-matched as possible and the mixed lymphocyte response (MLR) should be absent. DNA typing techniques have obviated the need for MLR testing in related donors. In the case of cadaveric donor kidneys, there is a direct relationship between the degree of HLA incompatibility and graft loss. For example, there is a projected 10-year graft survival rate of 27 percent if there are five HLA mismatches, but a 52 percent rate if there is only one mismatch. Chronic rejection is frequently due to nephrosclerosis, often initially characterized by proliferation of the intima (with eventual fibrosis) in the renal vasculature. Prophylaxis against rejection includes the use of cyclosporine A, which inhibits production of the immunostimulatory molecule IL-2 by helper-inducer T lymphocytes and the mercaptopurine analogue azathioprine. Azathioprine is metabolized by the purine degradative pathway to uric acid via the action of xanthine oxidase. Thus,

coadministration of the xanthine oxidase inhibitor allopurinol could interfere with drug catabolism and lead to a dangerously toxic effect of a given dose of azathioprine.

316. **The answer is A-Y, B-N, C-Y, D-Y, E-N.** *(Chap 245. Coe, N Engl J Med 327:1141–1152, 1992.)* The clinical scenario is certainly consistent with distention/irritation of the renal collecting system due to stone passage. Since about 75 percent of all renal stones are caused by either calcium oxalate or calcium phosphate, it is likely that the scout film of the abdomen will be positive. While surgical removal (either directly or by retrograde passage of a basket) was the primary approach in the treatment of a renal stone that led to intractable pain, obstruction, bleeding, or infection, lithotripsy (stone dissolution by sound waves) is becoming the preferred alternative. Ultrasound can be applied directly via a cystoscopically placed transducer, via percutaneous flank incision, or by extracorporeal means. The composition of the kidney stone should be directly assessed, if possible. Outpatient evaluation should consist of measurements of serum electrolytes, creatinine, uric acid, serum and urine calcium, and urine oxalate and citrate. In this fashion one will screen for idiopathic hypercalciuria (the most common reason for nephrolithiasis), primary hyperparathyroidism, hyperuricosuria, distal renal tubular acidosis, and hyperoxaluria (associated with fat malabsorption, including that due to ileal resection or bypass). If the patient is found to have idiopathic hypercalciuria, thiazide diuretics are a reasonable therapeutic approach because they lower calcium excretion.

317–319. **The answers are 317-A, 318-C, 319-D.** *(Chap 46.)* All the sets of laboratory values presented in the question indicate renal insufficiency with metabolic acidosis. Calculation of unmeasured anions (anion gap) is helpful in determining the etiology of the acidosis. Ethylene glycol ingestion, for example, not only causes acute renal failure but leads to rapid accumulation of metabolic acids. Acidosis is disproportionate to the degree of renal insufficiency and is characterized by a high anion gap (choice A). Amphotericin B also causes renal insufficiency with disproportionate metabolic acidosis. Acidosis, however, is due to a distal tubular acidification defect (distal, or type 1, renal tubular acidosis) and is characterized by hyperchloremia, a normal anion gap, and inability to lower the urine pH (choice C). Urinary potassium loss also may be excessive. With moderate renal insufficiency caused by glomerulonephritis, metabolic acidosis is usually mild and the anion gap is only slightly, if at all, elevated (choice D).

The set of laboratory data in choice E illustrates moderate renal insufficiency with disproportionate hyperkalemia and hyperchloremic acidosis, so-called type IV renal tubular acidosis. A number of causes of renal insufficiency, most notably diabetic nephropathy but usually not acute glomerulonephritis, can produce these findings. The laboratory values in choice B illustrate an apparent reduction of the anion gap, which has been reported most frequently in association with multiple myeloma. The apparent reduction in unmeasured anions is due to the presence of abnormal circulating paraprotein that bears a positive charge.

Disorders of the Alimentary Tract and Hepatobiliary System

DIRECTIONS: Each question below contains five suggested responses. Choose the **one best** response to each question.

320. A 56-year-old woman has had profuse, watery diarrhea for 3 months. Laboratory studies of fecal water show the following:

Sodium: 39 mmol/L
Potassium: 96 mmol/L
Chloride: 15 mmol/L
Bicarbonate: 40 mmol/L
Osmolality: 270 mosmol/kgH$_2$O (serum osmolality: 280 mosmol/kgH$_2$O)

The most likely diagnosis is

(A) villous adenoma
(B) lactose intolerance
(C) laxative abuse
(D) pancreatic insufficiency
(E) nontropical sprue

321. A 56-year-old man presents to his internist with jaundice. The patient is receiving no medication and his only symptomatic complaint is mild fatigue over the past 2 months. Physical examination is remarkable only for the presence of scleral icterus. The patient has no significant past medical history. Analysis of serum chemistry reveals the following:

SGOT: 0.58 μkat/L (35 U/L)
SGPT: 0.58 μkat/L (35 U/L)
Total bilirubin: 91.7 μmol/L (7 mg/dL)
Direct bilirubin: 85.5 μmol/L (5 mg/dL)
Alkaline phosphatase: 12 μkat/L (720 U/L)

Which of the following is the next most appropriate diagnostic step?

(A) CT of the abdomen
(B) Liver biopsy
(C) Review of peripheral blood smear
(D) Endoscopic retrograde cholangiopancreatography (ERCP)
(E) No further evaluation necessary; the patient has Dubin-Johnson syndrome

322. A 24-year-old patient known to be infected with type 1 human immunodeficiency virus (HIV-1) presents with a 2-week history of intermittent bloody diarrhea, urgency, abdominal pain, and malaise. Stool culture for enteropathogenic organisms is negative and analysis for ova and parasites is similarly unrevealing. The patient is taking no medication. The diarrheal symptoms do not respond to a course of trimethoprim-sulfamethoxazole. Colonoscopic examination reveals multiple areas of ulceration and mucosal erosion. Biopsy reveals the presence of cells containing a large, densely staining nucleus and abundant intracytoplasmic inclusions. The most appropriate therapy for this patient is

(A) pentamidine
(B) pyrimethamine
(C) ganciclovir
(D) acyclovir
(E) isoniazid

323. All the following can inhibit secretion of gastric acid EXCEPT

(A) reduction of the intragastric pH below 3.0
(B) somatostatin
(C) secretin
(D) histamine
(E) presence of fat in the duodenum

324. All the following statements regarding the association of *Helicobacter* (formerly *Campylobacter*) *pylori* and gastritis are true EXCEPT

(A) growth of *H. pylori* in the stomach is believed to be a cause of chronic gastritis, whereas growth in the duodenum is not clearly implicated in the pathogenesis of duodenal ulcer
(B) *H. pylori* is a gram-negative bacillus that invades the gastric mucosa, thereby producing mucosal inflammation
(C) *H. pylori* can be identified by its ability to cleave urea
(D) eradication of the bacteria results in histologic improvement of gastric mucosa
(E) the antibiotics ampicillin or metronidazole can eradicate *H. pylori*

325. A 57-year-old man seeks attention in the emergency department for weakness and melena, which he has had for 3 days. He says he has not had significant abdominal pain and had no prior gastrointestinal bleeding. On examination he is disheveled and unshaven, appears older than his stated age, and has a 20 mmHg orthostatic drop in blood pressure. Findings include bilateral temporal wasting, anicteric and pale conjunctivae, spider angiomas on his upper torso, muscle wasting, hepatosplenomegaly, and hyperactive bowel sounds without abdominal tenderness to palpation. Stool is melenic. Nasogastric aspiration reveals "coffee-grounds" material, which quickly clears with lavage. Hematocrit is 30 percent and mean corpuscular volume is 105 fL. Saline gastric lavage is initiated. The appropriate next step in the management of this man's illness would be to

(A) perform gastroscopy
(B) pass a Sengstaken-Blakemore tube and begin an intravenous infusion of vasopressin (Pitressin)
(C) order an upper gastrointestinal series
(D) order immediate visceral angiography
(E) insert a large-bore intravenous line and type and cross-match the man's blood

326. A patient with ascites undergoes a diagnostic paracentesis that reveals milky, opaque fluid. The protein content of the fluid is 25 g/dL and the cell count includes 500 red blood cells per microliter and 1500 white cells (predominantly lymphocytes) per microliter; the triglyceride concentration is 1500 mg/dL. Which of the following entities would most likely account for these findings?

(A) Tuberculosis
(B) Alcoholic cirrhosis
(C) Bacterial peritonitis
(D) Ovarian carcinoma
(E) Nephrotic syndrome

327. A 45-year-old man says that for the past year he occasionally has regurgitated food particles eaten several days earlier. His wife complains that his breath has been foul-smelling. He has had occasional dysphagia for solid foods. The most likely diagnosis is

(A) gastric outlet obstruction
(B) scleroderma
(C) achalasia
(D) Zenker's diverticulum
(E) diabetic gastroparesis

328. During the last year, a 55-year-old man has experienced vague postprandial epigastric fullness. For the last several months, he has been anorectic and has lost 4.5 kg (10 lb). Physical examination is unrevealing except for faintly guaiac-positive stool. Hematocrit is 26 percent. A representative x-ray from his upper gastrointestinal series is reproduced below. The man's physician should now

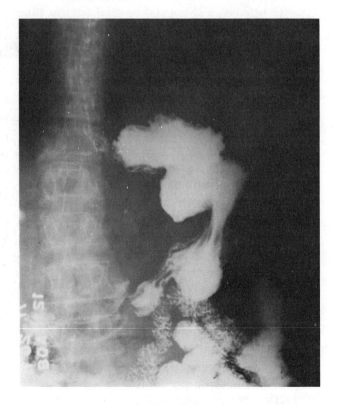

(A) prescribe ranitidine
(B) prescribe sucralfate
(C) perform a double-contrast upper gastrointestinal series
(D) perform gastroscopy
(E) recommend total gastrectomy

329. A 42-year-old woman presents with a complaint of watery diarrhea and abdominal pain that has occurred intermittently over the past 4 years. After the passage of three or four loose stools in the morning, she feels well for the rest of the day and never has nocturnal diarrhea. Physical examination reveals an anxious woman with a tender left lower abdominal quadrant and no fecal material in the rectum; the results are otherwise normal. Sigmoidoscopic examination discloses excess mucus, but the mucosa appears normal. Barium enema is normal except for sigmoid spasticity, and examination of a stool specimen reveals well-formed feces that are negative for blood, pathogenic bacteria, and parasites. Results of thyroid studies are normal. A trial of milk restriction results in no change in symptoms.

At this point the physician should

(A) consider a trial of diphenoxylate or loperamide to control symptomatic diarrhea
(B) tell the patient that her symptoms are largely emotional in origin
(C) consider a trial of psyllium to increase stool bulk
(D) obtain stool electrolytes and osmolality
(E) perform a jejunal aspirate and analyze the fluid for parasites

330. A 65-year-old man presents with a feeling of abdominal fullness. Physical examination reveals a distended abdomen and flank dullness that shifts with change in position, as well as a firm periumbilical nodule. Which of the following disorders is most likely to account for these findings?

(A) Alcoholic cirrhosis
(B) Tuberculous peritonitis
(C) Pancreatitis with pseudocyst
(D) Carcinoma of the colon
(E) Nephrotic syndrome

331. When operation is performed for suspected appendicitis and that diagnosis proves incorrect, the most common condition discovered is

(A) mesenteric lymphadenitis
(B) pelvic inflammatory disease
(C) acute gastroenteritis
(D) ruptured ovarian cyst
(E) no organic disease

332. All the following statements about achalasia are true EXCEPT

(A) the underlying abnormality appears to be defective innervation of the esophageal body and lower esophageal sphincter
(B) dysphagia, chest pain, and regurgitation are the predominant symptoms
(C) chest x-rays often reveal a large gastric air bubble
(D) manometry reveals a normal or elevated pressure of the lower esophageal sphincter
(E) nifedipine is effective in controlling symptoms in many patients

333. A 45-year-old man presented with sharp epigastric pain relieved by antacids and food. Barium study of the upper gastrointestinal tract reveals a crater in the proximal portion of the duodenal bulb. Which of the following statements concerning therapeutic alternatives is correct?

(A) Atropine or related anticholinergic agents are effective in improving symptoms
(B) Sucralfate is effective in eradication of *Helicobacter pylori* colonization
(C) Cimetidine or other H_2-receptor antagonists are more effective than sulcralfate in promoting healing
(D) Sucralfate can significantly reduce the bioavailability of fluoroquinolone antibiotics
(E) Omeprazole, a specific inhibitor of parietal cell H^+, K^+-ATPase, is contraindicated in routine situations because of its carcinogenic potential

334. A 75-year-old woman with a history of aspirin-induced gastritis 5 years ago now has severe knee and hip pain thought to be due to osteoarthritis. She requires treatment with nonsteroidal anti-inflammatory agents. Which of the following agents would be most helpful for prophylaxis against recurrent gastrointestinal bleeding?

(A) Omeprazole
(B) Misoprostol
(C) Nizatidine
(D) Sucralfate
(E) Atropine

335. Each condition listed below is associated with an increased risk of cancer of the esophagus. Which one is most closely linked to *adenocarcinoma* of the esophagus?

(A) Achalasia
(B) Smoking
(C) Barrett's esophagus
(D) Tylosis
(E) Alcoholism

336. Four months ago, a 36-year-old man with a peptic ulcer underwent a Billroth II anastomosis, antrectomy, vagotomy, and gastrojejunostomy. He now returns for evaluation of a stomal (anastomic) ulcer. Fasting serum gastrin level is 350 ng/L; 5 min after intravenous infusion of secretin the serum gastrin level is 100 ng/L. The man should be advised that the most appropriate treatment for his condition is

(A) total vagotomy
(B) total gastrectomy
(C) resection of the distal antrum attached to the duodenal stump
(D) laparotomy to search for a gastrin-producing tumor
(E) medical therapy with liquid antacids

337. A 59-year-old man presents with fatigue, epigastric pain, early satiety, and iron-deficiency anemia. Upper gastrointestinal endoscopy reveals diffuse thickening throughout the entire stomach with some extension into the duodenum. Biopsy is undertaken. Review of the specimen reveals infiltration with malignant-appearing lymphocytes. Which of the following statements concerning the current situation is correct?

(A) The patient has a greater than average likelihood of having blood group A

(B) The patient should receive combination chemotherapy with 5-fluorouracil, doxorubicin, and mitomycin C

(C) The prognosis would have been better if the biopsy had revealed neoplastic signet-ring cells

(D) Chemotherapy is absolutely contraindicated because of the risk of bleeding and perforation

(E) Immunoperoxidase studies would probably reveal evidence of B-cell derivation

338. A patient who presented with painful and tender lower extremities underwent an extensive workup. He ultimately improved after being placed on a gluten-free diet, though he had no significant complaints of diarrhea. What was the probable cause of the musculoskeletal complaints in this patient?

(A) Vitamin D deficiency
(B) Vitamin B_{12} deficiency
(C) IgA deficiency
(D) Iron deficiency
(E) Improvement in severe anxiety

339. All the following statements regarding eosinophilic enteritis are true EXCEPT

(A) peripheral blood eosinophilia is present

(B) it may affect the stomach, small intestine, and colon

(C) the majority of patients have a history of food allergies or asthma

(D) treatment with corticosteroids is often effective

(E) it may be difficult to distinguish from regional enteritis

340. Which of the following diagnostic studies for malabsorption is usually normal in persons who have bacterial overgrowth syndrome?

(A) Fecal fat quantitation (24 h)

(B) Stage II Schilling test (intrinsic factor given with vitamin B_{12})

(C) D-Xylose absorption test

(D) Lactulose breath test

(E) Quantitative cultures of jejunal aspirates

341. A 30-year-old man complains of abdominal cramps, bloating, and diarrhea. He believes these symptoms are exacerbated after ingestion of dairy products. He is otherwise well and has no abnormalities on physical or laboratory examination. Which is the most specific and sensitive measurement to diagnose this patient's condition?

(A) Breath hydrogen after ingestion of 50 g lactose

(B) Blood glucose after ingestion of 100 g lactose

(C) Breath labeled carbon dioxide after ingestion of oral glycine-1-[^{14}C] glycocholate

(D) Urine xylose after ingestion of 25 g D-xylose

(E) Vitamin A serum level

342. A 72-year-old woman with known mitral stenosis and atrial fibrillation presents with severe abdominal pain. The pain began fairly suddenly 24 h ago and was located in the periumbilical region; however, today the pain is throughout the entire abdomen. Other than the aforementioned cardiac disease, the past medical history is unremarkable. Her only medication is digoxin 0.25 mg/d. Physical examination reveals an anxious patient with a temperature of 38.3°C (101°F) orally, blood pressure of 100/60, pulse of 120, and respiratory rate of 26. Her skin is cold and clammy. The oral mucosa is dry. Cardiac auscultation is remarkable for a grade 2/4 diastolic rumble. Bowel sounds are normal. There is mild abdominal distention and tenderness without rebound. Stool is guaiac-positive but not grossly bloody or melenic. Initial laboratory evaluation reveals a WBC of 16,000/μL with a differential of 75 percent neutrophils, 10 percent bands, 10 percent lymphocytes, and 5 percent monocytes; hematocrit of 42 percent; and platelet count of 522,000/mL. Plain film of the abdomen reveals air-fluid levels. The most appropriate diagnostic maneuver at this time is

(A) exploratory laparotomy
(B) laparoscopy
(C) angiography
(D) CT of the abdomen
(E) upper GI series with small bowel follow-through

343. For the last 6 months, a 50-year-old man has had diarrhea and migratory arthralgias and has lost 9.1 kg (20 lb). An upper gastrointestinal barium study shows a malabsorption pattern in the small bowel. Stool fat content is 35 g per 24 h. Following oral administration of 25 g of D-xylose, a 5-h urine collection contains 0.8 g of D-xylose. A peroral small-bowel biopsy reveals subtotal villus atrophy, dilated lymphatics, and infiltration of the lamina propria with macrophages that stain positively with periodic acid Schiff (PAS) stain. The man's physician should now

(A) start him on a gluten-free diet
(B) prescribe prednisone, 60 mg/d and tapered over 2 months
(C) prescribe prednisone, 60 mg/d indefinitely
(D) prescribe trimethoprim-sulfamethoxazole for at least 1 year
(E) recommend an exploratory laparotomy with splenectomy and biopsy of retroperitoneal nodes

344. A 62-year-old physician was well until 3 weeks ago when she developed a urinary tract infection. She was treated with ampicillin for 10 days, taking her last dose 7 days ago. Four days ago, she developed abdominal pain, fever, and bloody diarrhea. On examination, she appears acutely ill; her temperature is 38.3°C (101°F) and her abdomen is diffusely tender. Sigmoidoscopy demonstrates a hyperemic mucosa studded with plaquelike lesions. Based on the most likely diagnosis, optimal therapy would include

(A) trimethoprim-sulfamethoxazole
(B) oral vancomycin
(C) sulfasalazine
(D) vascular reconstruction
(E) corticosteroids

345. A 70-year-old Irish consular official seeks local medical attention for diarrhea and weight loss, which have been present for 2 years. He says he has always been in good health "even though I'm the runt of the litter" (he is the smallest of eight siblings). Laboratory studies include normal complete blood cell count and serum electrolyte concentrations. Serum D-xylose concentration is 0.76 mmol/L (15 mg/dL) 2 h after an oral challenge, and 24-h fecal fat determination is 12 g on a 100-g fat diet. A representative biopsy specimen of his jejunum is shown below. Which of the following statements about the man's illness is correct?

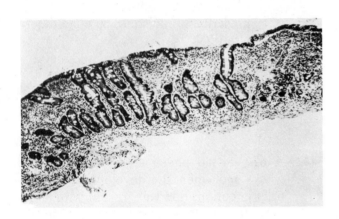

(A) This condition is believed to be due to a gram-negative bacillus
(B) Abdominal pain, arthralgia, low-grade fever, and lymphadenopathy are frequently present
(C) Corticosteroid therapy is the treatment of choice
(D) Adherence to a strict gluten-free diet usually results in normalization of malabsorption tests and reversal of jejunal pathology
(E) A rebiopsy after gluten challenge is indicated at this time

346. Which of the following statements concerning screening for colorectal cancer is correct?

(A) Patients who have a positive fecal Hemoccult test while on a low-meat diet are likely to have colorectal carcinoma
(B) The vast majority of patients with documented colorectal cancers have a positive fecal Hemoccult test
(C) No randomized studies of Hemoccult screening have documented a significant reduction in mortality from colorectal cancer in annually screened persons
(D) Present American Cancer Society recommendations include Hemoccult screening beginning at age 50 and sigmoidoscopic examination every 3 to 5 years beginning at age 50 for persons at average risk
(E) Rehydration of Hemoccult slides has no effect on the positivity rate

347. A 53-year-old man with rectal bleeding was found to have adenocarcinoma 2 cm below the peritoneal reflection. After a negative metastatic workup, the patient underwent resection of the tumor with primary reanastomosis. Pathologic examination revealed a moderately well-differentiated adenocarcinoma of the rectum with 2 out of 10 adjacent lymph nodes that contained cancer. The patient has no other medical problems. Optimal therapy at this point should include

(A) pelvic radiation therapy
(B) a chemotherapy regimen containing 5-fluorouracil
(C) a combination of pelvic irradiation and a chemotherapy regimen containing 5-fluorouracil
(D) a chemotherapy regimen containing 5-fluorouracil plus levamisole
(E) observation alone

348. A 28-year-old man has had diarrhea and crampy abdominal pain of the right lower quadrant for the last 4 weeks. During the last 10 days, he also has had episodic low-grade fever, abdominal distention, and anorexia without vomiting but leading to a weight loss of 3.2 kg (7 lb). On examination, he is mildly uncomfortable. Vital signs are temperature, 37.8°C (100.1°F); pulse, 100 beats per minute; and blood pressure, 110/60 mmHg. His sclerae are anicteric, and there is no palpable lymphadenopathy. A tender, indistinct fullness is palpable in the right lower quadrant of the abdomen, but otherwise the abdomen is soft and without rebound tenderness or palpable hepatosplenomegaly. Rectal examination reveals no masses or focal tenderness, but the stool is guaiac-positive. Laboratory values include a hematocrit of 30 percent and a white blood cell count of 11,300/mm³ with a shift to the left. Flat-plate and upright x-rays of the abdomen show some air-filled loops of small bowel but no air-fluid levels. Sigmoidoscopy is unremarkable. On barium enema examination, barium fails to reflux into the terminal ileum, but the colon is otherwise normal. A representative film from a small-bowel barium examination is shown below.

Which of the following disorders is most consistent with the clinical picture described?

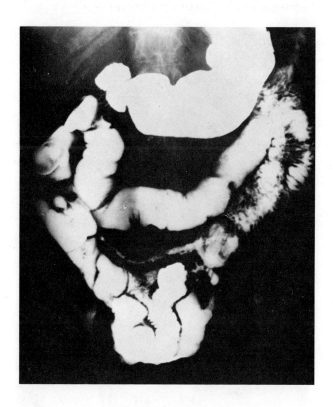

(A) Perforated appendix with appendiceal abscess
(B) Whipple's disease
(C) Regional enteritis
(D) Adenocarcinoma of the small intestine
(E) Lymphoma of the small intestine

349. A 20-year-old man was found to have ulcerative proctitis 2 years ago. Mild rectal bleeding was well controlled on daily steroid enemas, which were discontinued a year ago. For the last 3 months, he has had increasingly frequent bloody diarrhea (now 6 to 10 times a day), lower abdominal cramps, low-grade fever, anorexia, and a 5-kg (11-lb) weight loss. Physical examination of this thin, pale young man, who appears acutely ill, reveals these vital signs: temperature, 37.8°C (100°F); pulse, 110 beats per minute; and blood pressure, 120/70 mmHg. The lower abdomen is mildly and diffusely tender, but there is no rebound tenderness and bowel sounds are active. Stool is grossly bloody. Sigmoidoscopy, limited to 10 cm because of discomfort, shows marked mucosal erythema and friability; diffuse ulceration is present, and an exudate contains pus and blood.

 Three hours after a barium enema, which shows ulcerations throughout the colon, the man's abdominal pain markedly worsens. Vital signs now are temperature, 39.6°C (103.2°F); pulse, 130 beats per minute; and blood pressure, 90/60 mmHg. On examination the abdomen is distended and diffusely tender with rebound; bowel sounds are infrequent. An abdominal flat-plate x-ray is pictured below.

 The most likely diagnosis for the disorder described above is

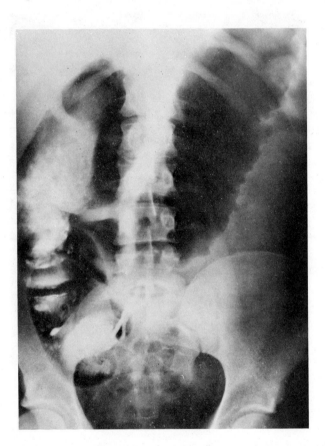

 (A) acute colonic perforation
 (B) inferior mesenteric artery occlusion
 (C) nonthrombotic mesenteric ischemia
 (D) volvulus
 (E) toxic megacolon

350. As a consequence of severe liver damage, hepatic amino acid handling is deranged. In this situation, plasma levels of which of the following are likely to be lower than normal?

(A) Ammonia (NH_3)
(B) Ammonium (NH_4^+)
(C) Alanine
(D) Urea
(E) Glycine

351. Which of the following drugs will be less potent in the presence of severe liver disease?

(A) Phenytoin
(B) Lidocaine
(C) Tetracycline
(D) Imipramine
(E) Propranolol

352. All the following are risk factors for development of cancer of the colon EXCEPT

(A) Crohn's colitis
(B) adenomatous polyps
(C) uterosigmoidostomy
(D) ulcerative colitis
(E) juvenile polyposis

353. All the following statements regarding primary biliary cirrhosis (PBC) are true EXCEPT

(A) a positive antimitochondrial antibody test is present in more than 90 percent of patients
(B) increased serum cryoprotein concentrations are frequently present
(C) the majority of patients are women
(D) administration of D-penicillamine appears to be an effective treatment
(E) rheumatoid arthritis, CRST syndrome, and scleroderma occur with increased frequency in patients with PBC

354. A 19-year-old female exchange student from London has had bouts of jaundice, fever, malaise, arthralgias, and marked elevation of hepatic transaminases over the last 6 months. The patient was not exposed to hepatotoxic drugs. Hypergammaglobulinemia has been noted. Serologic evaluation for infection with hepatitis A, B, and C has been negative, as have tests for systemic lupus. Liver biopsy now reveals bridging necrosis. Which of the following tests will be most helpful in confirming the diagnosis?

(A) Rheumatoid factor
(B) Hemoglobin electrophoresis
(C) Antibodies to liver and kidney microsomal antigens
(D) Antibodies to hepatitis D virus
(E) Antibodies to hepatitis E virus

355. Which of the following is an important physiologic function of bile acids?

(A) Conjugation with toxic substances, thereby allowing their excretion
(B) Allowing the excretion of hemoglobin breakdown products
(C) Aiding the absorption of vitamin B_{12}
(D) Facilitating absorption of dietary fats
(E) Maintaining appropriate intestinal pH

356. The most common organism isolated from the ascitic fluid of patients with spontaneous bacterial peritonitis is

(A) *Streptococcus pneumoniae*
(B) *Staphylococcus aureus*
(C) *Escherichia coli*
(D) *Bacteroides fragilis*
(E) enterococcus

357. A 37-year-old man with chronic alcoholism is admitted to the hospital with acute pancreatitis. On the third hospital day, sudden, complete blindness develops in the left eye. The most likely explanation is

(A) alcohol withdrawal symptoms
(B) transient ischemic attack (transient monocular blindness)
(C) occlusion of the retinal vein
(D) acute glaucoma
(E) Purtscher's retinopathy

358. In which one of the following situations would therapy with oral chenodeoxycholic acid be most effective in dissolving the gallstone(s)?

(A) A 27-year-old Asian woman with thalassemia
(B) A 49-year-old woman with two 2-cm stones
(C) A 60-year-old man with gallstones visible on chest x-ray
(D) A 45-year-old woman with a history of gallstone pancreatitis and a residual 1-cm radiolucent gallstone
(E) A 55-year-old man with a history of biliary colic, several small gallstones seen on ultrasonography, and a poorly opacified gallbladder following oral cholecystography

359. Which of the following could falsely depress the serum amylase level in a patient suspected of having acute pancreatitis?

(A) Hypertriglyceridemia
(B) Hypercholesterolemia
(C) Hypocalcemia
(D) Associated pleural effusion
(E) Associated intestinal infarction

360. Mechanical obstruction of the colon is most commonly caused by

(A) adhesions
(B) carcinoma
(C) volvulus
(D) hernia
(E) sigmoid diverticulitis

361. In which of the following causes of fatty liver is microvesicular fat seen in biopsy specimens of liver?

(A) Jejunoileal bypass for morbid obesity
(B) Acute fatty liver of pregnancy
(C) Total parenteral nutrition
(D) Prolonged intravenous hyperalimentation
(E) Carbon tetrachloride poisoning

362. Magnetic resonance imaging (MRI) of the liver can be particularly helpful in all the following conditions EXCEPT

(A) hereditary hemochromatosis
(B) Wilson's disease
(C) thalassemia intermedia
(D) halothane hepatitis
(E) chronic exposure to vinyl chloride

363. Of the following agents that can account for drug-induced hepatitis, which one produces liver injury in a predictable and dose-dependent fashion?

(A) Halothane
(B) Chlorpromazine
(C) Methyldopa
(D) Acetaminophen
(E) Erythromycin

364. In a patient with hepatic cirrhosis, hepatic encephalopathy can be precipitated by all the following factors EXCEPT

(A) gastrointestinal bleeding
(B) metabolic acidosis
(C) renal insufficiency
(D) vomiting
(E) viral hepatitis

365. One month ago, a 21-year-old woman was begun on daily isoniazid therapy because of a positive tuberculin skin test. She now feels well and her physical examination is unremarkable. Routine laboratory data include the following: serum alanine aminotransferase (ALT), 2.5 μkat/L (150 Karmen units/mL); total bilirubin, 17 μmol/L (1.0 mg/dL); and alkaline phosphatase, 25 units. The most appropriate action by the woman's physician would be to order

(A) another antituberculous drug
(B) corticosteroids
(C) a liver biopsy
(D) an ultrasound of the gallbladder
(E) continuation of isoniazid therapy

366. A 45-year-old man with Laennec's cirrhosis and a history of hepatic encephalopathy comes to the local emergency room because of alcoholic intoxication. Physical examination is remarkable for palmar erythema, spider angiomas, and bilateral gynecomastia. Liver span is 8 cm and the edge cannot be felt; a spleen tip, however, is palpable. Stool is guaiac-negative. He has no asterixis. Laboratory studies include the following:

Hematocrit: 38 percent
Mean corpuscular volume: 104 fL
White blood cell count: 4000/mm³
Platelet count: 97,000/mm³
Prothrombin time: 17.5 s
Total serum bilirubin: 14 μmol/L
  (0.8 mg/dL)
Serum aspartate aminotransferase (AST):
  0.5 μkat/L (30 U/L)
Serum alkaline phosphatase: 1.0 μkat/L
  (60 U/L)

The man is given intravenous hydration and vitamin and mineral supplements, including folic acid (1 mg), thiamine (100 mg), magnesium (2 g), and vitamin K (10 mg). After spending the night in the hospital's detoxification unit, he awakens sober and alert. Repeat prothrombin time is 12 s.

The most likely explanation for the elevation in the man's initial prothrombin time is

(A) alcoholic hepatitis
(B) folate deficiency
(C) intestinal malabsorption
(D) disseminated intravascular coagulation
(E) laboratory error

367. A 67-year-old woman, who has previously been healthy, undergoes emergency surgery for a ruptured abdominal aortic aneurysm. Intraoperatively she requires 8 units of packed red blood cells to maintain her blood pressure and hematocrit. Following surgery she is hemodynamically stable. On the third postoperative day she appears jaundiced, but abdominal examination is unremarkable and she is afebrile. Total serum bilirubin concentration at this time is 141 μmol/L (8.3 mg/dL) (direct, 107 μmol/L [6.3 mg/dL]). Serum alkaline phosphatase level is 6 μkat/L (360 U/L), and serum AST level is 0.85 μkat/L (51 Karmen units/mL). The most likely explanation for the woman's jaundice is

(A) a stone in the common bile duct
(B) halothane hepatitis
(C) posttransfusion hepatitis
(D) acute hepatic infarct
(E) benign intrahepatic cholestasis

368. A 35-year-old former hemodialysis nurse is seen because of a 6-month history of fatigue and amenorrhea. On examination she has scleral icterus, a mildly tender liver, and a tibial rash consistent with erythema nodosum. ALT and AST levels are both in the range of 1.5 μkat/L (100 U/L) and bilirubin is 51.3 μmol/L (3 mg/dL), while alkaline phosphatase and serum albumin levels are normal. Hepatitis serologic testing detects HBsAg and IgG anti-HBcAg. Liver biopsy discloses a mononuclear cell portal infiltrate and hepatocyte destruction at the periphery of lobules.

Which of the following therapeutic strategies is best?

(A) Administration of low-dose cyclophosphamide, 50 mg/d for 2 months
(B) Administration of prednisone, 20 to 40 mg/d for 2 months and then taper-based on response
(C) Administration of prednisone, 10 mg every other day for 3 months
(D) Administration of acyclovir, 400 mg every 6 h for 2 weeks
(E) Administration of interferon-α, 10 million units three times per week for 4 months

369. A 50-year-old man with a history of organomegaly and an elevated hematocrit without apparent secondary cause was well until the sudden onset of pain of the right upper quadrant. On examination the patient is afebrile and has clear lungs, normal cardiac function, an abdominal fluid wave, splenomegaly, and a markedly enlarged liver with a palpable, very tender edge. Liver function tests are normal except for mild elevation of hepatic transaminases.

   Which of the following is the most appropriate procedure for purposes of establishing a diagnosis?

   (A) CT scan of the liver
   (B) Abdominal ultrasound
   (C) Radionuclide liver-spleen scan
   (D) Hepatic venography
   (E) Paracentesis

370. Chronic active hepatitis is most reliably distinguished from chronic persistent hepatitis by the presence of

   (A) extrahepatic manifestations
   (B) hepatitis B surface antigen in the serum
   (C) antibody to hepatitis B core antigen in the serum
   (D) a significant titer of anti-smooth-muscle antibody
   (E) characteristic liver histology

371. Cholecystectomy is advisable in all the following patients EXCEPT

   (A) a patient with the calcified outline of the gallbladder visible on plain abdominal x-ray
   (B) a patient hospitalized for treatment of biliary colic four times in the last 2 months
   (C) a patient with a history of a recent episode of acute cholecystitis who responded favorably to a 7-day course of intravenous antibiotics
   (D) a diabetic patient without abdominal symptoms in whom gallstones were incidentally noted on ultrasound done to assess renal size
   (E) a patient with a history of pancreatitis caused by gallstone

372. A 52-year-old woman is hospitalized for medical management of severe alcoholic hepatitis. On the ninth hospital day she develops a temperature of 38.3°C (101°F) and generalized abdominal discomfort. Abdominal examination reveals a fluid wave and significant and diffuse abdominal tenderness without guarding; hepatosplenomegaly is present but is unchanged from the admission examination. Rectal and pelvic examinations reveal no area of localized tenderness; stool guaiac testing is positive. Hematocrit is 27 percent, white blood cell count is 12,000/mm³, and liver function tests are unchanged from admission—total serum bilirubin, 214 μmol/L (12.5 mg/dL); serum AST, 2.5 μkat/L (150 Karmen units/mL); and serum alkaline phosphatase, 3.0 μkat/L (180 U/L).

   The procedure most likely to yield diagnostic information in this case would be

   (A) serum amylase determination
   (B) blood culture
   (C) supine and upright x-rays of the abdomen
   (D) abdominal sonography
   (E) paracentesis

373. A 38-year-old woman is hospitalized for an upper gastrointestinal hemorrhage. Following an uneventful recovery, an upper gastrointestinal series (part of which is reproduced below) is obtained. The abnormality demonstrated in the x-ray suggests which of the following diagnoses?

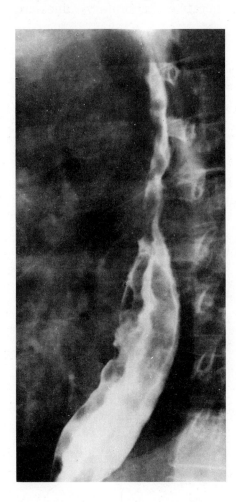

(A) Erosive gastritis
(B) Laennec's cirrhosis
(C) Hiatal hernia
(D) Gastric ulcer
(E) Reflux esophagitis

374. All the following conditions are known to predispose to the formation of cholesterol gallstones EXCEPT

(A) obesity
(B) hypercholesterolemia
(C) clofibrate therapy
(D) oral contraceptive therapy
(E) surgical resection of the ileum

375. A 58-year-old man with biopsy-proven Laennec's cirrhosis is hospitalized because of massive ascites and pedal edema. There is no evidence of respiratory compromise or hepatic encephalopathy. Initial laboratory values are as follows:

Serum electrolytes (mmol/L): Na^+ 130; K^+ 3.6; Cl^- 85; HCO_3^- 30
Serum creatinine: 88 μmol/L (1.0 mg/dL)
Blood urea nitrogen: 6.4 μmol/L (18 mg/dL)

Bed rest, sodium and water restriction, and the administration of spironolactone (50 mg/d) produce no significant weight change after 5 days. Which of the following therapeutic measures would be most appropriate at this time?

(A) Intravenous furosemide, 80 mg now
(B) Oral spironolactone, 100 mg/d
(C) Oral acetazolamide, 250 mg/d
(D) Placement of a peritoneovenous (LeVeen) shunt
(E) Therapeutic paracentesis

376. A 64-year-old man with insulin-dependent adult-onset diabetes mellitus seeks emergency medical treatment after 2 days of increasingly severe abdominal pain of the right upper quadrant, which has spread over the entire abdomen and is associated with nausea, vomiting, fever, and chills. On examination, he is alert and oriented but appears to be quite acutely distressed. Vital signs are temperature, 39.4°C (103°F); pulse, 140 beats per minute; and blood pressure, 100/60 mmHg. His sclerae are mildly icteric. His abdomen is diffusely tender with marked guarding in the right upper quadrant; there is no palpable hepatosplenomegaly, and there are no audible bowel sounds. Rectal examination reveals no focal tenderness; stool is guaiac-negative. Laboratory values are as follows:

Hematocrit: 34 percent
White blood cell count: 22,500/mm^3 with a marked left shift
Plasma glucose: 17.8 mmol/L (325 mg/dL)
Blood urea nitrogen: 10.5 μmol/L (30 mg/dL)
Serum AST: 2.1 μkat/L (125 Karmen units/mL)
Serum alkaline phosphatase: 210 units
Serum amylase: 3.3 μkat/L (200 U/dL)

His abdominal flat-plate x-ray is shown below. During the first 4 h of hospitalization, the man's condition is stabilized somewhat with the administration of intravenous fluids and insulin. A nasogastric tube is inserted, blood cultures are drawn, and he is begun on broad-spectrum antibiotics.

The most appropriate management at this point would be to order

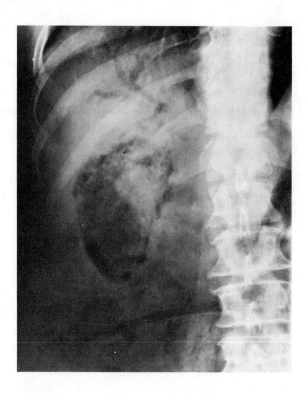

(A) conservative medical measures only for the next 48 to 72 h
(B) an abdominal ultrasound examination
(C) an upper gastrointestinal examination with Gastrografin dye
(D) endoscopic retrograde cholangiopancreatography
(E) preparations for an emergency laparotomy

377. A 65-year-old man with long-standing, stable, biopsy-proven postnecrotic cirrhosis develops abdominal pain of the right upper quadrant and abdominal swelling. He is afebrile. Palmar erythema, spider telangiectasias, and mild jaundice are noted on physical examination. His abdomen is distended, shifting dullness is present, a tender, firm liver edge is felt 3 fingerbreadths below the right costal margin, and a spleen tip is palpable. A faint bruit is heard over the liver. Laboratory values include the following:

Hematocrit: 34 percent
White blood cell count: 4300/mm³
Platelet count: 104,000/mm³
Serum albumin: 26 g/L (2.6 g/dL)
Serum globulins: 46 g/L (4.6 g/dL)
Alkaline phosphatase: 8.0 μkat/L
  (480 U/L)

Paracentesis reveals blood-tinged fluid. The serum marker most specifically associated with this man's condition is

(A) antinuclear antibody
(B) alpha fetoprotein
(C) antimitochondrial antibody
(D) 5'-nucleotidase
(E) chorionic gonadotropin

378. Administration of which of the following drugs or classes of drugs has been shown to prolong survival in persons with acute pancreatitis?

(A) Cimetidine
(B) Aprotinin (Trasylol)
(C) Antibiotics
(D) Anticholinergics
(E) None of the above

379. Complications of chronic pancreatitis include all the following EXCEPT

(A) gastric varices
(B) erythema nodosum
(C) vitamin B_{12} malabsorption
(D) pleural effusion
(E) jaundice

380. All the following factors portend a poor survival rate during an attack of acute pancreatitis EXCEPT

(A) hyperbilirubinemia
(B) hypoalbuminemia
(C) hypocalcemia
(D) hypoxemia
(E) discolored peritoneal fluid

381. A 52-year-old woman has hepatomegaly. Percutaneous liver biopsy reveals "adenocarcinoma," but the woman refuses further evaluation or treatment. A year later she presents with weight loss (13.6 kg, 30 lb) and a skin rash that has waxed and waned. Examination shows angular stomatitis and a firm, enlarged liver. An erythematous, bullous, necrotic skin rash (Color Plate A) is present on the face, perineum, and legs. Sonography reveals an enlarged pancreas. Hematologic testing shows the woman to be anemic.

The diagnostic test of choice would be

(A) serum amylase determination
(B) plasma glucagon determination
(C) plasma vasoactive intestinal polypeptide (VIP) determination
(D) plasma gastrin determination
(E) pancreatic arteriography

382. A 35-year-old woman with a history of acute lymphoblastic leukemia is seen 7 weeks after receiving an allogeneic bone marrow transplant. Routine prophylaxis for graft-versus-host disease with corticosteroids and methotrexate is being administered. She complains of midsternal pain upon swallowing. Biopsy of one of the lesions noted on endoscopy (Color Plate B) would reveal

(A) lymphoblasts on a Wright's-stained smear
(B) multinucleated giant cells on Wright's staining
(C) hyphal forms on silver staining
(D) small cysts on silver staining
(E) overgrowth of bacteria on Gram's stain

383. Chronic reflux esophagitis is LEAST likely to result in the development of

    (A) gastrointestinal bleeding
    (B) an esophageal peptic stricture
    (C) a lower esophageal ring
    (D) Barrett's esophagus (esophagus lined by columnar epithelium)
    (E) adenocarcinoma

384. A patient with scleral icterus and a positive reaction for bilirubin by urine dipstick testing could have which of the following disorders?

    (A) Autoimmune hemolytic anemia
    (B) Dubin-Johnson syndrome
    (C) Crigler-Najjar type II disorder
    (D) Thalassemia intermedia
    (E) Gilbert's syndrome

385. Which one of these extraintestinal complications of inflammatory bowel disease is LEAST likely to be associated with ulcerative colitis?

    (A) Pericholangitis
    (B) Pyoderma gangrenosum
    (C) Arthritis
    (D) Uveitis
    (E) Oxalate kidney stones

386. The following statements describing Meckel's diverticulum are true EXCEPT

    (A) it is the most frequent congenital anomaly of the digestive tract
    (B) mechanical obstruction due to intussusception may occur
    (C) in young adults, inflammatory complications may produce a clinical syndrome indistinguishable from acute appendicitis
    (D) it is usually present in the jejunum
    (E) technetium scans are valuable in the diagnosis of those diverticula associated with gastrointestinal bleeding

387. Which one of the following statements about hepatitis B *e* antigen (HBeAg) is LEAST accurate?

    (A) HBeAg can be detected transiently in the sera of patients ill with acute hepatitis B infection
    (B) The presence of HBeAg in the serum is correlated with infectiousness
    (C) The absence of HBeAg in the serum rules out chronic infection caused by the hepatitis B virus
    (D) HBeAg is immunologically distinct from HBsAg but is genetically related to HBcAg
    (E) The disappearance of HBeAg from the serum may be a harbinger of resolution of acute hepatitis B infection

DIRECTIONS: Each question below contains five suggested responses. For **each** of the **five** responses listed with every question, you are to respond either YES (Y) or NO (N). In a given item **all, some, or none** of the alternatives may be correct.

388. True statements regarding delta hepatitis virus (HDV) include

(A) HDV is a defective RNA virus
(B) HDV can infect only persons infected with HBV
(C) the HDV genome is partially homologous with hepatitis B virus (HBV) DNA
(D) HDV infection has been found only in limited areas of the world
(E) simultaneous infection with HDV and HBV results in an increased risk of development of chronic hepatitis

389. Causes of upper gastrointestinal bleeding that usually are missed by routine upper gastrointestinal x-rays but can be diagnosed by endoscopy include

(A) Mallory-Weiss tears
(B) duodenal ulcers
(C) gastric ulcers
(D) erosive gastritis
(E) Osler-Rendu-Weber syndrome

390. True statements about the management of variceal hemorrhage include which of the following?

(A) Because of the risk of perforation, endoscopic sclerotherapy should be reserved for patients who rebleed after surgery
(B) Peripheral vein infusion of vasopressin is as effective as superior mesenteric artery infusion in controlling variceal hemorrhage
(C) Propranolol reduces the risk of bleeding in patients with large varices
(D) Elective portacaval shunt surgery prevents recurrent variceal hemorrhage but does not improve life expectancy
(E) The selective distal splenorenal shunt appears to be associated with a lower incidence of postoperative hepatic encephalopathy than is the portacaval shunt

391. True statements regarding the prophylaxis of viral hepatitis include which of the following?

(A) Although immune globulin (IG) is effective in preventing clinically apparent type A hepatitis, not all IG preparations have adequate anti-HAV titers to be protective
(B) If given soon enough after exposure to hepatitis B, hepatitis immune globulin (HBIG) is effective in preventing infection
(C) HBIG and hepatitis B vaccine can be effectively administered simultaneously
(D) Hepatitis B vaccine is effective in preventing delta hepatitis infection in persons who are not HBsAg carriers
(E) IG prophylaxis after needle-stick, sexual, or perinatal exposure to hepatitis C is effective in preventing infection

392. A "bald" tongue (i.e., one devoid of papillae) may be observed in which of the following clinical scenarios?

(A) A 45-year-old man with recent onset of glucose intolerance and change in shoe size
(B) An 18-year-old man with abnormal facies, developmental delay, and myeloblasts noted on peripheral blood smear
(C) A 55-year-old woman with painful joints, eye irritation, and dental caries
(D) A 30-year-old man from Africa with recent mental deterioration, gummatous infiltration of the palate, and a positive rapid plasma reagin (RPR) test
(E) A 25-year-old man with macrocytic anemia and a history of major abdominal surgery

393. Which of the following antiemetics will act on the chemoreceptor trigger zone in the brain?

    (A) Ondansetron
    (B) Metoclopramide
    (C) Prochlorperazine
    (D) Scopolamine
    (E) Diphenhydramine

394. Correct statements concerning the diagnosis of the Zollinger-Ellison syndrome (gastrinoma) include which of the following?

    (A) It should be considered in the differential diagnosis of chronic diarrhea
    (B) It should be considered in the presence of large mucosal folds observed at radiographic examination of the upper gastrointestinal tract
    (C) Endoscopic retrograde pancreatico-duodenography is helpful in identifying gastrinomas missed on selective arteriography or CT
    (D) A patient with recurrent duodenal ulcer whose fasting gastrin is 50 ng/L (repeat 100 ng/L) should undergo a secretin test
    (E) A gastrin level measured 10 min after secretin injection will be 200 ng/L greater than the preinjection level

395. True statements concerning the short bowel syndrome include which of the following?

    (A) Following massive small-bowel resection, a transient syndrome of gastric hypersecretion may develop
    (B) If more than 100 cm of ileum have been resected, dietary fat intake should be reduced to 40 g/d
    (C) Ileal malabsorption of bile salts results in enhanced fluid and electrolyte absorption in the colon
    (D) Antiperistaltic agents would aid fluid and electrolyte absorption
    (E) Loss of ileal tissue is better tolerated than loss of an equal length of jejunal tissue

396. The medical therapy of Crohn's disease can be described by which of the following statements?

    (A) Metronidazole is useful if the perineal area is involved
    (B) Azathioprine may reduce steroid requirements
    (C) Corticosteroids are more effective in the treatment of Crohn's disease of the small intestine than in the treatment of Crohn's disease of the colon
    (D) In persons in whom a remission in disease activity has been achieved, sulfasalazine decreases the frequency of relapse
    (E) Sulfasalazine is contraindicated in the treatment of pregnant women who have Crohn's disease

397. A 40-year-old man has a history of ulcerative colitis. Features of his illness that would contribute to an increased risk of developing colon cancer include

    (A) disease duration of more than 10 years
    (B) history of toxic megacolon
    (C) presence of pancolitis (total colonic involvement)
    (D) presence of pseudopolyps on colonoscopy
    (E) high steroid requirements

398. Subacute ischemic colitis can be described by which of the following statements?

    (A) The usual presenting symptom is severe abdominal pain
    (B) Rectal bleeding may be the presenting symptom
    (C) Involvement of the rectum is uncommon
    (D) Symptoms and signs of nonocclusive ischemic colitis resolve in 2 to 4 weeks
    (E) Angiography is the definitive diagnostic procedure

399. True statements regarding acute bleeding from colonic diverticula include which of the following?

(A) Diverticulitis usually is present
(B) The source of hemorrhage is more likely to be on the right side than on the left side of the colon
(C) Bleeding usually abates spontaneously
(D) Angiographic detection of bleeding usually is unsuccessful
(E) It is the most common cause of acute lower GI bleeding in the elderly

400. Percutaneous needle liver biopsy would be indicated in a diagnostic workup for

(A) unexplained hepatosplenomegaly
(B) persistently abnormal liver function tests
(C) suspected hepatic angioma
(D) suspected miliary tuberculosis
(E) suspected obstruction of the common bile duct

401. Which of the following conditions would likely be associated with the set of serum values presented below?

Total bilirubin: 34 μmol/L (2 mg/dL)
AST: 1.0 μkat/L (60 U/L)
Alkaline phosphatase: 8.0 μkat/L (480 U/L)

(A) Primary biliary cirrhosis
(B) Stricture of the common bile duct
(C) Acute viral hepatitis
(D) Acetaminophen overdose
(E) Chlorpromazine therapy

402. Adenomatous polyps of the colon are correctly characterized by which of the following statements?

(A) Most adenomatous polyps are clinically silent
(B) Polyps represent a marker for the development of colon cancer in adjacent mucosa
(C) The size of an adenomatous polyp correlates with the risk of malignancy
(D) Villous adenomas are more likely than tubular polyps to be malignant
(E) Pedunculated polyps have a greater malignant potential than sessile polyps

403. Acute viral hepatitis can be described by which of the following statements?

(A) There is a direct correlation between peak rise in AST and ALT and the degree of hepatocellular damage
(B) A serum bilirubin concentration greater than 340 μmol/L (20 mg/dL), in the absence of hemolysis, is a poor prognostic sign
(C) A serum sickness-like syndrome may precede the onset of clinical jaundice caused by hepatitis B virus infection
(D) The presenting symptoms and signs are useful in predicting the specific etiologic agent responsible
(E) Steroid therapy has been shown to shorten the clinical course of the illness

404. An 18-year-old man is evaluated because of weight loss and diarrhea. On examination he was found to have pedal edema and decreased breath sounds at the right lung base. A thoracentesis reveals milky fluid. Subsequent laboratory workup reveals lymphocytopenia, hypoproteinemia, and hypogammaglobulinemia. Which of the following features could also be expected with this condition?

(A) Abnormal peripheral lymphatics
(B) Dilated and telangiectatic lymphatic vessels in the lamina propria on small-bowel biopsy
(C) Response to lactose-free diet
(D) Response to low-fat diet supplemented by medium-chain triglycerides
(E) 1 g D-xylose in 5-h urine collection after 25 g oral D-xylose

405. A patient with newly diagnosed tropical sprue could have which of the following extragastrointestinal manifestations of malabsorption?

(A) Megaloblastic anemia
(B) Night blindness
(C) Purpura
(D) Tetany
(E) Pyoderma gangrenosum

406. Correct statements concerning sulfasalazine therapy for inflammatory bowel disease include

   (A) sulfasalazine is a drug that requires cleavage by colonic bacteria to be effective
   (B) the active moiety is sulfapyridine, which inhibits the *Helicobacter* (formerly *Campylobacter*) bacteria believed to cause the colitis
   (C) it must be used along with steroids to provide effective treatment for an acute attack
   (D) the active moiety can be given by enema and provides an effective treatment
   (E) chronic use of sulfasalazine may reduce recurrences in patients with ulcerative colitis

407. Gilbert's syndrome is characterized by which of the following statements?

   (A) The serum total bilirubin is predominantly unconjugated and rarely exceeds 85 μmol/L (5 mg/dL)
   (B) Fasting increases the serum bilirubin concentration
   (C) It appears to be inherited in an autosomal recessive pattern
   (D) Serum bilirubin concentration increases after the administration of phenobarbital
   (E) Examination by light microscopy of liver biopsy specimens discloses normal results

408. Correct statements concerning the hereditary polyposis syndromes include which of the following?

   (A) Gardner's syndrome is characterized by multiple hamartomatous polyps in the large and small intestines
   (B) In Peutz-Jeghers syndrome adenomatous polyps in the large and small intestine have a high rate of malignant degeneration
   (C) Turcot's syndrome is similar to familial colonic polyposis except that malignant brain tumors frequently accompany the polyposis
   (D) Familial colonic polyposis is inherited in an autosomal dominant fashion
   (E) Patients with familial colonic polyposis have a 100 percent incidence of colon cancer by age 40

409. Reye's syndrome often is associated with

   (A) marked hyperbilirubinemia
   (B) ingestion of salicylate
   (C) hyperglycemia
   (D) elevated serum levels of aminotransferase
   (E) recent viral illness

410. An increased incidence of hepatocellular carcinoma is found in which of the following disorders?

   (A) Hemochromatosis
   (B) α_1-Antitrypsin deficiency
   (C) Long-term ingestion of aflatoxin
   (D) Chronic hepatitis B virus infection
   (E) Alcoholic liver disease

411. Which of the following serologic patterns would be consistent with acute hepatitis B infection?

	HBsAg	Anti-HBs	Anti-HBc	HBeAg	Anti-HBeAg
(A)	+	−	IgM	+	−
(B)	+	−	IgG	+	−
(C)	−	−	IgM	−	−
(D)	+	−	IgG	−	+
(E)	−	+	IgG	−	−

412. A patient undergoes a liver biopsy for chronic abnormalities on liver function tests. On pathologic review, multiple granulomas are found. Correct statements concerning this patient's condition include

(A) an empirical trial of steroids should be instituted
(B) sarcoidosis is a possible etiology
(C) a careful drug-exposure history should be obtained
(D) schistosomiasis is a possible etiology
(E) the absence of caseating granulomas rules out miliary tuberculosis

413. A 65-year-old man presents because his wife notes that his eyes are becoming yellow. On further questioning, the patient complains of epigastric discomfort, dark urine, light stools, and pruritus. Past medical history and physical examination are unremarkable. Laboratory tests confirm the clinical impression of an elevation in the serum level of conjugated bilirubin. Abdominal ultrasound demonstrates a mass in the head of the pancreas and enlargement of the common bile duct. Chest x-ray and abdominal-pelvic CT disclose no additional abnormalities. A CT-guided needle biopsy of the mass obtains tissue that, on pathologic examination, reveals neutrophils and fibrous elements.

Which of the following procedures would be reasonable at this point?

(A) Another attempt at CT-guided needle biopsy
(B) Endoscopic retrograde cholangiopancreatography (ERCP)
(C) Celiac angiography
(D) Repeat CT scan in 2 to 3 months
(E) Percutaneous placement of biliary stent

DIRECTIONS: The following group of questions consists of lettered headings followed by a set of numbered items. For each numbered item select the **one** lettered heading with which it is **most** closely associated. Each lettered heading may be used **once, more than once, or not at all.**

Questions 414–417

Match each of the case histories of esophageal disease (see facing page) with the barium swallow x-ray with which it is most likely to be associated.

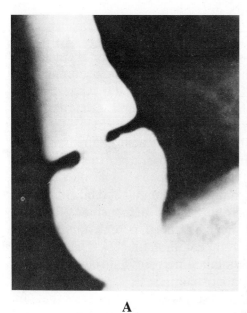

A

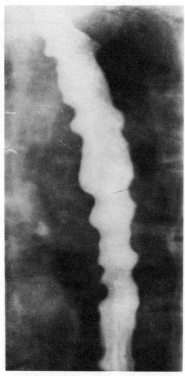

B

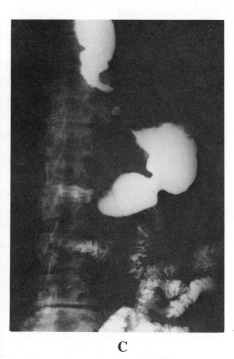

C

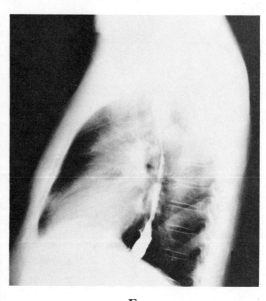

D

E

(A) Radiograph A
(B) Radiograph B
(C) Radiograph C
(D) Radiograph D
(E) Radiograph E

414. A 40-year-old truck driver has had occasional dysphagia for solid foods for the last 5 years

415. A 61-year-old bartender has had frequent heartburn for the last 4 years and dysphagia for solid foods for the last 3 months

416. A 55-year-old alcoholic man has had mild dysphagia for solid foods for the last month, during which time he has lost 5 kg (11 lb)

417. A 34-year-old accountant has occasional dysphagia for solid foods and frequent retrosternal chest pain that radiates to the back, occurs at rest, and lasts several minutes

Disorders of the Alimentary Tract and Hepatobiliary System

Answers

320. The answer is A. *(Chap 39. Field, N Engl J Med 321:800, 1989.)* In the case described, the osmolality of fecal water is approximately equal to serum osmolality. Furthermore, there is no osmotic "gap" in the fecal water—the osmolality of the fecal water can be accounted for by the stool electrolyte composition: $[2 \times ([Na^+] + [K^+])] = [2 \times (39 + 96)] = 270$. A villous adenoma of the colon typically produces a secretory diarrhea. Lactose intolerance, nontropical sprue, and excessive use of milk of magnesia produce osmotic diarrheas with osmotic "gaps" caused by lactose, carbohydrates, and magnesium, respectively. Pancreatic insufficiency causes steatorrhea, not watery diarrhea.

321. The answer is A. *(Chap 42. Frank, JAMA 262:3031, 1989.)* Initial considerations in evaluating a patient with jaundice require a determination of whether or not the patient has primarily unconjugated hyperbilirubinemia or conjugated hyperbilirubinemia, in which case more than 50 percent of the serum bilirubin is direct-reacting. Since this patient has clear-cut conjugated hyperbilirubinemia, he may have the (solubilized) bilirubin detectable in the urine. The major differential diagnosis in this case is between impaired hepatocyte bilirubin excretion and extrahepatic biliary obstruction. In the former case, interference with the biliary excretion of bilirubin that has been previously conjugated by hepatocytes leads to entry of this pigment into the systemic circulation. Such intrahepatic obstruction may occur in drug reactions, alcoholic hepatitis, the third trimester of pregnancy, the postoperative state, and viral or autoimmune hepatitis. In the case of the Dubin-Johnson and Rotor syndromes, the conjugated hyperbilirubinemia is due to a congenital defect in bilirubin excretion and is generally not associated with abnormalities of alkaline phosphatase or hepatic aminotransferases. Patients who have conjugated hyperbilirubinemia and abnormal liver enzymes generally fall into two groups, those whose aminotransferase elevation is dominant and who are suspected of having a hepatocellular disorder and those with primary elevation of alkaline phosphatase and who are likely to have either intra- or extrahepatic biliary obstruction. In the latter group of patients, it is imperative to rule out extrahepatic obstruction by means of ultrasonography of the right upper quadrant or abdominal CT. If the biliary ducts are not dilated on radiologic evaluation, the next most appropriate procedure would be either a percutaneous transhepatic cholangiogram or endoscopic retrograde cholangiopancreatography.

322. The answer is C. *(Chaps 39, 279. Goodgame, Ann Intern Med 119:924, 1993.)* Diarrhea in patients with AIDS may be due to many microbiologic agents. Patients infected with HIV-1 are at risk of infection with nonopportunistic pathogens such as *Salmonella, Shigella, Campylobacter, Entamoeba, Chlamydia, Neisseria gonorrhoeae, Treponema pallidum,* and *Giardia lamblia* and are also at risk for infections that occur in the presence of immunodeficiency. Infectious agents in the latter category include protozoa such as *Cryptosporidium, Isospora belli,* or *Blastocystis;* bacteria such as *Mycobacterium avium-intracellulare;* and viral pathogens such as cytomegalovirus (CMV), herpes simplex virus, adenovirus, and HIV itself. CMV infection of the gastrointestinal tract may present with upper GI symptoms, nausea, vomiting, abdominal pain, or symptoms of ulcerative colitis such as bloody diarrhea. Diagnosis of CMV infection, which almost certainly represents reinfection or reactivation since affected persons are virtually always previously exposed to CMV, can be diagnosed by finding typical cytomegalic cells on histopathologic analysis. Such cells, evidence of the CMV-mediated cytopathic effect, are characterized by being large (25 to 35 μm) with a basophilic internuclear inclusion (sometimes surrounded by a clear halo—the "owl's eye" effect) and frequently associated with clusters of intracytoplasmic inclusions. Serious CMV-mediated gastroenteritis should be treated with ganciclovir, which may result in weight gain and improved quality of life. Foscarnet, an inhibitor of viral DNA polymerase, may be useful in cases of ganciclovir failure or intolerance. Antibacterial antibiotics, antifungal agents, antituberculous drugs, and acyclovir have no role in histologically proven CMV colitis.

323. The answer is D. *(Chap 252.)* Physiologic feedback loops mediate inhibition of gastrin release, thereby inhibiting secretion of acid in the stomach; the two most important are acidic gastric pH and presence of fat or hypertonic fluids in the duodenum. Acid-induced release of somatostatin by antral endocrine cells may mediate, in a paracrine fashion, inhibition of secretion of gastrin and activity of parietal cells. Secretin is released in the presence of acid in the upper small intestine and can also inhibit secretion of gastric acid. Other peptides found in the small intestine that may play a role in the inhibition of secretion of gastric acid include gastric inhibitory peptide, vasoactive intestinal peptide, enteroglucagon, neurotensin, peptide YY, and urogastrone. Histamine, presumably released by the mast cells lying adjacent to the acid secretory parietal cells in the gastric mucosa, acts together with gastrin and acetylcholine to stimulate release of acid.

324. The answer is B. *(Chap 252. Graham, Ann Intern Med 116:705, 1992.)* Gastric colonization with the short gram-negative bacillus *Helicobacter* (formerly *Campylobacter*) *pylori* is thought to be the principal cause of active chronic gastritis, which is characterized by a neutrophilic exudate in, but not ulceration of, the gastric mucosa. The bacteria do not invade the mucosa, but rather grow in the deep mucus gel layer and synthesize glycoprotein-destroying proteases and phospholipases, thereby contributing to mucosal injury. Though *H. pylori* colonization is associated with gastric and duodenal ulcers, causality remains unproven. However, virtually 100 percent of patients with active chronic gastritis harbor a dense gastric infiltration with this organism. *H. pylori* may be identified in gastric biopsy samples by histology (the bacteria are Giemsa-positive), culture, or urease activity. Colloidal bismuth compounds can eradicate the organism by unknown means; treatment with ampicillin and metronidazole is also associated with eradication of *H. pylori* with concomitant disappearance of the inflammatory changes in the gastric mucosa.

325. The answer is E. *(Chap 41.)* The presence of coffee-grounds material in a nasogastric aspirate from a person with melena indicates recent bleeding of the upper gastrointestinal tract. In a patient with obvious signs of cirrhosis, esophageal varices must be considered in the differential diagnosis of upper gastrointestinal bleeding; other possible diagnoses include peptic ulcer, gastroduodenitis, esophagitis, and Mallory-Weiss tear. Before diagnostic procedures, such as endoscopy or upper gastrointestinal series, are undertaken, the placement of a large-bore intravenous line and commencement of volume replacement therapy are mandatory in order to prevent hypotension. Moreover, blood should be typed and cross-matched in case of further bleeding. Diagnostic angiography is indicated only when brisk bleeding prevents diagnosis by endoscopy or barium study. Specific therapy for variceal bleeding—i.e., passage of a Sengstaken-Blakemore tube and intravenous infusion of vasopressin—should be considered if diagnostic studies reveal bleeding varices.

326. The answer is A. *(Chap 44.)* A diagnostic paracentesis in which 50 to 100 mL of fluid is removed is the central test in the routine evaluation of a patient with ascites of new onset. Routine tests include examination of the gross appearance of the fluid, protein content, cell count, white cell differential, Gram stain, acid-fast stain, and microbiologic cultures. The plasma-ascites albumin gradient may be helpful in characterizing ascites. If the difference between the plasma albumin and ascitic fluid is less than 1.1 g/dL, then conditions other than uncomplicated cirrhosis should be considered. Chylous ascites indicates that a turbid, milky, or creamy peritoneal fluid has been obtained, usually due to the presence of thoracic or intestinal lymph. Such a fluid shows fat globules on microscopic examination and an increased triglyceride content (greater than 1000 mg/dL) on chemical analysis. This condition results from lymphatic obstruction, most commonly due to trauma (especially lymphoma), tuberculosis, or filariasis. Nephrotic syndrome may also be associated with apparent chylous ascites, but the lymphocyte count is usually much lower than 250/mL.

327. The answer is D. *(Chap 251.)* A Zenker's diverticulum typically causes halitosis and regurgitation of saliva and food particles consumed several days earlier. When a Zenker's diverticulum fills with food, it may produce dysphagia by compressing the esophagus. Gastric outlet obstruction can cause bloating and regurgitation of newly ingested food. Gastrointestinal disorders associated with scleroderma include esophageal reflux, the development of wide-mouthed colonic diverticula, and stasis with bacterial overgrowth. Achalasia typically presents with dysphagia for both solids and liquids. Gastric retention caused by the autonomic neuropathy of diabetes mellitus usually results in postprandial epigastric discomfort and bloating.

328. The answer is D. *(Chaps 252, 253.)* The x-ray presented shows a large malignant-appearing gastric ulcer on the lesser curvature of the stomach. Because the differentiation between benign and malignant gastric ulcer by x-ray is not infallible (there are as many as 25 percent false positives and negatives), the diagnosis of gastric cancer should be confirmed by fiberoptic gastroscopy with brush cytology and at least six biopsies from the ulcer margin. Gastroscopy is useful in diagnosing primary gastric lymphoma, which is associated with a much better 5-year survival rate than is adenocarcinoma. Double-contrast radiographic techniques help to detect small lesions by improving mucosal detail but do not generally improve accuracy in distinguishing benign from malignant ulcers.

329. The answer is A. *(Chap 256. Lynn, N Engl J Med 329:1940–1945, 1993.)* This presentation is classic for one of the three clinical variants of the irritable bowel syndrome, each associated with abnormal colonic motility and increased visceral perception. Other groups have chronic abdominal pain and constipation or alternating constipation and diarrhea. The chronic nature of the condition and the presence of formed stool militate against a workup for secretory or osmotic diarrhea. Giardiasis, while typically occult and requiring jejunal sampling for diagnosis, usually presents with belching and pain, not diarrhea of 4 years' duration. The absence of discernible significant organic pathology should not prompt a discussion with the patient that centers on a psychogenic cause of her problem; such an approach will frequently lead to alienation of the patient. Instead, an effort to effect safe symptomatic improvement of the diarrhea with antispasmodics is worthwhile. Psyllium to increase stool bulk is a good choice for patients with irritable bowel syndrome who complain of constipation.

330. The answer is D. *(Chap 43.)* In addition to diagnostic paracentesis, an important part of the evaluation for ascites of new onset includes a careful physical examination. Evidence for cirrhosis, such as palmar erythema and spider angiomas, should be sought. Supraclavicular adenopathy (Virchow's node) or a hard periumbilical node (Sister Mary Joseph's nodule) suggests metastatic carcinoma arising from a pelvic or gastrointestinal primary site.

331. The answer is A. *(Chap 259.)* Virtually any condition that can lead to abdominal pain needs to be included in the differential diagnosis of appendicitis. Diagnostic accuracy is about 75 percent. Although acute diverticulitis, cholecystitis, perforated ulcer, pancreatitis, obstruction, renal stone, and pyelonephritis can present diagnostic difficulties, the most frequent findings at operation when appendicitis is incorrectly diagnosed are (in order of frequency) mesenteric lymphadenitis, no organic disease, acute pelvic inflammatory disease, ruptured ovarian cyst, and acute gastroenteritis. Mesenteric lymphadenitis indicates the presence of enlarged, inflamed lymph nodes at the mesenteric root; *Yersinia* species have been cultured from nodal specimens obtained at operation in some patients with this condition.

332. The answer is C. *(Chap 251.)* Achalasia is a motor disorder of esophageal smooth muscle in which the lower esophageal sphincter (LES) does not relax properly in response to swallowing and normal esophageal peristalsis is replaced by abnormal contractions. Manometry reveals a normal or elevated LES pressure and a reduced or absent swallow-induced relaxation. A decreased number of ganglion cells is noted in the esophageal body and LES of patients with achalasia, suggesting that defective innervation of these areas is the underlying abnormality. Dysphagia, chest pain, and regurgitation are the predominant symptoms. The chest x-ray often reveals absence of the gastric air bubble and the barium swallow reveals a dilated esophagus. Calcium-channel antagonists such as nifedipine relax smooth muscle and have been effective in treating some patients. However, the mainstay of therapy remains pneumatic dilation.

333. The answer is D. *(Chap 252. McCarthy, N Engl J Med 325:1017, 1991.)* A physician has many alternatives when deciding upon a therapeutic course in a patient with radiographically or endoscopically proven duodenal ulcer. Therapy is based on neutralization of gastric acids by antacids, the inhibition of gastric acid secretion by antisecretory agents such as H_2-receptor antagonists, prostaglandins (PGE_1, PGE_2), and proton pump inhibitors (e.g., omeprazole). Drugs such as sucralfate act locally by impeding diffusion of hydrogen ions to the base of the ulcer and by binding other injurious molecules. Colloidal bismuth stimulates gastric mucosal secretion of prostaglandins and glycoprotein mucus, as well as eradicates *H. pylori* colonization. Treatment for 4 to 6 weeks with any individual member of any of the above classes will probably be sufficient to induce healing in most patients. For the average patient, maintenance therapy is not required. While there is no evidence that dietary changes are important, elimination of cigarette smoking should be undertaken. There is no evidence, for example, that cimetidine or any other related H_2-receptor antagonist is superior to sucralfate in promoting ulcer healing. Side effects among the various drug classes differ. Sucralfate is associated with a very low rate of side effects; however, it can reduce the bioavailability of the fluoroquinolone antibiotics, so these drugs should not be used concomitantly.

334. The answer is B. *(Chap 252. Walt, N Engl J Med 327:1575, 1992.)* Gastric mucosal injury, potentially resulting in ulcers and erosive gastritis, may be produced by aspirin and nonsteroidal anti-inflammatory agents including indomethacin, ibuprofen, and naproxen. These agents may be directly toxic to the gastric mucosa by depleting protective endogenous mucosal prostaglandins. Moreover, they more directly interrupt the mucosal barrier, thereby allowing back-diffusion of hydrogen ions as well as reducing gastric mucus secretion and increasing gastric acid secretion. The prostaglandin E_1 analogue misoprostol is effective in preventing ulcers and gastritis caused by nonsteroidal anti-inflammatory drugs. Its mechanism of action is believed to be stimulation of gastric mucus and duodenal bicarbonate secretion, as well as the maintenance of the gastric mucosal barrier via epithelial cell restitution.

335. The answer is C. *(Chap 253.)* Squamous cell cancer of the esophagus accounts for approximately 10,000 deaths annually in the U.S. Worldwide, incidences vary greatly, but it is particularly common in a belt from the Caspian Sea to northern China. In the United States, epidemiologic studies have linked smoking and alcohol to squamous cell cancer of the esophagus and may explain the association of this tumor with head and neck carcinoma. Exposure to agents that damage the mucosa (e.g., very hot tea, lye, radiation) or ingestion of carcinogens such as nitrites, smoked opiates, or fungal toxins is associated with an increased risk of esophageal carcinoma. The long-term stasis associated with achalasia leads to chronic irritation of the esophagus, which is thought to predispose to cancer formation. Tylosis is a genetically acquired disease characterized by thickening of the skin of the hands and feet and is associated with squamous cell cancer of the esophagus. Chronic gastric reflux (Barrett's esophagus) is associated with adenocarcinoma but not squamous cell carcinoma of the esophagus.

336. The answer is C. *(Chap 252.)* The causes of stomal (anastomotic) ulceration following peptic ulcer surgery include incomplete vagotomy, retained gastric antrum, the Zollinger-Ellison syndrome (gastrinoma), poor gastric emptying, and ingestion of ulcerogenic drugs. In the case presented, if the previous antrectomy had been complete, the serum gastrin level should not be elevated. An elevated serum gastrin level that declines after intravenous administration of secretin is characteristic of a retained gastric antrum attached to the duodenal stump. Neither frequent antacid therapy nor a total vagotomy is effective in healing a stomal ulcer; thus, resection of the retained antrum is indicated. In the Zollinger-Ellison syndrome, the serum gastrin level paradoxically increases after intravenous infusion of secretin.

337. The answer is E. *(Chap 253. Haber, Semin Oncol 15:154, 1988.)* Malignant neoplasms of the stomach typically present with epigastric pain, postprandial fullness, and weight loss or fatigue. Iron-deficiency anemia may also be seen. Histologically, 90 percent of stomach cancers are adenocarcinomas and 10 percent are due to non-Hodgkin's lymphomas or leiomyosarcomas. Risks for the development of gastric adenocarcinoma include decreased gastric acidity, prior antrectomy (latency period of 15 to 20 years), atrophic gastritis, and presence of blood group A. The aforementioned risk factors are not associated with the development of primary gastric lymphoma, a more treatable disease than adenocarcinoma. The only real chance for a cure with adenocarcinoma is complete surgical removal of the tumor and resection of adjacent lymph nodes. The use of adjuvant chemotherapy or radiation therapy or both following complete resections in adenocarcinoma seems to offer little benefit compared with surgery alone. Moreover, the use of these modalities in cases where resection was only partial is controversial, although combination chemotherapy with a regimen such as 5-fluorouracil, doxorubicin, and mitomycin C will lead to partial responses in up to 50 percent of the cases. On the other hand, complete removal of the tumor in patients with gastric lymphoma results in a 5-year survival rate of 40 to 60 percent (compared with 25 to 30 percent in adenocarcinoma). Combination chemotherapy with regimens such as CHOP (cyclophosphamide, doxorubicin, vincristine, and prednisone), used in more typical disseminated non-Hodgkin's lymphomas, may well be a useful adjunct in the postsurgical setting and may even be able to substitute for surgery. The latter point is a subject of much debate; however, fears that presurgical chemotherapy would lead to an inordinant risk of bleeding or perforation seem unfounded based on recent studies.

338. The answer is A. *(Chap 254.)* Though most patients with celiac sprue will have a typical malabsorptive syndrome characterized by bloating, diarrhea, and weight loss, other presentations include iron-deficiency anemia; abnormal bleeding due to hypoprothrombinemia; metabolic bone disease typified by bone pain, bony tenderness, demineralization of bone, and compression fractures; and emotional disturbances brought on by weight loss of uncertain etiology. Response to a gluten-free diet in the presence of documented malabsorption and the typical flattened villi on small bowel biopsy would establish the diagnosis. The etiology of the osteomalacia is a combination of calcium malabsorption due to lack of absorptive surface for vitamin D in the distal small bowel as well as the absence of vitamin D required for optimal bone mineralization. Established associations between celiac sprue and diabetes mellitus, selected IgA deficiency, and lymphocytic colitis have been previously documented.

339. The answer is C. *(Chap 254.)*   Eosinophilic enteritis is a disorder of the stomach, small intestine, or colon or all three in which some part of the gut wall is infiltrated by eosinophils. The diagnosis also requires the presence of peripheral blood eosinophilia. Although early reports emphasized the presence of food allergies, less than half the patients have a history of food allergies or asthma. The presence of anemia, Hemoccult-positive stools, abnormalities of the ileum and cecum on barium radiographic studies, and a favorable response to administration of steroids may make eosinophilic enteritis difficult to distinguish from Crohn's disease. Although no controlled trials of corticosteroid therapy have been performed, symptoms usually respond to short-term corticosteroid therapy.

340. The answer is C. *(Chap 254.)*   Malabsorption due to bacterial overgrowth results from bacterial utilization of ingested vitamins and the deconjugation of bile salts by bacteria in the proximal jejunum. Deconjugated bile salts do not form micelles in the jejunum, and long-chain fatty acids cannot be absorbed. The bacteria also separate ingested vitamin B_{12} from intrinsic factor, thus interfering with its absorption from the ileum. The absorption of simple carbohydrates generally is not impaired, though complex carbohydrates may be metabolized by bacteria. Thus, persons with bacterial overgrowth have steatorrhea, an abnormal Schilling test (even with administration of intrinsic factor), increased metabolism of nonabsorbable carbohydrates (e.g., lactulose), and increased bacterial concentrations in jejunal aspirates. Absorption of D-xylose, a simple carbohydrate, is often normal.

341. The answer is A. *(Chap 254.)*   The incidence of isolated lactase deficiency is about 10 percent in the adult white population but higher in black Americans and Asians. Patients with acquired lactase deficiency have failure of normal hydrolysis of disaccharides in the brush border of intestinal epithelial cells. Common symptoms include abdominal cramps, bloating, and diarrhea after the ingestion of milk or dairy products. Since the lactose is not hydrolyzed and absorbed, an osmotic effect shifts fluid into the lumen. The symptoms are not due to an allergic reaction, insofar as blood glucose fails to rise normally after an ingestion of an oral dose of lactose. However, this test is plagued by frequent false positive and false negative results. Measurement of hydrogen released after ingestion of 50 g lactose is more sensitive and specific. Hydrogen release due to the action of colonic bacteria on unabsorbed lactose causes a rapid rise in breath hydrogen, indicative of a failure to absorb the disaccharide. Interestingly, patients with lactase deficiency may tolerate yogurt because of the presence of bacterial-derived lactases.

342. The answer is C. *(Chap 256.)*   Occlusive acute ischemia of the small intestine may result from an arterial thrombus or embolus in the celiac or superior mesenteric arteries and occurs most commonly in patients with atrial fibrillation, artificial heart valves, or valvular heart disease. Arterial thrombosis is associated with extensive atherosclerosis, low cardiac output, or both. Acute mesenteric ischemia, such as might be caused by an embolus originating in the dilated left atrium of a patient with rheumatic valvular disease, produces colicky periumbilical pain that changes to diffuse and constant discomfort. Vomiting and diarrhea may also occur. Abdominal examination reveals mild tenderness and distention, but is often not dramatic even in the face of intestinal necrosis. Mild gastrointestinal bleeding, rather than massive hemorrhage, is the rule. Abdominal films disclose air-fluid levels and distention. Barium study, if undertaken, will reveal nonspecific dilation, poor motility, and thick mucosal folds ("thumb printing") of the small intestine. Gangrene may occur with more dramatic manifestations of peritonitis, sepsis, and shock 24 to 72 h after the initial insult. When acute mesenteric ischemia is suspected, patients should undergo immediate celiac and mesenteric angiography to localize the embolus and then embolectomy should be performed. However, in many cases the ischemic duration has been prolonged and, at the time of surgery, resection of a segment of small bowel may be necessary. Moreover, many patients who require surgery to correct the complications of acute mesenteric ischemia are poor operative risks due to age, dehydration, sepsis, and comorbid disease.

343. The answer is D. *(Chap 254. Relman, N Engl J Med 327:293–301, 1992.)* The man described in the question has Whipple's disease, a bowel disorder associated with dilated gut lymphatics and characterized by weight loss, abdominal pain, diarrhea, malabsorption, central nervous system manifestations, and arthralgias. Electron microscopy has revealed the presence of bacilliform bodies in the lamina propria; these rod-shaped structures, which are located within or adjacent to macrophages that contain PAS-positive granules, have been identified as the gram-negative actinomycete *Tropheryma whippelii*. The treatment of choice is at least 1 year of therapy with antibiotics; trimethoprim-sulfamethoxazole is the first-line therapy. Clinical recovery is accompanied by the disappearance of the bacilliform bodies.

344. The answer is B. *(Chap 255.)* Sigmoidoscopic demonstration of a hyperemic mucosa studded with plaquelike lesions is characteristic of pseudomembranous (antibiotic-associated) colitis, which is caused by the enterotoxin of *Clostridium difficile*. Although symptoms commonly develop while the offending antibiotic is still being taken, the syndrome may not become evident until several days or weeks after completion of therapy. Ischemic colitis may cause bloody diarrhea but not the mucosal lesions described. Amebic or *Shigella* infestation is associated with punched-out ulcerations of the mucosa. Toxic megacolon is a complication of active colitis. Treatment is primarily directed at eradicating the bacteria with oral vancomycin or the less expensive metronidazole.

345. The answer is D. *(Chap 254. Trier, N Engl J Med 325:1709–1719, 1991.)* The histologic specimen pictured in the question shows villous atrophy, crypt hyperplasia, and inflammation typical of intestinal changes in nontropical sprue (celiac disease), an illness with a high incidence in Ireland. The disease, due to gluten (water-insoluble wheat protein)-mediated intestinal damage, is associated with an increased incidence of histocompatibility antigens HLA-DR3 and HLA-DQw2. Although two-thirds of symptomatic cases present in childhood, the onset of clinical symptoms of malabsorption may occur at any age. Persons with subclinical sprue during adolescence may have mild growth retardation and may be smaller than their siblings. Because the villous absorptive surface is markedly reduced in affected persons, an acquired lactase deficiency is often present and causes symptoms of milk intolerance. A strict gluten-free diet or use of corticosteroids in refractory disease usually relieves symptoms and signs of malabsorption and promotes restoration of normal jejunal histology. Failure to respond to a gluten-free diet suggests alternative diagnoses such as intestinal lymphoma, and gluten challenge followed by biopsy is indicated. A malabsorptive syndrome associated with abdominal pain, arthralgias, low-grade fever, and lymphadenopathy is not typical of celiac disease and should suggest another diagnosis, such as Whipple's disease or intestinal lymphoma.

346. The answer is D. *(Chap 257. Mandel, N Engl J Med 328:1365–1371, 1993.)* The goal of screening for colorectal cancer is to detect surgically curable neoplasms. Though rigid or flexible sigmoidoscopy clearly has a role in early detection of distal colon cancers, the overall benefit or cost/benefit of routine screening in this fashion has yet to be established. Most efforts have been in the area of Hemoccult testing for occult fecal blood. The following features complicate the use of this modality: (1) approximately 50 percent of those with documented colorectal cancers have a negative Hemoccult test; (2) asymptomatic cancers are found in only 10 percent of those who test positive (although benign polyps will be detected in an additional 20 to 30 percent); and (3) those with a positive test are subjected to additional uncomfortable and expensive procedures including sigmoidoscopy, barium enema, and colonoscopy. Nonetheless, a recently reported study from the University of Minnesota documented a statistically significant reduction in mortality in a group of patients undergoing annual Hemoccult screening compared with a randomized control group who received routine care. A cost-effectiveness analysis of this study has not yet been performed. The present American Cancer Society recommendations are somewhat more aggressive than the available data would completely support: annual digital rectal examinations beginning at age 40, annual fecal Hemoccult screening beginning at age 50, and sigmoidoscopy (preferably flexible) every 3 to 5 years, beginning at age 50 for asymptomatic persons at average risk. Of course, those patients with a positive family history or other high-risk features in whom the probability of colorectal cancer is higher than that in the average population should be more aggressively screened.

347. The answer is C. *(Chap 258. Crook, N Engl J Med 324:709, 1991.)* Total resection of the primary tumor is the treatment of choice for both colon and rectal carcinoma. Assuming that metastases are ruled out, the presence or absence of extension into the muscularis mucosa or the presence of carcinoma in regional lymph nodes is an important prognostic feature. For example, those with regional lymph node involvement have a 30 to 60 percent 5-year survival, whereas those whose cancer extends into the muscularis but not to the mucosa and who do not have positive lymph nodes have an 85 percent 5-year survival. 5-Fluorouracil (5-FU) is the most active single agent in treating advanced colorectal cancer, but adjuvant chemotherapy with 5-FU in high-risk (serosal or nodal involvement) patients has not shown a statistically meaningful reduction in the rate of recurrence. On the other hand, recent randomized trials have indicated a survival benefit if 5-FU is administered in combination with the antihelminthic agent levamisole in patients with node-positive tumors. Furthermore, radiation therapy to the pelvis can significantly lower the probability of local recurrence in patients with high-risk rectal carcinoma. Data from several controlled studies indicate that postoperative radiation therapy combined with chemotherapy (including 5-FU) appears to reduce the likelihood of local recurrences and to increase the potential for long-term survival without recurrence. In this setting, chemotherapy may be acting as a radiation sensitizer, since chemotherapy alone in these patients seems to have little beneficial effect.

348. The answer is C. *(Chap 255.)* Radiographic demonstration of luminal narrowing, mucosal ulceration, and cobblestoning in the ileum is compatible with a diagnosis of regional enteritis. In Whipple's disease, x-rays characteristically show marked thickening of mucosal folds in the duodenum and jejunum. On barium enema, an appendiceal abscess usually presents as a mass indenting the cecal tip. Adenocarcinoma of the small bowel usually occurs as an ulcerated mass lesion in the duodenum. Infiltrating lymphomas of the distal bowel may be difficult to distinguish from regional enteritis radiographically, but stenotic bowel segments would not suggest lymphoma.

349. The answer is E. *(Chap 255.)* The clinical history and x-ray presented in the question are consistent with toxic megacolon in association with severe ulcerative colitis. Toxic megacolon is most likely to occur when hypomotility agents, such as diphenoxylate or loperamide, are given to persons with severe colitis, or when such persons undergo a barium-enema radiographic procedure. In the case presented, a barium enema was not only dangerous but, in fact, unnecessary, because the presence of diarrhea and signs of systemic illness indicated that the disease no longer was limited to the rectum. Colonic perforation may also be associated with severe ulcerative colitis; the presence of subdiaphragmatic air on abdominal x-rays would be suggestive.

350. The answer is D. *(Chap 264.)*   Amino acids (except for the branched-chain amino acids leucine, isoleucine, and valine) are taken up by the liver via the portal circulation and are metabolized to urea. Severe liver damage disrupts normal amino acid metabolism and is reflected in elevated serum levels of non-branched-chain amino acids. Since urea cannot be produced, ammonia cannot be handled. Elevated levels of serum ammonia certainly play a large role in the development of hepatic encephalopathy in liver failure and portal hypertension. Therefore, levels of ammonia and, in the case of alkylosis, ammonium ion rise at the expense of urea. Other mechanisms leading to increased blood ammonia levels include excessive amounts of intestinal nitrogen (e.g., due to bleeding); decreased intestinal motility allowing greater bacterial deamination of amino acids; depressed renal function leading to an increase in blood urea nitrogen and a greater opportunity for bacterial urease to convert this to ammonia; alkalosis, which will preferentially lead the NH_4^+/NH_3 equilibrium in favor of ammonia; and portal hypertension, which will allow ammonia from the gut to bypass hepatic detoxification.

351. The answer is D. *(Chap 264.)*   Hepatic enzymes play a critical role in the metabolism of many drugs and hormones. So-called phase I reactions result in modification of reactive groups by oxidation, reduction, hydroxylation, sulfoxidation, deamination, dealkylation, or methylation. The microsomal P450 system is an example of an enzymatic system that carries out some of these reactions, usually leading to drug inactivation. Therefore, in the case of severe liver disease and suppressed availability of such detoxifying enzymes, drug clearance will decrease. The following drugs require dosage adjustments in patients with liver disease: phenytoin, phenobarbital, acetaminophen, glucocorticoids, lidocaine, quinidine, propranolol, nafcillin, chloramphenicol, tetracycline, trimethoprim, and rifampin. On the other hand, certain drugs, such as cyclophosphamide and the antidepressant imipramine, require conversion to their active moieties by this enzyme system. Phase II reactions, generally resulting in a more soluble compound allowing biliary or renal excretion, include conversion of substances to their glucuronide or sulfate derivatives.

352. The answer is E. *(Chap 257. Aaltonen, Science 260:812, 1993.)*   The specific cause of colon cancer is unknown, although recent studies reveal an excess of genetic allele loss in advanced colonic neoplasia. However, certain diseases are known to increase the risk of development of cancer of the colon. Crohn's colitis is associated with an increased risk of colon cancer, although the risk is less than that for patients with ulcerative colitis. Colon cancer has been observed to occur with increased frequency in patients with uterine cancer. Patients with adenomatous polyps are at higher risk for the subsequent development of colon cancer than is the general population. Therefore, such patients should have periodic follow-up examinations. As many as 25 percent of patients with colorectal carcinoma have a family history of this disease; recent reports suggest the role of a gene on chromosome 2, which codes for a gene involved in DNA repair, in many of these cases. The polyps in juvenile polyposis are hamartomatous and have no malignant potential. Colonic neoplasms at a site distal to the ureteral implant have been noted to occur 15 to 30 years after uterosigmoidostomy.

353. The answer is D. *(Chap 268.)*   Primary biliary cirrhosis (PBC) is a disease of unknown etiology, but the frequent association with autoimmune disorders such as rheumatoid arthritis, CRST syndrome, scleroderma, and sicca syndrome has suggested that an abnormal immune response plays an etiologic role. The disease typically affects middle-aged women and runs a slowly progressive course, with death resulting from hepatic insufficiency occurring within 10 years of diagnosis. A positive antimitochondrial antibody test is relatively sensitive and specific for PBC, occurring in greater than 90 percent of patients. Other serum abnormalities include increased alkaline phosphatase and 5′-nucleotidase activities and the presence of cryoproteins. Treatment is entirely supportive. Neither corticosteroids nor D-penicillamine has proved to be effective. Colchicine, methotrexate, ursodiol, and cyclosporine may each have a role in slowing the progression of disease. Impaired bile excretion may lead to sequelae associated with malabsorption of the fat-soluble vitamins A, D, E, and K.

354. The answer is C. *(Chap 267.)* Autoimmune hepatitis is a serious disorder characterized by progressive hepatic inflammation with a 6-month mortality of 40 percent. Typical cases have features of autoimmunity such as arthritis, vasculitis, or sicca syndrome. Serologic correlates include hypergammaglobulinemia (generally >2.5 g/dL), rheumatoid factor, and circulating autoantibodies (i.e., antinuclear, smooth muscle, and thyroid). There are several variants: (1) type 1, the classic syndrome seen in young women with lupoid features and circulating ANA; (2) type 2a, also seen in young women (mainly from western Europe) but associated with high titers of antibodies to liver and kidney microsomal antigens (LKM-1) and responsive to corticosteroids; and (3) type 2b, which occurs in older (Mediterranean) men and is associated with low LKM-1 levels and interferon responsiveness. Rheumatoid factor elevation is nonspecific and not helpful in establishing the diagnosis. Hepatitis D infection would require prior infection with hepatitis B. Hepatitis E is rare in western Europe and never progresses to chronicity.

355. The answer is D. *(Chap 272.)* Synthesized from hepatic cholesterol, the primary bile acids cholic and chenodeoxycholic acid are conjugated with glycine or taurine and excreted into the bile. Other secondary bile acids may be formed in the intestine by the action of colonic bacteria. One of the most important characteristics of bile acids is their detergent properties, which allow them to form molecular aggregates with cholesterol termed *micelles*. Cholesterol is poorly soluble in water; its solubility in bile is dependent both on the lipid concentration and the relevant amount of bile acids and lecithin. Bile acids are also required for the normal intestinal absorption of dietary fats by a similar micellar transport mechanism. Finally, bile acids are important in facilitating water and electrolyte transport in the intestine. In order to maintain the reusable pool of bile acids, the molecules are actively reabsorbed in the distal ileum, taken up in the portal bloodstream, and returned to hepatocytes for reconjugation and resecretion. Compared with a normal-size bile acid pool of 2 to 4 g, the daily fecal loss of bile acids is only in the range of 0.5 g.

356. The answer is C. *(Chap 268. Crossley, Gut 26:325, 1985.)* Spontaneous bacterial peritonitis refers to the development of acute bacterial peritonitis without an obvious primary source of infection. The diagnosis can be suspected on clinical grounds and supported by an elevated leukocyte count in ascitic fluid. However, confirmation of the diagnosis can be made only by bacterial culture. In the United States, *Escherichia coli* is the leading cause of spontaneous bacterial peritonitis and is isolated from approximately 30 percent of patients. *Streptococcus pneumoniae* and *Klebsiella* species are the second and third most commonly isolated organisms. Therefore, when the diagnosis is suspected based on neutrophil count in ascitic fluid of >250 μL, empiric therapy with cefatoxime or ampicillin and an aminoglycoside is frequently instituted.

357. The answer is E. *(Chap 274.)* Purtscher's retinopathy is a relatively rare but devastating complication of acute pancreatitis. It is characterized by sudden loss of vision and the presence of cotton-wool spots and hemorrhages in the area of the optic disc and macula. The cause is thought to be occlusion of the posterior retinal artery by aggregated granulocytes.

358. The answer is D. *(Chap 272.)* Selected patients with gallstones may respond well to treatment with oral chenodeoxycholic acid, its related molecule ursodeoxycholic acid, or both. Patients who are candidates for such therapy must have either cholesterol or mixed radiolucent gallstones. Secondly, gallstones greater than 1.5 cm in diameter or those in gallbladders failing to opacify following oral cholecystography will be very unlikely to respond to dissolution therapy. Chenodeoxycholic acid is thought to work by decreasing HMG-CoA reductase activity and thereby hepatically secreted cholesterol. Deoxycholic acid works by a similar mechanism, as well as by retarding cholesterol crystal nucleation. Up to 2 years of therapy with these agents is often required to dissolve a gallstone; after withdrawal, there is a recurrence rate of up to 30 to 50 percent. The same group of patients who are candidates for medical therapy to dissolve gallstones are also generally the patients who are candidates for gallstone lithotripsy, a method of fragmenting stones by extracorporeal shock waves.

359. The answer is A. *(Chap 273.)*   The serum amylase is an effective screening test for acute pancreatitis. Levels greater than 300 U/dL make the diagnosis extremely likely, especially if intestinal perforation and infarction are excluded (both of these conditions can raise the serum amylase). In all but 15 percent of patients with acute pancreatitis, the serum amylase level is elevated within 24 h and begins to decline by 3 to 5 days in the absence of extensive pancreatic necrosis, partial infarction, or pseudocyst formation. Reasons for normal values could be a delay in obtaining the blood test, the presence of chronic rather than acute pancreatitis, or the presence of hypertriglyceridemia. Both serum amylase and lipase (perhaps the single best enzyme to diagnose acute pancreatitis) will be falsely low in patients with hypertriglyceridemia. Serum trypsinogen may have theoretical advantages over amylase and lipase, insofar as the pancreas is the only source of this enzyme.

360. The answer is B. *(Chap 258.)*   Carcinoma of the colon is the most common cause of mechanical obstruction of the colon and is followed in frequency by sigmoid diverticulitis and volvulus. These three causes account for 90 percent of cases of colonic obstruction. Adhesions and hernias cause about 75 percent of cases of small-intestine obstruction but are uncommon causes of colonic obstruction.

361. The answer is B. *(Chap 270.)*   Fatty liver refers to the infiltration of hepatocytes by triglyceride. Typically, the fat accumulates in large cytoplasmic droplets. However, in acute fatty liver of pregnancy and in Reye's syndrome, the fat is contained in small vacuoles and is termed *microvesicular fat.* The reason for the specific morphologic appearance of fat in these two disorders is unknown, but it provides a useful histologic differential point.

362. The answer is D. *(Chap 262.)*   MRI may be more sensitive than CT in evaluating hepatic mass lesions. Vascular lesions such as benign hemangiomas or malignant angiosarcomas caused by chronic exposure to vinyl chloride are well-detected by MRI. At this time the value of MRI in most diffuse hepatic parenchymal diseases, such as drug-induced or infectious hepatitis or cirrhosis, is unclear. On the other hand, MRI is quite useful for monitoring diseases characterized by the hepatic deposition of metals such as copper (Wilson's disease) or iron (hemochromatosis or conditions associated with secondary iron overload, such as thalassemia intermedia).

363. The answer is D. *(Chap 266.)*   Acetaminophen hepatotoxicity is mediated by a toxic metabolite formed by the hepatic cytochrome P450 system. Glutathione is responsible for detoxifying the metabolite, but when stores of this scavenger are depleted, hepatocyte necrosis may ensue. Thus, acetaminophen is a direct hepatotoxin; a single dose of 10 to 15 g will produce evidence of liver injury and doses above 25 g can be fatal. Such injury can be ameliorated somewhat by timely administration (<24 h after overdose) of a glutathione-restoring sulfhydryl compound such as *N*-acetylcysteine. Many other agents produce hepatic injury in an idiosyncratic fashion due to hypersensitivity (halothane, methyldopa, chlorpromazine), genetic variations in the handling of drug metabolites (isoniazid, diphenylhydantoin), or unknown mechanisms.

364. The answer is B. *(Chaps 265, 268.)*   Gastrointestinal bleeding, which causes an increase in the production of ammonia and other nitrogenous substances in the colon, is a common predisposing factor to hepatic encephalopathy in persons with cirrhosis. Hypokalemic alkalosis, caused by excessive diuresis or vomiting, may precipitate hepatic encephalopathy by increasing the ratio of ammonia to ammonium; gut and renal absorption of ammonia increases, and more ammonia enters the brain. Acidosis has the opposite effect. Deterioration of liver function, such as in viral hepatitis, can precipitate encephalopathy in cirrhotic persons. If worsening renal function produces an increase in blood urea nitrogen, there is additional availability for NH_3 production via the action of gut bacterial urease on urea.

365. The answer is E.   *(Chap 266.)*   About 10 percent of persons treated with isoniazid develop mild elevations of serum aminotransferase levels during the first few weeks of therapy. These levels usually return to normal despite continued use of isoniazid. About 1 percent of persons with elevated aminotransferase levels develop symptoms of hepatitis and are at high risk for developing fatal hepatic failure. The older the patient, the higher the risk of isoniazid hepatitis; thus, because the patient described in this question is young and asymptomatic, isoniazid can safely be continued, as long as she is watched for symptoms of hepatitis. A liver biopsy would not be indicated at this time.

366. The answer is C.   *(Chaps 254, 268.)*   Alcohol produces impairment in the absorption of many nutrients, including vitamin K. (The use of neomycin in the treatment of hepatic encephalopathy also can lead to a decrease in vitamin K.) When hypoprothrombinemia in a person with liver disease is easily corrected by parenteral vitamin K administration, decreased intestinal absorption of vitamin K should be suspected. Coagulopathy resulting from impaired hepatic function, such as in alcoholic hepatitis, is unlikely to be corrected by exogenous vitamin K. Although the patient discussed in the question is probably deficient in folate, as evidenced by the high mean corpuscular volume, folic acid administration has no effect on prothrombin time. Exogenous vitamin K would not correct the hypoprothrombinemia associated with disseminated intravascular coagulation.

367. The answer is E.   *(Chap 265.)*   Benign postoperative intrahepatic cholestasis can develop as a consequence of major surgery for a catastrophic event in which hypotension, extensive blood loss into tissues, and massive blood replacement are notable. Factors contributing to jaundice include the pigment load from transfusions, decreased liver function due to hypotension, and decreased renal bilirubin excretion due to tubular necrosis. Jaundice becomes evident on the second or third postoperative day, with bilirubin levels (mainly levels of conjugated bilirubin) peaking by the tenth day. Serum alkaline phosphatase concentration may be elevated up to tenfold, but aspartate aminotransferase (AST) levels are only mildly elevated. Hepatitis, choledocholithiasis, and hepatic infarct are unlikely diagnoses in the absence of abdominal tenderness, fever, or a significant rise in AST levels. The incubation period of posttransfusion hepatitis is 7 weeks, making this diagnosis unlikely.

368. The answer is E.   *(Chap 267. Perrillo, N Engl J Med 323:295, 1990.)*   Glucocorticoid therapy has been shown to prolong survival in patients with chronic active hepatitis of nonviral etiology. This patient, who has evidence of chronic hepatitis B infection as the cause of her chronic active hepatitis (this diagnosis has been made because of piecemeal necrosis on liver biopsy), would not benefit from administration of steroids. Though many agents have been tried in chronic active viral hepatitis, none have thus far been shown to be effective in the majority of patients. A 4-month course of interferon-α is associated with a 40 percent seroconversion rate from HBeAg positivity to detectable levels of anti-HBe. Interferon therapy is also beneficial in patients with chronic hepatitis C infection.

369. The answer is D.   *(Chap 270.)*   Primary erythrocytosis with organomegaly strongly suggests the diagnosis of polycythemia rubra vera. One well-recognized complication of this condition is hypercoagulability, with a particular propensity toward hepatic vein thrombosis. Such an occlusion would lead to the Budd-Chiari syndrome characterized by a grossly enlarged, tender liver with severe ascites. In addition to hepatic vein thrombosis secondary to a hypercoagulable state, such a syndrome could result from idiopathic causes, hepatic invasion by tumor, or the venoocclusive disease associated with chemotherapy or radiation. Once right-sided heart failure is excluded clinically, the diagnosis is best established by hepatic venography or liver biopsy showing sinusoidal dilatation.

370. The answer is E.   *(Chap 267.)*   Although chronic active hepatitis may be associated with extraintestinal manifestations (e.g., arthritis) and the presence in the serum of autoantibodies (e.g., anti-smooth-muscle antibody), these factors are not invariably present. The distinction between chronic active and chronic persistent hepatitis can only be established by liver biopsy. In chronic active hepatitis there is piecemeal necrosis (erosion of the limiting plate of hepatocytes surrounding the portal triads), hepatocellular regeneration, and extension of inflammation into the liver lobule, features not seen in chronic persistent hepatitis. Both diseases may be associated with serologic evidence of hepatitis B infection.

371. The answer is D.   *(Chap 272. Ransohoff, Gastroenterology 92:1588, 1987.)*   The risk of subsequent complications or symptoms in a patient with silent, or asymptomatic, gallstones is less than 1 to 2 percent per year. A prolonged period of being asymptomatic suggests that the risk of subsequent gallbladder-related problems is quite low; few patients develop complications without prior warning symptoms. Thus, it is no longer recommended that diabetics with silent gallstones undergo prophylactic cholecystectomies. If symptoms of biliary colic (an aching or pressure in the epigastrium or right upper quadrant, often with vomiting) occur with a frequency or severity great enough to disrupt the patient's normal routine, then cholecystectomy should be performed. Surgery should also be undertaken in patients who have experienced a prior complication of gallstone disease, such as pancreatitis, acute cholecystitis, or gallstone fistula or ileus. Finally, certain underlying gallbladder conditions predispose to subsequent complications and should be treated with cholecystectomy. Such conditions include calcified or porcelain gallbladder, which is associated with the development of gallbladder carcinoma, cholesterosis (lipid deposition in the lamina propria of the gallbladder wall), and adenomyomatosis (benign nodular proliferation of gallbladder surface epithelium).

372. The answer is E.   *(Chap 268.)*   Persons who have cirrhosis, particularly alcoholic cirrhosis and ascites, may develop acute bacterial peritonitis without a clearly definable precipitating event. The clinical presentation of spontaneous bacterial peritonitis may be subtle, such as fever of unknown origin and mild abdominal pain, and be attributed to other causes. Diagnosis is based on a careful examination of ascitic fluid obtained by paracentesis and should include cell count, Gram's stain, and culture.

373. The answer is B.   *(Chaps 41, 268.)*   The x-ray presented in the question demonstrates esophageal varices, which are associated with portal hypertension. Of the diseases listed, only Laennec's cirrhosis would lead directly to portal hypertension. Although the other lesions might be associated with upper gastrointestinal bleeding, none would be expected to produce varices.

374. The answer is B.   *(Chap 272.)*   Obesity, clofibrate therapy, age, and oral contraceptive therapy predispose to gallstone formation by increasing biliary cholesterol excretion. Extensive ileal resection leads to malabsorption of bile salts, depletion of the bile acid pool, and an inability to micellize cholesterol, resulting in an increased risk of gallstone formation. No correlation exists between serum cholesterol concentration and biliary cholesterol secretion; consequently, hypercholesterolemia per se does not predispose to cholelithiasis. Other important predisposing factors to the formation of cholesterol gallstones include gallbladder hypomotility due to prolonged parenteral nutrition, fasting, or pregnancy.

375. The answer is E.   *(Chap 268.)*   If fluid and sodium restriction is unsuccessful in the mobilization of ascitic fluid, cautious diuresis is indicated; spironolactone, rather than furosemide or acetazolamide, would be the drug of choice. Aggressive diuretic therapy can lead to volume depletion, azotemia, electrolyte disturbances, and hepatic encephalopathy. Therapeutic paracentesis (4 to 6

L) is now felt to be effective, especially if albumin is infused to avoid exacerbation of intravascular depletion. The peritoneovenous (LeVeen) shunt should be reserved for cases of intractable ascites; its use is accompanied by significant complications, including infection and disseminated intravascular coagulation.

376. The answer is E. *(Chap 272.)*   The radiograph reproduced in the question shows emphysematous cholecystitis, a form of acute cholecystitis in which the gallbladder, its wall, and sometimes even the bile ducts contain gas secondary to infection by gas-producing bacteria. This condition occurs most frequently in elderly men and diabetic persons. The morbidity and mortality associated with emphysematous cholecystitis exceed those of acute cholecystitis. Once preoperative preparations are complete, laparotomy and cholecystectomy should be performed promptly.

377. The answer is B. *(Chap 269.)*   The clinical constellation of tender hepatomegaly, a bruit in the right upper quadrant of the abdomen, bloody ascites, and very elevated alkaline phosphatase occurring in a patient with previously stable cirrhosis is characteristic of primary hepatocellular carcinoma. This disease typically is associated with very high levels of alpha fetoprotein, a unique and specific fetal alpha$_1$ globulin. Rarely, ectopic hormones, such as chorionic gonadotropin, are found in the serum of patients with hepatocellular carcinoma. The enzyme 5'-nucleotidase may be elevated in any condition associated with hepatocellular damage. Antimitochondrial antibodies are found in primary biliary cirrhosis and are not typical of primary hepatocellular carcinoma.

378. The answer is E. *(Chap 274.)*   Conventional therapy for acute pancreatitis includes analgesia, intravenous volume replacement, and abstinence from oral intake to "rest" the pancreas. Controlled trials have not demonstrated any benefit to symptomatic recovery or survival rate by administration of cimetidine, aprotinin (an inhibitor of pancreatic enzyme release), antibiotics, or glucagon. However, antibiotics are beneficial when secondary infection supervenes (e.g., abscess, phlegmon, or ascending cholangitis). Anticholinergic agents have not been shown to be beneficial and may worsen tachycardia, bowel hypomotility, and oliguria.

379. The answer is B. *(Chap 274.)*   Vitamin B$_{12}$ (cobalamin) malabsorption is commonly associated with chronic pancreatitis. The mechanism of vitamin B$_{12}$ malabsorption is thought to be excessive binding of the vitamin by non-intrinsic-factor binding proteins, which normally are destroyed by pancreatic proteases. Consequently, the condition is corrected by administration of pancreatic enzymes. Gastric varices, which may bleed, are caused by splenic vein thrombosis due to inflammation of the tail of the pancreas. Pleural effusions, most notably left-sided, can result from leaking pseudocysts or a pancreatic-pleural fistula; effusion fluid has a high amylase content. Jaundice results from compression of the common bile duct caused by edema or inflammation in the head of the pancreas. Although persons with chronic pancreatitis may develop tender red nodules on the legs, these are due to subcutaneous fat necrosis and not to erythema nodosum.

380. The answer is A. *(Chap 274. Agarwal, Am J Gastroenterol 86:1385, 1991.)*   Serum bilirubin elevations >68 μmol/L (>4.0 mg/dL) occur in about 10 percent of patients with acute pancreatitis, are usually transient, and do not portend a poor prognosis unless accompanied by very high levels of serum lactic dehydrogenase. The finding of hypoxemia, often heralding the development of the adult respiratory distress syndrome, is ominous. Hypocalcemia (<1.96 mmol/L [<8 mg/dL]), which possibly indicates interperitoneal fatty acid saponification of calcium, is also a grave prognostic sign. Hypoalbuminemia and massive requirement for colloid replacement suggest profound peripancreatic disease as does the presence of discolored or hemorrhagic fluid obtained at paracentesis. Other risk factors for high mortality during an attack of acute pancreatitis include older age, hypotension, leukocytosis, hyperglycemia, fall in hematocrit, and azotemia.

381. The answer is B. *(Chap 276.)* The combination of weight loss, anemia, and a bullous skin eruption in a patient with hepatic metastases and evidence of a pancreatic lesion is highly suggestive of a glucagonoma. This tumor of pancreatic alpha cells is usually malignant; metastasizes early; often occurs in middle-aged women; and is accompanied by hyperglycemia, painful stomatitis and cheilosis, hypoaminoacidemia, and a characteristic skin rash—necrolytic migratory erythema. With appropriate histologic techniques, the diagnosis of a pancreatic alpha-cell tumor can be established by liver biopsy, but marked plasma hyperglucagonemia is pathognomonic. Arteriography may demonstrate a pancreatic tumor but is not diagnostic. Treatment is early surgical removal; chemotherapy of metastatic disease is usually ineffective.

382. The answer is C. *(Chaps 250, 251.)* Though candidal infection is a frequent cause of esophagitis, typically manifested by dysphagia, it may be seen with immunodeficiency states such as AIDS, with use of immunosuppressive agents including glucocorticoids, and with use of broad-spectrum antibiotics. Esophagitis may also be seen in diabetics, patients with systemic lupus erythematosus, and those who have experienced corrosive esophageal injury. Oral thrush is a helpful, but not invariant coexisting finding. Candidal esophagitis may be complicated by bleeding, perforation, stricture, or systemic invasion. Upper gastrointestinal radiography may reveal multiple nodular filling defects. Endoscopic evaluation typically reveals a whitish exudate in the setting of underlying erythematous mucosa. Definitive diagnosis would require demonstration of yeast or hyphal forms on Gram's, periodic acid-Schiff, or silver stains. Uncomplicated cases of candidal esophagitis respond well to fluconazole, which is preferred to ketoconazole because of reduced bioavailability of the latter compound at increased gastric pH.

383. The answer is C. *(Chap 251.)* Chronic acid-induced (reflux) esophagitis may cause bleeding from diffuse erosions or discrete ulcerations. Peptic damage to the submucosa can result in fibrosis and subsequent stricture. Barrett's esophagus is formed as destroyed squamous epithelium is replaced by columnar epithelium, usually similar to that of the adjacent gastric mucosa. Adenocarcinoma may develop in 2 to 5 percent of persons with a Barrett's esophagus. A lower esophageal ring is a structural lesion that is not related to reflux esophagitis.

384. The answer is B. *(Chaps 42, 265.)* A simple and important method to determine whether the cause of jaundice is conjugated or unconjugated hyperbilirubinemia is measurement of urinary excretion of bilirubin. Under normal circumstances the urine contains no bilirubin since the unconjugated, water-soluble bilirubin, which accounts for 96 percent of the bilirubin in serum, is tightly bound to albumin and is not filtered by the glomeruli. Even in cases of unconjugated hyperbilirubinemia due to overproduction (as in hemolysis or the ineffective erythropoiesis characteristic of certain hemoglobinopathies) or due to decreased conjugation, there is no urinary excretion of bilirubin. Congenital deficiencies of the glucuronyl transferase enzyme responsible for converting bilirubin into its soluble form include Gilbert's syndrome and Crigler-Najjar types I and II (in type I disease, the transferase enzyme is totally absent). In cases of conjugated hyperbilirubinemia, in which more than 50 percent of the serum bilirubin is composed of the conjugated type, enough bilirubin remains unbound that filtration of this substance occurs and the urine dipstick becomes positive. In addition to extrahepatic obstruction, causes of conjugated hyperbilirubinemia include defects in hepatic excretion of a congenital (e.g., Dubin-Johnson or Rotor syndromes) or an acquired (hepatocellular disease or estrogen use) nature.

385. The answer is E. *(Chap 255.)* Most extraintestinal disorders of inflammatory bowel disease are associated with both Crohn's disease and ulcerative colitis, including pericholangitis, uveitis, and a variety of skin and joint manifestations. Complications that are unique to Crohn's disease because of inflammation of the terminal ileum include hypocalcemia, which is caused by malabsorption of vitamin D, and the formation of urinary oxalate stones, which results from increased colonic absorption of dietary oxalate. Owing to bile-salt malabsorption caused by ileal disease, cholesterol gallstones tend to form in persons with regional enteritis.

386. The answer is D. *(Chap 256.)* Meckel's diverticulum is the most frequently occurring congenital anomaly of the gastrointestinal tract and is found in 2 percent of adult autopsies. The diverticulum may contain ectopic gastric mucosa, and local acid secretion may produce ileal ulceration and lower gastrointestinal bleeding. In young adults, Meckel's diverticulitis can mimic acute appendicitis. Technetium, taken up by diverticular gastric mucosa, can detect the lesion, which is easily missed on conventional barium x-rays. Gastrointestinal obstruction may occur if the diverticulum intussuscepts or twists on a fibrous remnant of the omphalomesenteric duct. Surgical excision is the treatment of any significant complication of a Meckel's diverticulum.

387. The answer is C. *(Chap 266.)* Hepatitis B *e* antigen (HBeAg) is a protein that is associated with the HBV core particle. HBeAg is a soluble protein found only in HBsAg-positive serum and is immunologically distinct from HBsAg as well as from intact HBcAg, an antigen expressed on the hepatitis B virus nucleocapsid core. Interestingly, both HBcAg and HBeAg are encoded on the so-called C-gene of the hepatitis B genome. Owing to the close association of HBeAg and HBsAg, the presence of HBeAg in the serum is linked with infectiousness, and the antigen is present during the viremic period of acute hepatitis B. Although HBeAg correlates well with viral replication, detection of HBeAg in serum has not been found to predict the subsequent development of chronic hepatitis B infection; equally, the absence of HBeAg in serum does not preclude the development of chronic hepatitis B infection. In acute hepatitis B, the disappearance of HBeAg from serum often presages resolution of the acute infection; however, HBeAg-negative persons should be considered infectious until antibody to HBsAg is no longer detected in the serum.

388. The answer is A-Y, B-Y, C-N, D-N, E-N. *(Chap 266. Hoofnagle, JAMA 261:1321, 1989.)* The delta agent hepatitis D virus (HDV) is a recently recognized defective RNA virus that coinfects with and requires the helper function of HBV for its replication and expression. Therefore, the duration of HDV infection is determined by and limited to the duration of HBV infection. Although the delta core is encapsulated by an outer coat of HBsAg, the delta antigen has no antigenic similarity to that of any of the HBV antigens, and the RNA genome is not homologous with HBV DNA. HDV infection has a worldwide distribution and exists in two epidemiologic patterns, endemic and epidemic. In endemic areas (Mediterranean countries) HDV infection is found among those with HBV infection and is transmitted predominantly by nonpercutaneous routes, such as close personal contact. In nonendemic areas, such as the United States or northern Europe, HDV infection is limited to persons with frequent exposure to blood products, such as intravenous drug addicts and hemophiliacs. In general, patients with simultaneous HBV and HDV infections do not have an increased risk of development of chronic hepatitis compared with patients with acute HBV infection alone. HDV superinfection of patients with chronic HBV infection carries an increased risk of fulminant hepatitis and death.

389. The answer is A-Y, B-N, C-N, D-Y, E-Y. *(Chap 250.)* Although upper gastrointestinal endoscopy is superior to radiographic techniques in its ability to identify superficial lesions of the esophagus, stomach, and duodenum, barium studies are able to detect a very high percentage of lesions that breach the mucosa. For example, most gastric and duodenal ulcers can be identified on an air-contrast upper gastrointestinal series. In contrast, erosive gastritis, the telangiectasias of Osler-Rendu-Weber syndrome, and small mucosal tears of the gastroesophageal junction (Mallory-Weiss tears) are missed with the best radiographic techniques but usually are found by routine endoscopy.

390. The answer is A-N, B-Y, C-Y, D-Y, E-Y. *(Chaps 41, 268. Terblanche, N Engl J Med 320:1393, 1989.)* Peripheral (intravenous) and central (superior mesenteric artery) infusions of vasopressin are equally effective in temporarily controlling variceal hemorrhage. For more permanent hemostasis, surgery may be required. Elective portacaval shunt surgery can prevent recurrent variceal bleeding, although the overall survival rate is not improved. The distal splenorenal shunt, when compared with the portacaval shunt, appears to have a lower incidence of postoperative encephalopathy; for either procedure, however, the presence of jaundice, ascites, or encephalopathy portends a less favorable operative outlook. Sclerotherapy is a promising newer technique that is an effective therapy to be employed, if available, prior to surgery. Beta blockade with propranolol, at doses sufficient to lower the resting heart rate by 25 percent, appears to reduce the incidence of recurrent variceal bleeding and may be an effective prophylactic agent in those who have large varices but have not yet bled.

391. The answer is A-N, B-N, C-Y, D-Y, E-N. *(Chap 266.)* The prevention of viral hepatitis is of particular importance because of the limited therapeutic options. The prophylactic approach varies with the type of hepatitis. All preparations of immune globulin (IG) contain sufficient titers of anti-HAV to prevent a clinically apparent type A hepatitis. If given early enough, infection will be prevented in approximately 80 percent of patients. For intimate contacts, 0.02 mL/kg of IG is recommended as soon as possible after exposure. The prevention of hepatitis B is based upon both passive immunoprophylaxis with hepatitis B immune globulin (HBIG) and hepatitis B vaccine. HBIG appears to be effective in reducing clinically apparent illness but does not appear to prevent infection. Hepatitis B vaccine has been shown to be highly effective in preventing HBV infection. Because only persons with HBV infection are susceptible to delta hepatitis, hepatitis B vaccine is effective in preventing delta infection in persons who are not carriers of HBsAg. There is no effective prophylaxis of HDV infection for those patients who are already HBsAg carriers. Although it has not been shown to be effective, many authorities recommend postexposure prophylaxis of hepatitis C with IG because it is safe and inexpensive and may be effective.

392. The answer is A-N, B-N, C-Y, D-Y, E-Y. *(Chap 36.)* An atrophic, or "bald," tongue may be seen in association with several hematologic disorders, including iron deficiency and B_{12} deficiency as in the patient with malabsorption due to prior ileal or gastric resection. Impaired salivary production, as in the case of the patient with Sjögren's syndrome, can lead to an increased incidence of dental caries as well as to a bald tongue. The oral gummatous lesions characteristic of tertiary syphilis may also be associated with glossitis and bald tongue. An enlarged (but normally papillated) tongue is associated with Down's syndrome (which carries an increased risk for the development of acute leukemia), infiltration with lymphoma or amyloid, and acromegaly, as exemplified by the man with enlarged feet and glucose intolerance (due to the hyperglycemic effects of growth hormone).

393. The answer is A-Y, B-Y, C-Y, D-N, E-N. *(Chap 38. Mitchelson, Drugs 43:443, 1992.)* Two areas in the central nervous system control the act of vomiting. The vomiting center in the lateral reticular formation in the medulla receives input from both the gastrointestinal tract and from higher centers in the brain and controls outflow to the phrenic nerve, spinal nerve, and vagus, each of which innervates muscles involved in retching. The chemoreceptor trigger zone located near the floor of the fourth ventricle can be activated by a host of stimuli or drugs including opiates, dopaminergics, digitalis, radiation, and varied metabolic toxins and abnormalities (e.g., uremia). Pathways emanating from the chemoreceptor trigger zone lead to the vomiting center, which directly controls the act of vomiting. Dopaminergic inhibitors, such as the phenothiazine derivative prochlorperazine, inhibit the dopamine receptors in the chemoreceptor trigger zone, thereby suppressing vomiting. Phenothiazine derivatives frequently are associated with troublesome anticholinergic side effects such as sedation, dry mouth, and hypotension. Metoclopramide is another dopamine antagonist that can affect central pathways, but it has the added benefit of a cholinergic effect that enhances gastric emptying. Antihistamines such as diphenhydramine and anticholinergics such as scopolamine do not act on the chemoreceptor trigger zone, but can be helpful in the control of vomiting caused by dysfunction of the inner ear. Ondansetron is particularly effective in the treatment of chemotherapy-induced nausea and vomiting. This relatively new agent is a serotonin antagonist that blocks receptors in the chemoreceptor trigger zone and gut.

394. The answer is A-Y, B-Y, C-N, D-N, E-Y. *(Chap 252.)* Most gastrinomas are found in the pancreas, often in multiple locations. In 20 to 60 percent of cases, gastrinomas are associated with other components of the multiple endocrine neoplasia (MEN) type I syndrome (neoplasms in the parathyroid or pituitary as well as the pancreas). The Zollinger-Ellison (Z-E) syndrome accounts for less than 1 percent of all peptic ulcers. About two-thirds of gastrinomas are malignant. The diagnosis should be suspected in cases of multiple, unusually located, recurrent, fulminant, or poorly responding peptic ulcers. On upper gastrointestinal examination, large mucosal folds are mainly noted in the stomach, but can also be observed at more distal sites. Diarrhea due to hypersecretion of acid or, less commonly, steatorrhea due to acid-mediated inactivation of pancreatic lipase may occur even in the absence of peptic ulcers. Endoscopic retrograde cholangiopancreatography (ERCP) is highly inferior to selective angiography or CT in identifying pancreatic gastrinomas, which are difficult to localize presurgically by any means. Elevated fasting levels of gastrin (>200 ng/L) are required for the diagnosis of gastrinoma; two normal levels in the absence of overwhelming evidence to the contrary essentially rule out the diagnosis. Positive responses to provocative tests include a paradoxical rise in serum gastrin by 200 ng/L after infusion of secretin, a rise in serum gastrin level by 400 ng/L after infusion of calcium gluconate, or a failure to rise above baseline after administration of a standard meal.

395. The answer is A-Y, B-Y, C-N, D-Y, E-N. *(Chap 254.)* Surgical resection of a significant portion of small intestine can result in a variety of clinical abnormalities, which are collectively referred to as the *short bowel syndrome*. By a mechanism as yet unelucidated, massive small-bowel resection can lead to transient gastric hypersecretion, which results in inactivation of pancreatic enzymes directly and in dilution of pancreatic secretions. The loss of ileal tissue, less well tolerated than removal of an equal length of jejunum, causes poor absorption of bile salts; depletion of the bile acid pool results in steatorrhea, which is best managed by a low-fat diet (40 g/d). Increased passage of bile acids into the colon stimulates a secretory diarrhea, which may respond to treatment with the bile salt–sequestering agent cholestyramine. Antiperistaltic agents, such as belladonna alkaloids and diphenoxylate, presumably enhance absorption by prolonging mucosal contact time and thus can benefit patients with the short bowel syndrome.

396. The answer is A-Y, B-Y, C-Y, D-N, E-N. *(Chap 255. Peppercorn, Ann Intern Med 112:50–60, 1990.)* Among the findings of the National Cooperative Crohn's Disease Study in 1979 were that corticosteroids are more efficacious in the treatment of Crohn's disease of the small intestine than in the treatment of Crohn's disease of the colon. However, steroids can mask a septic deterioration and must be used cautiously. Azathioprine and mercaptopurine may be useful corticosteroid-sparing agents. Sulfasalazine was found to be effective in the therapy of active colonic disease, but neither sulfasalazine nor corticosteroids decrease the frequency of recurrence once remission has been achieved. Both drugs may be used safely in treating pregnant women. In more recent studies, metronidazole, which is not useful in ulcerative colitis, has been reported to be useful in the treatment of perineal and colitic manifestations of Crohn's disease.

397. The answer is A-Y, B-N, C-Y, D-N, E-N. *(Chap 255.)*   Risk factors for the development of colon carcinoma in persons who have ulcerative colitis include presence of the disease for more than 10 years, extensive mucosal involvement (pancolitis), and a family history of carcinoma of the colon. The risk of cancer in persons with pancolitis is estimated to be 12 percent at 15 years, 23 percent at 20 years, and 42 percent at 24 years. Neither a history of toxic megacolon nor the prolonged use of high-dose steroids increases the risk of cancer. Pseudopolyps, although frequently associated with severe disease, are not precancerous lesions.

398. The answer is A-N, B-Y, C-Y, D-Y, E-N. *(Chap 255.)*   Ischemic colitis most often occurs in elderly persons who have vascular disease. Areas of the colon with extensive collateral circulation, such as the rectum, usually are spared. Angiography of arteries and veins rarely is indicated for diagnosis or therapy because vessel occlusions are almost never detected. Even though acute ischemic colitis may present with rectal bleeding and lower abdominal pain, most cases do not present with the severity of signs and symptoms suggestive of an acute abdomen. This disease usually does not recur, and symptoms tend to resolve in 2 to 4 weeks. Ischemic colitis is sometimes diagnosed retrospectively as the cause of a colonic stricture.

399. The answer is A-N, B-Y, C-Y, D-N, E-Y. *(Chap 256.)*   Acute hemorrhage from colonic diverticula is the most common cause of lower gastrointestinal bleeding among elderly persons. Although diverticula are more common in the left side of the colon, bleeding tends to originate from the ascending (right) colon. Bleeding usually stops with bed rest and transfusion; however, when conservative measures fail to curb hemorrhage, intraarterial infusion of vasoconstrictive medications, introduced during angiography, can be effective. Although acute diverticulitis may be associated with occult bleeding, gross hemorrhage rarely occurs.

400. The answer is A-Y, B-Y, C-N, D-Y, E-N. *(Chap 263.)*   Unexplained hepatosplenomegaly and unexplained persistence of elevated liver function tests are the principal indications for percutaneous needle liver biopsy. The presence of these phenomena suggests a diagnosis either of diffuse parenchymal disease of the liver, which occurs with drug reactions and metabolic liver disease, or of multiple focal lesions, which are caused by granulomatous or metastatic disease. The diagnosis of miliary tuberculosis, for example, can often be made by liver biopsy (more than 40 percent of all cases have a positive liver biopsy). A focal defect identified on liver scan also can be evaluated by percutaneous liver biopsy, often with sonographic guidance of the needle. A percutaneous liver biopsy should never be performed, however, when a vascular lesion of the liver, such as an angioma, is suspected. Although liver biopsy can confirm the presence of suspected biliary obstruction, ultrasonography, computerized tomography, and transhepatic or endoscopic cholangiography are better techniques for determining the cause of common bile duct obstruction.

401. The answer is A-Y, B-Y, C-N, D-N, E-Y. *(Chap 263.)*   Elevated levels of serum alkaline phosphatase (of hepatic origin) generally reflect impaired hepatic excretory function. Thus, the concentration of this enzyme may be elevated in persons with incomplete extrahepatic biliary obstruction (e.g., bile duct stricture) or intrahepatic cholestasis (e.g., chlorpromazine-induced cholestasis or early primary biliary cirrhosis); in all three of these examples, serum bilirubin concentration is only slightly elevated. Both acute viral hepatitis and acetaminophen hepatotoxicity are associated with extensive hepatocellular damage and frequently produce peak serum aspartate aminotransferase levels of above 8.33 μkat/L (500 U/L).

402. The answer is A-Y, B-N, C-Y, D-Y, E-N. *(Chap 257.)*   Adenomatous polyps of the colon are very common in the general population, and the incidence increases with age. They are usually detected by screening barium enemas or colonoscopy performed as part of an evaluation of occult gastrointestinal blood loss. A small minority of polyps cause bleeding or obstruction. The majority of polyps occur in the rectosigmoid colon. An increasing size and flatness (rather than extension from a stalk) correlate with an increased risk of malignancy. Polyps less than 1.5 cm have a 1 percent chance of containing malignant cells; >10 percent of polyps greater than 2 cm contain malignant cells. Though few polyps become cancers, recent data suggest that aggressively removing all colorectal adenomas can dramatically reduce the incidence of invasive carcinoma of the colon. There are three histologic types of polyps: tubular, tubulovillous, and villous. Of these, villous adenomas tend to be the largest and have the greatest risk of malignancy. Because polyps with carcinoma in situ do not metastasize, colonoscopic resection is considered curative. However, affected patients must be examined carefully for synchronous lesions and followed for recurrent disease.

403. **The answer is A-N, B-Y, C-Y, D-N, E-N.** *(Chap 266.)* Viral hepatitis may be associated with peak serum levels of the serum aminotransferases AST and ALT of 68 μkat/L (4000 IU) or more; however, the acute level of these enzymes is poorly correlated with the degree of hepatocellular damage. A prolonged prothrombin time, hypoalbuminemia, hypoglycemia, and marked hyperbilirubinemia portend a poor prognosis. A serum sickness-like syndrome is associated with hepatitis B infection and occurs in 5 to 10 percent of affected persons. The etiologic agent cannot be surmised accurately from the presenting symptoms and signs in most persons. Steroid therapy has no value in the treatment of acute viral hepatitis.

404. **The answer is A-Y, B-Y, C-N, D-Y, E-N.** *(Chap 254.)* Patients with intestinal lymphangiectasia—characterized by protein-losing enteropathy, hypoproteinemia, hypogammaglobulinemia, edema, chylous effusions, fat malabsorption, and lymphocytopenia—typically present in childhood or young adulthood. The generalized congenital disorder of lymphatic development includes the dilated lymph vessels typically seen on small-bowel biopsy. The abnormal lymphatics are presumed to rupture into the bowel lumen, which leads directly to hypoproteinemia and steatorrhea. Absorption of carbohydrates such as D-xylose and lactose that are not dependent upon lymphatics is typically preserved. The decreased lymph flow associated with a low-fat diet supplemented by medium-chain triglycerides (transported by the portal vein rather than the lymph) results in significant clinical improvement.

405. **The answer is A-Y, B-Y, C-Y, D-Y, E-N.** *(Chap 254.)* Tropical sprue is a malabsorptive disease of unclear etiology that may be due to a nutritional deficiency, a microorganism, or a toxin elaborated by a microorganism. Malabsorption of at least two nutrients is the rule. Patients commonly malabsorb iron, vitamin B_{12}, xylose (carbohydrates), and fat. Consequently, megaloblastic anemia and problems associated with the absorption of the fat-soluble vitamins A (night blindness), D (hypocalcemia possibly with tetany), and K (hypoprothrombinemia and purpura) may be seen. In the setting of prolonged calorie malnutrition, a state of secondary hypopituitarism may be manifested by decreased libido. The diagnosis of tropical sprue is supported by a jejunal biopsy that discloses shortened and thickened villi, increased crypt height, and infiltration of mononuclear cells in the lamina propria. In addition to a trial of antibiotic therapy (sulfonamide or tetracycline), treatment with vitamin B_{12}, folate, and antibiotics should be undertaken. Pyoderma gangrenosum is an ulcerative skin lesion found in patients with inflammatory bowel disease.

406. **The answer is A-Y, B-N, C-N, D-Y, E-Y.** *(Chap 255. Podolsky, N Engl J Med 325:928, 1008, 1991.)* Sulfasalazine (Azulfidine) as a single agent is an effective treatment for an acute attack of inflammatory bowel disease of mild-to-moderate severity. In ulcerative colitis, controlled trials have shown that chronic use can decrease subsequent attack rates. Sulfasalazine is cleaved by intestinal bacteria to the inactive moiety sulfapyridine, which is rapidly excreted in the urine, and into the active compound 5-aminosalicylate, which is thought to work in part via inhibition of prostaglandin synthesis in the colon. The latter agent, though expensive, can be administered effectively by enemas, allowing use by patients who are poorly tolerant of oral sulfasalazine because of hypersensitivity reactions such as rash, arthritis, or pleuritis.

407. The answer is A-Y, B-Y, C-N, D-N, E-Y. *(Chaps 42, 265.)* Gilbert's syndrome is a benign disorder in which a partial deficiency of bilirubin glucuronyl transferase leads to mild unconjugated hyperbilirubinemia. The serum total bilirubin concentrations fluctuate between 17 μmol/L (1 mg/dL) and 51 μmol/L (3 mg/dL) and rarely exceed 86 μmol/L (5 mg/dL). No clear pattern of inheritance has been identified. Fasting reliably raises the serum bilirubin concentration and is a useful diagnostic test. Phenobarbital, which enhances glucuronyl transferase activity, results in a decrease in serum bilirubin concentration. Although a liver biopsy is not required for the diagnosis, liver biopsy specimens are normal when examined by light microscopy.

408. The answer is A-N, B-N, C-Y, D-Y, E-Y. *(Chap 257. Kinzler, Science 251:1366, 1991.)* Familial polyposis of the colon is a rare condition inherited in an autosomal dominant fashion through loss of function of a tumor-suppressor gene (APC) on the long arm of chromosome 5. It is characterized by adenomatous polyps throughout the colon. A total proctocolectomy can eliminate the certain risk of cancer by age 40. Peutz-Jeghers syndrome is characterized by hamartomatous polyps (without risk of malignant degeneration) in the stomach and all intestinal sites. In Gardner's syndrome adenomatous polyps line the large and small intestine; in addition to a high risk of colon cancer, such patients are plagued with multiple benign tumors including osteomas, fibromas, and lipomas. Turcot's syndrome refers to the constellation of adenomatous colonic polyps and malignant brain tumors.

409. The answer is A-N, B-Y, C-N, D-Y, E-Y. *(Chap 270.)* Reye's syndrome typically occurs in children recovering from a viral illness. There is often a history of ingestion of aspirin during the viral illness. Marked elevations in the serum levels of aminotransferase and ammonia as well as in prothrombin time are usually present, and affected children often develop hypoglycemic episodes. Despite these biochemical and physiologic signs of deranged hepatic function, jaundice is usually minimal. Mortality is approximately 50 percent.

410. The answer is A-Y, B-Y, C-Y, D-Y, E-Y. *(Chap 269. Okuda, Hepatology, 15:948, 1992.)* Chronic liver disease of any etiology is associated with an increased incidence of hepatocellular carcinoma (HCC). Thus, patients with alcoholic liver disease, hemochromatosis, and α_1-antitrypsin deficiency are all at increased risk of development of HCC. Worldwide, chronic hepatitis B virus infection is an important cause of chronic liver disease and subsequent HCC. Mycotoxins such as aflatoxin are found in foodstuffs in many parts of the world and are thought to be carcinogenic.

411. The answer is A-Y, B-N, C-Y, D-Y, E-N. *(Chap 266.)* The diagnosis of acute hepatitis B infection can be made by the detection of HBsAg in serum, unless there is the simultaneous presence of IgG anti-HBc, which indicates chronic infection. The only exception to the latter rule is in the case of late acute (or early chronic) infection when anti-HBe is present as well as HBsAg and the anti-HBcAg has already converted from the IgM to IgG. HBeAg is a marker of infectivity, either in acute or chronic infection. Positivity for both IgG anti-HBcAg and anti-HBsAg indicates recovery from prior infection (anti-HBeAg may be positive or negative in this case). An additional caveat is the relatively uncommon situation during acute infection when the level of HBsAg is too low to be detected, but the presence of IgM anti-HBcAg establishes the diagnosis.

412. The answer is A-N, B-Y, C-Y, D-Y, E-N. *(Chap 270.)* Granulomas can be found on liver biopsy in cases of fever of unknown origin or during evaluation of patients who have abnormalities of unclear etiology on liver function tests. Though mild transaminase abnormalities may occur, hepatic dysfunction is usually restricted to mild elevations of the alkaline phosphatase. In approximately 20 percent of cases it is not possible to identify a systemic cause of the hepatic granulomas. In such a situation, and only if a diagnosis of miliary tuberculosis is rigorously excluded (even including an initial empirical trial of antituberculous therapy), a trial of steroids could be considered. Though tuberculosis is the etiology in the majority of cases when caseating lesions are present, the absence of caseating granulomas does not exclude tuberculosis. Systemic granulomatous diseases other than tuberculosis that may involve the liver include schistosomiasis, histoplasmosis, brucellosis, berylliosis, sarcoidosis, and drug reactions.

413. The answer is A-N, B-Y, C-Y, D-N, E-N. *(Chap 275. Warshaw, N Engl J Med 326:455–465, 1992.)* The clinical history is highly suggestive of carcinoma of the head of the pancreas. The failure to obtain diagnostic tissue at needle biopsy is not unusual because of surrounding inflammation, edema, and fibrosis. Even though well over 90 percent of patients with pancreatic cancer cannot be cured surgically, an attempt at such a procedure is appropriate, particularly for lesions in the pancreatic head, which tend to present earlier because they produce extrahepatic biliary obstruction and because of the frequent confusion with other more curable lesions in this location (duodenal, ampullary, and distal bile duct tumors). Therefore, such a patient should undergo a preoperative celiac angiogram to rule out vascular invasion by tumor and ensure resectability. It would not be unreasonable to attempt a preoperative diagnosis via ERCP, although the yield will be small. Repeating a needle biopsy is unlikely to achieve diagnostic results. Neither watchful follow-up nor palliative biliary stent therapy is appropriate until a tissue diagnosis of cancer and a determination of unresectability have been made.

414–417. The answers are 414-A, 415-E, 416-D, 417-B. *(Chaps 37, 251.)* The presence for several years of dysphagia for solid food indicates a benign disease and is characteristic of a lower esophageal (Schatzki) ring (radiograph A). This lesion appears as a thin, weblike constriction near the lower esophageal sphincter. Even though the ring is congenital, dysphagia, which typically is episodic, may not occur until middle age.

Dysphagia for solid foods following a long history of heartburn suggests the development of a peptic stricture (radiograph E). (However, peptic stricture can develop in persons who do not have a history of heartburn.) On barium swallow, peptic strictures usually are seen to be 1 to 3 cm long and located near the squamocolumnar junction. Longer strictures may result from persistent vomiting or prolonged nasogastric intubation.

Rapidly progressive dysphagia and weight loss are characteristic of esophageal carcinoma (radiograph D). Dysphagia begins with solid foods but may progress to include liquids. Alcohol and tobacco use can be important predisposing factors. Barium swallow may show an ulcerating, infiltrating, or polypoid lesion.

Dysphagia caused by diffuse esophageal spasm (radiograph B) may occur with or without chest pain and often involves both solids and liquids. The chest pain, which may mimic the pain of myocardial ischemia, usually occurs at rest or on swallowing. Barium swallow shows uncoordinated, simultaneous contractions that may create a "corkscrew" configuration.

Radiograph C shows features typical of achalasia. A "beaklike" tapering of the distal esophagus and proximal dilation are prominent features. Affected persons characteristically present with painless dysphagia for solids and liquids.

Immunologic, Allergic, and Rheumatic Disorders

DIRECTIONS: Each question below contains five suggested responses. Choose the **one best** response to each question.

418. Of the following, which is expressed *earliest* in B-cell development?

    (A) Surface immunoglobulin D
    (B) Surface immunoglobulin G
    (C) Surface immunoglobulin M
    (D) Cytoplasmic μ chains
    (E) Fc receptors

419. The hyperviscosity syndrome is most characteristic of which of the following plasma cell disorders?

    (A) Multiple myeloma
    (B) Heavy chain disease
    (C) Indolent myeloma
    (D) Waldenström's macroglobulinemia
    (E) Primary amyloidosis

420. The postulated mechanism of action of nonsteroidal anti-inflammatory drugs (NSAIDs) is

    (A) inhibition of leukotriene formation due to inhibition of its synthesis from arachidonic acid
    (B) inhibition of prostaglandin formation due to inhibition of its synthesis from arachidonic acid
    (C) inhibition of arachidonic acid liberation from membrane phospholipids
    (D) direct inhibition of histamine released by mast cells
    (E) direct inhibition of mast cell activation

421. A 29-year-old man with episodic abdominal pain and stress-induced edema of the lips, tongue, and occasionally larynx is likely to have low functional or absolute levels of which of the following proteins?

    (A) C5A (complement cascade)
    (B) IgE
    (C) T-cell receptor, alpha chain
    (D) Cyclooxygenase
    (E) C1 esterase inhibitor

422. A 35-year-old woman comes to the local health clinic because for the last 6 months she has had recurrent urticarial lesions, which occasionally leave a residual discoloration. She also has had arthralgias. Sedimentation rate obtained now is 85 mm/h. The procedure most likely to yield the correct diagnosis in the case would be

    (A) a battery of wheal-and-flare allergy skin tests
    (B) measurement of total serum immunoglobulin E (IgE) concentration
    (C) measurement of C1 esterase inhibitor activity
    (D) skin biopsy
    (E) patch testing

423. A 23-year-old man seeks medical attention for perennial nasal congestion and post-nasal discharge. He states he does not have asthma, eczema, conjunctivitis, or a family history of allergic disease. His nasal secretions are rich in eosinophils. The test most likely to yield a specific diagnosis in this setting is

(A) serum IgE level (competitive radio-immunosorbent technique)
(B) serum IgE level (radiodiffusion technique)
(C) elimination diet test
(D) skin testing
(E) sinus x-rays

424. Large granular lymphocytes carry out which of the following physiologic functions?

(A) Non-antibody-mediated killing of target cells
(B) Antigen presentation to T-lymphocytes
(C) Direct tissue damage in the presence of IgE
(D) Stimulation of hematopoietic development
(E) Assistance in T-cell memory

425. A patient undergoing evaluation for possible infection with *M. tuberculosis* develops a skin wheal 48 h after intradermal placement of TB purified-protein derivative (PPD). Which of the following cellular events accounts for these findings?

(A) IL-7-induced B-cell activation and secretion of antibodies
(B) IL-3-mediated B-cell activation and induction of help for T-cell activation
(C) Monocyte-derived IL-6 activation of T cells
(D) Complement-mediated endothelial cell damage
(E) CD44-mediated monocyte adhesion to endothelial cells

426. A 47-year-old man has had fever, weight loss, arthralgias, pleuritic chest pain, and midabdominal pain for the last 2 months. One week ago he noticed difficulty dorsiflexing his right great toe. Blood pressure is 150/95 mmHg (he has always been normotensive), and laboratory studies reveal anemia of chronic disease, high erythrocyte sedimentation rate, and polymorphonuclear leukocytosis. The chest x-ray is clear. The most likely diagnosis is

(A) giant cell arteritis
(B) allergic granulomatosis
(C) Wegener's granulomatosis
(D) polyarteritis nodosa
(E) hypersensitivity vasculitis

427. Which of the following statements regarding the renal involvement associated with systemic lupus erythematosus is true?

(A) Clinically apparent renal disease occurs in 90 percent of affected persons
(B) Interstitial nephritis is a rare finding on renal biopsy
(C) Renal biopsy is not initially necessary in patients with deteriorating renal function and active urine sediment
(D) Renal disease is uncommon in patients with high-titer anti-double-stranded DNA antibodies
(E) Urinalysis in affected persons usually reveals proteinuria but little sediment and no red blood cells

428. A 25-year-old woman presents with a history of recurrent expectoration of foul-smelling sputum and intermittent fevers. Chest x-ray discloses characteristic "tram-tracking" bronchial thickening. Physical examination reveals coarse rhonchi in the right chest and splenomegaly. Blood test results are normal except for low levels of serum IgG and IgA. Her past medical history is remarkable for frequent upper respiratory infections and for a history of diarrhea 3 years ago due to *Giardia lamblia* infection. The most appropriate therapy would be

(A) corticosteroids
(B) corticosteroids and an alkylating agent
(C) monthly intravenous immunoglobulin
(D) splenectomy
(E) bone marrow transplantation

429. Which of the following is the most important distinguishing feature between HIV-1 and other retroviruses?

(A) Ability to bind to CD4-positive human T lymphocytes
(B) Numerous glycoproteins in its lipid membrane
(C) Use of host reverse transcriptase
(D) Complexity of genome
(E) Ability to transform human cells

430. All the following are immunologic abnormalities detected in patients with acquired immunodeficiency syndrome (AIDS) EXCEPT

(A) deficient T-lymphocyte response to antigenic and mitogenic stimulation
(B) decreased serum levels of immunoglobulins
(C) depletion of CD4$^+$ lymphocytes
(D) normal numbers of CD8$^+$ lymphocytes
(E) defective natural killer cell function

431. All the following statements concerning the HLA-D region on the sixth human chromosome are correct EXCEPT

(A) it is located outside the major histocompatibility gene complex
(B) it encodes proteins involved in the mixed lymphocyte response
(C) it encodes proteins expressed only on certain immune effector or closely related cells
(D) siblings matched for HLA-A, -B, and -C antigens will usually be matched at the D region
(E) it is located close to genes encoding for complement components

432. Which of the following statements best describes the role of polymerase chain reaction (PCR) in the diagnosis of HIV infection?

(A) It should be used if the western blot is indeterminate
(B) It is a useful screening test
(C) It should be used if two consecutive serologic tests (ELISA) are positive
(D) It should be used if the initial serologic test is positive, but the second is negative
(E) It has no real role

433. An HIV-infected patient known to have a circulating CD4-positive T-lymphocyte count of 300/μL is found to have a platelet count of 10,000/μL. The white count and hematocrit are not similarly deranged and there is no bleeding. The patient has never had any manifestations of AIDS. Which of the following statements best describes the patient's current situation?

(A) It is likely that severe bleeding will be the cause of significant morbidity or mortality for this patient
(B) Bone marrow examination would reveal a decreased number of megakaryocytes
(C) High-dose intravenous immunoglobulin is likely to induce a long-lasting remission
(D) Zidovudine is the treatment of choice
(E) Splenectomy should now be performed

434. All the following statements concerning the ataxia-telangiectasia syndrome are correct EXCEPT

   (A) it is inherited in an autosomal recessive manner

   (B) the cause is adenosine deaminase deficiency

   (C) malignancy is a common cause of death

   (D) bronchiectasis may occur

   (E) both humoral and cellular limbs of the immune system are affected

435. All the following statements regarding the epidemiology of HIV infection are correct EXCEPT

   (A) the occupational risk of HIV infection among health care workers is small (<0.5 percent per exposure) but real

   (B) over 1 per 1000 U.S. military recruits are infected

   (C) most U.S. cases of AIDS are now in the high-risk group of intravenous drug abusers

   (D) the chance that a single donor blood unit will contain HIV is between 1:40,000 and 1:250,000

   (E) most pediatric cases arise because of in utero transmission from an infected mother

436. Which of the following statements regarding central nervous system disease in patients with HIV infection is correct?

   (A) The most common cause of central nervous system disease is the AIDS dementia complex

   (B) The most common cause of seizures is cryptococcal meningoencephalitis

   (C) Antiretroviral agents have no role

   (D) The most common finding on MRI is multiple white matter lesions

   (E) Actual histologic evidence of direct HIV involvement is rare

437. Which of the following statements concerning Kaposi's sarcoma in patients with HIV infection is correct?

   (A) Most patients develop Kaposi's sarcoma at some point during the disease process

   (B) Lymph node involvement portends a poor prognosis

   (C) The most important determinant of response to interferon therapy is the tumor burden

   (D) Pulmonary involvement is usually manifested by apical infiltrates

   (E) Kaposi's sarcoma is more common in homosexuals than in intravenous drug abusers

438. A 32-year-old HIV-infected homosexual man complains of increasing dyspnea, fever, and a nonproductive cough. His peripheral CD4+ T-lymphocyte count is 100/μL. Each of the following pathogens is associated with this patient's illness EXCEPT

   (A) *Pneumocystis carinii*

   (B) cytomegalovirus

   (C) *Mycoplasma pneumoniae*

   (D) *Cryptococcus neoformans*

   (E) *Mycobacterium tuberculosis*

439. All the following are compatible with illness induced by therapeutic administration of antithymocyte globulin EXCEPT

   (A) malaise and fever 2 to 3 days after beginning initial therapy

   (B) lymphadenopathy

   (C) depressed CH_{50} level

   (D) positive C1q binding assay

   (E) fever

440. Not including *Pneumocystis carinii* pneumonia and tuberculosis, proven prophylactic therapy for which of the following infections exists for HIV-infected patients with CD4-positive T-lymphocyte counts less than 100/μL?

   (A) *Cytomegalovirus*

   (B) *Herpes simplex*

   (C) *Myobacterium avium-intracellulare*

   (D) *Cryptosporidia*

   (E) *Salmonella*

441. Which of the following is the LEAST common immunologic manifestation of HIV infection?

    (A) Cutaneous reactions to drugs
    (B) Anaphylactic reactions to drugs
    (C) Anticardiolipin antibodies
    (D) Oligoarticular arthritis
    (E) Fibromyalgia

442. A woman who has rheumatoid arthritis suddenly develops pain and swelling in the right calf. The most likely diagnosis is

    (A) ruptured plantaris tendon
    (B) pes anserinus bursitis
    (C) ruptured popliteal cyst
    (D) thrombophlebitis
    (E) Achilles tendonitis

443. All the following are considered to be disease-modifying agents in the treatment of rheumatoid arthritis EXCEPT

    (A) gold
    (B) prednisone
    (C) D-penicillamine
    (D) sulfasalazine
    (E) hydroxychloroquine

444. Which histologic subtype of lymphoma occurs most commonly in patients infected with HIV?

    (A) Immunoblastic (large cell) lymphoma
    (B) Small, noncleaved (Burkitt's) lymphoma
    (C) Small, cleaved (follicular) lymphoma
    (D) Primary central nervous system lymphoma
    (E) Hodgkin's disease, mixed cellularity

445. A 68-year-old woman presents to her internist for a routine checkup. Her physical examination is normal and routine laboratory evaluation is also normal except for an elevated total protein of 90 g/L (9.0 g/dL). Further workup includes the following: serum protein electrophoresis that reveals an M spike (proven to be IgG-κ on immunoelectrophoresis) of 19 g/L (1.9 g/dL), an unremarkable urine protein electrophoresis, bone marrow aspirate and biopsy that discloses normal hematopoiesis and 3 percent bone marrow plasma cells, and a negative skeletal survey. The proper course of action at this point is to

    (A) obtain quantitative immunoglobulin levels
    (B) obtain beta-microglobulin level
    (C) begin therapy with melphalan and prednisone
    (D) begin therapy with high-dose prednisone
    (E) reassure the patient; no additional action is required at this time

446. Which of the following systemic manifestations is LEAST characteristic of early adult rheumatoid arthritis?

    (A) High fever
    (B) Weight loss
    (C) Muscle wasting
    (D) Vague musculoskeletal symptoms
    (E) Fatigue

447. Which of the following conditions is LEAST likely to occur in late extraarticular seropositive rheumatoid arthritis?

    (A) Neutropenia
    (B) Dry eyes
    (C) Leg ulcers
    (D) Sensorimotor polyneuropathy
    (E) Hepatitis

448. Within minutes after injection of radiocontrast at the time of abdominal CT, a patient develops urticaria, flushing, and congestion of tongue and larynx. Respiratory stridor develops and intubation is emergently required. The mechanism of this event is

(A) direct activation of mediator release from mast cells or basophils or both
(B) IgE-mediated reaction against protein-hapten conjugates
(C) IgE-mediated reaction against native proteins
(D) deficiency of C1 esterase inhibitor
(E) inherited inability to normally catabolize the radiocontrast agent

449. A 35-year-old woman relates a 1-year history of recurrent crops of small, reddish-brown pruritic skin bumps. She also notes facial flushing, lightheadedness, and lower abdominal pain. Pressure on one of these skin lesions results in increased itching and redness. Some attacks are brought on by the use of alcohol or nonsteroidal anti-inflammatory agents. An upper GI series reveals an ulcer crater in the duodenal bulb. Skin biopsy would reveal

(A) aggregates of neutrophils in small venules
(B) mast cell infiltration
(C) hyperkeratosis and infiltration of lymphocytes into the dermis
(D) malignant-appearing neovascularization
(E) normal findings

450. In which of the following clinical situations would a diagnosis of ankylosing spondylitis most likely be correct?

(A) For the last 10 years, a 28-year-old man has had low back pain and stiffness, worse at night and relieved with activity
(B) For the last 5 years, a 32-year-old man has had low back pain made worse with activity but improved with bed rest
(C) For the last 10 years, a 34-year-old man has had intermittent bouts of mild low back pain; now, however, he suddenly is unable to dorsiflex his right great toe
(D) For the last 10 years, a 65-year-old man has had low back pain radiating down both posterior thighs to the knees
(E) For the last 15 years, a 72-year-old man has had progressive low back pain made worse with walking but improved with rest and leaning forward

451. Arthritis associated with psoriasis can be manifest in several different ways. Each of the following is characteristic of psoriatic arthritis EXCEPT

(A) asymmetric oligoarticular arthritis
(B) rheumatoid factor–positive symmetric polyarthritis
(C) arthritis of distal interphalangeal joints
(D) severe destructive polyarthritis (arthritis mutilans)
(E) spondylitis and sacroiliitis with or without peripheral arthritis

452. A 26-year-old woman with systemic lupus erythematosus (SLE) is noted to have a prolonged partial thromboplastin time. This abnormality is associated with

    (A) leukopenia
    (B) drug-induced lupus
    (C) central nervous system vasculitis
    (D) central nervous system hemorrhage
    (E) deep venous thrombosis

453. A patient with diffuse cutaneous scleroderma (systemic sclerosis) who had been stable for several years is recently noted to have hypertension. This patient is at significant risk of dying from

    (A) thrombotic stroke
    (B) central nervous system hemorrhage
    (C) renal failure
    (D) pulmonary hypertension
    (E) pulmonary fibrosis

454. For the last two years, a 27-year-old man has had recurrent episodes of asymmetric inflammatory oligoarticular arthritis involving his knees, ankles, and elbows lasting from 2 to 4 weeks. He also states he has had recurrent, painful "canker sores" in his mouth for the last 10 years. Now, he presents with fever, arthritis, mild abdominal pain, severe headache, and superficial thrombophlebitis in the left leg. The most likely diagnosis in this man is

    (A) regional enteritis
    (B) systemic lupus erythematosus
    (C) Behçet's syndrome
    (D) Whipple's disease
    (E) ulcerative colitis

455. A 37-year-old woman with Raynaud's phenomenon complains of progressive weakness with inability to arise out of a sitting position without assistance. On examination, the patient has swollen "sausagelike" fingers, alopecia, erythematous patches on the knuckles, facial telangiectasias, and proximal muscle weakness. Laboratory evaluation includes a normal CBC and serum chemistries, except for creatine phosphokinase 4.5 μkat/L (270 U/L) and aldolase 500 nkat/L (30 U/L). The following serologic profile is found: rheumatoid factor is positive at 1:1600; ANA is also positive at 1:1600 with a speckled pattern and very high titers of antibodies against the ribonuclease-sensitive ribonucleoprotein component of extractable nuclear antigen. This patient probably has

    (A) early rheumatoid arthritis
    (B) systemic sclerosis
    (C) systemic lupus erythematosus
    (D) dermatomyositis
    (E) mixed connective tissue disease

456. An 18-year-old man presents with abdominal pain, nausea, and vomiting. He also notes the onset of a rash and painful joints. Physical examination is remarkable for the presence of palpable purpura distributed over the buttocks and lower extremities as well as guaiac-positive stool. Laboratory evaluation is remarkable for urinalysis that discloses mild proteinuria and red blood cell casts. Other serum studies are normal. Skin biopsy would likely reveal

    (A) necrotizing angiitis
    (B) eosinophilic angiitis
    (C) leukocytoclastic vasculitis
    (D) extravasated red blood cells without vasculitis
    (E) mast cell infiltration

457. All the following physical findings may be seen in osteoarthritis EXCEPT

    (A) Heberden's nodes
    (B) Bouchard's nodes
    (C) bony crepitus on joint movement
    (D) boutonnière deformity
    (E) positive "shrug" sign

458. A 50-year-old woman has had Raynaud's phenomenon of the hands for 15 years. The condition has become worse during the last year, and she has developed arthralgias and arthritis involving the hands and wrists as well as mild sclerodactyly and difficulty swallowing solid foods. Laboratory studies reveal a positive serum antinuclear antibody assay at a dilution of 1:160. Anticentromere antibodies are present in high titers; antiribonucleoprotein antibodies are not detectable. The most likely diagnosis of this woman's disorder is

    (A) systemic sclerosis
    (B) mixed connective-tissue disease
    (C) overlap syndrome
    (D) dermatomyositis
    (E) systemic lupus erythematosus

459. A 25-year-old man has had pain and swelling in the right knee for the last year. He is otherwise well and gives no history of trauma. X-rays show several erosions at the margin of the right knee joint. Aspiration of the joint yields 25 mL of dark-brown synovial fluid of good viscosity. The most likely diagnosis is

    (A) atypical rheumatoid arthritis
    (B) incomplete Reiter's syndrome
    (C) hemangioma
    (D) osteochondritis dissecans
    (E) pigmented villonodular synovitis

460. A 52-year-old previously well man who has had hoarseness as well as intermittent pain and swelling in his right knee and left foot over the past few months presents now because of pain and swelling in both ears. On examination he has conjunctivitis and beefy red skin over the ears and bridge of the nose, although the earlobes appear normal. His most likely diagnosis is

    (A) Cogan's syndrome
    (B) Reiter's syndrome
    (C) relapsing polychondritis
    (D) rheumatoid arthritis
    (E) squamous carcinoma

461. True statements about human T cells include which of the following?

    (A) They are the principal cells in the cortical "germinal centers" and medullary cords of lymph nodes
    (B) They carry membrane-bound IgD on their surface
    (C) They constitute 70 to 80 percent of circulating blood lymphocytes
    (D) They arise from stem cells in the thymus
    (E) They are the main effectors of antibody-dependent, cell-mediated cytotoxicity

462. Human immunoglobulin A (IgA) can be described by which of the following statements?

    (A) It is the predominant immunoglobulin in plasma
    (B) It exists in four subclasses, of which IgA2 is predominant
    (C) It can prevent attachment of microorganisms to epithelial cell membranes
    (D) It is prominent early in the immune response and is the major class of antibody in cold agglutinins
    (E) It has the shortest half-life of the five classes of immunoglobulin

463. A 27-year-old woman with systemic lupus erythematosus is in remission; current treatment is azathioprine, 75 mg/d, and prednisone, 5 mg/d. Last year she had a life-threatening exacerbation of her disease. She now strongly desires to become pregnant. Which of the following is the LEAST appropriate action?

(A) Advise her that the risk of spontaneous abortion is high
(B) Warn her that exacerbations can occur in the first trimester and in the postpartum period
(C) Tell her it is unlikely a newborn will have lupus
(D) Advise that fetal loss rates are higher if anticardiolipin antibodies are detected in her serum
(E) Stop the prednisone just before she attempts to become pregnant

464. Which of the following is LEAST likely to be seen in Sjögren's syndrome?

(A) Dental caries
(B) Corneal ulceration
(C) Renal tubular acidosis
(D) Lymphoma
(E) Cardiac fibrosis

465. A strong association exists between the HLA-B27 histocompatibility antigen and ankylosing spondylitis. This association is best characterized by which of the following statements?

(A) A positive HLA-B27 determination in a person with low back pain can verify a diagnosis of ankylosing spondylitis
(B) Half of all HLA-B27-positive persons have sacroiliitis or spondylitis
(C) Persons who are black or of Asian heritage have a higher prevalence of both ankylosing spondylitis and HLA-B27 antigen
(D) Up to 10 percent of cases of ankylosing spondylitis are not associated with HLA-B27 antigen
(E) The concordance rate in identical twins is nearly 100 percent

466. Patients who are HLA-B27-positive may develop constitutional symptoms, tendonitis, mucocutaneous lesions, and uveitis after infections with all the following organisms EXCEPT

(A) enteropathogenic *Escherichia coli*
(B) *Salmonella*
(C) *Shigella*
(D) *Yersinia*
(E) *Campylobacter*

DIRECTIONS: Each question below contains five suggested responses. For **each** of the **five** responses listed with every question, you are to respond either YES (Y) or NO (N). In a given item **all, some, or none of the alternatives** may be correct.

467. True statements about human B lympho-cytes include which of the following?

    (A) They represent less than 25 percent of lymphocytes in peripheral blood
    (B) They require the presence of antigen for maturation
    (C) Maturity is heralded by the presence of IgD on the cell surface
    (D) They have membrane receptors for the Fc portion of IgG
    (E) They have membrane receptors for the (activated) C3 component of complement

468. A physician working on a Hopi Indian res-ervation in New Mexico develops a flulike illness with the additional features of cough; conjunctivitis; painful, red lesions on his legs; and a painful, swollen right knee. Correct statements regarding this patient's arthritis include

    (A) culturing the joint fluid will probably yield the diagnosis
    (B) serology may be helpful in establish-ing the diagnosis
    (C) the arthritis could have arisen from hematogenous seeding
    (D) the arthritis could be a sterile mani-festation of acute hypersensitivity
    (E) the arthritis could have arisen from adjacent osteomyelitis

469. Correct statements regarding T-cell immu-nophenotype include which of the follow-ing?

    (A) The T-cell antigen receptor is the ear-liest surface marker of T-cell lineage
    (B) The expressions of CD4 (T4) and CD8 (T8) surface antigens are mu-tually exclusive
    (C) The T-cell adhesion molecule, CD2 (T11), accounts for the ability of T cells to form rosettes with sheep red blood cells
    (D) The T-cell antigen receptor complex consists of a signal-transducing moiety and an antigen-recognition moiety
    (E) Mature T cells display surface pro-teins that are members of the immu-noglobulin gene superfamily

470. Persons who are diagnosed as having Di George's syndrome usually have

    (A) hypocalcemic tetany
    (B) hypothyroidism
    (C) T-cell deficiency
    (D) hypogammaglobulinemia
    (E) congenital heart disease

471. Correct statements about isolated immunoglobulin A deficiency include which of the following?

(A) The incidence of atopic disease is high
(B) The risk of adverse reactions to transfusions is increased
(C) The incidence of autoimmune disease is increased
(D) Secretory IgA levels usually are normal
(E) The reduced number of IgA-bearing B cells accounts for the reduced serum IgA levels

472. True statements regarding immune-complex disease include which of the following?

(A) Normally, most immune complexes are removed by the reticuloendothelial system
(B) Signs and symptoms stem from the deposition of immune complexes in tissues other than those of the reticuloendothelial system
(C) Persistence of immune complexes in the circulation seems to be a requirement for the development of renal manifestations
(D) Renal lesions depend on antigen-antibody combinations in which antigen is in slight excess
(E) The rash of cutaneous necrotizing vasculitis may be an example of immune-complex disease

473. True statements regarding HLA class I molecules include

(A) they consist of four polypeptide chains
(B) they include a beta$_2$-microglobulin subunit
(C) they share less than 25 percent homology with one another
(D) they are distributed unevenly from one racial group to another
(E) they are expressed on all cells except mature red blood cells

474. Correct statements regarding the treatment of patients with HIV infection include which of the following?

(A) Zidovudine (AZT) therapy has been proved beneficial in those patients with <500 CD4 (T4)-positive lymphocytes, even if they are asymptomatic
(B) AZT is ineffective in treating HIV-related neurologic symptoms
(C) Myelosuppression is the most common and important side effect of AZT
(D) AZT is an antiretroviral drug by virtue of its ability to selectively inhibit viral DNA polymerase
(E) Aerosolized pentamidine is an effective prophylactic treatment for recurrent *Pneumocystis* pneumonia, but its use has been associated with some cases of extrapulmonary *P. carinii* infection

475. A 63-year-old woman with a history of rheumatoid arthritis since age 42 is seen for the first time by a new physician. The patient has been doing poorly of late. Though her joint disease has not been a problem, she has lost weight and has been plagued by chronic foul-smelling diarrhea, easy bruising, profound fatigue, and peripheral edema. On examination she has waxy skin plaques clustered in the axillary folds, a large tongue, a quiet precordium, hepatosplenomegaly, guaiac-positive stool, and peripheral neuropathy. Laboratory evaluation includes the findings of proteinuria (5 g/d), normal serum chemistry except slightly low albumin and slightly elevated alkaline phosphatase, and low-voltage QRS complexes on electrocardiography. In order to expeditiously diagnose the problem, one could

(A) perform a bone marrow aspirate and biopsy
(B) obtain three serial sputum samples for acid-fast bacillus (AFB) culture
(C) perform an abdominal CT examination
(D) obtain an abdominal subcutaneous fat pad aspirate
(E) perform a rectal biopsy

476. Drug-induced systemic lupus erythematosus (SLE) can be characterized by which of the following statements?

(A) Twenty percent of patients receiving procainamide develop drug-induced lupus

(B) Nephritis is a frequent consequence of hydralazine-induced lupus

(C) Most patients on hydralazine develop a positive antinuclear antibody (ANA) test; however, only 10 percent suffer from lupuslike symptoms

(D) If patients with drug-induced lupus fail to respond within several weeks of discontinuing the offending agent, a trial of corticosteroids is indicated

(E) If a patient with drug-induced lupus has persistent symptoms for longer than 6 months, an anti-ds antibody and CH_{50} levels should be drawn

477. Correct statements concerning the use of nonsteroidal anti-inflammatory drugs (NSAIDs) in the treatment of rheumatoid arthritis include which of the following?

(A) The mechanism of action of NSAIDs is the blockade of 5-lipoxygenase

(B) The newer NSAIDs are more efficacious than aspirin

(C) The newer NSAIDs induce platelet dysfunction

(D) NSAIDs can exacerbate allergic rhinitis and asthma

(E) The mechanism of NSAID-induced azotemia is unrelated to these drugs' ability to disrupt arachidonic acid metabolism

478. True statements about sarcoidosis include which of the following?

(A) Accumulation of suppressor-cytotoxic T lymphocytes occurs in sites of disease activity

(B) The ratio of black to white patients in the United States may exceed 10:1

(C) Chest radiography and pulmonary function testing are sensitive means of evaluating the intensity of pulmonary inflammation

(D) Transbronchial biopsy may reveal granulomata in a high percentage of patients and is a useful means of diagnosis

(E) Asymptomatic hilar adenopathy accounts for 10 to 20 percent of cases of sarcoidosis in the United States

479. Accurate statements about rheumatoid factors include which of the following?

(A) They are antibodies to the Fc fragment of immunoglobulin G

(B) They are associated with several conditions in which there is chronic antigenic stimulation

(C) Their presence in the serum of persons with rheumatoid arthritis correlates with a worse prognosis than that for persons with seronegative disease

(D) Their presence correlates with articular manifestations of rheumatoid arthritis

(E) They frequently do not appear in the serum of persons with rheumatoid arthritis until late in the course of the illness

480. The diagnosis of many rheumatic diseases, including rheumatoid arthritis, is based entirely on clinical grounds. Clinical characteristics associated with rheumatoid arthritis include

(A) prolonged morning stiffness
(B) migratory polyarthritis
(C) arthritis involving the distal interphalangeal joints
(D) arthritis of the cervical spine
(E) carpal tunnel syndrome

481. A 27-year-old man presents because of a painful, swollen knee and ankle of 2 weeks' duration. He has never had joint disease prior to this time. The patient also complains of low back pain and a recent history of clear penile discharge. On examination he has vesicles (some of which have crusted over) on the palms, soles, and glans penis; injected conjunctivae; a swollen right index finger; and arthritis of the right knee and left ankle. Correct statements regarding this patient include

(A) he will probably benefit from indomethacin
(B) his joint disease will probably improve after a course of tetracycline
(C) he is probably HLA-B27-positive
(D) x-ray of the pelvis would probably demonstrate blurring of the sacroiliac joint
(E) his erythrocyte sedimentation rate is likely to be elevated

482. A 40-year-old woman presents with purulent nasal discharge, cough, hemoptysis, and dyspnea. Chest x-ray reveals bilateral nodules; creatinine and erythrocyte sedimentation are elevated; urinalysis reveals hematuria and proteinuria. Accurate statements regarding this woman's condition include

(A) she probably has circulating anti-basement membrane antibodies
(B) she probably has circulating antineutrophil antibodies
(C) necrotizing granulomatous vasculitis would probably be found if a lung biopsy was carried out
(D) glucocorticoids and cyclophosphamide should be administered
(E) even with appropriate therapy, her prognosis is poor

483. Development of the x-ray findings shown below is linked on occasion to the presence of which of the following disorders?

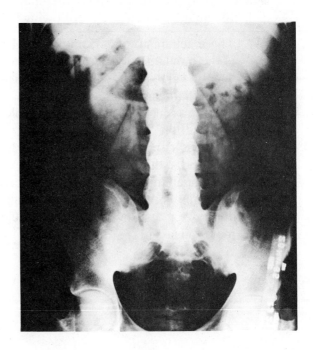

(A) Kidney stones
(B) Aortic insufficiency
(C) Peripheral neuropathy
(D) Uveitis
(E) Quadriplegia

484. The arthritis associated with the deposition of calcium pyrophosphate dihydrate crystals is accurately described by which of the following statements?

(A) Calcium pyrophosphate dihydrate crystals are thought to form from supersaturated solutions of calcium phosphate in synovial fluid

(B) Calcium pyrophosphate dihydrate crystals appear under polarized light as elongated rods with strong negative birefringence

(C) Clinical manifestations usually are limited to the knee joints

(D) Most affected persons have radiographic evidence of chondrocalcinosis

(E) Clinical syndromes caused by deposition of calcium pyrophosphate dihydrate crystals can mimic degenerative joint disease

485. Acute sarcoidosis is characterized by which of the following syndromes?

(A) Cough, hemoptysis, and interstitial pulmonary involvement

(B) Myopathy, keratotic skin lesions on the palms and soles, and arthralgias

(C) Fever, pulmonary stenotic murmur, and nailbed lesions

(D) Erythema nodosum, arthralgias, and hilar adenopathy

(E) Fever, parotid enlargement, uveitis, and facial nerve palsy

486. Familial Mediterranean fever (FMF) is correctly characterized by which of the following statements?

(A) Fifty percent of patients have no family history of the disease

(B) Chest pain is unusual

(C) Colchicine is likely to be beneficial

(D) Levels of dopamine beta-hydroxylase are increased

(E) Amyloidosis is a common complication throughout the world

487. A 52-year-old woman presents with nasal discharge and stuffiness, difficulty in breathing through the nose, and sinus pain. ENT examination reveals ulcers on the nasal septum and perforation of the soft palate. There is no history of prior illness or drug abuse. Biopsy of involved material under anesthesia reveals noncaseating granulomatous inflammation with necrotic debris. No malignant cells, vasculitis, or microorganisms are noted. Correct statements concerning this patient's condition include which of the following?

(A) The history and findings are consistent with Wegener's granulomatosis

(B) If she is not appropriately treated, the disease will probably be fatal

(C) The treatment of choice is radiation therapy

(D) The disease, if unchecked, can progress to involve the mediastinum and lungs

(E) Optimal treatment should involve surgical debridement

DIRECTIONS: The group of questions below consists of five lettered headings followed by a set of numbered items. For each numbered item select the **one** lettered heading with which it is **most** closely associated. Each lettered heading may be used **once, more than once, or not at all.**

Questions 488–491

For each diagnosis that follows, select the synovial fluid findings with which it is most likely to be associated.

(A) Fluid, clear and viscous; white blood cell count, 400/mm³; no crystals
(B) Fluid, cloudy and watery; white blood cell count, 8000/mm³; no crystals
(C) Fluid, dark brown and viscous; white blood cell count, 1200/mm³; no crystals
(D) Fluid, cloudy and watery; white blood cell count, 12,000/mm³; crystals, needlelike and strongly negatively birefringent
(E) Fluid, cloudy and watery; white blood cell count, 4800/mm³; crystals, rhomboidal and weakly positively birefringent

488.   Pigmented villonodular synovitis

489.   Calcium pyrophosphate deposition disease

490.   Gout

491.   Degenerative joint disease

Immunologic, Allergic, and Rheumatic Disorders

Answers

418. The answer is D. *(Chap 277.)* Lymphoid cells, including both T and B lymphocytes, arise from hematopoietic stem cells. Those cells destined to enter the B-cell lineage arise continuously in the bone marrow. The earliest cells destined to become B cells express surface CD10 (CALLA, J-5) protein, an endopeptidase thought to inactivate certain peptide hormones. These pre-B cells are large lymphoid cells containing cytoplasmic μ chains, the heavy chain of immunoglobulin M (IgM), as detected by immunofluorescence. Cytoplasmic light chains are not present, and pre-B cells lack membrane-bound IgM or immunoglobulin of any other class. In the process of B-cell maturation, smaller lymphoid cells will appear that bear a narrow rim of cytoplasmic IgM; later, cells with membrane-bound IgM develop.

419. The answer is D. *(Chap 280.)* Plasma cell diseases are a group of conditions in which a clone of cells capable of synthesizing and secreting immunoglobulins, or the heavy- or light-chain component of these molecules, proliferates abnormally. IgG immunoglobulins are the most common class produced in such diseases. Also, free light chains usually are produced in excess and are detected in urine as Bence Jones protein. Multiple myeloma is the most common plasma cell neoplasm. Its classic presentation includes bone pain, anemia, hypercalcemia, renal failure, and recurrent infections in an elderly person. Diagnosis is best made by looking for a homogeneous globulin peak on electrophoresis of serum, urine, or both. Waldenström's macroglobulinemia is a related condition in which the monoclonal immunoglobulin is of the IgM class. Because IgM is so large (it circulates as a pentamer), it is restricted to the bloodstream and in high concentrations tends to cause hyperviscosity of the blood. Other features differentiating Waldenström's macroglobulinemia from multiple myeloma are enlargement of lymph nodes and spleen and occasional transformation to chronic lymphocytic leukemia or lymphocytic lymphoma.

420. The answer is B. *(Chap 70.)* Eicosanoids refer to all metabolites of both the cyclooxygenase and lipoxygenase pathways of arachidonic acid metabolism. Eicosanoids, including the prostaglandins, thromboxane, and leukotrienes, act as local modulators of biochemical activity in the tissues in which they are formed and have generally short circulatory half-lives. As such, they function in a paracrine fashion and are considered to be autocoids, not hormones. Different members of this family have an impact on a host of physiologic functions including lipolysis, water balance, platelet aggregation, and gastrointestinal effects. The synthesis of these compounds begins from the cleavage of arachidonic acid from membrane phospholipids by phospholipase A_2 (or possibly phospholipase C). Free arachidonic acid can then be oxygenated by cyclooxygenase or lipoxygenase. Cyclooxygenase enzyme action, which can be inhibited by salicylates or NSAIDs, results in the formation of cyclic endoperoxides, which are metabolized either to prostaglandins or to thromboxane. On the other hand, lipoxygenase, for which no clinically important inhibitors exist, catalyzes the formation of hydroperoxyeicosatetraenoic acid (HPETE), the precursor of leukotriene formation. Glucocorticoids are believed to inhibit the formation of eicosanoids by inhibiting phospholipase A_2. By inhibiting the synthesis of inflammatory prostaglandins and thromboxane through their inhibitory action on cyclooxygenase, the NSAIDs are effective in treating the pain and discomfort associated with inflammation.

421. The answer is E. *(Chap 277. Frank, N Engl J Med 316:1525–1530, 1987.)* Complement activity, resulting from the sequential interaction of a large number of plasma and cell-membrane proteins, plays an important role in the inflammatory response. The classical pathway of complement activation is initiated by an antibody-antigen interaction. The first complement component (C1, a complex composed of three proteins) binds to immune complexes with activation mediated by C1q. Active C1 then initiates the cleavage and concomitant activation of components C4 and C2. The activated C1 is destroyed by a plasma protease inhibitor termed C1 esterase inhibitor. This molecule also regulates clotting factors XI and kallikrein. Patients with deficiency of C1q esterase inhibitor may develop angioedema, sometimes leading to death via asphyxia. Attacks may be precipitated by stress or trauma. In addition to low antigenic or functional levels of C1 esterase inhibitor, patients with this autosomal dominant condition may have normal levels of C1 and C3, but low levels of C4 and C2. Danazol therapy produces a striking increase in the level of this important inhibitor and alleviates symptoms in many patients. An acquired form of angioedema due to C1 esterase inhibitor deficiency has been described in patients with autoimmune or malignant disease.

422. The answer is D. *(Chap 282.)* Urticaria and angioedema are common disorders, affecting approximately 20 percent of the population. In acute urticarial angioedema, attacks of swelling are of less than 6 weeks' duration; chronic urticarial angioedema is by definition more long-standing. Urticaria usually is pruritic and affects the trunk and proximal extremities. Angioedema is generally less pruritic and affects the hands, feet, genitalia, and face. The woman described in the question has chronic urticaria, which probably is due to a cutaneous necrotizing vasculitis. The clues to the diagnosis are the arthralgias, presence of residual skin discoloration, and elevated sedimentation rate—these would be uncharacteristic of other urticarial diseases. Diagnosis can be confirmed by skin biopsy. Chronic urticaria is rarely of allergic cause; hence, allergy skin tests and measurement of total immunoglobulin E levels are not helpful. Measurement of C1 esterase inhibitor activity is useful in diagnosing hereditary angioedema, a disease not associated with urticaria. Patch tests are used to diagnose contact dermatitis.

423. The answer is D. *(Chap 282. Naclerio, N Engl J Med 325:860–869, 1991.)* Allergic rhinitis can be either seasonal as a result of pollen exposure or perennial as a result of exposure to dust or mold spores (or both). In these IgE-mediated reactions to inhaled foreign substances, nasal eosinophilia is common. Vasomotor rhinitis is a chronic, nonallergic condition in which vasomotor control in the nasal membranes is altered. Irritating stimuli, such as odors, fumes, and changes in humidity and barometric pressure, can cause nasal obstruction and discharge in affected persons, and nasal eosinophilia is not noted. Because the man described in the question has either perennial allergic rhinitis due to dust or mold-spore allergy or eosinophilic nonallergic rhinitis, skin testing for responses to suspected allergens should be diagnostic. Though total serum IgE may be elevated, demonstration of specificity is critical. Specificity can be demonstrated by binding to a antigen and detected by uptake of radiolabeled anti-IgE (radioallergosorbent technique; RAST). RAST is more difficult than skin testing due to the requirement for defined antigens and standardization. Pollen skin tests are unlikely to be helpful because of the perennial nature of the condition described. An elimination diet can be used diagnostically or therapeutically in persons with suspected food allergy; however, food allergy rarely causes rhinitis. Sinus x-rays, whether positive or negative, would not reveal the underlying cause of the rhinitis.

424. The answer is A. *(Chap 277. Robertson, Blood 76:2421, 1990.)*   Previously termed "null cells," large granular lymphocytes (LGL) constitute about 5 to 10 percent of peripheral blood lymphocytes. These cells express surface receptors for the Fc portion of IgE (CD16) and proliferate in response to interleukin 2 (IL-2). Subsets of LGL mediate both antibody-dependent cellular cytotoxicity (the binding of an antibody-coated target cell to an Fc receptor-bearing effector cell resulting in lysis of the target) as well as natural killer cell activity. Natural killer (NK) cell activity, believed to be important in antitumor activity and transplant rejection, represents nonimmune and non-antibody-mediated killing of target cells. Natural killer cells activated by IL-2 (LAK cells) infused into patients with renal cell carcinoma and further stimulated with IL-2 have resulted in clinical responses. NK cells bear a surface molecule termed CD56 (also known as N-CAM or NKH-1), a 140,000-kd protein that may mediate NK cell adhesion.

425. The answer is C. *(Chap 277.)*   Reactions are initiated by mononuclear leukocytes and require 48 to 72 h to evidence a response after antigen exposure. Such delayed-type hypersensitivity reactions are best exemplified by local reactions to skin challenge in persons previously exposed to the test antigen. The cellular events resulting in such hypersensitivity responses are centered around T cells (particularly lymphokine-secreting TH-1-helper T cells) and macrophages. Antigen processed by monocytes-macrophages is presented to specific T cells. Macrophages secrete interleukin 1 and interleukin 6 to clonally amplify the specific T cell and also secrete lymphokines such as IL-2 and gamma interferon to recruit additional T cells and macrophages to participate in the inflammatory response. Macrophages recruited in this fashion may undergo epithelioid cell transformation to form giant cells, perhaps in response to IL-4 and interferon-γ. In addition to mycobacterial infections, diseases in which delayed-type hypersensitivity is important include histoplasmosis, chlamydial infections, schistosomiasis, and berylliosis.

426. The answer is D. *(Chap 291.)*   Polyarteritis nodosa is a vasculitis of medium-sized vessels. Early systemic features include fever, weakness, anorexia, weight loss, myalgias, and arthralgias (though severe and persistent arthritis is uncommon). Pericarditis and pleuritis also can occur. Mononeuritis multiplex develops because of involvement of the vasa nervorum; it is reflected in the man described by the sudden loss of the ability to dorsiflex his right great toe. Abdominal pain occurs in 60 to 70 percent of affected persons and is related to disease involvement of mesenteric arteries. Hypertension develops from arterial occlusion and occurs before renal involvement. Laboratory findings of elevated erythrocyte sedimentation rate, anemia of chronic disease, and polymorphonuclear leukocytosis all occur with polyarteritis nodosa. Pulmonary involvement is unusual and serves to distinguish this entity clinically from allergic granulomatosis and Wegener's granulomatosis. Hypersensitivity vasculitis is a term applied to small-vessel vasculitides associated with a range of findings from purely cutaneous disease to minimal skin disease but life-threatening involvement of major organs. Giant cell arteritis involves the aorta and other great vessels, producing constitutional symptoms and large-vessel occlusion in young women (Takayasu's disease) and in the elderly (temporal arteritis, polymyalgia rheumatica).

427. The answer is C. *(Chap 284. Balow, Ann Intern Med 106:79, 1987.)* Renal disease is clinically evident in about half those persons with systemic lupus erythematosus (SLE). However, nearly all persons with SLE have some evidence of renal disease on renal biopsy. Renal disease associated with SLE includes both glomerulonephritis and interstitial nephritis. Glomerular disease has been classified into membranous nephritis and mesangial, focal, and diffuse glomerulonephritis. Immune-complex interstitial nephritis occurs most commonly in persons who have diffuse glomerulonephritis. Urinalysis performed for persons with active renal disease usually reveals microscopic hematuria, red cell casts, and proteinuria; the exception is membranous lupus nephritis, in which proteinuria is the dominant finding. Drug-induced lupus rarely leads to renal disease. Anti-dsDNA antibodies at high titer are associated with severe nephritis. Renal biopsy is not necessary in SLE patients whose renal function is rapidly deteriorating when they have an active sediment. If such patients fail to respond to the prompt initiation of glucocorticoid therapy demanded in such a situation, then biopsy should be undertaken. Patients with mild clinical disease should have a biopsy to determine if they have active, severe, inflammatory lesions, which might respond to therapy.

428. The answer is C. *(Chap 278. Sneller, Ann Intern Med 118:720–730, 1993.)* Common variable immunodeficiency represents a heterogeneous group of adults who have in common deficiencies of all major immunoglobulin classes. The defect is believed to be due to an abnormality in B-cell maturation, though most of these patients tend to have normal levels of clonally diverse B lymphocytes. The B cells can recognize antigen and proliferate, but fail to differentiate to the immunoglobulin-secreting stage. Associated with this abnormality is nodular lymphoid hyperplasia in various organs (including the gut) and splenomegaly. This panhypogammaglobulinemic disorder should be suspected in adults with chronic pulmonary infections, unexplained bronchiectasis (like the case presented in this example), chronic giardiasis, malabsorption, and atrophic gastritis. Patients develop intestinal neoplasms at increased frequency. They also develop autoimmune conditions, such as Coombs-positive hemolytic anemia and idiopathic thrombocytopenic purpura. There is some suggestion that, in addition to failure of B cells to secrete immunoglobulin, T cells have an impaired ability to release lymphokines. The mainstay of therapy for common variable immunodeficiency is to increase the antibody content by administration of intravenous immunoglobulin concentrates. The goal is to increase the IgG level to 5 g/L, which can generally be accomplished by monthly administration of 200 to 400 mg/kg of intravenous immunoglobulin. True anaphylactic reactions to immunoglobulin treatment are rare.

429. The answer is D. *(Chaps 151, 279. Greene, N Engl J Med 321:308–316, 1991.)* The etiologic agent of AIDS, HIV-1, is a member of the lentivirus subfamily of retroviruses that infect humans. There are four human retroviruses, including HTLV-I and HTLV-II, which can transform human cells in tissue culture. HTLV-I is the etiologic agent of acute T-cell leukemia/lymphoma and tropical spastic paraparesis. This virus, like HIV-1, also infects CD4-positive T lymphocytes. However, HIV is remarkable in that it contains six genes in addition to the three typical genes, *gag, pol,* and *env,* contained in the genome of other retroviruses. The *gag* gene encodes glycoproteins in the viral coat. The *pol* gene encodes reverse transcriptase as well as other enzymes necessary for integration of the viral genome into the host chromosome. The *env* gene encodes a viral coat protein that mediates CD4 binding and membrane fusion. Other genes include the *vif* gene, which promotes infectivity of cell-free virus, the *vpr* gene, which is a weak transcriptional activator, and the *tat* gene, which codes for a protein that binds to transactivating sequences. It is hoped that functions mediated by some of these HIV-1-specific genes might be appropriate loci for the design of thera-peutic strategies. In addition to T cells and monocytes, HIV-1 may also infect bone marrow pro-genitors, gut epithelium, and glial cells. Infection of these cells may contribute to the hematologic abnormalities, diarrhea-wasting syndrome, and progressive dementia observed in patients infected with HIV-1.

430. The answer is B. *(Chap 279. Pantaleo, N Engl J Med 328:327, 1993.)* AIDS is characterized by the infection of CD4$^+$ lymphocytes by the AIDS retrovirus (HIV-1) with subsequent deficiency in numbers and functions of this T-cell subpopulation, which includes the important helper-inducer cells necessary for production of a variety of immune responses. Thus, there is a defect in the response of T cells to soluble antigen and to mitogenic substances such as phytohemagglutinin and concanavalin A. Natural killer cell function is abnormal and may be augmented in vitro by addition of the lymphokine interleukin 2. There is polyclonal activation of B lymphocytes with a resultant increase in serum immunoglobulin levels and occasional production of autoantibodies.

431. The answer is A. *(Chap 64.)* The major histocompatibility gene complex (MHC), located on the short arm of chromosome 6, contains genes involved in the recognition of self, antigen presentation to T and B cells, and the rejection of tissue allografts. Ubiquitously expressed class I molecules are the products of the HLA-A, -B, and -C genes. Also in the MHC, the HLA-D region, separated from the ABC genes by an area responsible for certain complement components (C2, C4B, Bf, C4A) and tumor necrosis factor, codes for class II molecules, which are only expressed on T cells, B cells, and monocytes (and their derivatives, such as Langerhans' skin cells). Class I molecules are responsible for the mixed lymphocyte reaction (MLR), which is important in determining com-patibility of donor and host tissues in a potential transplant situation. Because the ABC and D regions are closely linked, recombination between these two areas is uncommon (approximately 2 percent). Thus, an ABC-matched sibling is usually, but not always, matched at the D locus as well. In addition to a recombination event, another reason for a positive MLR in an HLA-ABC matched sibling pair is histoincompatibility at minor loci, which are located throughout the genome.

432. The answer is A. *(Chap 279.)* The standard serologic test for HIV infection, the enzyme-linked immunosorbent assay (ELISA), has a sensitivity of over 99.5 percent. However, this test is not particularly specific in that low-risk patients are subject to a false positive rate of over 10 percent. If the ELISA test is indeterminate or positive, the test should be repeated. If the repeat is positive or indeterminate, one should proceed to the next step, which is a western blot test. If the repeat ELISA is negative, then the person can be assumed not to have HIV infection. A western blot test involves the reaction of the serum with a strip impregnated with HIV-1 antigens. Binding of anti-bodies in the patient's serum to the antigens on the strip is detected with an enzyme-conjugated anti-human antibody. A positive western blot test requires the detection of antibodies to several HIV-1 gene products. If the western blot is indeterminate, perhaps due to infection in evolution or due to cross-reacting antibodies in the patient's serum, one should proceed to a PCR test and repeat the western blot in 1 month. If the PCR is negative and there is no progression on the western blot, the diagnosis of HIV infection is ruled out. The PCR test is extraordinarily sensitive, but the false-positive rate would be too high for use as a cost-efficient screening test. A DNA PCR test for HIV involves the isolation of DNA from blood mononuclear cells and incubation with primers from both the *gag* and LTR regions, followed by amplification and hybridization to detect HIV proviral DNA. An RNA PCR test can be used to monitor the level of HIV genome present in plasma (i.e., before cell entry and reverse transcription of the RNA genome).

433. **The answer is D.** *(Chap 279.)*   In patients infected with HIV, symptoms and signs of clinical illness typically begin once the CD4-positive T-lymphocyte count falls beneath 500 cells/μL. Clinical characteristics of early symptomatic disease include generalized lymphadenopathy, thrush, oral hairy leukoplakia, herpes zoster, molluscum contagiosum, and thrombocytopenia. While thrombocytopenia is common in patients whose CD4-positive T-cell counts are less than 400/μL, it rarely represents a serious clinical problem. Counts are generally above 50,000, and even in those whose counts are lower, bleeding is rare unless the count is below 10,000. The pathogenesis of thrombocytopenia in those with HIV infection appears to be similar to that of idiopathic thrombocytopenic purpura (ITP). Bone marrow examination, which should be done to rule out other causes of thrombocytopenia, reveals normal or increased numbers of megakaryocytes. Moreover, immune complexes containing anti-gp120 antibodies have been noted on the surface of platelets. Secondly, many patients with HIV infection have antiplatelet antibodies. The therapeutic strategy for HIV-associated thrombocytopenia is similar to that for ITP. High-dose intravenous immunoglobulin or glucocorticoids can induce a short-term response; however, since the antiretroviral agent zidovudine can induce a longer-lasting response in over 70 percent of patients with HIV-associated thrombocytopenia, it is considered the treatment of choice. In those refractory to medical management, splenectomy is a viable alternative. It is important to administer pneumococcal polysaccharide vaccine (and vaccines for *Haemophilus influenzae* and meningococcus as well) to those about to undergo splenectomy because of the propensity of HIV-infected persons to develop serious infections with encapsulated organisms.

434. **The answer is B.** *(Chap 278. Rosen, N Engl J Med 311:235, 300, 1984.)*   Ataxia-telangiectasia is an autosomal recessive primary immunodeficiency disorder associated with abnormal thymic development, progressive cerebellar ataxia, and oculocutaneous telangiectasia. The responsible gene, located on chromosome 11, leads to a generalized defect in the ability to repair damage to DNA. Such a defect accounts for the frequent occurrence of malignancies, particularly lymphomas, and the exquisite sensitivity to therapeutic irradiation. There is evidence for both humoral and cellular immunodeficiency; most patients have depressed IgA and IgE levels as well as cutaneous anergy. Sinopulmonary infections are common with severe resultant respiratory insufficiency, often associated with bronchiectasis. Adenosine deaminase deficiency is associated not with ataxia-telangiectasia but with severe combined immunodeficiency.

435. **The answer is C.** *(Chap 279.)*   Among the U.S. cases of AIDS in adults, 60 percent are in homosexual men who do not use intravenous drugs; however, attack rates have precipitously declined in the homosexual community, probably owing to behavior modification. On the other hand, infections continue to rise among intravenous drug users. Because of blood donor screening and heat treatment of factor VIII concentrates, the rate of seroconversion in hemophiliacs is dropping. Blood donor screening reduces the risk of exposure to HIV in a single unit of blood to between 1/40,000 and 1/250,000. Pediatric AIDS arises mainly in infants born to mothers who are intravenous drug users or sexual partners of intravenous drug users. The remainder of pediatric AIDS patients are hemophiliacs or recipients of blood transfusions. The overall prevalence of HIV infection is quite low: about 0.04 percent of blood donors, who are a low-risk group because of the voluntary exclusion of high-risk individuals, to 0.15 percent of U.S. military recruits, a group relatively high in risk because of sexual activity and socioeconomic status. There is a small but real risk of seroconversion in those who are exposed to HIV-contaminated materials at the work place; less than 0.5 percent of those who have sustained penetrating injuries or whose mucosae have been splashed with blood from AIDS patients have become infected.

436. **The answer is A.** *(Chap 279.)*   Most patients with HIV infection evidence clinical disease of the central nervous system (CNS) at some point in their course. Cerebrospinal fluid findings are ab-

normal in approximately 90 percent of patients, even during asymptomatic states of infection. Such abnormalities include pleocytosis, isolation of virus and antiviral antibodies, and elevated CSF protein. The most common CNS disease in HIV-infected persons is the AIDS dementia complex, which refers to a syndrome of signs and symptoms that generally occurs late in the course of disease. In addition to dementia, patients may have various additional problems such as unsteady gait and poor balance or behavior problems such as apathy and lack of initiative. The precise cause of the AIDS dementia complex is unclear, but it is probably due to direct effects of HIV infection in the CNS. Eighty to ninety percent of patients with HIV infection can be shown to have some degree of histologic evidence of CNS involvement. The radiologic correlate of AIDS dementia complex is general atrophy, ventricular dilation, and bright spots on T2-weighted MRI images. The ring-enhancing lesions in toxoplasmosis are seen in about 15 percent of all HIV-infected patients with CNS disease and are the second most common cause of seizures after the AIDS dementia complex. The third most common cause of seizures is cryptococcal meningitis. Progressive multifocal leukoencephalopathy is relatively unusual and produces multiple white-matter lesions on T2-weighted MRI images. Neurosyphilis, CNS lymphoma, and tuberculous meningitis are other less common CNS diseases in patients with HIV infection. Antiretroviral treatment has been associated with some improvement in patients with the AIDS dementia complex and therefore merits a therapeutic trial in patients so afflicted.

437. The answer is E. *(Chap 279.)* Kaposi's sarcoma is probably more a consequence of disordered cytokine regulation than it is clonally derived true cancer, since the tumor respects tissue planes and is rarely invasive. Interestingly, the incidence of Kaposi's sarcoma in those diagnosed with AIDS is declining. At least in part, this decrease is due to the fact that AIDS-related Kaposi's sarcoma occurs predominantly in homosexual men, rather than in those with AIDS from other risk groups. Secondly, certain epidemiologic data suggest that a sexually transmitted cofactor plays a role in the development of this neoplasm. With safer sex practices in the homosexual community, especially in New York and Los Angeles, the transmission of this putative cofactor and the risk of Kaposi's have declined. The Kaposi's lesions typically appear as reddish-purple nodules on sun-exposed areas, but the lymph nodes, gastrointestinal tract, and lungs may also be affected. In contrast to many other malignancies, the presence of lymph node involvement is not a marker of advanced disease, since it may indicate relatively intact immune function. In those with pulmonary involvement, the chest x-ray usually shows bilateral lower lobe infiltrates. Most AIDS patients with Kaposi's sarcoma die not as a consequence of their malignancy, but rather from opportunistic infections. Therefore, cytotoxic and immunosuppressive chemotherapy should be used with care. Interferon-α is an effective treatment, but only for those whose CD4 + T-lymphocyte count is still relatively preserved. The interferon-α response rate ranges from 80 percent in those whose CD4-positive T cells are greater than 600/μL to 10 percent for patients with under 150 CD4-positive T cells/μL.

438. The answer is C. *(Chap 279.)* Based on the expanded definition of AIDS to include any HIV-infected person whose CD4 + T-cell count is <200/μL, the clinical situation suggests the diagnosis of the acquired immunodeficiency syndrome (AIDS). *M. pneumoniae,* while a frequent cause of mild community-acquired pneumonia in the otherwise normal host, is not commonly associated with AIDS. *P. carinii,* a protozoal pathogen, is the most frequent cause of respiratory disease in the AIDS patient; it affects approximately 60 percent of such patients some time during the course of their illness. Both cytomegalovirus and *C. neoformans* are less common but significant respiratory pathogens in this patient population. Tuberculosis must always be considered in an AIDS patient with pulmonary symptoms. Tuberculous dissemination occurs frequently.

439. The answer is A. *(Chap 283. Lawly, N Engl J Med 311:1407, 1984.)* The administration of horse antithymocyte globulin (ATG) to patients with aplastic anemia or as an immunosuppressant after bone marrow transplant can lead to a clinical syndrome identical to that of classic serum sickness and one that approximates animal models of immune complex disease. Eight to thirteen days after beginning therapy with ATG, the clinical features begin with fever, malaise, rash (often urticarial), arthralgias, nausea, melena, lymphadenopathy, and proteinuria. There are high levels of circulating immune complexes; more precise quantitation rests on one of a number of generally inconclusive assays, including the Raji cell assay (lymphoblastoid line that binds to C3) and C1q binding assay (first complement subcomponent). With all these circulating immune complexes containing their Fc receptors, the complement system is overactivated, so there are accompanying decreases in C3, C4, and CH_{50}.

440. The answer is C. *(Chap 279.)* The ideal approach to the management of HIV infection would be prevention by alteration of behavior or through the development of a vaccine. However, it is possible to enhance the quality and quantity of life with antiretroviral agents such as zidovudine as well as by attempting to prevent secondary infections, which are a significant cause of morbidity and mortality. Once the CD4-positive T-lymphocyte count drops below 200/μL, prophylaxis against *Pneumocystis carinii* pneumonia should begin with administration of trimethoprim-sulfamethoxazole at a dose of one double-strength tablet twice a day. PPD-positive patients should receive a 1-year course of isoniazid. *Mycobacterium avium-intracellulare* (MAI) infection is very common among HIV-infected patients whose CD4-positive T-cell counts are below 100/μL. Based on a clinical trial that demonstrated that rifabutin (100 mg/d) was effective in delaying the onset of MAI bacteremia by an average of 6 months, this drug has been licensed for primary prophylactic therapy. Many authorities recommend primary prophylaxis with fluconazole against fungal infections, though formal definition of the benefit of such an approach remains to be shown.

441. The answer is B. *(Chap 279. Kaye, Ann Intern Med 11:158, 1989.)* In contrast to the profound immunodeficiency that characterizes most manifestations of AIDS, a host of immunologic and rheumatologic disorders are common in patients with HIV infection. Certainly the most common such reaction is cutaneously manifested sensitivity to the antibiotics required for treatment of the secondary infections so common in these patients. Sixty-five percent of patients who receive trimethoprim-sulfamethoxazole develop an erythematous morbilliform pruritic eruption. Fortunately, anaphylaxis is very rare, and desensitization is possible. Patients infected with HIV may develop diseases that resemble classic autoimmune diseases in non-HIV-infected persons. A variant of Sjögren's syndrome characterized by dry eyes, dry mouth, and lymphocytic infiltrates of the salivary gland and lung may be seen. HIV-associated arthropathy is characterized by a nonerosive oligoarticular arthritis that generally involves the large joints. Widespread musculoskeletal pain of at least 3 months' duration with tender points, typical of fibromyalgia, may occur in up to 10 percent of HIV-infected IV drug abusers. Reactive arthritides, such as Reiter's syndrome or psoriatic arthritis, have also been described.

442. The answer is C. *(Chap 285.)* Persons who have rheumatoid arthritis can develop popliteal cysts as a complication of synovitis of the knee. Popliteal cysts can expand upward into the thigh or downward into the calf. Rupture of a popliteal cyst produces sudden pain and swelling; because these symptoms resemble those of thrombophlebitis—though perhaps more dramatic in onset—an arthrogram may be needed to confirm the diagnosis. Although rupture of the plantaris tendon can occur in persons exposed to mechanical trauma, it would not be the most likely diagnosis for the woman described in the question. The anserine bursa is located on the medial aspect of the knee joint and not in the calf. Achilles tendonitis should not cause pain and swelling of the calf.

443. The answer is B. *(Chap 285. Harris, N Engl J Med 322:1277–1289, 1990.)*   The so-called disease-modifying drugs used in the treatment of rheumatoid arthritis include gold compounds, D-penicillamine, sulfasalazine, and antimalarials. They are minimally anti-inflammatory and take weeks or months to induce a remission; therefore, nonsteroidals must be continued during their administration. Toxicities of these drugs, which are substantial, mandate careful consideration prior to their use and careful follow-up during maintenance. The indications to employ one of these disease-modifying agents are unclear, but one should consider these agents when symptoms cannot be controlled after several months' trial of nonsteroidals. Glucocorticoids have not been shown to modify the course of rheumatoid arthritis and have substantial long-term side effects, although they clearly can provide short-term control.

444. The answer is A. *(Chap 279.)*   Lymphoma generally does not occur until the CD4-positive T-lymphocyte count falls beneath 200/μL. This contrasts with Kaposi's sarcoma, which occurs at a relatively constant rate throughout the course of the illness. The lymphomas are generally B cell in origin, may contain Epstein-Barr virus DNA in the malignant cell genome, and may be either monoclonal or oligoclonal. Intermediate to high-grade lymphomas account for 80 percent of lymphomas in patients with AIDS. Three-fourths of these are either large cell or immunoblastic lymphomas. The remainder of systemic high-grade lymphomas are small, noncleaved cell (Burkitt's) lymphomas, which demonstrate the characteristic translocation between chromosome 8 and chromosome 14 or 22. Primary CNS lymphoma accounts for about 20 percent of lymphoma in HIV-infected patients. CNS lymphomas tend to occur at an even lower CD4-positive T-cell count than do the aforementioned peripheral lymphomas. Primary CNS lymphoma may present with focal neurologic deficits; radiologic evaluation may reveal up to three 5-cm lesions. Results with the multiagent chemotherapy used to treat similar lymphomas in non-HIV-infected persons have been quite disappointing. The median survival is 10 months for systemic HIV-related lymphoma and 2 to 4 months for those with primary CNS lymphoma. Hodgkin's disease, particularly the mixed cellularity or lymphocyte-depleted subtypes, may also occur, and, unlike the high cure rates for patients with Hodgkin's disease in general, the median survival for those with HIV infection and Hodgkin's disease is only 12 to 15 months.

445. The answer is E. *(Chap 280. Barlogie, Blood 73:865, 1989.)*   The diagnosis of multiple myeloma rests on bone marrow plasmacytosis (greater than 10 percent of the cells should be malignant-appearing plasma cells), lytic bone lesions, and a serum or urine M component. The M component represents either complete or partial antibody molecules synthesized by a monoclonal proliferation of plasma cells. Patients with myeloma may have a host of clinical problems related to the plasma cell neoplasm and its secreted products. Skeletal destruction can produce hypercalcemia, pathologic fractures, spinal cord compression, bone pain, and lytic bone lesions. Renal failure is common and may be due to light-chain deposition in renal tubules, amyloidosis, or calcium or urate nephropathy. Cytopenias due to bone marrow infiltration are typical. Infection with encapsulated microorganisms occurs because of associated hypogammaglobulinemia, believed to be due to B-cell dysregulation. However, certain patients have a serum M spike but no such clinical problems and do not have an excessive number of bone marrow plasma cells. These individuals have benign monoclonal gammopathy, also called monoclonal gammopathy of uncertain significance (MGUS). MGUS patients are generally over age 50. Their M spike is less than 20 g/L (2.0 g/dL) and they do not have Bence Jones proteinuria. These patients require no therapy and should merely be followed over time since only about 11 percent go on to develop frank myeloma.

446. The answer is A. *(Chap 285.)*   Systemic manifestations in early rheumatoid arthritis may be severe, but are frequently nonspecific. Such nonspecific constitutional symptoms require a period of observation before synovitis supervenes and the diagnosis becomes clear. Weight loss and muscle wasting may be as severe as in persons who have a malignancy or primary muscle disease. In about 10 percent of patients, the disease begins in a more fulminant fashion with the rapid onset of polyarthritis associated with fever, lymphadenopathy, and splenomegaly.

447. The answer is E. *(Chap 285.)*   Many of the systemic manifestations of late rheumatoid arthritis are related to the presence of rheumatoid factors in high titer in the serum. Joint disease, paradoxically, may not be active during this stage of the illness. Nail-fold thrombi, leg ulcers, and sensorimotor polyneuropathy are all manifestations of rheumatoid vasculitis and presumably are related to the effect of immune complexes containing rheumatoid factors. High levels of immune complexes are detected by immune-complex assays done at this stage of disease. Felty's syndrome, characterized by neutropenia and splenomegaly, occurs late in the course of rheumatoid arthritis and is related to the presence of high titers of rheumatoid factors. Many affected persons also have rheumatoid vasculitis. Fifteen to twenty percent of patients with rheumatoid arthritis develop Sjögren's syndrome with associated dry eyes. Hepatitis is not a common feature of late extraarticular seropositive rheumatoid arthritis.

448. The answer is A. *(Chap 282. Bochner, N Engl J Med 324:1785–1790, 1991.)*   Anaphylaxis is the word used to describe the rapid and generalized immunologically mediated events characterized clinically by cutaneous wheals and upper or lower airway obstruction (or both) after exposure to a specific antigen. The angioedema and urticaria that occur during anaphylaxis are believed to be due to the release of mast cell (and possibly basophil) mediators (histamine and serum proteases from preformed granules, arachidonic acid metabolites such as leukotrienes, and cytokines including, but not limited to tumor necrosis factor-α, interferon-γ, and interleukin 1). The mechanism of this release depends on the inciting agent. For example, anaphylaxis in response to bee stings, foods, and heterologous serum (e.g., tetanus antitoxin) is believed to be on the basis of IgE-mediated reaction against the relevant protein. On the other hand, anaphylaxis to penicillin and other antibiotics is due to IgE recognition of protein-hapten conjugants. Dialysis-induced anaphylaxis is due to complement activation. Finally, radiocontrast media directly activate mast cells or basophils or both to release the mediators of anaphylaxis.

449. The answer is B. *(Chap 282.)*   Most patients with systemic mastocytosis have an indolent syndrome characterized by mast cell infiltration of the skin, gastrointestinal mucosa, liver, and spleen. Cutaneous manifestations include the small, reddish-brown macules or papules, termed urticaria pigmentosa, which would be characterized histopathologically as having excess numbers of mast cells. These lesions are associated with Darier's sign, in which urticaria and erythema develop in response to trauma. Histamine-mediated hypersecretion of gastric acid accounts for an increased incidence of gastritis and peptic ulcers in patients with systemic mastocytosis. Bone pain, organomegaly, or lymphadenopathy may also be seen. In addition to documentation of mast cells in various organs, biochemical confirmation can be made by urine collection for histamine metabolites or by measuring increased blood levels of histamine or mast cell–derived neutral protease tryptase. The spectrum of mast cell disease ranges from indolent to more aggressive varieties characterized by mast cell infiltration of liver and spleen and in some cases the invariably fatal development of mast cell leukemia.

450. The answer is A. *(Chap 289.)*   The diagnosis of ankylosing spondylitis is made on clinical grounds. Historical features suggesting inflammatory back disease include pain and prolonged stiffness that are worse at night and during rest periods and characteristically relieved with activity. In contrast, mechanical low back pain usually is eased with bed rest and made worse with activity, such as sitting, standing, walking, and lifting. Signs of nerve-root compression are not part of the clinical spectrum of ankylosing spondylitis. Ankylosing spondylitis usually presents before the age of 40 years; on the other hand, degenerative joint disease and degenerative disk disease are common causes of back pain in the elderly. Back pain made worse with walking and improved with rest and lumbar flexion is characteristic of the pseudoclaudication syndrome associated with lumbar spinal stenosis.

451. The answer is B. *(Chap 298.)*   Five different clinical syndromes of psoriatic arthritis have been described. The most common (70 percent of cases) is an asymmetric oligoarticular arthritis. A second group produces arthritis mainly in distal interphalangeal joints and is associated with severe psoriatic nail changes. Psoriatic spondylitis is similar to the spondylitis of Reiter's syndrome. Rheumatoid factor–negative symmetric polyarthritis also is associated with psoriasis, and this condition can look very much like rheumatoid arthritis. About 5 percent of patients with psoriatic arthritis have a destructive variety called "arthritis mutilans." Persons who have psoriasis and rheumatoid factor–positive symmetric polyarthritis are thought to have both psoriasis and rheumatoid arthritis.

452. The answer is E. *(Chap 284.)*   Patients with SLE may have a host of autoantibodies. Virtually all have antinuclear antibodies directed at multiple nuclear and cytoplasmic antigens. Approximately 50 percent have an anticardiolipin antibody, which is associated with a prolonged partial thromboplastin time and false positive serologic tests for syphilis. This so-called lupus anticoagulant may be manifested by thrombocytopenia, venous or arterial clotting, recurrent fetal loss, and valvular heart disease. Though thrombotic problems are most common, if the antibody is associated with hypoprothrombinemia, severe thrombocytopenia, or antibodies to clotting factors (usually VIII or IX), bleeding may result. Confirmation that the partial thromboplastin time is prolonged on the basis of a lupus anticoagulant may be proved by failure of normal plasma to correct the defect.

453. The answer is C. *(Chap 286.)*   Patients with the more malignant variant of systemic sclerosis (scleroderma) have diffuse cutaneous disease characterized by skin thickening in the extremities, face, and trunk. It is the subset of patients, in contrast to those with limited cutaneous disease who often have the CREST syndrome, who are at risk for developing kidney and other visceral disease. Hypertension heralds the onset of a renal crisis manifested by malignant hypertension, encephalopathy, retinopathy, seizures, and left ventricular failure. The renin-angiotensin system is markedly activated; therefore, angiotensin-converting enzyme inhibitors are particularly effective. Even patients who require dialysis may reverse course and have a slow return of renal function after the passage of several months. Patients with systemic sclerosis may also develop esophageal dysfunction, hypomotility of the small intestine (which can produce pain and malabsorption), pulmonary fibrosis sometimes progressing to pulmonary hypertension, and heart failure due to myocardial fibrosis.

454. The answer is C. *(Chap 290.)*   Behçet's syndrome, a recurrent disease of unknown cause, is characterized by painful oral and genital ulcers, eye inflammation, arthritis, central nervous system symptoms, thrombophlebitis, fever, and abdominal symptoms. The combination of fever, aphthous ulcers, arthritis, and abdominal pain may mimic inflammatory bowel disease, although central nervous system involvement (e.g., severe headache) and thrombophlebitis would make this diagnosis less likely. Whipple's disease is associated with arthritis, abdominal pain, and central nervous system disease, but not with aphthous ulcers and thrombophlebitis; also, Whipple's disease usually affects middle-aged men. Fever, arthritis, abdominal pain, and headache would be compatible with a diagnosis of systemic lupus erythematosus. However, the mucosal lesions of lupus are painless and occur on the hard and soft palate, and thrombophlebitis is not a characteristic feature. The diagnosis of Behçet's disease now requires the presence of recurrent oral ulcers plus two of the following: recurrent genital ulcerations, eye lesions, skin lesions or a positive pathergy test (inflammatory reactivity to scratches or intradermal saline).

455. The answer is E. *(Chap 287.)*   Mixed connective tissue disease (MCTD) is a syndrome characterized by high titers of circulating antibodies to the ribonucleoprotein component of extractable nuclear antigen in association with clinical features similar to those of SLE, systemic sclerosis, polymyositis, and rheumatoid arthritis. The average patient with MCTD is a middle-aged woman with Raynaud's phenomenon who also has polyarthritis, sclerodactyly (including swollen hands), esophageal dysfunction, pulmonary fibrosis, and inflammatory myopathy. Cutaneous manifestations include telangiectasias on the face and hands, alopecia, a lupuslike heliotropic rash, and erythematous patches over the knuckles. Myopathy may involve severe weakness of proximal muscles associated with high levels of creatine phosphokinase and aldolase. Both pulmonary involvement and esophageal dysmotility are common, but frequently asymptomatic until quite advanced. Almost all patients have high titers of rheumatoid factor and antinuclear antibodies. Such antibodies are directed toward the ribonuclease-sensitive ribonucleoprotein component of extractable nuclear antigen.

456. The answer is C. *(Chap 291.)*   Hypersensitivity vasculitis refers to a group of disorders presumed to be associated with a reaction to an antigen such as an infectious agent or drug. The common denominator of this group is the involvement of small vessels, especially postcapillary venules. Vasculitis is leukocytoclastic, meaning that nuclear debris remaining from neutrophilic infiltration is present. In the subacute or chronic stages, mononuclear cells predominate. Henoch-Schönlein purpura is caused by immune complexes containing IgA antibody, which may be due to a reaction to drugs, certain foods, insect bites, or immunization. Such complexes are deposited in the skin, gastrointestinal mucosal vessels, and glomeruli. The disease is characterized by arthralgias, glomerulonephritis, and gastrointestinal signs and symptoms (particularly nausea, vomiting, diarrhea, constipation, or passage of blood and mucus per rectum). However, the most characteristic finding is palpable purpura on the buttocks and lower extremities. Though the disease is usually self-limited, it can progress to a chronic form. Patients occasionally require glucocorticoid therapy.

457. The answer is D. *(Chap 296.)*   Osteoarthritis, the most common joint disease, is diagnosed on the basis of clinical and laboratory features. One of the earliest x-ray findings is joint space narrowing as periarticular cartilage is lost. A joint involved with osteoarthritis may be tender or slightly swollen; significant effusions are rare. The sensation of bone rubbing against bone (bony crepitus) may be elicited upon movement of an affected joint. Bony prominences on both the distal interphalangeal joints (Heberden's nodes) and the proximal interphalangeal joints (Bouchard's nodes) are commonly seen. Osteoarthritis in the patellofemoral joint may manifest as a positive "shrug" sign, i.e., pain when the patella is manually compressed against the femur when the quadriceps contracts. In contrast, rheumatoid arthritis (RA) commonly involves the proximal interphalangeal joint. Moreover, destruction of ligaments and tendons seen in RA may result in characteristic hand changes such as hyperextension of the proximal interphalangeal joints with compensatory flexion of the distal interphalangeal joints (swan-neck deformity) or flexion deformity of the proximal interphalangeals and extension of the distal interphalangeals (boutonnière deformity).

458. The answer is A. *(Chaps 286, 287.)*   Systemic sclerosis can be classified into two variants depending on whether scleroderma is present only in the fingers (sclerodactyly) or whether it is also present proximal to the metacarpophalangeal joints. The former disorder is associated with a constellation of findings labeled the *CREST syndrome: C*alcinosis, *R*aynaud's phenomenon, *e*sophageal dysmotility, *s*clerodactyly, and *t*elangiectasia. Although once thought not to be associated with significant internal organ involvement, the CREST variant of systemic sclerosis has occurred in association with the development of pulmonary arterial hypertension or biliary cirrhosis. The fluorescent antinuclear antibody (ANA) test is positive in 40 to 80 percent of persons with systemic sclerosis. Antibodies are produced to deoxyribonucleoprotein, nucleolar, centromere, and topoisomerase 1 antigens.

Mixed connective-tissue disease is the overlap of three rheumatic disease syndromes: systemic lupus erythematosus (SLE), polymyositis, and the CREST variant of systemic sclerosis. It is associated with high titers of antinuclear antibodies directed against the extractable nuclear antigen ribonucleoprotein. Arthritis and a positive ANA are not sufficient to make a diagnosis of SLE. Overlap syndromes are diseases that fulfill diagnostic criteria for two rheumatic diseases. In the case described, symptoms and signs were insufficient to fulfill the diagnostic criteria for more than one rheumatic syndrome.

459. The answer is E.   *(Chap 299.)*   Pigmented villonodular synovitis, the cause of which is unknown, is a disorder of young adults that usually affects one joint only, frequently a knee. There is recurrent bleeding into the affected joint; the synovial fluid of that joint often contains blood and typically is dark brown in color, an indication of past bleeding from the synovium. The enlarged villi covering the synovium are made up of large numbers of round and polyhedral cells. Hemosiderin granules and cholesterol crystals can be identified in synovial cell cytoplasm as well as in interstitial spaces. Bone adjacent to the affected synovium can show evidence of erosion; however, invasion of other tissues does not occur. Treatment is complete synovectomy. Hemangioma usually presents in childhood.

460. The answer is C.   *(Chap 299. Michet, Rheum Dis Clin North Am 16:441, 1990.)*   Relapsing polychondritis is an inflammatory disorder that affects cartilage in the ear, nose, larynx, and tracheobronchial tree. This intermittent, yet sometimes progressive disorder can also be associated with ocular manifestations, aortic regurgitation, and premonitory asymmetric oligoarthritis affecting some large and small peripheral joints. Diagnosis of relapsing polychondritis can be made in the presence of the aforementioned clinical features; biopsy of affected tissues displaying cartilage destruction would be confirmatory, but is usually unnecessary. Patients with Wegener's granulomatosis may have nasal, but not auricular involvement. Cogan's syndrome may include ocular and auditory problems, but does not involve the external ear. There was no urethritis or skin lesions in this case to suggest Reiter's syndrome. The arthritis in rheumatoid disease tends to be symmetric and erosive. Squamous cell carcinoma would be unlikely to involve both ears and the larynx simultaneously.

461. The answer is C.   *(Chap 277.)*   T lymphocytes are the principal mediators of cellular immunity and also serve important helper and suppressor functions in the regulation of antibody synthesis by B lymphocytes. In humans, they have the property of forming rosettes with sheep erythrocytes (E-rosettes), and they lack readily detectable immunoglobulin of any class on their membranes. Although the maturation of T cells is thymus-dependent, the cells arise from precursors in bone marrow. T cells constitute about 70 to 80 percent of blood lymphocytes; they comprise greater than three-quarters of thymus lymphocytes but less than one-quarter of bone marrow lymphocytes. In lymph nodes, they are found in paracortical areas. Specific monoclonal antibodies have been developed to characterize various subsets of T cells—cells that carry a CD4+ surface antigen are helper cells, and those with a CD8+ antigen function as cytotoxic-suppressor cells. Antibody-dependent cell-mediated cytotoxicity is a property of a class of non-B, non-T lymphocytes called large granular lymphocytes (LGL cells). Antibody-dependent cell-mediated cytotoxicity can also be mediated by monocyte-macrophages and neutrophils.

462. The answer is C. *(Chap 277.)* Immunoglobulin A is the predominant immunoglobulin in body secretions (IgG is predominant in serum). Each secretory IgA molecule is a dimer consisting of a secretory component and a J chain. The secretory component, a protein of molecular weight 70,000, is synthesized by epithelial cells and facilitates IgA transport across mucosal tissues. The J chain is a small glycopeptide that aids the polymerization of immunoglobulins. IgA exists as two subclasses: IgA1 (75 percent of the total) and IgA2 (25 percent but more prevalent in secretions). IgA provides defense against local infections in the respiratory, gastrointestinal, and genitourinary tracts and prevents access of foreign substances to the general systemic immune system. It also can prevent virus binding to epithelial cells. IgM, not IgA, is the principal immunoglobulin in the primary immune response and is the usual antibody in cold agglutinins. The half-life of IgA is about 6 days; IgE has the shortest half-life, approximately 2 to 2.5 days.

463. The answer is C. *(Chap 284.)* Although most clinicians believe that women with systemic lupus erythematosus should not become pregnant if they have active disease or advanced renal or cardiac disease, the presence of SLE itself is not an absolute contraindication to pregnancy. The outcome of pregnancy is best for those women in remission at the time of conception. Even in women with quiescent disease, exacerbations may occur (usually in the first trimester and in the immediate postpartum period), and 25 to 40 percent of pregnancies end in spontaneous abortion. Fetal loss rates are higher in patients with lupus anticoagulant or anticardiolipin antibodies. Flare-ups should be anticipated and vigorously treated with steroids. Steroids given throughout pregnancy also usually have no adverse effects on the child. In the case presented, the fact that the woman had a life-threatening bout of disease a year ago would argue against stopping her drugs at this time. Neonatal lupus, which is manifested by thrombocytopenia, rash, and heart block, is rare but can occur in mothers with anti-Ro antibodies.

464. The answer is E. *(Chap 288.)* Sjögren's syndrome, an autoimmune destruction of the exocrine glands, can be primary or it can occur in association with rheumatoid arthritis, SLE, or systemic sclerosis. A mononuclear cell infiltrate, which can be seen in virtually any organ, is pathognomonic if found in the salivary gland in association with keratoconjunctivitis sicca (conjunctival and corneal dryness) and xerostomia (lack of salivation). Since minor salivary glands will be obtained in a lip biopsy, such a procedure can be diagnostic. Severe dryness of the mouth can lead to an increased incidence of dental caries. Corneal dryness may be severe enough to result in ulceration. The most common form of renal involvement (seen in 40 percent of patients with primary Sjögren's) is an interstitial nephritis resulting in renal tubular acidosis. Hypersensitivity vasculitis, manifested by palpable purpura of the lower extremities, is not uncommon. Sensory neuropathies, interstitial pneumonitis, and autoimmune thyroid disease may also accompany primary Sjögren's syndrome. Finally, pseudolymphoma, characterized by lymphadenopathy and enlargement of the parotid gland, and frank non-Hodgkin's lymphoma may occur. Cardiac disease is very rare in Sjögren's syndrome.

465. The answer is D. *(Chap 289.)* The diagnosis of ankylosing spondylitis is based on characteristic history and physical examination. A determination of HLA-B27 status does not help in the diagnosis of ankylosing spondylitis. Seven percent of the normal white population in the United States are positive for HLA-B27, and 5 to 10 percent of persons with bona fide ankylosing spondylitis are negative for HLA-B27. It has been shown that 20 percent of HLA-B27-positive persons who are first-degree relatives of cases have evidence of ankylosing spondylitis. Blacks and Asians have a lower prevalence of HLA-B27 antigenicity and a lower prevalence of ankylosing spondylitis. The concordance rate in identical twins is 60 percent or less, indicating that environmental factors also play a role in disease pathogenesis.

466. The answer is A. *(Chap 289.)*   In the United States and Great Britain, postdysenteric Reiter's syndrome occurs much less frequently than postvenereal Reiter's syndrome. *Salmonella, Shigella, Yersinia,* and, more recently, *Campylobacter* enteric infections have been associated with the development of the disorder. Urethritis occurs in both forms of the disease, though it is more common in the postvenereal type. Reactive arthritis must be distinguished from disseminated gonococcal infection, to which it bears similarities.

467. The answer is A-Y, B-N, C-Y, D-Y, E-Y. *(Chap 277.)*   The lymphoid system can be divided into two functionally distinct compartments: the thymus-dependent T-cell compartment, and the "bursal-equivalent" B-cell compartment. B cells are the precursors of plasma cells; their primary role is to produce immunoglobulins. B lymphocytes in humans and most other mammalian species are characterized by the presence of readily detectable surface immunoglobulins. Most B cells have a receptor specific for the Fc portion of immunoglobulin, and some B cells have receptors for complement proteins, including the activated fragments C3b (CD35) and C3d (CD21). Pre-B cells arise in the bone marrow continuously throughout life. Such pre-B cells, which mature in an antigen-independent fashion, are characterized by the presence of cytoplasmic IgM. Upon further development immature B cells, which express IgM on their cell surface, occur. Mature B cells migrate out of the bone marrow and express surface IgD as well as either IgM, IgG, IgA, or IgE. The antigen-dependent phase of B-cell development may then occur with memory B-cell induction and the formation of the immunoglobulin-secreting plasma cell. Mature B cells constitute about 15 percent of peripheral blood lymphocytes, 50 percent of splenic lymphocytes, and 10 percent of bone marrow lymphocytes.

468. The answer is A-N, B-Y, C-Y, D-Y, E-Y. *(Chaps 91, 163.)*   The patient has desert fever, a syndrome caused by coccidioidomycosis infection, which is endemic in the southwest United States. This syndrome is largely an acute hypersensitivity reaction to the primary pulmonary infection, which is symptomatic in only 40 percent of affected persons. Manifestations of hypersensitivity may include erythema nodosum, erythema multiforme, arthralgia, arthritis, conjunctivitis, and episcleritis. However, disseminated coccidioidomycosis may occur during the primary infection and could result in osteomyelitis (which may seed an adjacent synovium directly), fungal arthritis, skin lesions, or CNS disease. Even in the case of hematogenously derived joint infection, synovial fluid cultures will rarely be positive; synovial biopsy for culture and histology may be required. Serologic tests, while possibly acutely negative in a patient with primary pulmonary infection only, can be quite helpful, particularly when there is disseminated involvement.

469. The answer is A-N, B-N, C-Y, D-Y, E-Y. *(Chap 277.)*   T-cell precursors leave the yolk sac, fetal liver, or bone marrow and migrate to the thymus, where they undergo further maturation. Even before T-cell receptor gene rearrangements occur, pre-T cells express the CD7 antigen, the earliest marker of T-cell lineage. After the CD2 adhesion molecule, which functions as the receptor for sheep red blood cells, is expressed on the cell surface, assembly of the T-cell receptor complex begins. This complex consists of the five proteins that make up the CD3 signal transduction moiety plus the two antigen-recognizing heterodimer molecules that form the actual T-cell antigen receptor. The proteins that can function as part of the T-cell antigen receptor all have a variable (produced by V-J recombination) and constant region and bear homology to the immunoglobulin heavy and light chains. Along with the histocompatibility proteins and the CD2, CD4, and CD8 molecules, the T-cell antigen receptor chains are members of the immunoglobulin gene superfamily, which provides the immunologic diversity required to distinguish self from nonself and recognize an inordinate number of foreign antigens. After CD3 T-cell receptor expression, but before suppressor or helper phenotype is determined, there is a thymic stage wherein both CD4 and CD8 antigens are expressed. Some lymphoblastic lymphomas arise at this stage of T-cell development.

470. The answer is A-Y, B-N, C-Y, D-N, E-Y. *(Chap 278.)*   Di George's syndrome, also called *congenital thymic aplasia,* is caused by abnormal development of the third and fourth pharyngeal pouches during the sixth to eighth weeks of intrauterine life. The structures arising from these pharyngeal evaginations are the thymus, the tissues of the lips and central portion of the face, the ear tubercle, the aortic arch, and the parathyroid glands. Consequently, a child demonstrating the classic presentation of Di George's syndrome has the following abnormalities: hypocalcemic tetany; congenital heart disease involving aortic arch structures; cellular immunodeficiency with a T lymphopenia, absence of a thymus, and failure of blood lymphocytes to respond to phytohemagglutinin and allogeneic cells; and an abnormal facies with low-set ears, "fish-shaped" mouth, and hypertelorism. Thyroid function is normal, and B-cell immunity as measured by immunoglobulin levels and antibody response to immunization usually is unimpaired. Treatment of Di George's syndrome is by transplant of a fetal thymus.

471. The answer is A-Y, B-Y, C-Y, D-N, E-N. *(Chap 278. Buckley, N Engl J Med 325:110, 1991.)*   Isolated IgA deficiency is the most common immunodeficiency disorder, with an incidence between 1:600 and 1:800. Affected persons have a normal or reduced number of B cells with surface IgA, but seem to have overabundant immature cells that coexpress IgA and IgM, suggesting a block in B-cell terminal differentiation. This presumption is substantiated by in vitro studies showing that lymphocytes from IgA-deficient persons can synthesize but are unable to secrete IgA. Both serum IgA and secretory IgA usually are reduced. Although IgA deficiency need not be associated with clinical disease, it frequently is. Recurrent sinopulmonary infection is most common. Allergy occurs with an incidence of 1:200 to 1:400, compared with 1:600 to 1:800 in the general population. Approximately 30 to 40 percent of IgA-deficient persons have antibodies directed against IgA, thus predisposing them to anaphylactoid reactions following the infusion of blood products unless the blood is obtained from IgA-deficient donors. Persons with isolated IgA deficiency are also at greater risk for developing autoimmune diseases, including lupus and rheumatoid arthritis. Immunoglobulin treatment will not restore IgA levels to normal and is of little value in this condition.

472. The answer is A-Y, B-Y, C-Y, D-Y, E-Y. *(Chap 283.)*   Most antigen-antibody complexes are cleared by cells of the reticuloendothelial system. It appears that in some conditions the reticuloendothelial system can be overwhelmed by immune complexes, thereby impeding the removal and leading to the deposition of immune complexes. Deposition of these complexes in tissues other than those of the reticuloendothelial system is responsible for the signs and symptoms of immune-complex disease. In animal models, the persistence of complexes is necessary for the development of renal disease; also, slight antigen excess has been found to predispose to the formation of antigen-antibody complexes, which persist in the circulation and lead to inflammatory illness. Immune complex–mediated vascular damage can lead to cutaneous necrotizing vasculitis. Electron microscopy reveals subendothelial immune complexes that presumably incite an array of inflammatory cells to migrate toward the vessel.

473. The answer is A-N, B-Y, C-N, D-Y, E-Y. *(Chap 64.)*   Class I HLA antigens are encoded at the A, B, and C loci of the human major histocompatibility complex on chromosome 6. Each such antigen consists of an 11.5-kilodalton (kd) beta$_2$-microglobulin subunit (also encoded in the HLA region) and a 44-kd chain with three separate domains that contain the antigenic specificity. Only certain areas of the heavy chain are diverse, so individual molecules share greater than 80 percent sequence homology. Class I molecules are expressed on all cells except mature red blood cells. These antigens are defined serologically and are useful in predicting results for organ transplants. Because class I antigens are not distributed evenly from one racial group to another, it can be more difficult for a person of African descent, for example, to procure a bone marrow donor from a registry where most of the potential donors descend from Northern Europe.

474. The answer is A-Y, B-N, C-Y, D-N, E-Y. *(Chap 279. Hirsch, N Engl J Med 328:1686, 1993.)* AZT inhibits viral reverse transcriptase, the enzyme required in all retroviruses because it converts viral RNA into DNA, which can then be integrated into the host's genome. AZT has been a major advance in the treatment of patients with HIV infection. Both asymptomatic and symptomatic patients with AIDS whose peripheral CD4+ (T4+) T-cell counts are less than 500 cells per microliter may benefit from treatment with 100 mg AZT five times daily. AZT treatment is associated with limited prolongation of survival and retardation of progression of disease in those with early disease. Moreover, impressive improvements in HIV-associated neurologic sequelae have been observed. The most common side effect, other than myelosuppression resulting in anemia and neutropenia, is gastrointestinal intolerance. Anemia may be ameliorated by the concomitant use of the recombinant growth factor erythropoietin. Once a patient contracts *P. carinii* pneumonia, aerosolized pentamidine 300 mg/month is effective prophylaxis, but it does result in an increased incidence of extrapulmonary infections.

475. The answer is A-N, B-N, C-N, D-Y, E-Y. *(Chap 281.)* This patient has many of the hallmarks of systemic amyloidosis. An abdominal fat pad aspirate or a rectal biopsy is the best way to make the diagnosis, although biopsy of any affected organ may be carried out. A positive Congo red histologic stain helps to establish the diagnosis. The classification of amyloid protein fibrils that are deposited in the tissues is based on their biochemical type. AL amyloid residues bear homology to immunoglobulin light chains and are seen in de novo or myeloma-associated disease. The AA type of amyloid, made up of a protein of 76 amino acids, is seen secondary to a host of chronic inflammatory conditions, including long-standing rheumatoid arthritis, tuberculosis, bronchiectasis, familial Mediterranean fever, and leprosy. Other types of amyloid proteins are seen in familial amyloid polyneuropathy, medullary carcinoma of the thyroid, and Alzheimer's disease (the beta, or A4, protein). Amyloidosis should be suspected in any patient with an underlying chronic inflammatory disease who develops hepatomegaly, splenomegaly, malabsorption, cardiac disease, or proteinuria. Cardiac disease usually consists of congestive heart failure with low QRS-complex voltage, arrhythmias, and exquisite sensitivity to digitalis. Waxy papules or plaques in the axillary folds may signal the deposition of amyloid in the skin; purpura after minor trauma is not uncommon. Gastrointestinal problems caused by amyloid include macroglossia, malabsorption, and bleeding. In addition to amyloid-induced synovitis, peripheral neuropathy and carpal tunnel syndrome may be seen.

476. The answer is A-Y, B-N, C-N, D-Y, E-Y. *(Chap 284.)* The most common cause of drug-induced SLE is procainamide, which produces a positive ANA in 75 percent of those who take it and a 20 percent incidence of clinical lupus. In contrast, hydralazine induces an ANA in 25 percent and a clinical lupus syndrome in 10 percent. Slow acetylators seem to have more problems with drug-induced autoimmune phenomena. Though up to 50 percent of those with drug-induced lupus have arthralgias, pleuropericarditis, or both, renal disease is rare. In an effort to distinguish drug-induced lupus (which should last less than 6 months) from de novo lupus (a disease uniquely positive for anti-dsDNA and anti-Sm), a complete ANA panel should be sent. Most patients will respond initially to withdrawal of the offending drug; if not, then a brief trial of steroids is indicated.

477. The answer is A-N, B-N, C-Y, D-Y, E-N. *(Chap 285. Brooks, N Engl J Med 324:1716–1725, 1991.)* NSAIDs, including aspirin, are effective agents in the treatment of symptomatic rheumatoid arthritis. However, none of the newer agents have been shown to be more effective than aspirin, though some do have fewer gastrointestinal side effects. All of these agents induce platelet dysfunction. Their mechanism of action is the blockage of the activity of the enzyme cyclooxygenase, which converts arachidonic acid into the inflammation-mediating prostaglandins. 5-Lipoxygenase, which is not inhibited by most NSAIDs, converts arachidonic acid into leukotrienes. It may be the dysregulation of normal arachidonic acid metabolism that leads to the occasional NSAID-induced worsening of allergic rhinitis and asthma. The absence of renal vasodilatory prostaglandins normally produced by the action of cyclooxygenase can lead to renal insufficiency, particularly in those with underlying renal vascular disease.

478. The answer is A-N, B-Y, C-N, D-Y, E-Y. *(Chap 292.)* Sarcoidosis is a systemic granulomatous inflammatory disorder that frequently involves the lungs, where it causes a typical interstitial lung disease that may be asymptomatic, may cause transient respiratory difficulties with or without hilar adenopathy, or may progress to end-stage pulmonary fibrosis. Extrapulmonary sarcoidosis may involve the eyes, skin, liver, bones, gastrointestinal tract, kidneys, nervous system, and heart. In the United States, 10 to 20 percent of cases consist of asymptomatic hilar adenopathy detected on chest radiographs taken for other reasons; these cases may constitute a higher fraction of the total in other countries where routine preemployment chest radiography is more widely practiced. The disease occurs more frequently among blacks than whites by a substantial margin. At sites of disease activity, such as the lung, there is an accumulation of activated helper-inducer (CD4+) lymphocytes, with release of immunologic mediators such as interleukin 2 and gamma-interferon, and resultant granuloma formation. In contrast to other interstitial lung diseases, the diagnosis may frequently be made by the demonstration of the characteristic granulomatous inflammation in tissue obtained by transbronchial biopsy. Prognosis depends on the risk of progression to advanced pulmonary fibrosis, and those persons with intense pulmonary inflammation may benefit from treatment with corticosteroids. Chest radiography and pulmonary function testing cannot distinguish accurately between active inflammation and established fibrosis; hence, most clinicians familiar with the disease utilize procedures such as bronchoalveolar lavage or gallium-67 scanning, or both, to assess the intensity of the alveolitis present. These procedures may be performed serially during the course of the patient's illness to follow the progress of the disease and response to therapy.

479. The answer is A-Y, B-Y, C-Y, D-N, E-N. *(Chap 285.)* Rheumatoid factors are antibodies to the Fc fragment of immunoglobulin G. They may be of the IgG, IgA, or IgM class; the widely used latex and sheep-cell agglutination tests detect rheumatoid factors primarily of the IgM class. Chronic antigenic stimulation is one of the processes important in the production of rheumatoid factors. Rheumatoid factors are associated not only with rheumatoid arthritis and other autoimmune diseases but also with lymphoreticular malignancies and chronic infections, such as subacute bacterial endocarditis. Rheumatoid factors are usually present within the first year of onset of rheumatoid arthritis; their presence correlates with the extraarticular manifestations of the disease. Patients with rheumatoid arthritis who have positive serologic tests for IgM rheumatoid factor have a worse prognosis than those who are seronegative.

480. The answer is A-Y, B-N, C-N, D-Y, E-Y. *(Chap 285.)* Joint stiffness in the morning or after periods of inactivity lasting more than 1 h is characteristic of inflammatory rheumatic disease. Arthritis characteristic of rheumatoid arthritis is persistent, remaining in the same joints for months. Migratory arthritis, in which short-lived arthritis symptoms in one joint subside as symptoms begin in another joint, is not characteristic of rheumatoid arthritis. Persons who have rheumatoid arthritis can have involvement of the cervical spine, the wrist joints, and all the small joints of the hand except the distal interphalangeal joints. Wrist-joint arthritis can lead to median-nerve entrapment (carpal tunnel syndrome).

481. The answer is A-Y, B-N, C-Y, D-N, E-Y. *(Chap 289.)* This patient has an acute inflammatory asymmetric polyarthritis associated with ocular (conjunctivitis, occasionally anterior uveitis) and cutaneous (keratoderma blennorrhagicum on palms and soles; circinate balanitis on the glans penis) disease. Moreover, he has had a recent episode of urethritis, possibly caused by chlamydia. He therefore has so-called reactive arthritis, also known as Reiter's syndrome. This entity can follow certain infectious illnesses, most notably dysentery or venereal disease usually in patients who are HLA-B27-positive. The constitutional symptoms associated with the acute illness can be severe. The erythrocyte sedimentation rate is frequently elevated. Sacroiliitis and spondyloarthropathy may be seen as late sequelae. Patients will respond to nonsteroidal agents, but there is little evidence to support the benefit of antibiotics, other than in eradicating chlamydia, if present.

482. The answer is A-N, B-Y, C-Y, D-Y, E-N. *(Chap 291. Hoffman, Ann Intern Med 116:488–498, 1992.)* This patient presents with findings characteristic of Wegener's granulomatosis. Sinus disease (manifested by bloody or purulent nasal discharge), pulmonary disease, and glomerulonephritis are seen in greater than 80 percent of affected patients. Sinus involvement would be unlikely in Goodpasture's syndrome, which is associated with anti-basement membrane antibodies. Other findings characteristic of Wegener's include ocular involvement, skin lesions, and nervous system manifestations (including cranial neuritis or mononeuritis multiplex), as well as elevated ESR, anemia, leukocytosis, and hypergammaglobulinemia. The diagnosis can be made by finding necrotizing granulomatous vasculitis in an involved site. Although the immunopathogenesis of this entity is unclear, antibodies to a neutrophil protein (found in the azurophilic granules) can be frequently found. The disease can be successfully treated in over 90 percent of patients with the use of glucocorticoids and cyclophosphamide. The glucocorticoids are gradually tapered and the cyclophosphamide, the mainstay of treatment, should be continued for about 1 year after complete remission.

483. The answer is A-N, B-Y, C-N, D-Y, E-Y. *(Chap 289.)* The x-ray shown in the question is compatible with a diagnosis of ankylosing spondylitis, a disease that shows striking concordance with the HLA-B27 antigen. Early radiographic evidence of sacroiliitis includes blurring of joint margins, irregular subchondral erosions, and sclerosis affecting both sides of the sacroiliac joint. With progression of the disease, the joint is lost completely. Radiographic findings of early spondylitis include straightening of the lumbar spine and squaring of the lumbar and thoracic vertebrae. Later, syndesmophytes appear along the lateral and anterior surfaces of the intervertebral disks and bridge adjacent vertebrae, creating the so-called bamboo spine. Complications of ankylosing spondylitis include uveitis (in 30 percent of affected persons) and aortic insufficiency (3 percent). The rigid spine is subject to fracture, most commonly in the cervical area, and this creates the potential for quadriplegia even after relatively minor trauma.

484. The answer is A-N, B-N, C-N, D-Y, E-Y. *(Chap 297.)* Synovial deposition of calcium pyrophosphate dihydrate crystals occurs in pseudogout, an inflammatory disorder producing arthritis in older persons. Crystals are thought to form on the surface of articular cartilage (chondrocalcinosis) and then are shed into synovial fluid; in gout, on the other hand, crystals are thought to arise from a supersaturated solution of sodium urate. Under polarized light, calcium pyrophosphate dihydrate crystals have a weak positive birefringence and can be difficult to see if not looked for carefully. Most affected persons have radiographic evidence of chondrocalcinosis. Common sites of involvement are the menisci of the knees, articular disk of the distal radioulnar joint, the symphysis pubis, and the annulus fibrosis of the intervertebral disks. Clinical syndromes other than pseudogout, among them pseudorheumatoid arthritis and pseudodegenerative joint disease, also involve deposition of calcium pyrophosphate crystals.

485. The answer is A-N, B-N, C-N, D-Y, E-Y. *(Chap 292.)* While 10 to 20 percent of patients with sarcoidosis present with asymptomatic disease found incidentally on chest x-ray and 40 to 70 percent have the characteristic insidious development of disease, the remainder present over the span of a few weeks. Constitutional and respiratory symptoms dominate the acute presentation. Two distinct patterns of acute sarcoidosis are recognized. Löfgren's syndrome, seen in Scandinavian, Irish, and Puerto Rican females, is characterized by erythema nodosum, arthralgias, and bilateral hilar lymphadenopathy. The constellation of findings in the Heerfordt-Waldenström syndrome consists of fever, parotid enlargement, anterior uveitis, and facial nerve palsy. Interstitial pulmonary involvement would be rare in acute sarcoidosis. Myopathy and skin lesions are most consistent with dermatomyositis. Although 5 percent of patients with sarcoidosis have cardiac abnormalities, valvular heart disease—other than occasional instances of papillary muscle dysfunction—is rare.

486. **The answer is A-Y, B-N, C-Y, D-Y, E-N.** *(Chap 293. Pras, N Engl J Med 326:1509–1513, 1992.)* Familial Mediterranean fever (FMF), or familial paroxysmal polyserositis, is an inherited disorder of unknown etiology. There is no pathognomonic finding, although in certain families the disease has been linked to the short arm of chromosome 16. Evidence of serosal inflammation should be documented. Recently, elevated levels of the enzyme dopamine beta-hydroxylase have been found in patients with this disorder. The relationship of such a finding to the pathophysiology of FMF is unknown; however, levels of this enzyme decline after therapy with colchicine, an agent that remarkably retards the frequency and severity of attacks. Attacks typically consist of fever and abdominal pain, although 75 percent of patients also have pleuritic chest pain or joint pain or both at some time. FMF-associated drug addiction is a more worrisome problem in the United States than is amyloidosis, which is reported in the Middle East. The reason for the unequal geographic incidence of amyloidosis is unknown. The disease is more frequently found in non-Ashkenazic Jews, Italians, and Arabs; however, approximately 50 percent of patients give no family history.

487. **The answer is A-N, B-Y, C-Y, D-N, E-N.** *(Chap 294.)* Patients with midline granuloma, characterized by local inflammation and destructive mutilation of head and neck tissues, may present with nasal and sinus symptoms. Ulcerations of the nasal septum and soft and hard palates are harbingers of very destructive processes in any area in the neck or above. Granulomatous infiltration and necrosis will be noted on pathologic examination of the involved areas. Radiation therapy is the treatment of choice and is successful in averting the almost certainly fatal course in untreated patients. Midline granuloma can be difficult to distinguish from cocaine-induced septal perforation, malignant lymphoma, and a host of chronic infections including histoplasmosis, blastomycosis, coccidioidomycosis, leprosy, tuberculosis, syphilis, and leishmaniasis. While Wegener's granulomatosis is associated with similar upper airway findings, the absence of vasculitis on biopsy, the absence of pulmonary and renal disease, and the presence of palatal perforation make the diagnosis of midline granuloma much more likely. Midline granuloma never involves structures below the neck.

488–491. **The answers are 488-C, 489-E, 490-D, 491-A.** *(Chaps 295, 299. Baker, N Engl J Med 329:1013–1020, 1993.)* The analysis of synovial fluid begins at the bedside. When fluid is withdrawn from a joint into a syringe, its clarity and color should be assessed. Cloudiness or turbidity is caused by the scattering of light as it is reflected off particles in the fluid; these particles are usually white blood cells, although crystals may also be present. The viscosity of synovial fluid is due to its hyaluronate content. In inflammatory joint disease, synovial fluid contains enzymes that break down hyaluronate and reduce fluid viscosity. In contrast, synovial fluid taken from a joint in a person with degenerative joint disease, a noninflammatory condition, would be expected to be clear and have good viscosity. The color of the fluid can indicate recent or old hemorrhage into the joint space. Pigmented villonodular synovitis is associated with noninflammatory fluid that is dark brown in color ("crankcase oil") as a result of repeated hemorrhage into the joint. Gout and calcium pyrophosphate deposition disease produce inflammatory synovial effusions, which are cloudy and watery. In addition, these disorders may be diagnosed by identification of crystals in the fluid—sodium urate crystals of gout are needlelike and strongly negatively birefringent, whereas calcium pyrophosphate crystals are rhomboidal and weakly positively birefringent.

Hematopoietic Disorders and Neoplasia

DIRECTIONS: Each question below contains five suggested responses. Select the **one best** response to each question.

492. All the following conditions impair the release of oxygen to body tissues EXCEPT

    (A) methemoglobinemia
    (B) carbon monoxide poisoning
    (C) hyperventilation
    (D) hypophosphatemia
    (E) acidosis

493. A 70-year-old man of Irish extraction returns to his physician for a routine check of his blood pressure. He is a vigorous, retired executive who except for mild hypertension is healthy. After his examination, as he is getting dressed, he states that his wife has been nagging him to mention a spot on his nose (as shown in Color Plate C). He is certain that this lesion, which has been present for several years, is of no significance. The most likely diagnosis for this lesion is

    (A) dermal nevus
    (B) sebaceous hyperplasia
    (C) clear cell acanthoma
    (D) xanthoma
    (E) basal cell carcinoma

494. A 52-year-old woman sees her physician for an "insurance physical." Physical examination reveals only a pigmented lesion (as shown in Color Plate D) present on one foot. The woman states that the lesion apparently was present at birth and does not itch or bleed; it is, however, not as homogeneous in color as it used to be. Which of the following statements about the condition described is true?

    (A) Bleeding and tenderness would be the first signs of malignant degeneration
    (B) It is unlikely that the lesion, present since birth, is malignant
    (C) It would be dangerous to perform an incisional biopsy of this lesion
    (D) Change in color of the lesion is a suspicious sign for potential malignancy
    (E) Early diagnosis of this lesion would not affect prognosis

495. A 58-year-old man presents with fatigue. His physical examination is normal except for the presence of splenomegaly. CBC discloses hematocrit, 29 percent; platelet count, 90,000/µL; WBC, 2700/µL; and an essential normal red cell morphology (differential 12 percent monocytes, 12 percent granulocytes, and 76 percent lymphocytes). A bone marrow aspirate and biopsy were performed. The aspirate was dry and the biopsy is pending. Based on the available information, the most likely diagnosis in this case is

(A) chronic lymphocytic leukemia
(B) hairy cell leukemia
(C) chronic myeloid leukemia
(D) myelofibrosis
(E) multiple myeloma

496. A 58-year-old chronic alcoholic and heavy smoker presents with a 3-cm, firm, right midcervical neck mass. Which of the following is the most appropriate approach at this time?

(A) Indirect laryngoscopy
(B) CT of the neck
(C) CT of the brain
(D) Excisional biopsy
(E) Needle biopsy

497. A 28-year-old man with newly diagnosed acute myelogenous leukemia spikes a temperature to 38.7°C (101.7°F) on the sixth day of induction therapy. He feels well and has no physical complaints. His only medicine is intravenous cytosine arabinoside, 140 mg every 12 h. Physical examination is unrevealing. His white blood count is 900/mm³, of which 10 percent are granulocytes and the rest mostly lymphocytes; platelet count is 24,000/mm³. Findings on chest x-ray and urinalysis are normal.

After obtaining appropriate cultures, the man's physician should

(A) observe closely for the development of a clinically evident source of fever
(B) begin antibiotic therapy with gentamicin and mezlocillin
(C) begin granulocyte transfusion and antibiotic therapy with gentamicin and mezlocillin
(D) begin gammaglobulin treatment and antibiotic therapy with gentamicin and mezlocillin
(E) begin antibiotic therapy with amphotericin, gentamicin, and mezlocillin

498. Coumarin-induced skin necrosis is occasionally associated with the institution of oral anticoagulants in patients with

(A) antithrombin III deficiency
(B) protein C deficiency
(C) protein S deficiency
(D) plasminogen deficiency
(E) dysfibrinogenemias

499. Patients who lack the plasma membrane receptor for the complement component C3bi (CR3) have which of the following clinical problems?

(A) Neutropenia
(B) Angioedema
(C) Gonococcal infections
(D) *Staphylococcus aureus* infections
(E) Viral infections

500. A 55-year-old woman presents to the emergency department because her family notes that she has yellow skin. The patient has lost 15 pounds over the past 3 months, but states that this is because she has been dieting in preparation for her daughter's wedding. Her past medical history is significant only for vitiligo. Her physical examination is unremarkable except for the presence of scleral icterus and a yellow tinge to the skin. Laboratory evaluation reveals hematocrit of 17 percent, WBC count of 2500/μL, and platelet count of 70,000/μL. Serum chemistries are normal except for direct bilirubin of 51 μmol/L (3 mg/dL) and indirect bilirubin of 12 μmol/L (0.7 mg/dL). The patient's reticulocyte count is 5 percent. MCV is 108 fL. Which one of the following additional laboratory findings would most likely be associated with this patient's clinical syndrome?

(A) Clonal chromosomal abnormalities on karyotypic analysis of the bone marrow
(B) Positive direct Coombs' test
(C) Extrahepatic biliary obstruction
(D) Decreased gastric fluid pH
(E) Antiparietal cell antibody

501. All the following hereditary syndromes are associated with the development of malignancies EXCEPT

(A) neurofibromatosis
(B) chronic granulomatous disease of childhood
(C) ataxia-telangiectasia
(D) familial polyposis coli
(E) Fanconi's anemia

502. Which of the following characteristics is more apt to be associated with Hodgkin's disease than with non-Hodgkin's lymphoma?

(A) "B" (constitutional) symptoms
(B) Involvement of Waldeyer's ring
(C) Extralymphatic presentation
(D) Dissemination at the time of diagnosis
(E) Approximately 40,000 new cases annually

503. A 27-year-old woman presents with stage II (breast and lymph node involvement) right breast cancer. Her family history is markedly positive for other tumors. One of her sisters developed an osteogenic sarcoma at age 17, her brother was diagnosed with acute leukemia at age 5, her mother died of breast cancer, and she has two uncles with soft-tissue sarcomas, both developing this disease when in their thirties. This patient's peripheral blood lymphocytes would be most likely to reveal which of the following abnormalities?

(A) Retinoblastoma gene mutation
(B) p53 gene mutation
(C) Translocation between chromosomes 9 and 22
(D) Translocation between chromosomes 8 and 14
(E) Mutations of epidermal growth factor receptor gene

504. A patient with a myelodysplastic syndrome (subtype, refractory anemia with ringed sideroblasts) has been transfusion-dependent for the past 2 years. The patient has received a total of 50 units of packed red blood cells. His physical examination is normal except for hyperpigmentation. Laboratory evaluation reveals mild glucose intolerance. He has failed a trial of erythropoietin.

Which of the following would be the most important therapeutic approach at this time?

(A) Granulocyte colony–stimulating factor
(B) Phlebotomy
(C) Ascorbic acid
(D) Desferrioxamine
(E) Hypertransfusion (maintain hematocrit at 40 percent)

505. A 26-year-old woman has painful mouth ulcers. Six weeks ago, she was started on propylthiouracil for hyperthyroidism. She is afebrile, and physical examination is unremarkable except for several small oral aphthous ulcers. White blood cell count is 200/mm³ (15 percent neutrophils, 80 percent lymphocytes, 5 percent monocytes); hemoglobin concentration, hematocrit, and platelet count are normal. The woman's physician should stop the propylthiouracil and

(A) schedule a follow-up outpatient appointment
(B) arrange for HLA typing of her siblings in preparation for bone marrow transplantation
(C) prescribe oral prednisone, 1 mg/kg
(D) hospitalize her for broad-spectrum antibiotic therapy
(E) hospitalize her for white blood cell transfusion

506. All the following may be found in the blood as a consequence of splenectomy EXCEPT

(A) erythrocytic Heinz bodies
(B) erythrocytic target forms
(C) erythrocytic Howell-Jolly bodies
(D) spherocytic red blood cells
(E) nucleated red blood cells

507. An 18-year-old black man undergoing a physical examination prior to playing college sports is found to have a normal CBC except that the MCV is 72 fL. Subsequent testing reveals a normal metabisulfite test and a normal hemoglobin electrophoresis. Which of the following conditions most likely accounts for these findings?

(A) Hemoglobin E trait
(B) Sickle C disease
(C) Sickle beta thalassemia
(D) Beta-thalassemia trait
(E) Alpha-thalassemia trait

508. A 30-year-old black woman with longstanding sickle cell anemia presents with severe pain in the chest and abdomen approximately 1 week after having an upper respiratory infection. No intrathoracic or intraabdominal pathology was immediately obvious on routine physical examination and laboratory evaluation. The most appropriate therapeutic intervention at this point is

(A) hypertransfusion
(B) hydration and narcotic analgesia
(C) hydroxyurea
(D) broad-spectrum antibiotics
(E) exploratory laparotomy

509. In persons who have chronic myelogenous leukemia, the translocation that accounts for the Philadelphia chromosome most commonly is found in

(A) all cells of the body
(B) all three hematopoietic cell lines but not in nonhematopoietic cells
(C) all cells of the granulocytic cell line but not in nongranulocytic cells
(D) all bone marrow stem cells but not in mature cells
(E) all bone marrow stem cells and certain mature granulocytes

510. Which of the following statements describes the relationship between testicular tumors and serum markers?

(A) Pure seminomas produce α-fetoprotein (AFP) or β-human chorionic gonadotropin (β-HCG) in more than 90 percent of cases
(B) More than 40 percent of nonseminomatous germ cell tumors produce no cell markers
(C) Both β-HCG and AFP should be measured in following the progress of a tumor
(D) Measurement of tumor markers the day following surgery for localized disease is useful in determining completeness of the resection
(E) β-HCG is limited in its usefulness as a marker, because it is identical to human luteinizing hormone

511. A 45-year-old man presents with fatigue. Two years ago the patient received six cycles of combination chemotherapy (each cycle consisted of cyclophosphamide, doxorubicin, vincristine, and prednisone) for non-Hodgkin's lymphoma in chest and abdominal sites. The patient entered complete remission and has been followed expectedly since that point. His last prior visit was 3 months ago at which time he had no evidence of recurrent lymphoma, felt well, and had a normal laboratory examination. At this time his physical examination is remarkable for a purple discoloration of the fingertips, ears, and nose. The patient is somewhat pale. There is no evidence for peripheral lymphadenopathy. Laboratory studies include the following: white count 10,000/μL (differential 60 percent neutrophils, 10 percent bands, 10 percent lymphocytes, 10 percent monocytes, 3 percent eosinophils, 1 percent basophils, 2 percent metamyelocytes, 1 percent myelocytes, and 1 nucleated red blood cell), hematocrit 28 percent, and platelet count 300,000/μL. The following results are also found: MCV 98 fL, lactic dehydrogenase 6.8 μkat/L (400 U/L), total bilirubin 51 μmol/L (3.0 mg/dL), and direct bilirubin 5.1 μmol/L (0.3 mg/dL). Review of the peripheral blood smear reveals clumped red cells. A routine direct Coombs' test is negative. Additional laboratory testing would most likely reveal

(A) positive direct Coombs' test (using anti-IgG antisera) if specimen is processed without allowing cooling
(B) positive indirect Coombs' test detected with anti-IgG antibodies
(C) circulating antibodies against Epstein-Barr virus
(D) circulating antibodies against fetal red blood cells
(E) circulating antibodies against *Mycoplasma pneumoniae*

512. A 50-year-old woman presents with bleeding gums. Other than petechiae, her physical examination is normal. She has not had any recent infections, nor has she been exposed to any drugs or industrial solvents. Hematologic laboratory values are as follows: hemoglobin 80 g/L (8 g/dL), hematocrit 24 percent, mean corpuscular volume (MCV) 101 fL, reticulocyte count 0.5 percent, WBC count 1500/μL (10 percent neutrophils), and platelet count 18,000/μL. Bone marrow examination is remarkable for a dry aspirate and a biopsy that discloses a severely hypocellular marrow with 90 percent fat infiltration. The remaining scant hematopoietic elements do not appear to be dysplastic. Further laboratory studies reveal the lack of antinuclear antibodies, normal sugar water and acid hemolysis tests, normal vitamin B_{12} levels, normal serum folate levels, and no evidence for antibodies to HIV.

The patient is placed on nandrolone decanoate for a period of 6 months without response. Which of the following is the most appropriate therapeutic approach at this time?

(A) Plasmapheresis
(B) Splenectomy
(C) Equine antithymocyte serum
(D) Erythropoietin
(E) Daunorubicin and cytosine arabinoside combination chemotherapy

513. A 25-year-old, previously healthy woman presents with jaundice, confusion, and fever. Initial physical examination is unremarkable except for scattered petechiae on the lower extremities, scleral icterus, and disorientation on mental status examination. Laboratory examination discloses the following: hematocrit, 27 percent; white cell count, 12,000/μL; platelet count, 10,000/μL; bilirubin, 85 μmol/L (5 mg/dL); direct bilirubin, 10 μmol/L (0.6 mg/dL); urea nitrogen, 21 mmol/L (60 mg/dL); creatinine, 400 μmol/L (4.5 mg/dL). Red blood cell smear discloses fragmented red blood cells and nucleated red blood cells. Prothrombin, thrombin, and partial thromboplastin times are all normal.

The most effective and appropriate therapeutic maneuver is likely to be

(A) plasmapheresis
(B) administration of aspirin
(C) administration of high-dose glucocorticoids
(D) administration of high-dose glucocorticoids plus cyclophosphamide
(E) splenectomy

514. Paroxysmal nocturnal hemoglobinuria is associated with all the following conditions EXCEPT

(A) elevation of leukocyte alkaline phosphatase levels
(B) aplastic anemia
(C) iron-deficiency anemia
(D) venous thrombosis
(E) acute leukemia

515. A 38-year-old woman presents with redness and burning in the distal extremities. She has no other complaints. She has never been pregnant. Physical examination is normal except for redness of the fingertips and splenomegaly. Laboratory examination reveals hematocrit 40 percent, WBC count 9000 with a normal differential, and platelet count of 950,000/μL. Other laboratory studies include reticulocyte count of 1 percent, bone marrow examination that discloses a hypercellular marrow with megakaryocytic hyperplasia and hyperlobated megakaryocytes, absent collagen deposition, and the presence of normal amounts of bone marrow iron. Cytogenetic studies reveal a normal female karyotype. A red cell mass study is normal. Which of the following statements concerning the patient's condition is true?

(A) Observation is indicated
(B) Splenectomy should be performed
(C) Oral administration of chlorambucil, 0.4 mg/kg daily for 5 days, should begin
(D) Aspirin, 2 tablets every 6 h, should be administered
(E) Hydroxyurea, 1000 mg daily orally, is indicated

516. The cytotoxic action of anticancer agents is thought to be defined by first-order kinetics, which means that these agents

(A) kill a constant fraction of tumor cells
(B) kill a constant number of tumor cells
(C) kill a number of tumor cells directly proportional to the time of exposure to the agent
(D) kill a number of tumor cells directly proportional to the molar concentration of the agent
(E) act directly on cells and do not require metabolism to an intermediate

517. A 42-year-old woman presents with epistaxis and gum bleeding. Physical examination is remarkable for a temperature of 38°C (100.4°F) and petechiae on the lower extremities. Laboratory evaluation includes a hematocrit of 29 percent, platelet count of 15,000/μL, and WBC of 2100/μL (differential including 22 percent blasts, 30 percent promyelocytes, 20 percent lymphocytes, 10 percent monocytes, 2 percent myelocytes and 3 percent metamyelocytes). PT is 15 s and PTT is 55 s. Bone marrow examination discloses a hypercellular marrow infiltrated with myeloblasts and heavily granulated promyelocytes. Myeloperoxidase stain of a bone marrow aspirate smear is markedly positive and demonstrates numerous intracellular rodlike forms. The patient is begun on all-*trans* retinoic acid. Which of the following is the most likely complication of this therapy?

(A) Worsening of disseminated intravascular coagulopathy
(B) Infection during neutropenia
(C) Respiratory distress
(D) Uric acid nephropathy
(E) Mucositis

518. All the following statements regarding toxic effects of chemotherapy are correct EXCEPT

(A) of all the antineoplastic agents, anthracyclines suppress bone marrow stem cells to the greatest degree
(B) vincristine is a relatively weak myelosuppressive agent and can be administered during periods of low blood counts
(C) cisplatin-induced nausea and vomiting can be controlled by metoclopramide or dexamethasone or both
(D) the use of melphalan (phenylalanine mustard) has been associated with secondary leukemia
(E) cisplatin can produce hypocalcemia by inducing renal electrolyte wasting

519. A 45-year-old man develops leukocytosis and fatigue. Workup reveals infiltration of the bone marrow with lymphoblasts. A sample of bone marrow is also sent for immunologic and cytogenetic analysis. Which of the following findings would be associated with the best prognosis?

(A) Common acute lymphocytic leukemia antigen (CALLA) CD10 positivity, normal cytogenetics
(B) CALLA CD10 positivity, t(9;22)
(C) Surface immunoglobulin positivity, t(8;14)
(D) My10 (CD34) positivity, normal cytogenetics
(E) My7 (CD13) positivity, t(4;11) translocation

520. In addition to a checkup including health counseling and examination of the oral cavity, thyroid gland, skin, lymph nodes, testes, and prostate, which of the following should be done annually in the fifth decade of life in the asymptomatic, average-risk man in order to promote the early detection of cancer?

(A) Colonoscopy
(B) Sigmoidoscopy
(C) Digital rectal examination with palpation of the prostate
(D) Digital rectal examination with palpation of the prostate and stool guaiac
(E) Digital rectal examination with palpation of the prostate, stool blood test, and chest x-ray

521. Iron deficiency is LEAST likely to result from

(A) lead poisoning
(B) hemodialysis
(C) chronic heart-valve hemolysis
(D) hereditary hemorrhagic telangiectasia
(E) idiopathic pulmonary hemosiderosis

522. A 72-year-old man who has become progressively more fatigued is found to be anemic. Hematologic laboratory values are as follows:

Hemoglobin: 100 g/L (10 g/dL)
Hematocrit: 27.5 percent
Mean corpuscular volume (MCV): 101 fL
Mean corpuscular hemoglobin (MCH): 30 pg
Mean corpuscular hemoglobin concentration (MCHC): 340 g/L (34 g/dL)
Reticulocyte count: 0.5 percent
White blood cell count: 7300/mm^3 (65 percent neutrophils)
Platelet count: 210,000/mm^3

The most likely diagnosis is

(A) acute leukemia
(B) aplastic anemia
(C) autoimmune hemolytic anemia
(D) iron deficiency
(E) myelodysplastic syndrome

523. Which of the following industrial toxins is associated with tumors of the liver?

(A) Asbestos
(B) Benzene
(C) Mustard
(D) Chromium
(E) Vinyl chloride

524. Proof that chronic myeloid leukemia is a clonal disease (neoplastic cells descending from a single cell) originated from studies of which of the following?

(A) Kappa and lambda light chain expression on cell surfaces
(B) N-*myc* amplification
(C) Isoenzyme analysis
(D) Detection of fusion protein
(E) Translocation between chromosomes 9 and 22

525. All the following predispose patients to an increased risk of developing malignant lymphoma EXCEPT

   (A) Chédiak-Higashi syndrome
   (B) AIDS
   (C) rheumatoid arthritis
   (D) multiple sclerosis
   (E) phenytoin

526. A 59-year-old postmenopausal woman underwent radical mastectomy 3 years ago for carcinoma of the breast. All nodes biopsied were negative, and the estrogen receptor status of the tumor was positive at 150 fmol/mg of cytosol protein. No further therapy was ordered. Now the woman presents with right upper leg pain. Plain films reveal a 3-cm lytic lesion in the right upper femur with cortical erosion, and a bone scan shows not only the femoral lesion but also three separate lesions in her ribs, two in her skull, and one in her pelvis. Chest x-ray is unremarkable, and liver function tests are normal.

   The most appropriate therapeutic option now would be

   (A) tamoxifen, 10 mg twice daily
   (B) tamoxifen, 10 mg twice daily, plus CMF combination chemotherapy (cyclophosphamide, methotrexate, and 5-fluorouracil)
   (C) tamoxifen, 10 mg twice daily, plus external-beam radiation to the femoral lesion
   (D) tamoxifen, 10 mg twice daily, plus prophylactic internal fixation of the right femur followed by external-beam radiation
   (E) tamoxifen, 10 mg twice daily, plus both CMF and external-beam radiation to the femoral lesion.

527. A 65-year-old man develops superficial thrombophlebitis in multiple sites including the arms and chest. He has had several episodes in the past couple of months, each of which lasted a few days. Which of the following neoplasms is most closely associated with this patient's clinical problem?
   (A) Prostate carcinoma
   (B) Lung carcinoma
   (C) Pancreatic carcinoma
   (D) Acute promyelocytic leukemia
   (E) Paroxysmal nocturnal hemoglobinuria

528. Which of the following has been described as a potential mechanism whereby cancer cells can become resistant to the cytotoxic effects of paclitaxel (Taxol)?

   (A) Increased drug inactivation
   (B) Increased activating enzyme
   (C) Increased target enzyme
   (D) Induction of multidrug resistance protein
   (E) Increased glutathione conjugation

529. Which of the following procedures would be most sensitive in detecting early iron overload?

   (A) Quantitative iron determination in a liver biopsy specimen
   (B) Urinary iron excretion in response to a test dose of desferrioxamine
   (C) Serum ferritin concentration
   (D) Serum iron concentration, total iron-binding capacity, and calculated transferring saturation
   (E) Iron stain of a bone marrow aspirate

530. Which of the following statements concerning the diagnosis of pernicious anemia is true?

(A) The presence of antiparietal-cell antibodies is diagnostic of pernicious anemia

(B) Hematologic response to folate therapy alone rules out pernicious anemia as the cause of megaloblastic anemia

(C) Hyperkalemia may be a consequence of vitamin B_{12} therapy

(D) Bone marrow examination would be expected to reveal marked depletion of erythrocyte precursors in persons with untreated pernicious anemia

(E) Serum gastrin levels usually are elevated in persons with pernicious anemia

531. A 45-year-old woman with metastatic breast cancer whose hepatic metastases have recently grown after initial shrinkage on a combination chemotherapeutic regimen consisting of cyclophosphamide, methotrexate, and 5-fluorouracil is now receiving paclitaxel infusion. Shortly after the infusion, the patient develops tightening in the throat, wheezing, hives, and a lowering of the blood pressure. Which of the following is the most appropriate therapeutic strategy when considering additional chemotherapy for this patient?

(A) Discontinue paclitaxel and substitute another chemotherapeutic agent

(B) Readminister the paclitaxel infusion over a longer period of time and use premedication

(C) Readminister the paclitaxel, but have a temporary cardiac pacemaker in place

(D) Desensitize the patient with exposure to small doses of paclitaxel prior to readministering the drug

(E) Readminister paclitaxel along with G-CSF

532. A 65-year-old woman with myelodysplastic syndrome, subtype refractory anemia, has required platelet transfusional therapy intermittently for the past year. She normally receives one bag (approximately 6 units) of irradiated single donor platelets obtained by a pheresis. Her platelet count today is 6000 and she is receiving a bag of platelets. At the conclusion of the transfusion, she develops a temperature to 39°C (102.2°F) and has rigor. She has had several similar reactions in the past several weeks. Her platelet count drawn 1 h after the platelet transfusion is 36,000/μL. Assuming that blood and platelet culture results are negative, which of the following would be the best way to reduce the likelihood of such febrile reactions in the future?

(A) Premedicate the patient with acetaminophen and diphenhydramine

(B) Administer CMV-negative platelets

(C) Administer HLA-identical platelets

(D) Administer leukocyte-reduced platelets

(E) Administer platelets from the patient's sibling

533. A 27-year-old man has a testicular mass. Chest x-ray reveals six discrete tumor nodules, and an abdominal CT scan shows enlarged paraaortic nodes. Serum α-fetoprotein level is elevated. He undergoes transinguinal orchiectomy, which reveals teratocarcinoma. Treatment is started with three cycles of combination chemotherapy consisting of bleomycin, etoposide, and *cis*-platinum; he tolerates the chemotherapy well. Four of the six lung nodules resolve completely, the paraaortic nodes disappear, and α-fetoprotein levels return to normal. The two remaining pulmonary nodules, one in each lung, have diminished in size to about 2 cm. The man receives a fourth cycle of the same drugs with no change in his clinical status.

At this stage, his physician should

(A) continue the same chemotherapy for one more cycle but increase the dosage of drugs by 50 percent
(B) switch to a new drug regimen
(C) perform thoracotomy in order to biopsy and remove the nodule on one side
(D) administer low-dose, whole-lung radiation
(E) administer high-dose spot radiation to the individual lung nodules

534. A 60-year-old man with known lung cancer has recently developed lower back pain. Physical examination, including careful neurologic examination, is normal. Plain films of the back reveal several blastic lesions around T12 and L1. The next step in the man's management should be

(A) careful observation and frequent neurologic examinations
(B) electromyography with nerve conduction studies
(C) lumbar puncture
(D) CT scan of the spine
(E) corticosteroid therapy

535. A 32-year-old man with acute myeloid leukemia in first remission undergoes an allogeneic bone marrow transplant with non-purged marrow from his HLA-identical sister. Prior to the administration of his sister's marrow, the patient underwent preparation with high-dose cyclophosphamide and total body irradiation. About 6 days after the administration of the graft, the patient feels quite ill. He develops a fever to 39°C (102.2°F) and begins to note a maculopapular skin rash over the arms and back. He has severe diarrhea and intermittent abdominal pain. Results of his liver function tests are markedly abnormal with elevation of the serum bilirubin, SGOT, and alkaline phosphatase. The most likely cause for this clinical syndrome is

(A) graft-versus-host disease
(B) cytomegalovirus infection
(C) autoimmune transfusion reaction
(D) bacterial sepsis
(E) venoocclusive disease of the liver

536. A 40-year-old woman undergoes her first mammogram. The study reveals a cluster of microcalcifications in the right breast. Needle biopsy reveals a focus of lobular carcinoma in situ (no invasion). At this point the patient should be offered

(A) quadrantectomy and lymph node dissection on the ipsilateral side
(B) quadrantectomy only
(C) right breast mastectomy with irradiation depending on lymph node status at the time of surgery
(D) irradiation therapy to the right breast
(E) either observation or bilateral simple mastectomies

537. A 45-year-old woman with long-standing rheumatoid arthritis is diagnosed as having "anemia of chronic disease." The predominant mechanism causing this type of anemia in persons with chronic inflammatory disorders is

(A) defective porphyrin synthesis
(B) impaired incorporation of iron into porphyrin
(C) intravascular hemolysis
(D) depressed erythroid maturation due to decreased erythropoietin production
(E) impaired transfer of reticuloendothelial storage iron to marrow erythroid precursors

538. Which of the following statements best characterizes the hemolysis associated with glucose-6-phosphate dehydrogenase (G6PD) deficiency?

(A) It is more severe in affected blacks than in affected persons of Mediterranean ancestry
(B) It is more severe in females than in males
(C) It causes the appearance of Heinz bodies on Wright staining of a peripheral smear
(D) It most often is precipitated by infection
(E) The best time to perform the diagnostic test is during a hemolytic crisis

539. A 65-year-old man with a benign past medical history presents to his internist for a routine medical checkup. His physical examination and laboratory studies are normal except for a serum prostate specific antigen value of 8 ng/mL (normal 0 to 3 ng/mL). Which of the following is a true statement about the man's condition?

(A) His likelihood of prostate cancer is 75 percent
(B) If he does have prostate cancer, the disease is likely confined to the gland
(C) Assuming there is no evidence of metastatic spread, the patient should undergo a radical prostatectomy
(D) Assuming there is no evidence of spread, the patient should receive radiation therapy to the prostate
(E) The patient should receive therapy with leuprolide and flutamide

540. A 31-year-old man noted a pigmented lesion on his right thigh. Biopsy revealed nodular melanoma with a depth of 4.2 mm. The lesion was carefully excised with a negative margin of about 2 cm. Metastatic workup and the remainder of the physical examination are unremarkable, including the absence of inguinal nodes. Of the following interventions, which is likely to reduce the risk of eventual metastases of malignant melanoma in this patient?

(A) Lymph node dissection of the right groin
(B) Administration of bacillus Calmette-Guérin (BCG) vaccine
(C) Intravenous administration of decarbazine (DTIC) chemotherapy
(D) Regional perfusion of the right limb with DTIC
(E) None of the above

541. The Health Insurance Plan of New York evaluated mammography as a screening tool for breast cancer in 62,000 persons. After an 18-year follow-up period, it was found that the screened population

(A) showed a reduction in mortality when all age groups were analyzed together

(B) showed a 30 percent reduction in mortality from breast cancer, compared with a control group, for women 35 to 50 years of age

(C) showed a 30 percent reduction in mortality from breast cancer for women at high risk for the development of breast cancer (i.e., women having prior breast cancer or an affected first-degree relative)

(D) demonstrated no change in mortality from breast cancer for women of any age group, despite the stage of cancer at diagnosis

(E) had an increased mortality from breast cancer probably due to the carcinogenic effects of radiation delivered during mammography

542. A 38-year-old premenopausal woman has a 3-cm mass in her left breast. Breast biopsy reveals infiltrating ductal carcinoma, and a left modified radical mastectomy is performed. The pathology report states that the primary tumor is estrogen-receptor–positive and that 4 of 28 lymph nodes identified are involved with tumor. Chest x-ray, bone scan, liver scan, and blood chemistries are all normal.

The most appropriate next step in the management of this patient would be

(A) antiestrogen therapy (e.g., tamoxifen)

(B) appropriate combination chemotherapy

(C) postoperative radiation therapy to the left chest wall and axilla

(D) bilateral oophorectomy

(E) follow-up in 2 months

543. A 55-year-old man complains of numbness in both legs and progressive inability to walk over the past 2 months. Physical examination is normal except for a decreased perception of light touch and pain in the lower extremities as well as bilateral leg weakness. There is no sensory level. Laboratory workup is remarkable for a hematocrit of 30 percent and elevated total protein. Serum protein electrophoresis reveals an M spike. The etiology of this patient's weakness is most likely

(A) necrosis of central nervous system gray and white matter

(B) inflammation of dorsal root ganglia

(C) loss of cerebellar Purkinje cells

(D) elaboration of tumor-associated protein that elicits an immune response that is cross-reactive with peripheral nerves

(E) tumor-elaborated immunoglobulin that is reacting with myelin components

544. A 45-year-old woman presents with an axillary mass. She has no other complaints. Her past medical history is benign and she is taking no medication. Physical examination is unremarkable except for the presence of a firm, nonmoveable mass of 4×3 cm in the left axilla. Biopsy of the mass reveals poorly differentiated malignant neoplasm without gland formation. Immunoperoxidase staining of the tumor is negative for cytokeratin and positive for the leukocyte common antigen. The most appropriate next step for this patient is

(A) modified radical mastectomy with axillary radiation therapy

(B) axillary radiation therapy

(C) administration of cyclophosphamide, methotrexate, and 5-fluorouracil

(D) administration of tamoxifen

(E) chest and abdominal CT

545. Most persons who have hemoglobin variants with high oxygen affinity will

    (A) adapt poorly to hypoxic conditions
    (B) demonstrate abnormal hemoglobin electrophoresis
    (C) have erythrocytosis
    (D) have abnormal morphology of red blood cells
    (E) have increased 2,3-diphosphoglycerate (2,3-DPG) concentrations in red blood cells

546. Evaluation of a person who has pure red blood cell aplasia would be expected to reveal

    (A) markedly hypocellular bone marrow
    (B) normochromic, normocytic red blood cells
    (C) increased iron turnover on ferrokinetic studies
    (D) a reticulocyte count greater than 2.0 percent
    (E) decreased urinary erythropoietin content

547. A 28-year-old man presents with chest pain. Chest x-ray reveals a large mediastinal mass. Abdominal CT reveals periaortic lymphadenopathy. Physical examination, including examination of the testes, is negative. Mediastinoscopic biopsy reveals poorly differentiated carcinoma. Which of the following laboratory tests would be most likely to be positive?

    (A) Prostate specific antigen (PSA)
    (B) beta human chorionic gonadotropin (βhCG)
    (C) Carcinoembryonic antigen (CEA)
    (D) CA-125
    (E) CA19-9

548. All the following are neoplasms of B-lymphocyte lineage EXCEPT

    (A) chronic lymphocytic leukemia
    (B) follicular lymphomas
    (C) Burkitt's lymphoma
    (D) mycosis fungoides
    (E) small lymphocytic (well-differentiated) lymphomas

549. Regarding local therapy of operable breast cancer, which of the following statements is accurate?

    (A) Axillary radiation therapy should follow modified radical mastectomy
    (B) Radiation therapy administered following breast-conserving surgery has no effect on the local recurrence rate
    (C) Radiation therapy administered following breast-conserving surgery has no effect on the overall survival rate
    (D) All patients with a small tumor do equally well with either lumpectomy plus radiation or modified radical mastectomy
    (E) Node dissection should be performed in all patients in order to reduce the chance of local spread

550. A 21-year-old woman who has had severe menorrhagia is referred by her gynecologist for evaluation of a possible systemic coagulopathy. A younger sister has been noted to bleed excessively after trauma. She takes no medications; physical examination is unremarkable. Initial laboratory results include the following: platelet count, 252,000/mm³; prothrombin time, 23.6 s (control 11.6 s); and partial thromboplastin time, 26.9 s (control 33.3 s). Further laboratory testing should include

    (A) determination of alpha$_2$-antiplasmin level
    (B) screening for inhibitors
    (C) determination of bleeding time
    (D) determination of factor VII level
    (E) determination of factor VIII level

551. Thrombocytosis would be LEAST likely to occur in persons who have

    (A) polycythemia vera
    (B) hemolytic-uremic syndrome
    (C) sickle cell (SS) disease
    (D) iron-deficiency anemia
    (E) ulcerative colitis

552. A 65-year-old woman with increasing abdominal pain is found to have a pelvic mass on physical examination. After appropriate staging studies she undergoes a laparotomy and is found to have serous carcinoma of the ovary with involvement of one ovary and several omental implants. She then undergoes a hysterectomy, bilateral salpingo-oophorectomy, liver biopsy, omentectomy, cytologic examination of abdominal washings, and extensive inspection. All evidence of disease is removed.

Assuming generally good health, an uneventful postoperative recovery, and lack of proximity to a center performing clinical trials, she should now receive

(A) no further therapy
(B) combination chemotherapy
(C) combination chemotherapy only if serum CA125 level is elevated
(D) intraperitoneal chemotherapy
(E) whole abdominal radiation therapy

553. Which of the following clinical scenarios is LEAST likely to describe a paraneoplastic syndrome resulting from small cell tumors of the lung?

(A) Weakness and fatigability, primarily of proximal muscles; electromyographic results show increasing amplitude of contraction with repetitive stimulation
(B) Cerebellar ataxia, dysarthria, deafness, pleocytosis of cerebrospinal fluid, and cerebellar atrophy on CT scan of the brain
(C) Moon facies, truncal striae, hypertension, hypokalemia, and hyperglycemia
(D) Hypercalcemia, polydipsia, polyuria, and mental status changes in the absence of bony metastases
(E) Mental status changes, muscle weakness, hyponatremia, and decreased serum osmolality with inappropriately elevated urine osmolality

554. A feature of idiopathic thrombocytopenic purpura common to both children *and* adults is

(A) occurrence after an antecedent viral illness
(B) presence of antibodies directed against target antigens on the glycoprotein IIb-IIIa complex
(C) absence of splenomegaly
(D) persistence of thrombocytopenia for more than 6 months
(E) necessity of splenectomy to ameliorate thrombocytopenia

555. A 16-year-old boy presented with deep vein thrombophlebitis and pulmonary embolism. There is no familial history of thromboembolic disease. The platelet count on admission was 325,000/mm^3; prothrombin time, 13.1 s (control 11.4 s); partial thromboplastin time, 55.0 s (control 27.9 s); and thrombin time, 14.5 s (control 15 s). The most likely reason for the thrombotic diathesis in this patient is the presence of

(A) dysfibrinogenemia
(B) congenital antithrombin III deficiency
(C) lupus anticoagulant
(D) factor XI deficiency
(E) protein C deficiency

556. Persons with polycythemia vera and a hematocrit greater than 45 percent are most likely to display which of the following?

(A) Increased levels of urinary erythropoietin
(B) Increased bone marrow iron stores
(C) Decreased carotid blood flow
(D) Hypocellular bone marrow
(E) Myelophthisic changes in their peripheral blood smear, including teardrop-shaped red blood cells and normoblasts

557. A young woman presents with bleeding after a dental extraction. She is found to have a bleeding time of greater than 20 min along with a normal prothrombin time and partial thromboplastin time. There is a familial history of bleeding, and the patient's laboratory evaluation reveals a normal platelet count. The factor VIII coagulant activity is 54 percent of normal, von Willebrand factor (vWF) antigen is 48 percent of normal, and ristocetin cofactor is 13 percent of normal. A normal spectrum of vWF multimers in the patient's plasma on SDS-agarose electrophoresis is noted. This patient's coagulopathy is primarily caused by

(A) defective release of vWF from endothelial cells
(B) inappropriate binding of vWF to platelets
(C) reduced synthesis of vWF by endothelial cells
(D) an inability to assemble high-molecular-weight multimers or premature catabolism of vWF
(E) an alteration in the platelet receptor for vWF

558. A 1-year-old boy bleeds significantly after an inguinal hernia repair. The patient has no siblings, and there is no familial history of a bleeding diathesis. Platelet count, bleeding time, prothrombin time, and partial thromboplastin time are all normal. The most likely diagnosis is

(A) prekallikrein deficiency
(B) factor XII deficiency
(C) factor XIII deficiency
(D) thrombasthenia
(E) protein S deficiency

559. A 75-year-old man presents with ischemic changes of the distal lower extremities. Physical examination reveals the presence of an abdominal mass. Laboratory evaluation discloses a hematocrit of 28 percent; platelet count, 90,000/mm³; prothrombin time, 16 s (control 12 s); and partial thromboplastin time, 55 s (control 30 s). The fibrinogen level was reduced to 1.0 g/L (100 mg/dL) and the level of fibrin split products was elevated to 160 mg/L (160 µg/mL). Which of the following is the most appropriate therapy?

(A) Plasma exchange transfusion
(B) Administration of cryoprecipitate
(C) Administration of aminocaproic acid (Amicar)
(D) Platelet transfusions
(E) Administration of fresh frozen plasma

560. Two years ago a 68-year-old man was found to have a prostate nodule on routine examination. Biopsy revealed poorly differentiated prostatic adenocarcinoma; staging studies failed to reveal any evidence of extraprostatic spread. Because of a desire to maintain potency, the patient opted for radiation therapy as primary treatment. Except for requiring lower extremity revascularization for intractable claudication, he did well until recently, when he developed pain in his right hip. Prostate specific antigen was elevated. Bone scan revealed areas of positive uptake in the pelvis and ribs (not present on the original staging study). The patient expresses a desire not to have a bilateral orchiectomy, "unless it would significantly improve my quality of life or survival compared with other therapies."

The most appropriate strategy at this point is to

(A) biopsy one of the bony lesions
(B) administer cisplatin and 5-fluorouracil
(C) administer leuprolide and flutamide
(D) administer diethylstilbestrol (DES) at low dose
(E) perform an orchiectomy

DIRECTIONS: Each question below contains five suggested responses. For **each** of the five responses listed with every question, you are to respond either YES (Y) or NO (N). In a given item **all, some, or none** of the alternatives may be correct.

561. Macrocytosis of red blood cells, in the absence of megaloblastic changes in the bone marrow, may be due to

(A) hypothyroidism
(B) malabsorption
(C) acute hemolysis
(D) total gastrectomy
(E) liver disease

562. Which of the following findings would distinguish β-thalassemia trait from iron deficiency?

(A) Microcytic red blood cells
(B) Absence of anemia
(C) Elevated hemoglobin A_2 level
(D) Normal transferrin saturation
(E) Normal serum ferritin concentration

563. Correct statements regarding growth factors include which of the following?

(A) Platelet-derived growth factor, produced exclusively by platelets, is primarily involved in hematopoiesis
(B) The epidermal growth factor receptor is a protooncogene
(C) The monocyte growth factor receptor is a molecule that catalyzes phosphorylation of certain proteins on tyrosine residues
(D) Granulocyte-macrophage colony–stimulating factor can stimulate proliferation of normal and leukemic myeloid cells
(E) Each hematopoietic growth factor acts primarily in a paracrine fashion (i.e., stimulates nearby cells)

564. True statements about doxorubicin (Adriamycin) cardiotoxicity include which of the following?

(A) Acute cardiotoxicity, which is characterized by arrhythmias and other abnormal electrocardiographic changes, is brief and rarely serious
(B) Chronic cardiotoxicity occurs in fewer than 3 percent of persons whose lifetime dose of doxorubicin is below 500 mg/m²
(C) Weekly doxorubicin therapy is better tolerated than the same total dose given every 3 weeks
(D) Congestive heart failure frequently develops 6 months or more after the last dose of doxorubicin
(E) Previous cardiac irradiation and exposure to cyclophosphamide or anthracycline antibiotics other than doxorubicin increase the risk of cardiotoxicity

565. Persons who have sickle cell trait (AS hemoglobinopathy) may have which of the following characteristics?

(A) Impaired growth and development in childhood
(B) Increased incidence of hematuria
(C) Impaired ability to concentrate urine
(D) Increased mortality in pregnancy
(E) Increased incidence of splenic infarction with high-altitude hypoxia

566. Adhesion of platelets to walls of injured blood vessels involves which of the following?

(A) Collagen
(B) Platelet glycoprotein Ia-IIa
(C) Platelet glycoprotein Ib-IX
(D) Platelet glycoprotein IIb-IIIa
(E) von Willebrand factor

567. Oncogenes implicated in the formation of human tumors by virtue of a chromosomal translocation include

(A) c-*myc*
(B) *Rb*-1
(C) c-*ras*^{H}
(D) c-*abl*
(E) *bcl*-2

568. Correct statements regarding the treatment of patients with non-Hodgkin's lymphoma include which of the following?

(A) Radiation therapy is curative for most patients with low-grade non-Hodgkin's lymphoma
(B) In those patients with low-grade lymphoma who require chemotherapy, only combinations of agents can change overall survival rate
(C) Over 75 percent of patients with intermediate-grade (e.g., diffuse large cell) lymphoma will achieve complete remission with combination chemotherapy
(D) Maintenance therapy (prolonged therapy after complete remission is achieved) improves survival in patients with diffuse large cell lymphoma
(E) Patients with non-Hodgkin's lymphoma who have AIDS have the same rate of response to chemotherapy as stage- and grade-matched patients without AIDS

569. A patient being treated for refractory anemia has required monthly transfusions of 2 units of packed red blood cells over the past several months. Three days after receiving 2 units of packed red blood cells for a hematocrit of 22 percent, the patient's hematocrit was 27 percent. One week after the transfusion the hematocrit is 22 percent; the patient feels ill, has a low-grade fever, and is mildly jaundiced. Correct statements about this situation include which of the following?

(A) This problem is probably due to leukocyte alloimmunization
(B) Intravascular hemolysis has probably occurred
(C) The Rh status of donor and recipient should be rechecked
(D) If the patient is Rh-negative, one should look for anti-Kell or anti-Duffy antibodies in the patient's serum
(E) A positive direct Coombs test is likely

570. True statements regarding *both* hemophilia A (factor VIII deficiency) and hemophilia B (factor IX deficiency) include

- (A) the defective gene is located on the X chromosome
- (B) the affected factors require vitamin K for biologic activity
- (C) the partial thromboplastin time is elevated, but the prothrombin time is normal
- (D) joint bleeding is common
- (E) the optimal therapy is fresh frozen plasma

571. True statements regarding ovarian cancer include

- (A) it is second to cervical carcinoma as the leading cause of cancer death from gynecologic malignancies
- (B) nulliparity is a risk factor
- (C) a history of breast cancer is a risk factor
- (D) stromal cell and germ cell tumors of the ovary are the most common histologic subtypes
- (E) histologic grade is an important prognostic factor

572. Correct statements concerning staging laparotomy for Hodgkin's disease include which of the following?

- (A) While those who have a large spleen preoperatively are virtually certain to have splenic involvement, a normal-size spleen requires assessment at laparotomy
- (B) If a staging laparotomy is planned, a lymphangiogram is useful
- (C) Laparotomy should nearly always be performed if positive findings would advance the stage of the disease
- (D) The spleen should nearly always be removed during staging laparotomy
- (E) Removal of the spleen at laparotomy is associated with better tolerance of chemotherapy

573. The absence of ristocetin-induced platelet aggregation is associated with which of the following clinical disorders?

- (A) Glanzmann's thrombasthenia
- (B) Bernard-Soulier syndrome
- (C) Aspirin ingestion
- (D) Storage pool disease
- (E) von Willebrand's disease

574. Myeloproliferative disorders characteristically are associated with which of the following potential complications?

- (A) Opportunistic infection
- (B) Carcinoma
- (C) Excessive bleeding
- (D) Thromboembolism
- (E) Acute myelogenous leukemia

575. Which of the following factors will influence the frequency of dissemination of cutaneous malignant melanoma?

- (A) Primary tumor site
- (B) Dermatologic level of invasion
- (C) Thickness of the primary lesion
- (D) Geographic area of residence
- (E) Presence of microscopic tumor satellites

576. Correct statements regarding carcinoma of the prostate include

- (A) histologic grade is an important prognostic indicator
- (B) most prostate cancers arise from the transitional cell epithelium
- (C) cancer of the prostate is the most common malignancy in men
- (D) cancer of the prostate may spread hematogenously, via lymphatics, or by direct extension
- (E) an elevated prostate specific antigen indicates metastatic disease

577. Stable-phase chronic myelogenous leukemia (CML) is associated with which of the following?

(A) Splenomegaly
(B) Basophilia
(C) Elevated leukocyte alkaline phosphatase
(D) Diagnostic bone marrow findings
(E) Favorable response to hydroxyurea, busulfan, or interferon-α

578. Characteristics of dysplastic nevi include which of the following?

(A) Dysplastic nevi serve only as markers for the risk of melanoma; melanomas arise only in apparently normal skin
(B) Dysplastic nevi tend to have a uniform appearance in a given individual
(C) Dysplastic nevi are usually more than 6 mm in diameter
(D) If two family members have melanoma, there is a 50 percent risk of developing melanoma in the patient with dysplastic nevi
(E) Patients commonly have nevi on areas not exposed to the sun

DIRECTIONS: The group of questions below consists of five lettered headings followed by a set of numbered items. For each numbered item select the **one** lettered heading with which it is **most** closely associated. Each lettered heading may be used **once, more than once, or not at all.**

Questions 579-582

Match each of the following chemotherapeutic agents to its appropriate mechanism of action.

(A) Inhibits DNA synthesis and reacts with DNA to cause strand scission
(B) Produces double-strand breaks due to interaction with topoisomerase II
(C) Blocks thymidylate synthase
(D) Produces metaphase arrest by direct binding to tubulin
(E) Causes depurination and miscoding errors by its alkylating action

579. Bleomycin

580. Doxorubicin

581. Vinblastine

582. 5-Fluorouracil

Hematopoietic Disorders and Neoplasia

Answers

492. The answer is E. *(Chaps 32, 302, 355.)* The affinity of the hemoglobin molecule for oxygen is altered primarily by blood pH, temperature, red blood cell concentration of 2,3-bisphosphoglycerate (2,3-BPG), and arterial carbon dioxide tension. Increased affinity, such as is produced by a rise in pH or a drop in 2,3-BPG, temperature, or P_{CO_2}, favors the transport of oxygen to body tissue. That is, under these conditions, at a given P_{O_2} a greater percentage of hemoglobin will be saturated with oxygen and more oxygen can be carried by the blood. Reduced affinity for oxygen favors unloading of oxygen from the hemoglobin molecule to the tissues—or, at a given P_{O_2} less oxygen will be bound to hemoglobin. Carbon monoxide exposure leading to the formation of carboxyhemoglobin shifts the oxygen dissociation curve to the left and thereby allows oxygen release only at relatively low oxygen tensions. Hyperventilation, by lowering P_{CO_2} and raising pH, and hypophosphatemia, by reducing levels of 2,3-BPG, both increase hemoglobin-oxygen affinity. Methemoglobin cannot carry oxygen, which results in a functional anemia and decreasing release of oxygen to the tissues.

493. The answer is E. *(Chap 324.)* Basal cell carcinoma is the most common malignancy in the United States. The typical appearance is that of a slowly enlarging, pearly translucent papule with rolled borders and overlying telangiectasias. As the lesion enlarges, central ulceration may occur (rodent ulcer). Sun-exposed areas are most commonly involved—about 90 percent of tumors occur on the head and neck—and fair-skinned persons are at greatest risk. Dermal nevi, which occur commonly on the faces of adults, lack the translucency seen in basal cell carcinoma. Sebaceous hyperplasia usually is smaller and has a distinct yellowish color. Diagnosis of basal cell carcinoma is easily established by punch or incisional biopsy.

494. The answer is D. *(Chap 325.)* The characteristics that distinguish superficial spreading malignant melanoma from a normal mole include irregularity of its border and variegation of color. Instead of the homogeneous color and regular borders of a "normal" mole, the lesion shows disorderliness and irregularity. The first changes noted by persons who develop melanoma in a preexisting mole are a "darkening" in color or a change in the borders of the lesion. Irregularity of the borders in an expanding, darkening mole is melanoma until proved otherwise; biopsy should be done promptly because early diagnosis and excision reduce the mortality.

495. The answer is B. *(Chap 372. Estey, Blood 79:882–887, 1992.)* Hairy cell leukemia is a neoplasm of mature B lymphocytes typically presenting with pancytopenia, splenomegaly, and a dry bone marrow aspirate. Patients with hairy cell leukemia are prone to infections with unusual microorganisms, such as atypical mycobacteria; they tend to be granulocytopenic and have a preponderance of mature-appearing lymphocytes in the peripheral blood that have, on close inspection or on ultrastructural analysis, multiple hairlike projections. Bone marrow biopsies typically yield a "fried egg" appearance in that the cells appear to be separated from one another, due to these projections and fixation artifacts generated from them. Immunophenotypically, hairy cells are characterized by the presence of markers of mature B cell derivation as well as the CD25 antigen, which is the interleukin-2 receptor. Fortunately, there are many treatment modalities available for patients with hairy cell leukemia. The current treatment of choice is a 7-day intravenous infusion of 2-chlorodeoxyadenosine. This single course of treatment results in complete remissions in approximately 70 percent of patients. Other effective modalities include splenectomy, interferon-α, or pentostatin (deoxycoformycin).

496. The answer is A. *(Chap 320. Vokes, N Engl J Med 328:184–194, 1993.)* Patients who are heavy smokers and drinkers are at increased risk to develop squamous cell carcinoma of the head and neck. In fact, the risk for those who both smoke and drink is multiplicatively increased compared with those who abuse just one of these substances. A firm neck mass in a patient with these habits should prompt an aggressive search for a primary lesion in the head and neck region. A neck mass in the midcervical chain in the presence of a normal physical examination (thereby excluding large tumors of the mouth or supraglottic region) could represent a metastasis from an infraglottic primary. Therefore, the best way to ascertain the diagnosis in this case is to perform a careful upper aerodigestive examination, which should begin with indirect laryngoscopy. CT of the neck, while helpful in delineating the extent of disease, would likely not reveal the primary. An incisional biopsy or fine-needle aspirate of the neck mass is contraindicated because of the difficulties this would present for subsequent radical neck dissection and because of the possibility of tumor seeding along the biopsy tract. Ideally, the diagnosis of malignancy in this case would be made by biopsy of the primary tumor, rather than of the putative lymph node metastases. This would allow optimal planning for local therapy. The standard approach to a primary head and neck squamous cell carcinoma with a large lymph node metastasis is radiation therapy or surgery or both. However, use of induction chemotherapy is being investigated as a possible means both to improve survival and to reduce the amount of disfiguring local therapy that would be required in such instances.

497. The answer is B. *(Chaps 81, 310. Pizzo, N Engl J Med 328:1323, 1993.)* If not attacked promptly, infection in neutropenic patients can be quickly fatal. Often, these patients display neither the signs nor the symptoms of infection. Fever should be regarded as an indication of infection, and antibiotic therapy should begin immediately after appropriate cultures are obtained. An effective initial antibiotic regimen would consist of an aminoglycoside antibiotic or third-generation cephalosporin and a semisynthetic antipseudomonal penicillin. Gammaglobulin is of little benefit in the treatment of cancer patients. Granulocyte transfusions may be of benefit in a few selected cases. Amphotericin B is appropriate if defervescence does not occur after several days of antibacterial antibiotics.

498. The answer is B. *(Chap 315.)* Several reports have recently described the association of coumarin-induced skin necrosis in patients with congenital protein C deficiency. The skin lesions occur on the breasts, buttocks, legs, and penis. They appear to be a result of diffuse thrombosis of the venules with interstitial bleeding. This condition is presumed to result from an imbalance in hemostatic mechanism activity favoring thrombosis during the early phases of coumarin administration. Protein C has a relatively short half-life within the circulation (about 14 h) compared with that of some of the vitamin K–dependent procoagulant clotting factors (factor X and prothrombin), and a rapid drop in its effective concentration could produce such a situation.

499. The answer is D.   *(Chap 59.)*   Abnormal neutrophil function is grouped into categories of adherence-aggregation defects, abnormal chemotaxis, or reduced microbicidal activity. An inherited (autosomal recessive) absence of plasma membrane receptor for the complement component C3bi results in insufficiently adherent neutrophils. This defect is caused by a mutation in the beta subunit of leukocyte adhesion molecules LFA-1, Mac-1, and gp150,95 coded for by a gene located on the long arm of chromosome 21. The most severe expression of this disease results in a failure to induce leukocyte adhesion molecules on most immune effector cells. In addition to decreased neutrophil adherence, aggregation and chemotaxis are also impaired. Patients therefore develop recurrent bacterial and fungal infections involving skin and oral or genitourinary mucosae. Because of a failure of normal leukocyte margination, the neutrophil count is typically elevated. The most common bacterial infections in patients with absent C3bi are caused by *Staphylococcus aureus* and enteric gram-negative bacteria. Inherited disorders characterized by impaired neutrophil migration include hyperimmunoglobulin E–recurrent infection (Job's) syndrome, Chédiak-Higashi syndrome, and specific neutrophil granule deficiency. Chronic granulomatous disease, a rare disorder characterized by abnormal microbicidal capability of neutrophils, is caused by lack of one of four NADPH oxidase subunits. This defect results in absent superoxide and H_2O_2 in neutrophils, which leads to impaired bacterial and fungal killing.

500. The answer is E.   *(Chaps 56, 304. Stabler, Blood 76:871–881, 1990.)*   While pancytopenia is frequently due to an intrinsic bone marrow abnormality, vitamin B_{12} and folate deficiency may also present low blood counts. The elevated red cell volume coupled with a low (corrected) reticulocyte count suggests a hypoproliferative megaloblastic anemia. The history of vitiligo represents one of the several autoimmune-type diseases associated with pernicious anemia (PA). Other such immunologically mediated diseases include Graves' disease, myxedema, thyroiditis, idiopathic adrenocortical insufficiency, and hypoparathyroidism. PA is a failure of gastric production of intrinsic factor due to autoimmune destruction of parietal cells, which prevents B_{12} absorption in the distal ileum. Antibody-mediated destruction of parietal cells results in achlorhydria (an abnormally high gastric pH). The hematologic abnormalities of PA include elevated MCV, decreased reticulocyte count, hypersegmented neutrophil nuclei, and megaloblastic changes in the bone marrow that can, if severe, be confused with acute leukemia. Extramedullary manifestations of PA include neurologic abnormalities typified by demyelinization of the posterior and lateral spinal columns of the spinal cord, resulting in numbness and parasthesias, weakness, and ataxia. Patients with megaloblastic anemia on the basis of deficiency of intrinsic factor respond to cyanocobalamin injections within several days. Hypokalemia may complicate the recovery phase.

501. The answer is B.   *(Chap 317.)*   Certain familial and genetic syndromes are associated with an increased propensity to development of malignant neoplasms. Ataxia-telangiectasia, an autosomal recessive condition characterized by abnormal cellular immunity, conjunctival telangiectasias, and progressive spinocerebellar atrophy, is also associated with lymphoma. Carcinoma of the colon develops in almost all persons with familial polyposis coli and is found at the time of initial diagnosis of the polyps in about 40 percent of cases. Fanconi's anemia is one of a group of familial disorders associated with cytogenetic abnormalities and an increased risk of development of cancer. Neurofibromas undergo sarcomatous change in approximately 10 percent of affected patients. Chronic granulomatous disease of childhood is a disorder of oxidative metabolism in phagocytes and is not associated with neoplasia.

502. The answer is A.   *(Chap 311.)*   Hodgkin's disease can be distinguished from non-Hodgkin's lymphomas (NHL) by a variety of characteristics. The "B" (or constitutional) symptoms described for Hodgkin's disease are less common in patients with NHL, although the presence of these symptoms is thought to influence the prognosis negatively. Involvement of Waldeyer's ring occurs more commonly in NHL than in Hodgkin's disease. Extralymphatic presentation is more frequent with NHL than with Hodgkin's disease, and NHL is more often disseminated at the time of diagnosis. There are 40,000 new cases of NHL annually, compared with 7500 for Hodgkin's disease.

503. The answer is B. *(Chap 63. Weinberg, Science 254:1138, 1991.)* The most common genetic alteration in human cancer is mutation or deletion of the p53 gene, which is found on the long arm of chromosome 17. Wild type p53 suppresses malignant transformation of cells in tissue culture. It appears to regulate cell cycle progression by holding cells at the G1-S boundary. Like the retinoblastoma tumor suppressor gene, p53 may be activated by protein products of transforming viruses. A rare autosomal dominant cancer syndrome, the Li-Fraumeni syndrome, is characterized by families with a very high incidence of a diverse spectrum of childhood and adult tumors, including breast cancer, soft-tissue sarcomas, brain tumors, bone sarcomas, leukemia, and adrenocortical carcinoma. Germ line mutations in the p53 gene have been found in several of these families. Since an abnormality of one allele of p53 is inherited, these patients are at risk of developing homozygous p53 loss and a predisposition to neoplastic transformation. Mutations of the p53 gene are also very common in sporadic human tumors.

504. The answer is D. *(Chap 303.)* Since each unit of transfused blood contains 200 to 250 mg of iron and normal iron excretion is only 1 mg/d, a patient receiving about 40 units of blood annually will accumulate about 8 g of iron, putting him or her at risk for problems related to transfusional iron overload. In addition to the requirement for many transfusions, the disorder must also have a long natural history to allow for the development of the clinical sequelae of chronic iron overload. Thalassemia major, myeloproliferative disorders, myelodysplastic syndromes (without excess myeloblasts), pure red cell aplasia, and moderately severe aplastic anemia are diseases that may be associated with transfusional iron overload. The spectrum of problems produced by iron deposition in tissues includes cardiac dysfunction (arrhythmias, conduction defects, and restrictive cardiomyopathy), hepatic cirrhosis, glucose intolerance, gonadal dysfunction, and hyperpigmentation due to increased melanin production secondary to dermal iron deposition. The only available treatment for transfusion-associated hemochromatosis (phlebotomy is not an option because of chronic anemia) is chelation with desferrioxamine, which must be given subcutaneously over 12 to 16 h per day by a portable pump. While oral ascorbic acid may enhance iron excretion in patients receiving desferrioxamine, it has no role as a monotherapy and may be associated with dangerous cardiac toxicity.

505. The answer is A. *(Chaps 59, 67.)* Severe neutropenia is a rare idiosyncratic reaction to certain drugs, including propylthiouracil. In addition to having sore throat and oral and anal mucosal ulcerations, affected persons are susceptible to overwhelming, life-threatening infections. However, in the absence of fever or clinical signs of infection, they should be followed as outpatients, saving them exposures to nosocomial pathogens in the hospital. Empirical use of broad-spectrum antibiotics without fever or other signs of infection is not advisable, and corticosteroid therapy is not useful. White blood cell transfusion can be accompanied by serious morbidity (i.e., pulmonary leukostasis) and should be reserved for persons with transient neutropenia and documented septicemia. Because severe drug-induced neutropenia is generally self-limited once use of the offending drug has been stopped, consideration of bone marrow transplantation is not justified.

506. The answer is D. *(Chap 58.)* The spleen is responsible for removing senescent red blood cells from the circulation. The older, less deformable red blood cells cannot pass through the slitlike passages in splenic sinuses and are phagocytosed by red pulp macrophages. In the absence of a spleen, particulate matter of the red blood cells, such as nuclear material (Howell-Jolly bodies) or hemoglobin (Heinz bodies), that is normally pinched off during passage of red blood cells through the spleen remains visible on examination of the peripheral smear. Red cells that escape the marrow with a nucleus still present and target forms with excess membrane are normally handled by the spleen as well. The spherocytic red cells characteristically produced by extravascular antibody-mediated hemolysis and splenic conditioning would not likely be observed after splenectomy.

507. The answer is E. *(Chap 306. Kazazian, Semin Hematol 27:209, 1990.)* Hemoglobinopathies are a diverse group of congenital disorders characterized by one or more mutations in one of the genes coding for hemoglobin chains. The clinical consequences can range from no effect to incompatibility with life. Microcytosis occurs in these conditions except for the silent alpha-thalassemia carrier state in which only one of the four alpha-thalassemia genes is deleted. Such persons have no hematologic abnormalities. Persons with deletion of two of the four alpha-chain genes (alpha-thalassemia trait) tend to have microcytic and slightly hypochromic red cells without significant hemolysis or anemia. Hemoglobin electrophoresis may be normal or may reveal a decreased amount of hemoglobin A_2. Deletion of three of the four alpha-chain genes, so-called hemoglobin H disease, is associated with significant anemia and with a production of hemoglobin H (beta-chain tetramers) on hemoglobin electrophoresis. There are only two genes coding for the beta-hemoglobin chain. Patients with abnormalities in one such chain have beta-thalassemia trait characterized by microcytosis, abnormal-appearing red cells, and an elevated level of hemoglobin A_2 or F or both on hemoglobin electrophoresis. Any patient who inherits at least one allele with a hemoglobin S mutation (sickle hemoglobin, valine to glutamic acid substitution at the sixth amino acid of the hemoglobin beta chain) will demonstrate red blood cell sickling under reduced oxygen tension, as is artificially produced by addition of an oxygen-consuming agent such as metabisulfite to the blood. Therefore, any patient with sickle cell trait, sickle cell anemia, or a compound heterozygote such as sickle beta-thalassemia or sickle C will have a positive metabisulfite test (and would also have a positive hemoglobin electrophoresis). Hemoglobin E is a very common hemoglobin variant that is highly prevalent in southeast Asia. Patients with this disorder have an abnormal hemoglobin electrophoresis, slightly macrocytic red cells, and target cells, but no anemia or other clinical manifestations unless they also inherit beta thalassemia.

508. The answer is B. *(Chap 306. Wayne, Blood 81:1109–1123, 1993.)* Most clinical problems arising in patients with sickle cell anemia are due to vasoocclusive phenomena caused by sickling of deoxygenated red blood cells in capillaries. Microinfarcts can occur suddenly and cause severe pain in almost any part of the body, although the abdomen, chest, back, and joints are most commonly affected. These crises may be precipitated by upper respiratory infection, cold weather, or dehydration. Unfortunately, it is often difficult to distinguish between a painful sickle abdominal crisis and an actual acute abdominal emergency. Pleuritic chest pain and fever may occur in the absence of an infiltrate. If an infiltrate does occur, distinguishing between pneumonia and pulmonary infarction is difficult, although culture and Gram stain of the sputum might be helpful in this regard. In addition to painful crises, microinfarcts can cause chronic damage in the lungs, kidneys, liver, skeleton, and skin. Painful crises should mandate the use of adequate analgesia, including narcotics, and hydration. Unfortunately, there is an increased risk of opiate addiction in this patient population. Oxygen is helpful if hypoxemia complicates a painful crisis. The role of transfusional therapy in sickle cell anemia is controversial. There is some evidence to suggest that use of aggressive transfusions may decrease the frequency of painful crises, but such an approach has little role in an ongoing crisis. Antibiotics should only be administered in the setting of documented infection.

509. The answer is B. *(Chap 309.)* In about 95 percent of persons who have chronic myelogenous leukemia, material comprising approximately one-half of the long arm of chromosome 22 is translocated to the end of chromosome 9. This abnormality, called the Philadelphia chromosome, can be found in all hematopoietic cell lines. It is thought to represent an acquired somatic cell mutation in the bone marrow, with preferential survival and proliferation of the affected cell clone. The pathogenesis of chronic myelogenous leukemia is therefore a paradigm for all cancers that are believed to arise from a single cell that gives rise to the malignant clone. Normal stem cells exist in the marrow of patients with cancer, but they are suppressed by the malignant cells.

510. The answer is C. *(Chaps 317, 322.)*   Ninety percent of persons with nonseminomatous germ cell tumors produce either α-fetoprotein (AFP) or β-HCG; in contrast, persons with pure seminomas usually produce neither. These tumor markers are present for some time after surgery—if the presurgical levels are high, 30 days or more may be required before meaningful postsurgical levels can be obtained. The half-lives of AFP and β-HCG are 6 days and 1 day, respectively. After treatment, unequal reduction of β-HCG and AFP may occur, suggesting that the two markers are synthesized by heterogeneous clones of cells within the tumor; thus, both markers should be followed. β-HCG is similar to luteinizing hormone except for its distinctive beta subunit.

511. The answer is D. *(Chap 307.)*   If patients develop circulating anti-IgM antibodies with specificity for polysaccharide antigens on red cell membranes, they may suffer from so-called cold-reactive hemolysis. The clinical manifestations of the presence of such antibodies are hemolysis, which is generally not severe, and a mild elevation of the reticulocyte count, agglutination of red cells, and an increased rate of hemolysis at temperatures below 37°C. A second clinical manifestation of cold hemolysis is the presence of acrocyanosis, characterized by marked purple discoloration of the extremities, ears, and nose during cooling. IgM antibodies may be missed if the blood is allowed to cool after it is drawn because of adsorption onto the patient's own red blood cells and subsequent removal as the blood clots. Therefore, the blood should be allowed to clot at a warm temperature. Serological analysis will reveal a positive direct Coombs' test if anti-C3 antisera is used. The activation of complement by the fixed IgM molecules results in the marked accumulation of the C3dg degradation product on the red cell surface, allowing detection in this fashion. The specificity of the cold agglutinin antibody may be helpful in that a reaction with adult red cells compared with fetal (cord) blood is more common in benign lymphoproliferative disorders. On the other hand, antibodies that react more strongly with fetal cells compared with adult cells are called anti-i and are generally seen in lymphomas and in infectious mononucleosis. The patient in this question may well have a recurrence of his lymphoma, which is presenting as a cold hemolytic disease because of the presence of monoclonal IgM antibody. This problem is best treated by successful anti-lymphoma therapy.

512. The answer is C. *(Chap 309.)*   Aplastic anemia may follow exposure to agents that are toxic to the bone marrow such as benzene, chloramphenicol, or gold, or it may occur in association with viral infections including hepatitis C, Epstein-Barr virus, and parvovirus, which may selectively impair erythroid maturation in patients with ongoing hemolysis. The course of the disease is determined by the severity of the aplasia. In this case the patient has anemia, severe thrombocytopenia, and neutropenia as well as a marrow that is almost totally infiltrated by fat. Vitamin deficiency, invasion of the bone marrow with a neoplasm, paroxysmal nocturnal hemoglobinuria, systemic lupus erythematosus, and AIDS have been appropriately ruled out. The best therapy for a patient with severe aplastic anemia is allogeneic bone marrow transplantation from a histocompatible donor, preferably a sibling. However, if the transplant option is not available, then in addition to receiving traditional use of blood products as part of a regimen of supportive care, patients should receive a trial of androgens for 3 to 6 months. Failing such therapy, patients with severe aplastic anemia and without a bone marrow transplant option should receive some form of immunosuppressive therapy, both because of the potential immune etiology of this disorder and the association of a 50 percent response rate with immunosuppressive agents. The most commonly used therapy is animal antisera to human lymphocytes. Such therapy may be complicated by serum sickness. High-dose glucocorticoids or cyclosporine may be associated with a similar response rate. Splenectomy has no role in the management of aplastic anemia and would be dangerous to perform in this pancytopenic patient. Insofar as aplastic anemia is not believed to be humorally mediated, plasmapheresis also has no role. The administration of chemotherapeutic agents to patients with limited marrow reserve is extremely dangerous and should not be considered.

513.   **The answer is A.**   *(Chap 307. Thompson, Blood 80:1890, 1992.)*   This young woman is suffering from a combination of hemolytic anemia with fragmented red cells in the absence of disseminated intravascular coagulation (DIC), thrombocytopenia, fever, mental status changes, and renal dysfunction, which is essentially pathognomonic of thrombotic thrombocytopenic purpura (TTP). The etiology of TTP is unknown, though immunologic and primary vasculopathic phenomena have been associated with this disorder. Pathologically, arteriolar hyalinization, which is also seen in DIC, may be noted. Seventy percent of patients with TTP improve with exchange transfusion or plasmapheresis. Glucocorticoids, antiplatelet agents, splenectomy, and vincristine have been of benefit to subsets of patients, but each is less effective and probably associated with a greater risk than therapeutic plasmapheresis.

514.   **The answer is A.**   *(Chap 307. Schreiber, N Engl J Med 309:723, 1983.)*   Paroxysmal nocturnal hemoglobinuria (PNH) is an acquired disease caused by injury to or mutation in the bone marrow stem-cell pool. PNH can develop following recovery from aplastic anemia, and pancytopenia becomes evident in many affected persons sometime during the course of their illness. Iron deficiency, resulting from urinary iron loss, is a frequent complication of the chronic, intermittent, intravascular hemolysis associated with PNH. Thrombosis is a major cause of morbidity and mortality. In a minority of affected patients, PNH transforms into acute myelogenous leukemia. Functional leukocyte defects have been demonstrated in the disease, and the leukocyte alkaline phosphatase level is typically reduced (as in chronic myelogenous leukemia). Diagnosis is made by demonstrating red cell hemolysis in acidified serum (Ham's test) or in the presence of a reduced ionic strength environment (sucrose lysis test).

515.   **The answer is E.**   *(Chap 309.)*   When a patient presents with thrombocytosis, it is important to determine if this abnormality is due to a myeloproliferative disorder or is reactive due to infection, malignancy, hemolytic anemia, the postoperative state, hemorrhage, iron deficiency, drug reaction, chronic inflammatory disease, response to exercise, recovery from myelosuppression, recovery from B_{12} deficiency, or even myelodysplastic syndrome (either 5q− syndrome or rare cases of sideroblastic anemia). Once secondary causes of thrombocytosis have been satisfactorily excluded, then it is important to delineate the specific myeloproliferative disorder. The red cell mass virtually excludes polycythemia vera and normal cytogenetics makes the diagnosis of chronic myelogenous leukemia most unlikely. Anemia, massive splenomegaly, teardrop red cell forms, or an elevated white count would advance consideration of agnogenic myeloid metaplasia/myelofibrosis. However, the bone marrow examination did not disclose excess collagen fibrosis. As such, the patient in this question has essential thrombocythemia. Patients with this disease may develop hemorrhage or thrombotic complications. Older patients have a higher risk of thrombosis; some younger patients can be observed. However, this patient is symptomatic due to erythromelalgia, the syndrome of redness and painful burning of the distal extremities caused by localized platelet aggregation. Chronic use of alkylating agents should be avoided due to the risk of leukemogenesis. Antiplatelet agents may protect against thrombosis but could lead to severe hemorrhage. Splenectomy would result in an even higher platelet count. The best treatment in this patient is probably the use of hydroxyurea at a dose titrated to lower the platelet count to below 500,000. Interferon-α may be a useful alternative for those patients unable to tolerate hydroxyurea.

516.   **The answer is A.**   *(Chap 318.)*   By following first-order kinetics, anticancer agents kill a constant fraction, rather than a constant number, of tumor cells. A course of therapy that has been shown to be capable of killing three orders of magnitude of cells (i.e., 3 logs) will do so regardless of total number of tumor cells. Because most chemotherapeutic agents have been found to reduce the number of tumor cells by only 1 to 3 logs, their effectiveness in treating cancers with a trillion cells (10^{12}) has been limited, unless the tumor burden is reduced first.

517. The answer is C. *(Chap 309. Warrell, N Engl J Med 329:1130, 1993.)*   Acute promyelocytic leukemia (M3 according to the FAB [French-American-British] classification system) is characterized by bone marrow infiltration with malignant-appearing promyelocytes. Distinctive features of this entity compared with other subtypes of de novo acute myeloid leukemia include the common presentation with leukopenia, the frequent development of disseminated intravascular coagulopathy (DIC) due to release of procoagulant granules from the promyelocytes, and the pathognomonic demonstration of a translocation between chromosomes 15 and 17 on cytogenetic analysis. This translocation juxtaposes sequences from the retinoic acid–receptor alpha gene on chromosome 17 with another DNA binding protein, called PML, on chromosome 17. The resultant fusion protein plays some role in preventing normal differentiation. Interestingly, even before the documentation of the genetic basis for this translocation, it was noted by investigators in China that the use of all-*trans* retinoic acid, an orally administered vitamin A derivative, lead to complete remissions in the vast majority of patients with APML. The mechanism of action of this drug appears to be induction of differentiation of the malignant clone. As such, patients enter remission slowly over a period of 30 to 60 days. DIC, typically made worse by chemotherapy, is rapidly ameliorated by all-*trans* retinoic acid. Other cytotoxic effects of chemotherapy, such as mucositis and myelosuppression, do not occur with all-*trans* retinoic acid. Common side effects include dry skin and peeling at the corners of the mouth. A life-threatening complication, occurring in about 20 percent of patients treated with all-*trans* retinoic acid, is the so-called retinoic acid syndrome, manifested by pulmonary infiltrates and incipient respiratory failure, sometimes associated with a high white count. Steroids, leukopheresis, and hydroxyurea have each been associated with some improvement. Patients maintained on all-*trans* retinoic acid alone will eventually relapse, so initial induction therapy with all-*trans* retinoic acid should be followed by consolidation chemotherapy.

518. The answer is A. *(Chap 318.)*   The most prominent general side effects of chemotherapy relate to the effect of these drugs on dividing cells, including myelosuppression, stomatitis, and alopecia. Certain drugs, such as L-asparaginase and vincristine, can be administered during periods of low white blood cell count because they are relatively nonmyelosuppressive. Alkylating agents, such as melphalan, cyclophosphamide, and nitrogen mustard, damage bone marrow stem cells, an effect associated with the development of secondary myelodysplastic syndromes and acute leukemias. Anthracyclines are myelosuppressive, but they inhibit more committed hematopoietic cells than do the alkylating agents. Cisplatin is quite emetogenic; however, vomiting can be managed successfully with the use of a number of agents, including dexamethasone and metoclopramide. Massive losses of potassium and magnesium (in turn leading to hypocalcemia) must be anticipated with the use of cisplatin because of drug-induced renal tubular damage.

519. The answer is A. *(Chap 309.)*   Adults with acute lymphocytic leukemia (ALL) do not respond nearly as well to chemotherapeutic programs as do children with the same disease. The reason for the inferior results in adults is not poor tolerance of chemotherapy. Instead, adults with ALL are more likely to present with a disease typified by adverse prognostic factors, usually indicating derivation from a more primitive hematopoietic stem cell. For example, Philadelphia chromosome–positive ALL—t(9;22)—is much more common in adults than in children. Adults are also more likely to have leukemic cells that bear either myeloid antigens or immunophenotypic evidence of derivation from a primitive stem cell (CD34 positivity). Balanced translocations in ALL, such as the t(4:11) associated with biphenotypic leukemia, also portend a poor prognosis. The most favorable subtype of ALL is that derived from a pre-B cell—CALLA (CD10) or B4 (CD19) positivity—with normal cytogenetics. However, for reasons that remain unclear, even this "favorable" prognostic subgroup is not associated with the high cure rate characteristic of children with the same immunophenotype and cytogenetics.

520. The answer is C. *(Chap 317.)*   Early detection of cancer is a major focus for the internist in evaluating his or her patients. Such detection depends on an awareness of the epidemiology of cancers and the sensitivity and specificity of any proposed test. It is recommended that each time a patient is seen by his or her physician, cancers of the oral cavity, thyroid, skin, lymph node, testes, and prostate be considered by performance of a careful physical examination. Between the ages of 20 and 39 the American Cancer Society recommends that such a physical examination be performed every 3 years. For men aged 40 to 49 a digital rectal examination with palpation of the prostate is recommended annually. For those aged 50 and older, the annual cancer-related checkup should include a digital rectal examination and palpation of the prostate as well as annual stool blood test plus sigmoidoscopy every 3 to 5 years. Screening for advanced prostate cancer by serologic measurement of the prostate specific antigen (PSA), while sometimes recommended for men over 50, remains controversial. It is important to recognize that for a screening test such as PSA to be effective, it must pick up disease in the curable stage. Chest radiography, for example, is not useful as a screening test for lung cancer in average-risk, asymptomatic patients because cancers that are picked up by this modality tend to be too far advanced for meaningful intervention. On the other hand, PSA detection might well pick up insignificant cancers. Finally, it is important to recognize that a more aggressive approach to the detection of cancer is appropriate if a patient has a symptom or an abnormal physical examination.

521. The answer is A. *(Chap 303.)*   Lead poisoning causes defective heme synthesis by interfering with a number of steps in the heme synthetic pathway. In severe cases, a hypochromic, microcytic anemia results. However, iron deficiency is not present, and serum iron levels may actually be increased in affected adults. Iron deficiency results from chronic, recurrent gastrointestinal bleeding in persons with hereditary hemorrhagic telangiectasia and from pulmonary bleeding in persons with idiopathic pulmonary hemosiderosis. Chronic heart-valve hemolysis leads to intravascular liberation of hemoglobin and iron depletion through hemoglobinuria and hemosiderinuria. Iron deficiency can occur from recurrent blood loss during hemodialysis. Iron-deficient persons hyperabsorb lead, so lead poisoning is more common in impoverished children who have iron deficiency and pica.

522. The answer is E. *(Chap 308.)*   A slightly increased mean corpuscular volume and an inappropriately low reticulocyte count are characteristic of a macrocytic, hypoproliferative anemia. Iron-deficiency anemia is accompanied by microcytic red blood cell indices, and autoimmune hemolytic anemia typically is associated with reticulocytosis, unless a coexisting process, such as folate deficiency, interferes with the bone marrow erythropoietic response. Aplastic anemia and acute leukemia are unlikely diagnoses if white blood cell count and platelet count are normal. A macrocytic, hypoproliferative anemia in the older man described in the question would most likely be due to a myelodysplastic syndrome. A bone marrow examination with iron stain would be required to define the precise subtype of this heterogeneous disorder, which is characterized by a stem cell defect leading to disordered hematopoietic maturation. Given the normal platelet count and white blood cell count, either refractory anemia or refractory anemia with ringed sideroblasts is the most likely subtype.

523. The answer is E. *(Chap 317.)*   It is now well recognized that many environmental and industrial exposures are associated with an increased risk of neoplasia. For example, tobacco smoking is associated with an increased likelihood of developing cancer of the oral cavity, lung, esophagus, kidney, bladder, and pancreas. In fact, due to the increased frequency of cigarette smoking among American women after World War II, beginning in 1988 female deaths from lung cancer exceeded the deaths from breast cancer. Occupational causes of cancer include arsenic-induced lung cancer, skin cancer, and liver cancer. Asbestos exposure is a well-recognized cause of mesothelioma. Benzene and perhaps other industrial solvents are associated with an increased risk of leukemia. Chromium compounds and benzidine are industrial carcinogens associated with lung cancer and bladder cancer, respectively. The use of mustard gas in the workplace is associated with an increased incidence of lung cancer. Finally, workers in the plastic industry exposed to vinyl chloride have been shown to develop angiosarcoma, a rare tumor of the liver.

524. The answer is C. *(Chap 317.)*   The essential pathophysiologic event in chronic myeloid leukemia (CML) is a chromosomal translocation between chromosomes 9 and 22 that juxtaposes sequences from the *c-abl* proto-oncogene on chromosome 9 with a fairly restricted region of another gene, *bcr,* on chromosome 22. Detection of a translocation between chromosomes 9 and 22 on karyotypic analysis of cells from blood or bone marrow establishes the diagnosis of CML and is found in approximately 95 percent of patients with this disease. The chromosomal translocation results in the transcription of a novel mRNA and the subsequent translocation of a fusion protein, *bcr-abl.* This fusion protein is believed to play a critical role in the growth advantage characteristic of CML stem cells. While it would not be possible to detect the Philadelphia chromosome in mature cells such as neutrophils, which do not divide and give rise to the required metaphases, it is theoretically possible to detect the fusion protein on all cells descending from malignant clones. However, the initial demonstration that CML was a clonal disease came from studies involving analysis of the glucose-6-phosphate dehydrogenase (G6PD) isoenzyme in females who are heterozygous for this X-chromosome-linked gene. As such, all somatic cells from patients who are G6PD heterozygotes express either an A or B isoform. Hematopoietic cells derived from a normal patient would express 50 percent A and 50 percent B. However, mature blood cells from patients with CML all display either A or B ontogeny. Gene amplification studies would not prove clonality, although that may correlate closely with clinical status. Finally, detection of kappa or lambda excess is very helpful in determination of clonality in B-cell malignancies.

525. The answer is D. *(Chap 311.)*   There is an increased incidence of lymphoma in diseases of inherited and acquired immunodeficiency as well as in certain autoimmune diseases. Thus, children with Chédiak-Higashi syndrome, a congenital disorder of neutrophil function with associated granulomatous infections, are at risk for subsequent lymphomas as well. Ataxia-telangiectasia and Wiskott-Aldrich syndromes also predispose to lymphoma. In addition to AIDS, in which the incidence of non-Hodgkin's lymphomas (especially primary lymphoma of the central nervous system) is high, patients with other acquired immunodeficiency states, including drug-induced immunosuppression, may also develop lymphoma. Sjögren's syndrome, rheumatoid arthritis, sprue, and systemic lupus are among those autoimmune diseases associated with an increased incidence of lymphoma, thereby suggesting a pathogenetic basis in immune dysregulation. Many patients receiving phenytoin will develop atypical lymphoid hyperplasia, but a few will go on to develop frank lymphoma even after the drug is stopped. Although a fatal course is possible, certain lymphoproliferative disorders associated with Epstein-Barr virus will regress if immunosuppression is discontinued.

526. The answer is D. *(Chap 319.)*   The appropriate systemic therapy for postmenopausal women with estrogen-receptor–positive breast cancer metastatic to bone is either tamoxifen, 10 mg twice daily, or diethylstilbestrol. Radiation therapy can relieve bone pain and may prevent fractures if used prophylactically to treat lesions of weight-bearing bones. For lytic lesions greater than 2.5 cm in diameter in weight-bearing bones, prophylactic internal fixation followed by radiation therapy is the treatment of choice, especially if the lesions involve the cortex.

527. The answer is C. *(Chap 317. Luzzatto, Semin Oncol 17:147–149, 1990.)* A unifying pathophysiologic explanation for the association between malignancy and thrombosis has not been developed; however, many factors may play a role in increasing the likelihood of abnormal clotting in cancer patients. Such factors include immobilization and bed rest, dysproteinemias producing hyperviscosity, abnormal platelet function in myeloproliferative disorders, tumor-associated low-grade DIC (disseminated intravascular coagulation), and cancer-mediated thrombocytosis. Unlike the case for patients with coagulopathies, there is no useful laboratory test that will identify the hypercoagulable state. Different types of malignancies may be associated with specific thrombotic syndromes. For example, migratory superficial thrombophlebitis (Trousseau's syndrome) in the absence of apparent predisposing factors is most frequently associated with gastrointestinal malignancies, particularly pancreatic carcinoma. Hepatic vein thrombosis (Budd-Chiari syndrome) and portal vein thrombosis are associated with myeloproliferative disorders such as paroxysmal nocturnal hemoglobinuria, essential thrombocythemia, and polycythemia vera.

528. The answer is D. *(Chap 318.)* Acquired or intrinsic drug resistance represents a major reason for the failure of chemotherapy in a wide variety of malignant tumors. As a tumor expands, the spontaneous mutation rate will inevitably produce cells with resistance to the various chemotherapeutic compounds. Secondly, even earlier in tumorigenesis, there may be a very high level of intrinsic resistance. Mechanisms of drug resistance are variable. Resistance to individual drugs can occur because of defective transport, such as loss of a folate transport protein that inhibits methotrexate uptake; decreased activating enzyme, such as decreased deoxycytidine kinase activity in patients with cytarabine resistance; increased drug inactivation, such as by the addition of reduced glutathione; or alteration in the target enzyme, such as a change in the enzyme thymidylate synthase that occurs in cells resistant to 5-FU (5-fluorouracil influence). Overexpression of a 170-kDa membrane glycoprotein (P-glycoprotein) is associated with resistance to a number of structurally unrelated (natural) chemotherapeutic agents, including anthracyclines, vinca alkyloids, epipodophyllotoxins, and paclitaxel. Additional mechanisms of multidrug resistance distinct from P-glycoprotein expression may include alteration of topoisomerase II expression or an enhanced reducing environment due to the increased availability of glutathione detoxifying pathways.

529. The answer is A. *(Chap 303. Bothwell, Semin Hematol 19:54, 1982.)* Serum iron and transferrin saturation, ferritin level, and desferrioxamine challenge are comparably sensitive, noninvasive tests of iron stores. They may all be normal in the early stages of iron overload, such as in precirrhotic affected family members of persons with idiopathic hemochromatosis. The most sensitive test for detecting early iron overload is a quantitative iron analysis, usually determined by atomic absorption spectroscopy, of a liver biopsy specimen.

530. The answer is E. *(Chap 304.)* Antiparietal-cell antibodies are detected in 90 percent of persons with pernicious anemia but also in persons with atrophic gastritis and 10 to 15 percent of an unselected patient population. Although folate in large doses can correct the megaloblastic anemia of pernicious anemia, it does not correct the neurologic abnormalities. Megaloblastic anemias are characterized by ineffective erythropoiesis and bone marrow erythroid hyperplasia. Hypergastrinemia accompanies the achlorhydria of pernicious anemia. Marrow morphology begins to improve within hours of parenteral B_{12} therapy; reticulocytosis peaks in 1 week. Life-threatening hypokalemia may occur early in the course of therapy.

531. The answer is B. *(Chap 318.)* Paclitaxel (taxol) is a newly discovered, highly effective chemotherapeutic agent in the plant alkaloid category. This drug is derived from the Pacific yew tree and functions by preventing microtubular disassembly. It displays particular promise in breast cancer, ovarian cancer, and head and neck carcinomas. However, paclitaxel infusion is often complicated by hypersensitivity reactions including hypotension, bronchospasm, and urticaria. Rather than an immunologic phenomenon, the basis for this reaction is felt to be the vehicle (Cremophor EL) in which the drug is dissolved. This problem may be ameliorated by prolonging the infusion for 24 h or more and using intensive premedicines including cimetidine, diphenhydramine, and steroids. Other acute toxicities associated with paclitaxel include AV block, bradyarrhythmias, and chest pain. Moreover, peripheral neuropathy may occur. Synthetic compounds are currently under development.

532. The answer is D. *(Chap 312. Heyman, Semin Oncol 17:198, 1990.)* Platelet transfusions are a mainstay of the therapy in the chronically thrombocytopenic patient. Automated platelet pheresis yields approximately 6 units of platelets (each unit is 6×10^{10} platelets) from an individual donor, and these may be stored at room temperature for approximately 5 days. Each unit should raise the platelet count by at least 5000 cells/μL. Therefore, this patient has responded appropriately to her transfusion, although she has had a significant febrile reaction. It is important to rule out bacterial contamination of the transfused platelets, but this is a very rare complication. More commonly, febrile reactions after receiving platelets are due to reaction to HLA antigens to which the patient has been sensitized. While such reactions might be circumvented by administering platelets from an HLA-compatible donor or sibling, given the appropriate rise in the platelet count after the transfusion, the easiest way to approach the current problem would be to administer leukocyte-reduced platelets. Currently available filters can reduce the leukocyte content (and thereby diminish the exposure to sensitizing alloantigens) by more than 99.9 percent. Another advantage of leukocyte-reduced products is reduction of the risk of CMV transmission. Though transfusion-associated graft-versus-host disease is not eliminated by leukocyte reduction, since there are still a few remaining allogeneic lymphocytes in such products, this dreaded complication can be eliminated by irradiating all blood products at a dose of 25 Gy.

533. The answer is C. *(Chap 322. Roth, Semin Oncol 19:117, 1992.)* Persons with disseminated teratocarcinoma treated with combination chemotherapy achieve complete remission in more than 70 percent of cases. Occasionally, residual masses remain after chemotherapy and on biopsy prove to be benign mature teratomas rather than residual malignant disease. In these cases, partial responders can be converted to complete responders—and even cured—by surgical removal of residual masses. If viable cancer is detected in the surgical specimen, then additional chemotherapy should be administered.

534. The answer is D. *(Chaps 317, 381.)* Epidural spinal cord compression is an important complication of metastatic cancer. Local or radicular pain is the most frequent and earliest clinical symptom; subsequently, weakness and bladder and bowel dysfunction can develop. The diagnosis, which should always be considered even if neurologic examination is normal, is confirmed by demonstrating a lesion on MRI or CT scan. Lumbar spinal taps should be avoided because herniation of the cord into a decompressed region can occur after withdrawal of fluid. Surgery usually is recommended for persons with rapidly progressive neurologic signs; radiation is useful in treating persons who have slowly progressive deficits due to radiosensitive tumors. Neither systemic chemotherapy nor corticosteroids should be employed in place of surgery or radiotherapy.

535. The answer is A. *(Chap 313.)* One of the most important complications of allogeneic bone marrow transplantation is acute graft-versus-host disease. This condition is believed to be due to a reaction by engrafted lymphoid cells, particularly T cells, against host tissues. Graft-versus-host disease is essentially not a complication of syngeneic (identical twin) or autologous transplants. Acute graft-versus-host disease typically involves the skin, gastrointestinal tract, and liver. Elevations of the alkaline phosphatase and jaundice are common. An elevated isolation of bilirubin and alkaline phosphatase and the onset of ascites would raise consideration of venoocclusive disease (VOD) of the liver. Such a problem would probably not be associated with a skin rash and diarrhea. Secondly, hepatic VOD is much more common when therapy with combined alkylating agents is used as the preparative regimen. Efforts to prevent acute graft-versus-host disease have centered upon the use of immunosuppressive agents including corticosteroids, methotrexate, and cyclosporine. Another approach is the use of T cell–depleted donor marrows. However, while T cell–depleted donor marrows will reduce the risk of severe graft-versus-host disease, preliminary data suggest that the rate of relapse may be lower in patients with graft-versus-host disease than in those without.

536. The answer is E. *(Chap 316. Harris, N Engl J Med 327:319–328, 390–398, 473–480, 1992.)* Given the increasing frequency of breast biopsy for patients with suspected breast cancer, the incidence of carcinoma in situ is increasing. There are two histologically distinct types of carcinoma in situ: ductal and lobular. Ductal carcinoma in situ may form palpable tumors and is frequently confined to one breast. This finding would be a marker for an increased risk of developing an invasive cancer. Although controversial, based on a recently published clinical trial, it appears that the optimal treatment for such patients is wide excision followed by radiation therapy. On the other hand, lobular carcinoma in situ does not form palpable tumors and tends to be a diffuse finding in both breasts. Without treatment the cumulative incidence of a breast cancer (in either breast) is about 25 percent with a latent period of 5 to 20 years. Most doctors now routinely offer patients with lobular carcinoma in situ one of two very different treatment options: careful observation or bilateral simple mastectomies with breast reconstruction. In the absence of more specific data as to the risk of eventual development of breast cancer in an individual patient, the final choice between these two options depends on the degree of comfort the patient has with careful follow-up.

537. The answer is E. *(Chap 305. Sears, Med Clin North Am 76:567, 1992.)* A mild-to-moderate degree of anemia often accompanies chronic infectious, inflammatory, or neoplastic diseases. Typically, the anemia of chronic disease is normochromic and normocytic to microcytic. Bone marrow examination reveals normal erythroid maturation. Neither significant disturbance of hemoglobin synthesis nor hemolysis occurs in this type of anemia. Affected persons usually have a low serum iron concentration and a low total transferrin level (resulting in essentially normal or only slightly decreased fractional transferrin saturation). Even though storage iron is abundant, there is a decreased amount of iron in erythroblasts, reflecting a defect in the transfer of reticuloendothelial iron to developing red blood cells.

538. The answer is D. *(Chap 307. Beutler, N Engl J Med 324:169, 1991.)* The gene for glucose-6-phosphate dehydrogenase (G6PD) is located on the X chromosome; thus, G6PD deficiency is a sex-linked trait. Hemolytic anemia occurs much more commonly in males than in heterozygote female carriers, who usually are asymptomatic. Of the more than 100 variants of G6PD, the most commonly encountered variant of clinical significance in the United States is the A− type, which is found in about 15 percent of black males. It generally causes less severe hemolysis than the

Mediterranean variant. Hemolysis usually is precipitated by an environmental oxidant stress, most commonly viral or bacterial infection. Certain drugs, such as antimalarial agents, sulfonamides, phenacetin, and vitamin K, also can trigger hemolysis. These oxidant stresses cause precipitation of hemoglobin because affected persons are unable to maintain adequate intracellular levels of reduced glutathione. Precipitated hemoglobin forms Heinz bodies that are visualized only with supravital stains; these inclusions cause premature destruction of the red cells. The diagnosis should be considered in any person experiencing a hemolytic episode. However, since decreased G6PD levels are found mainly in older cells, a false negative test may be obtained during a hemolytic crisis, and the test should be repeated upon recovery.

539. The answer is B. *(Chap 323. Andriole, J Clin Oncol 10:1205–1207, 1992.)* Prostate specific antigen (PSA) determinations are assuming an increasingly important role in the diagnosis, screening, and staging of men with prostate cancer. Patients with urinary symptoms found to have an elevated level of serum prostate specific antigen have a 60 percent likelihood of having prostate cancer. About 16 percent of patients with prostate cancer have an elevated level of serum PSA as their sole diagnostic abnormality. However, additional studies need to be done to precisely delineate the role of prostate specific antigen evaluation in screening. Fewer than 10 percent of ambulatory volunteers older than 50 years have elevated serum PSA values. A serum PSA between 4 and 10 ng/mL indicates that cancer is 25 percent likely, whereas values greater than 10 ng/mL increase the likelihood of cancer to about 60 percent. About 20 percent of those with an elevated PSA (alone) compared with 10 percent of those with a suspicious digital rectal examination (alone) will have prostate cancer. The vast majority of cancers that are detected by screening for prostate specific antigen are localized clinically and therefore have an excellent chance of being cured with either radiation or surgery. Moreover, few tumors detected by PSA screening are incidental since most have a high volume or a worrisome Gleason score (indicating a poor prognosis based on histologic grade). On the other hand, additional studies demonstrating a screening-induced decrease in cancer-related mortality are necessary in order to convince all that screening for prostate cancer with PSA determinations is beneficial. A clear use for serum PSA determination is in postoperative evaluation. If the postoperative serum PSA value is detectable, the presence of residual tumor is likely. A rising PSA value after definitive radiation therapy indicates a high likelihood of eventual metastatic spread. The use of systemic chemotherapy for metastatic prostate cancer should be reserved for those patients with certain evidence of metastatic disease.

540. The answer is E. *(Chap 325. Koh, N Engl J Med 325:171–182, 1991.)* One of the most important prognostic factors for the risk of ultimate dissemination of localized melanoma is the thickness of the original lesion. Patients with a melanoma of greater than 4 mm in depth have less than a 50 percent 5-year survival. Other prognostic factors for low-stage (no clinically involved lymph nodes or metastases) melanoma include the presence of an ulcerative tumor, the mitotic rate, and the presence of microscopic tumor satellites. Recent studies suggest that relatively narrow margins (between 1 and 3 cm) are adequate to reduce the risk of local recurrence. The efficacy of elective regional lymph node dissection in those with clinically negative nodes remains controversial; the procedure should not be routinely done, particularly in the groin where the procedure is associated with a significant morbidity. Moreover, those with thick lesions have such a high risk of metastases that benefit from an elective node dissection is unlikely. Ideally, for patients free of disease after local resection but at high risk of subsequent metastases, an adjuvant therapy could be employed to erradicate micrometastases, thereby improving survival. Unfortunately, all tested strategies including systemic chemotherapy, regional limb perfusion chemotherapy, nonspecific immunotherapy, and radiation therapy have failed to show a benefit. Preliminary data from recent trials suggest that interferon-α may reduce the incidence of metastases in high-risk lesions, but additional follow-up is required.

541. The answer is A. *(Chap 319. Chu, J Natl Cancer Inst 80:1125, 1988.)* The Health Insurance Plan of New York evaluated mammography as a screening tool in 62,000 persons. Their screening procedure included physical examination as well. Though an earlier report had demonstrated a benefit for screening only in those over age 50, a more recent analysis with an 18-year follow-up describes a statistically significant 24 percent reduction in mortality for all age groups. While the high frequency of physical examinations in the HIP study may have been the most important factor in reducing mortality, a Swedish trial more clearly demonstrated the benefits of screening mammograms, at least in patients over age 50.

542. The answer is B. *(Chap 319. Early Breast Cancer Trialists' Collaborative Group, Lancet 339:71, 1992.)* For premenopausal women who have stage II carcinoma of the breast (axillary metastases only), the drug regimen combining cyclophosphamide, methotrexate, and 5-fluorouracil (CMF), when employed as an adjuvant therapy, leads to a statistically significant reduction in the recurrence rate. It is the treatment of choice following mastectomy in this group of women. Mortality after 5 years is decreased approximately 30 percent in women treated with CMF. Median survival is prolonged by approximately 3 years with CMF treatment.

543. The answer is E. *(Chap 328. Posner, Neurol Clin 9:919, 1991.)* A relatively common subtype of paraneoplastic neurologic syndromes is that which affects peripheral nerves. Subacute sensory neuronopathy, characterized by paresthesias and pain in the distal limbs with truncal sensory ataxia, is associated with axonal degeneration with relative myelin sparing. The most common type of paraneoplastic neuropathy is a mixed sensory and motor axonopathy. Symptoms may include muscle wasting, weakness, distal paresthesia, and occasionally pain. Pathologically, this disease is characterized by noninflammatory degeneration of axons with mild myelin loss and may be associated with small cell carcinoma of the lung, breast carcinoma, gastric carcinoma, Hodgkin's disease, lymphoma, and multiple myeloma. Another type of neuropathy associated with Waldenström's microglobulinemia or in certain patients with benign monoclonal gammopathy is the elaboration of IgM that reacts with a myelin-associated glycoprotein in peripheral nerves. Such an antibody tends to disrupt sensory rather than motor neurons. Another demyelinating neuropathy associated with IgG myeloma is predominantly motor, indolent, and not associated with an anti-myelin-associated glycoprotein antibody, although demyelinization is still the primary pathology. Patients with monoclonal gammopathies who develop neuropathy also include those with the POEMS syndrome, characterized by polyneuropathy, organomegaly, endocrinopathy, M-protein secretion, and skin changes. Any patient with a demyelinative myopathy secondary to monoclonal immunoglobulin protein may respond to immunosuppressive therapy.

544. The answer is E. *(Chap 326. Horning, J Clin Oncol 17:1281, 1989.)* In general, women who present with an isolated axillary mass that proves to be adenocarcinoma or poorly differentiated carcinoma should receive treatment appropriate for stage II breast cancer. They should receive either a modified radical mastectomy or breast irradiation for purposes of decreasing local recurrence followed by adjuvant systemic therapy with chemotherapy or tamoxifen or both, depending on menopausal status and the hormone receptor status of the tumor. However, patients whose routine pathology reveals either poorly differentiated adenocarcinoma or poorly differentiated malignancy deserve a careful pathologic review to determine if there are any findings compatible with a specific organ of origin. In this case, the absence of cytokeratin filaments argues against the diagnosis of breast carcinoma; on the other hand, the leukocyte common antigen positivity is highly consistent with a lymphoid neoplasm. The patient would be expected to respond to therapy as if she had a more straightforward presentation of lymphoma. To determine the optimal therapy for such a patient, the disease should be staged as in any non-Hodgkin's lymphoma. Therefore, CT of the chest and abdomen should be performed to determine whether there are additional sites of disease.

545. The answer is C. *(Chap 306.)*　　Several hemoglobin variants have an increased affinity for oxygen. This abnormality causes defective oxygen unloading to tissues, leading to erythropoietin-mediated erythrocytosis. Because reduced tissue oxygen delivery usually is compensated for fully by the development of erythrocytosis, levels of red-cell 2,3-diphosphoglycerate (2,3-DPG) are normal. Routine hemoglobin electrophoresis is normal in about one-third of these variants, and red blood cell morphology is not altered. Affected persons are not at a disadvantage when exposed to hypoxic conditions.

546. The answer is B. *(Chaps 56, 302, 308.)*　　Pure red blood cell aplasia is characterized by a normochromic, normocytic anemia and little production of reticulocytes. Erythroblasts are selectively absent from the bone marrow of affected persons. The production of white blood cells and platelets is preserved. In contrast to aplastic anemia, the bone marrow in persons with pure red blood cell aplasia is normocellular or even hypercellular. Iron kinetic studies reveal prolonged clearance of plasma iron and reduced turnover of iron. Levels of erythropoietin usually are markedly elevated.

547. The answer is B. *(Chap 326. Hainsworth, N Engl J Med 329:257–263, 1993.)*　　Approximately 10 percent of all cancer patients present in such a manner that assignment of the organ of origin of the tumor is unclear. Most patients who present in this fashion will have neoplasms that are poorly responsive to systemic therapy. However, it is important to recognize certain subgroups in whom a specific approach to treatment might be beneficial or even associated with long-term disease-free survival. One such group has what has been termed the *unrecognized extragonadal germ cell cancer syndrome.* This includes those patients displaying one or more of the following features: age less than 50; tumor involving midline structures, lung, or parenchymal lymph nodes; an elevated serum alpha fetoprotein or βhCG level; or evidence of rapid tumor growth. If patients with these features do not have any histologic or immunohistochemical features suggesting a primary site, then strong consideration should be given to treatment with a cisplatin-based chemotherapy regimen (as would be used for germ cell cancer). Approximately 20 percent of patients presenting in this fashion may be cured with the use of cisplatin, bleomycin, and VP-16 chemotherapy.

548. The answer is D. *(Chap 311.)*　　Neoplasms may be classified as to their cell of origin by the use of antisera and monoclonal antibodies against certain cell surface phenotypic markers and, more recently, by the use of DNA probes for immunoglobulin genes and genes for the beta chain of the T-cell receptor. The malignant cell in chronic lymphocytic leukemia (CLL) is a morphologically normal but functionally abnormal B lymphocyte. Follicular lymphomas arise from the proliferative part of the B-cell system (the lymphoid follicle), while the diffuse, small lymphocytic lymphomas (identical to CLL) are derived from the secretory compartment of the medullary cords. The Burkitt's lymphoma cell is a malignant cell of B-lymphocyte lineage; in many cases it bears a characteristic chromosomal translocation—t(8;14). In contrast to these B-cell neoplasms, mycosis fungoides is a peripheral T-cell lymphoma in which helper-cell function and phenotype have been identified.

549. The answer is C. *(Chap 319. Fisher, N Engl J Med 320:822, 1989.)*   Other than in the performance of early local therapy based on mammographic detection, no surgical or radiotherapeutic procedure has been shown to affect survival. In other words, survival is determined by the extent and response of systemic disease. The decision between lumpectomy plus radiation therapy and modified radical mastectomy therefore rests on which modality offers the best chance for local control. Although no survival benefit can be shown, radiation therapy should be administered along with lumpectomy because at least one study has documented a higher recurrent rate in those treated with lumpectomy alone (28 percent) compared with lumpectomy plus radiotherapy (5 percent). In most cases, local control can be achieved equally well with either approach. However, certain subgroups—especially those with extensive intraductal carcinoma or with positive lumpectomy resection margins—will experience a higher local recurrence rate if breast conservation is employed. Axillary lymph node dissection is appropriate in all patients for diagnostic (in order to determine the appropriate systemic therapy), not therapeutic, purposes.

550. The answer is D. *(Chaps 57, 315.)*   A marked prolongation of the prothrombin time with a normal partial thromboplastin time localizes the hemostatic defect to the extrinsic limb of the coagulation cascade. Congenital factor VII deficiency is a rare, autosomal recessive disorder. Factor VIII deficiency and the presence of specific inhibitors directed toward a coagulation factor (most commonly factor VIII) would be associated with a prolongation of the partial thromboplastin time. Nonspecific inhibitors (lupus anticoagulants) most commonly are associated with prolongation of the partial thromboplastin time and occasionally with prolongation of the prothrombin time (particularly when hypoprothrombinemia is present). Patients with alpha$_2$-antiplasmin deficiency have a bleeding disorder associated with accelerated clot lysis. Both the prothrombin time and the partial thromboplastin time are normal in these persons.

551. The answer is B. *(Chaps 314, 315.)*   The hemolytic-uremic syndrome occurs predominantly in children and is related to thrombotic thrombocytopenic purpura. It is characterized by microangiopathic hemolytic anemia and thrombocytopenia. Polycythemia vera, as well as the other myeloproliferative disorders, often is associated with thrombocytosis. Thrombocytosis also is a long-term sequela of splenectomy or splenic infarction (e.g., in sickle cell disease) and chronic inflammatory states (e.g., inflammatory bowel disease). For reasons that are unclear, thrombocytosis frequently is associated with iron deficiency.

552. The answer is B. *(Chap 321. Swenerton, J Clin Oncol 10:718, 1992.)*   The overall 5-year survival of those with disease that extends beyond the ovaries is 40 percent; however, some patients who are able to undergo complete or nearly complete initial cytoreductive surgery may be cured with combination chemotherapy. Presumably such therapy eradicates residual subclinical disease, which is invariably present despite the apparently complete resection. Although the optimal regimen has not been established, effective drugs include taxol, cisplatin, cyclophosphamide, hexamethylmelamine, and doxorubicin. Since some patients may have recurrent disease without an elevation of CA125, which is a useful antigen in monitoring response to therapy in those who have elevated levels, the delay of therapy pending a rise in this level would not be prudent. Clear survival benefits have yet to be shown for the fairly toxic regimen of whole abdominal radiation therapy. Intraperitoneal chemotherapy holds promise in the eradication of minimal disease, but its role needs to be defined by further clinical trials.

553. The answer is D. *(Chaps 327,328.)* Small cell neoplasms of the lung are associated with a wide variety of paraneoplastic syndromes, some of which are humorally mediated, while others are of unknown pathophysiology. The Lambert-Eaton myasthenic syndrome, which is associated with proximal muscle weakness and characteristic electromyographic findings, is linked almost exclusively with small cell tumors. Subacute cortical cerebellar degeneration, as exemplified by the findings outlined in scenario B, is associated with small cell tumors and some cases of ovarian cancer, carcinoma of the breast, and Hodgkin's disease. Cushing's syndrome due to hypersecretion of glucocorticoids and the syndrome of inappropriate secretion of antidiuretic hormone are also associated with small cell lung tumors, in addition to other cancers. Hypercalcemia is infrequently associated with small cell neoplasms, but it is not an infrequent manifestation of squamous and large cell lung tumors, in which cases it may be a result of secretion of substances with parathyroid hormone-like activity or of another factor associated with the humoral hypercalcemia of malignancy.

554. The answer is C. *(Chap 314.)* The onset of severe thrombocytopenia after an antecedent viral illness is common in children with a diagnosis of idiopathic thrombocytopenic purpura (ITP). Unlike childhood ITP, adult ITP tends to be a chronic disease in which spontaneous remissions are rare, and a majority of patients will have a fall in their platelet count after the withdrawal of corticosteroids, necessitating elective splenectomy. The presence of antibodies directed against target antigens on the glycoprotein IIb-IIIa or Ib-IX complex has been noted in some adults with chronic ITP but not in children. Splenomegaly is not a feature of ITP; it is a common finding in patients with secondary thrombocytopenia.

555. The answer is C. *(Chap 316. Feinstein, Blood 80:859, 1992.)* The presence of nonspecific anticoagulants (lupus type) may predispose patients to thrombosis and is also associated with habitual abortions in some women. Patients with congenital dysfibrinogenemias may have variable results on screening coagulation tests. They often have slight prolongations in the prothrombin times or partial thromboplastin times, prolonged thrombin times, and a disparity between functional and immunologic assays of fibrinogen. Despite these abnormalities, patients may have either no symptoms or moderate bleeding, and a few dysfibrinogenemias have been associated with hypercoagulability. Congenital deficiencies of antithrombin III and protein C are familial thrombotic disorders and are not associated with abnormalities of the various clotting times. Factor XI deficiency is an autosomal recessive disorder often associated with bleeding following trauma or during the perioperative period.

556. The answer is C. *(Chap 309.)* Persons with polycythemia vera and a hematocrit greater than 45 percent usually have diminished cerebral blood flow and are particularly at risk for developing thrombotic complications. Functional platelet abnormalities may cause both thrombotic and bleeding problems (the gastrointestinal tract is a common site of bleeding), and affected persons frequently are iron-deficient even at the time of presentation. Erythropoietin production is suppressed in polycythemia vera, a disease characterized by loss of normal control of erythroid stem-cell proliferation. The bone marrow is hypercellular, with hyperplasia of all marrow elements. Therapy is aimed at reducing the hematocrit below 45 percent.

557. **The answer is A.** *(Chap 314.)* Electrophoretic analysis has allowed the delineation of three major types of defects in von Willebrand's disease (vWD). The most common abnormality (type I disease) is characterized by a moderate decrease in the plasma level of von Willebrand factor (vWF antigen) resulting from defective release of the protein from endothelial cells. There are usually concordant reductions in antihemophilic factor or factor VIII coagulant activity as well as ristocetin cofactor activity.

The various forms of type II disease are characterized by normal or near normal levels of dysfunctional protein. In both types IIa and IIb, there is a loss of high-molecular-weight multimers on SDS-agarose electrophoresis. In type IIa patients, the pattern is caused by either an inability to assemble the larger multimers or by premature catabolism in the circulation. In contrast, patients with type IIb have inappropriate binding of the abnormal, larger vWF forms to platelets, which results in the formation of intravascular platelet aggregates. These are rapidly cleared from the circulation, which causes mild, cyclic thrombocytopenia.

A severe recessive form of vWD (type III disease) results from reduced synthesis of vWF by endothelial cells. A hyperactive platelet receptor (glycoprotein Ib) with increased affinity for larger vWF multimers is the defect in so-called platelet-type vWD, or pseudo-vWD. The gene encoding vWF has been cloned and localized to chromosome 12.

558. **The answer is C.** *(Chaps 57, 315.)* Factor XIII deficiency may be inherited or acquired and frequently causes severe bleeding problems. In this disorder, the bleeding time, prothrombin time, and partial thromboplastin time (PTT) are all normal. The screening test for factor XIII deficiency is a clot solubility in urea assay. Persons with deficiencies of factor XII (Hageman factor) or pre-kallikrein often have dramatic prolongations of the PTT, but do not have bleeding problems even with surgery or trauma. The presence of a normal bleeding time excludes thrombasthenia, an inherited disorder in which there is defective-platelet aggregation in response to agonists that require fibrinogen binding, such as adenosine diphosphate, thrombin, or epinephrine. Protein S is a vitamin K–dependent plasma protein and a cofactor for the expression of the anticoagulant activity of activated protein C. Familial protein S deficiency is associated with a thrombotic diathesis.

559. **The answer is E.** *(Chap 315.)* This patient has chronic disseminated intravascular coagulation in association with an abdominal aortic aneurysm. The prothrombin time and partial thromboplastin time are prolonged and the fibrinogen level is decreased on the basis of consumption. Appropriate therapy would include administration of fresh frozen plasma, while cryoprecipitate, a source of only factor VIII and fibrinogen, would be inadequate. Plasma exchange transfusions are the treatment of choice for thrombotic thrombocytopenic purpura. Aminocaproic acid (Amicar) is contraindicated in this setting, because it inhibits fibrinolysis and can therefore potentially induce thrombosis. The degree of thrombocytopenia is not of sufficient severity to require platelet transfusions.

560. **The answer is C.** *(Chap 323. Crawford, N Engl J Med 321:419, 1989.)* Given the poorly differentiated histology at presentation with the associated high risk of recurrence and the characteristic indicators of metastatic prostate cancer, biopsy is unnecessary. Since the patient has symptomatic disease, he should be started on androgen deprivation therapy, which is likely to cause a decrease in his pain. An equivalent response rate has been demonstrated with bilateral orchiectomy, diethylstilbestrol, and luteinizing hormone releasing hormone (LHRH) analogues such as leuprolide. Given his desire not to have an orchiectomy and his vascular disease, LHRH analogues would be the best approach. A recent study has documented a benefit to providing "total androgen blockade" with flutamide plus leuprolide compared with leuprolide alone. Prostatic carcinoma is poorly responsive to chemotherapy.

561. The answer is A-Y, B-N, C-Y, D-N, E-Y. *(Chaps 56, 304.)* Macrocytosis of red blood cells may be caused by defective DNA synthesis (i.e., megaloblastic anemias), among other factors. Reticulocytosis due to either blood loss or hemolysis may be associated with macrocytic indices because reticulocytes are about 20 percent larger than mature red blood cells. Increased surface area of red cell membranes due to increased membrane cholesterol incorporation occurs in liver disease and obstructive jaundice. In hypothyroidism, nonmegaloblastic macrocytic anemia develops; the cause is unclear. Vitamin B_{12} and folate deficiency states, following total gastrectomy or accompanying malabsorption syndromes, cause megaloblastic anemia.

562. The answer is A-N, B-N, C-Y, D-Y, E-Y. *(Chaps 302, 303.)* Iron deficiency frequently is confused with thalassemia trait, both α and β, in that all three of these conditions are characterized by a microcytic anemia. Iron stores, as reflected by transferrin saturation, serum ferritin level, and bone marrow iron staining, are depleted in iron deficiency but normal in both types of thalassemia trait. Hemoglobin electrophoresis reveals an increased hemoglobin A_2 level in β-thalassemia trait but subnormal levels in iron deficiency and α-thalassemia trait. (In the presence of concomitant iron deficiency, hemoglobin A_2 levels may be normal in persons with β thalassemia, but levels rise once iron stores are replenished.)

563. The answer is A-N, B-Y, C-Y, D-Y, E-N. *(Chap 301. Slamon, Science 244:707, 1989.)* Growth factors are believed to play a role in the pathogenesis of many diseases, both neoplastic and non-neoplastic. Platelet-derived growth factor is a 32-kDa heterodimer elaborated by a number of cells, including platelets, endothelial cells, smooth muscle-like cells, and activated macrophages. This molecule stimulates fibroblast proliferation and may aid in wound healing, but it may also be involved in atherosclerosis and in the pathogenesis of certain malignancies. Epidermal growth factor stimulates the proliferation of epithelial cells and fibroblasts. The epidermal growth factor receptor bears significant homology to the v-*erb*B viral transforming gene and to the HER-2/*neu* proto-oncogene, which is amplified in certain aggressive breast and ovarian tumors. Hematopoietic growth factors include CSF-1 (macrophage colony–stimulating factor), GM-CSF (granulocyte-macrophage colony–stimulating factor), G-CSF (granulocyte colony–stimulating factor), IL-3 (multipotent colony–stimulating factor), and erythropoietin (red blood cell–stimulating factor). Except for erythropoietin, which is made in the kidney in response to hypoxia and stimulates erythroid activity in the fashion of a classic hormone, the hematopoietic growth factors are believed to act mainly on adjacent cells (paracrine stimulation). GM-CSF and G-CSF may be helpful in augmenting recovery from chemotherapy-induced myelosuppression and other neutropenic states, but must be used with care in those with leukemia since it has been demonstrated that certain myeloid leukemias can also proliferate in response to these factors. The c-*fms* tyrosine kinase proto-oncogene codes for the transmembrane CSF-1 receptor.

564. The answer is A-Y, B-Y, C-Y, D-Y, E-Y. *(Chap 318.)* Two types of cardiotoxicity are associated with doxorubicin (Adriamycin) therapy. Acute cardiotoxicity produces electrocardiographic abnormalities, such as arrhythmias, but rarely is serious. Chronic cardiotoxicity, which rarely develops with total doxorubicin doses less than 500 mg/m$_2$, leads to congestive heart failure; it occurs with increased frequency in persons who also have received cardiac irradiation, cyclophosphamide, or anthracycline compounds other than doxorubicin. Up to half of all cases of cardiotoxicity occur 6 months or more after completion of therapy. Efforts to limit cardiotoxicity and thereby enable the administration of a higher total dose of anthracycline include weekly or continuous intravenous schedules, anthracycline analogues, and cardioprotective agents that limit free-radical–induced myocardial damage.

565. The answer is A-N, B-Y, C-Y, D-N, E-Y. *(Chap 306.)*   Hematuria and hyposthenuria both are increased in incidence in sickle cell trait; the mechanism of both abnormalities probably is related to the relatively hypertonic, acidic, and hypoxic conditions of the renal medulla, which predispose to local sickling. Splenic infarction may develop at altitudes above approximately 3000 meters (10,000 feet) during flights in unpressurized airplanes. A prospective study of matched pairs of individuals has shown no deficits in standard measurements of growth and development in children with sickle cell trait when compared with other children. Mortality during pregnancy is not affected appreciably by sickle cell trait.

566. The answer is A-Y, B-Y, C-Y, D-N, E-Y. *(Chaps 57, 314.)*   The formation of a platelet plug at the site of vascular injury (i.e., primary hemostasis) requires adhesion of platelets, release of granules, and aggregation of platelets. The first of these three processes depends on the binding of platelets to deepithelialized vessel walls through an interaction between basement membrane collagen and the collagen receptor, composed of platelet glycoproteins Ia and IIa. This link is stabilized by the binding of von Willebrand factor, a multimeric adhesive glycoprotein, to platelet glycoprotein Ib-IX. The adherent platelets then release a host of mediators that serve to promote secretion of granules of platelets, aggregation of platelets, and activation of the coagulation cascade. Dense granules of platelets release adenosine diphosphate, which allows fibrinogen to serve as a bridge between platelets via platelet glycoprotein IIb-IIIa so that aggregation may occur.

567. The answer is A-Y, B-N, C-N, D-Y, E-Y. *(Chaps 62, 63. Bishop, Science 235:305, 1987.)*   Proto-oncogenes, cellular homologues to viral genes capable of inducing malignant transformation, generally play a role in normal cell growth. Mutations or changed position on the genome, however, can lead to altered expression or function and concomitant malignant transformation. The translocation of chromosomes 8 and 14 in Burkitt's lymphoma brings the c-*myc* locus on chromosome 8 and the immunoglobulin heavy chain gene locus on chromosome 14 into close proximity, thereby dysregulating c-*myc* expression. The abnormal regulation of the c-*myc* nuclear-associated proto-oncogene involved in DNA synthesis may play a role in the pathogenesis of this tumor. Virtually every patient with chronic myelogenous leukemia has a translocation between chromosomes 9 and 22 (producing the Philadelphia chromosome) that brings a portion of the c-*abl* tyrosine kinase proto-oncogene next to a region called *bcr,* creating a fusion protein with similar properties to those of the v-*abl* oncogene. Low-grade follicular lymphomas frequently display a 14–18 translocation that brings an immunoglobulin gene locus adjacent to a region of unknown function, *bcl*-2, on chromosome 18. Activating point mutations in members of the *ras* gene family have been found in myeloid leukemias and in other tumors. Loss of heterozygosity (i.e., no functional copies of the normal gene remain) for the so-called antioncogene (recessive oncogene) *Rb*-1 on chromosome 13 is associated with familial retinoblastoma. Recently, recessive oncogenes, likely to play an important role in human neoplasia, have been described in association with other tumors, including colonic carcinoma, Wilms' tumor, and renal cell carcinoma.

568. The answer is A-N, B-N, C-Y, D-N, E-N. *(Chap 311. Armitage, N Engl J Med 328:1023, 1993.)*   Stage (extent of disease) and tumor grade (histologic appearance) are the most important factors for determining treatment of the non-Hodgkin's lymphomas. Since 80 to 90 percent of patients with low-grade lymphomas—small lymphocytic (diffuse, well-differentiated lymphocytic) or follicular, small cleaved cell (nodular, poorly differentiated lymphocytic)—present with disseminated disease, radiation therapy essentially can never be considered curative. On the other hand, such diseases behave in an indolent fashion and can be treated effectively in a palliative manner with single-agent alkylator therapy; the use of more aggressive combination regimens produces a higher complete response rate, but has never been conclusively shown to affect the natural history of the disease. Most patients with diffuse large cell lymphoma, the most common intermediate-grade histology, achieve complete remission and many can be cured with combination chemotherapy regimens, including cyclophosphamide, doxorubicin, vincristine, and corticosteroids (and possibly also etoposide or methotrexate, among others). Prolonged (greater than 1 year) maintenance therapy is of no value. A lymphoma presenting in a patient with AIDS has a much lower chance (less than 25 percent complete response rate) of responding to combination chemotherapy than does a lymphoma of similar histologic appearance in an immunocompetent patient.

569. **The answer is A-N, B-N, C-Y, D-Y, E-Y.** *(Chap 312.)*   The clinical scenario is consistent with a delayed transfusion reaction. Immediate transfusion reactions, which are most commonly due to ABO incompatibility and result from clerical error, are associated with intravascular hemolysis (anti-A and anti-B antibodies fix complement) manifested by lumbar pain, hemoglobinemia, and shock. Fever, malaise, and a drop in hematocrit with findings compatible with extravascular hemolysis (microspherocytes, indirect hyperbilirubinemia) 1 week after red cell transfusion are typical of a delayed transfusion reaction, which is usually mediated by antibodies to Rh (or if the recipient is Rh-negative, by anti-Duffy, anti-Kidd, or anti-Kell antibodies). A previous transfusion may have been the precursor of the clinically relevant anamnestic response. These antibodies likely coat the donor red cells, thereby producing a positive direct Coombs test. Less commonly the donor's plasma could contain antibodies that would react with the recipient's cells. Sensitization to the alloantigens on donor leukocytes transfused along with the red cells could account for fever, but not hemolysis.

570. **The answer is A-Y, B-N, C-Y, D-Y, E-N.** *(Chap 315.)*   Hemophilia A and B are clinically indistinguishable, X-linked disorders that cause bleeding into soft tissues, muscles, and weight-bearing joints. In both disorders, all tests of coagulation are normal except for an elevation of the partial thromboplastin time. Specific-factor assays are required to define a specific disorder. Factor VIII is a 265-kilodalton (kDa) protein that regulates the activation of factor X by intrinsic pathway proteases. Factor IX, which unlike factor VIII requires vitamin K–dependent, posttranslational modification, is a 55-kDa proenzyme converted to activated factor IXa by factor XIa. Factor IXa activates factor X with the participation of factor VIII. The distinction between these two entities is important because the therapy is different. The therapy of choice in hemophilia A (without a serum inhibitor) is factor VIII concentrate or cryoprecipitate. Recently developed monoclonally purified or recombinantly derived formulations of factor VIII should be used to minimize the risk of AIDS, other viral infections, and exposure to irrelevant proteins. Either fresh frozen plasma or prothrombin complex proteins should be used to treat hemophilia B. The latter product, which carries the special risk of unbridled activation of the coagulation system and thrombotic complications, may not be needed in the future because of the projected availability of a recombinant factor IX preparation.

571. **The answer is A-N, B-Y, C-Y, D-N, E-Y.** *(Chap 321.)*   Though the incidence of ovarian carcinoma is low, the propensity to present at an advanced stage (only 25 percent of patients have disease limited to one or both ovaries) helps to explain why this disease is the most common cause of death among all gynecologic malignancies. Only about 15 percent of ovarian cancers arise from nonepithelial elements. Epithelial tumors are most common in peri- or postmenopausal women, especially nulliparous women or those with few children. Prior breast cancer increases the risk of developing ovarian cancer by two- to fourfold. An advanced stage and a larger size of residual tumor after initial surgery carry an adverse prognosis, as do poorly differentiated ovarian carcinomas, which have a 5-year survival of well under 20 percent.

572. The answer is A-N, B-Y, C-N, D-Y, E-N. *(Chap 311. Urba, N Engl J Med 326:678, 1992.)* Staging laparotomy for persons who have Hodgkin's disease carries a mortality of 1.5 percent and a complication rate of 12 percent. It should not be considered a routine procedure but should be performed if the result would change the treatment plan, not just the stage of the disease. Staging laparotomy should include careful needle and wedge biopsies of the liver lobes and edge, biopsy of retroperitoneal lymph nodes identified by preoperative lymphangiography, and biopsies of any suspicious area. The spleen should be removed for complete pathologic examination; however, splenectomy does not improve tolerance to chemotherapy. Based on clinical assessment of spleen size alone, the false positive and false negative rates for splenic involvement with Hodgkin's disease are 25 and 35 percent, respectively. Lymphangiograms done before laparotomy can be used to guide the surgeon to biopsy potentially involved nodes.

573. The answer is A-N, B-Y, C-N, D-N, E-Y. *(Chaps 57, 314.)* The interaction of von Willebrand's factor (vWF) with the platelet is most readily studied in vitro by measuring the effect of the antibiotic ristocetin on platelet aggregation. Patients whose platelets are not aggregated by ristocetin either lack vWF activity (most persons with von Willebrand's disease except those with the type IIb variant) or the platelet receptor for vWF (glycoprotein Ib). The latter situation is found in the Bernard-Soulier syndrome, a rare clinical condition also characterized by reduced levels of several other platelet membrane proteins, mild thrombocytopenia, and large, lymphocytoid platelets. Platelets from patients with Glanzmann's thrombasthenia are deficient in the glycoprotein IIb-IIIa complex. This receptor serves as the binding site for fibrinogen in platelet-platelet interactions. Hence, thrombasthenic platelets adhere normally and will agglutinate with ristocetin but will not aggregate with any of the agonists that require fibrinogen binding, such as adenosine diphosphate (ADP), thrombin, or epinephrine. Aspirin specifically acetylates the platelet cyclooxygenase enzyme and decreases the production of thromboxane A_2. This results in a defect in secondary platelet aggregation in response to agonists such as ADP and epinephrine. A similar situation is found in persons with storage pool disease whose platelet granules lack reasonable stores of ADP and serotonin.

574. The answer is A-N, B-N, C-Y, D-Y, E-Y. *(Chap 309.)* The myeloproliferative disorders (polycythemia vera, essential thrombocythemia, chronic myelogenous leukemia, myeloid metaplasia, and myelofibrosis) are a group of related diseases of the bone marrow stem cell. All cell lines—erythroid, myeloid, and megakaryocytic—are affected. Several functional platelet defects have been identified in these disorders and result paradoxically in both bleeding and thromboembolic complications, which are the major cause of morbidity and mortality. All myeloproliferative disorders may develop into acute leukemia, especially if alkylating agents are used in treatment. Although abnormal white blood cell function also may be associated with these disorders, opportunistic infections generally are not encountered.

575. The answer is A-Y, B-Y, C-Y, D-N, E-Y. *(Chap 325.)* Primary malignant melanoma of the skin is the leading cause of death among all diseases arising in the skin. A number of factors have been identified that correlate with increased or decreased likelihood of dissemination. The most common site for melanoma in males is the torso, and lesions occurring on the torso offer a worse prognosis than do those occurring on a lower extremity. Both dermatologic level of invasion and thickness of the primary lesion are predictive of dissemination and, hence, of survival. For example, melanomas less than 0.76 mm thick are almost always surgically cured; those that penetrate ≥ 3.65 mm have a 60 percent rate of distant metastases. While geographic area of residence is an important determinant of risk of development of melanoma, with incidence of disease higher in latitudes with greater sun exposure, it does not appear to affect risk of dissemination in those with clinically localized disease. The presence of an ulcer in the primary tumor, mitotic rate, and the demonstration of tumor satellites (microscopic foci of tumor distinct from the primary tumor in the reticular dermis or subcutaneous fat) are also prognostic factors.

576. The answer is A-Y, B-N, C-Y, D-Y, E-N. *(Chap 323.)* Foci of prostatic carcinoma are frequently noted at autopsy, but only about one-third of such cases are clinically apparent. Nonetheless, prostatic carcinoma is the most common cancer type in men and the second leading cause of male cancer deaths in those over age 55. Ninety-five percent of prostate cancers are adenocarcinomas. The grade of cellular differentiation is an extremely important prognostic variable; a higher Gleason grade (ranging from 2 to 10) indicates a biologically more aggressive tumor. Though the prostate capsule is a natural barrier to spread, dissemination may occur directly to the seminal vesicles and bladder floor, via lymphatics to the obturator, iliac, presacral, or paraaortic nodes, or hematogenously—usually to the bones, especially the pelvis and lumbar vertebrae. Staging consists of clinical examination of the prostate, pelvic CT or MRI, bone scan (with correlative x-rays for positive areas), and detection of serum markers, including acid phosphatase and the more sensitive prostate specific antigen (PSA). An elevated PSA is not pathognomonic for metastatic disease, but it is more common in those with spread to the bones. Though CT scans are helpful, the only certain way to determine local and regional lymph node spread is via surgical staging.

577. The answer is A-Y, B-Y, C-N, D-N, E-Y. *(Chap 309. Talpaz, Ann Intern Med 114:532, 1991.)* Chronic myelogenous leukemia (CML), a myeloproliferative disorder in which bone marrow stem cells are affected, can be diagnosed on clinical grounds alone. A bone marrow examination disclosing myeloid hyperplasia with basophilia would be supportive but not diagnostic. Every patient with CML has a Philadelphia chromosome (translocation between the long arms of chromosomes 22 and 9), which may be identified by either cytogenetic or molecular analysis. In addition to the cytogenetic abnormality, stable-phase CML is characterized by leukocytosis with a left shift, basophilia, splenomegaly, and a low leukocyte alkaline phosphatase (high in reactive leukocytosis and in agnogenic myeloid metaplasia). The duration of the stable phase is variable, but the disease always progresses on to blast crisis, unless interrupted by an allogeneic bone marrow transplant. The leukocytosis and metabolic symptoms of stable-phase CML can be controlled with a number of agents, including hydroxyurea, busulfan, and interferon-α. Results with interferon-α treatment suggest that the percentage of cells containing Philadelphia chromosome may be reduced.

578. The answer is A-N, B-N, C-Y, D-Y, E-Y. *(Chap 325. Rigel, Cancer 63:386, 1989.)* A distinctive pigmented lesion, the dysplastic nevus, occurs in families with a high incidence of melanoma. The recognition of this syndrome is important because the patient and family members can undergo intense dermatologic follow-up with early detection of malignant lesions. Patients with dysplastic nevi and two family members with melanoma have a 50 percent lifetime risk of developing melanoma. Dysplastic nevi tend to have irregular borders and be variable in color and shape on a given individual. They are usually large (minimum diameter of 6 mm) compared with benign nevi. The back is the most common site of dysplastic nevi, but they may also be seen on the scalp, buttocks, and breast. Though dysplastic nevi do serve as markers for the development of melanoma on normal skin, they also serve as precursor lesions, which makes it vital to watch each dysplastic nevus carefully.

579-582. The answers are 579-A, 580-B, 581-D, 582-C. *(Chap 318.)* Bleomycin is an antibiotic complex consisting of seven structurally related polypeptides. It both inhibits DNA synthesis and reacts with DNA by free radical generation to cause strand scission. Indications for the use of bleomycin include lymphomas and tumors of the head and neck, skin, testes, and penis. Doxorubicin (Adriamycin), another antitumor antibiotic, inhibits DNA synthesis and DNA-dependent RNA synthesis. It acts by binding with DNA and causing untwisting of the helix, which facilitates intercalation. However, the mechanism of its cytotoxicity is probably due to the prevention of topoisomerase II action. Doxorubicin is useful in treating a wide variety of tumors.

5-Fluorouracil, a pyrimidine analogue, is converted to fluorodeoxyuridine monophosphate, which blocks thymidylate synthase, an enzyme important in the synthesis of thymidylate and DNA. Used topically, 5-fluorouracil is effective in treating certain neoplastic skin disorders, including superficial basal cell carcinoma. Recent studies suggest potentiation of 5-fluorouracil action by leucovorin, which induces tighter binding to thymidylate synthase.

Vinblastine and vincristine are plant alkaloids. They cause metaphase arrest in dividing cells by binding directly to tubulin; in addition, they interfere with the assembly of spindle proteins. Vinblastine is used in the treatment of persons who have Hodgkin's disease and testicular cancer.

Endocrine, Metabolic, and Genetic Disorders

DIRECTIONS: Each question below contains four or five suggested responses. Select the **one best** response to each question

583. The use of repeated phlebotomy in the treatment of persons with symptomatic hemochromatosis may be expected to result in

   (A) increased skin pigmentation
   (B) improved cardiac function
   (C) return of secondary sex characteristics
   (D) decreased joint pain
   (E) an unchanged 5-year survival rate

584. A 19-year-old man has had a 5-year history of hyperglycemic episodes and glycosuria. However, he has never been hospitalized for diabetic ketoacidosis. Which of the following statements regarding the mode of inheritance of his disease is correct?

   (A) This disease is inherited in an autosomal recessive fashion
   (B) If the patient has children, they will have an approximately 50 percent chance of developing diabetes
   (C) The diabetic susceptibility gene in this patient resides on human chromosome 6
   (D) The patient is likely to carry one of a limited number of HLA-D locus alleles
   (E) The patient has an unusual susceptibility to a viral infection

585. Which of the following statements correctly characterizes the hormonal and metabolic changes in a patient with non-insulin-dependent diabetes mellitus who ingests a carbohydrate meal?

   (A) A higher than normal amount of glucose is released from the liver
   (B) The rate of glucose oxidation is high
   (C) There is a greater than normal rise in early insulin secretion
   (D) Glucagon secretion is impaired
   (E) Glycogen synthesis is increased

586. All the following are features of X-linked recessive disorders EXCEPT

   (A) for an affected female to be born, the father must be affected
   (B) affected males transmit the disease to their sons in 50 percent of cases
   (C) male offspring of female carriers have a 50 percent chance of being affected
   (D) all female offspring of affected males are carriers
   (E) the pedigree pattern tends to be oblique (uncles and nephews) rather than vertical (parents and children) or horizontal (siblings)

277

587. A 27-year-old hiker is bitten on the wrist by a coral snake. Within minutes, he notes numbness and tingling in the vicinity of the bite. He reaches an emergency department within 60 min of the bite, and other than minimal local swelling and fang marks on his hand, physical examination is normal. The most important measure in the treatment of this man would be to

(A) perform cutdown and suction of the bite site
(B) put ice on the bite area to neutralize the venom
(C) give coral-snake antivenin intravenously
(D) perform a wide surgical debridement of the bite site
(E) reassure him that there is no significant risk with bites of a coral snake and that the numbness will soon disappear

588. Which of the following statements concerning intensive insulin therapy for diabetes (use of an external insulin pump or three or more daily insulin injections guided by frequent blood glucose monitoring) is correct?

(A) All patients with diabetes mellitus should receive such therapy
(B) It has been definitively shown that compared with standard therapy such intensive therapy reduces the likelihood of retinopathy in patients with insulin-dependent diabetes mellitus
(C) Such therapy will consistently return the blood glucose to normal levels, but a reduction of long-term complications has not been demonstrated
(D) With careful monitoring, an increase in the number of hypoglycemic episodes is avoided
(E) Intensive insulin therapy failed to reduce the level of glycosylated hemoglobin

589. A 55-year-old obese man with a history of non-insulin-dependent diabetes mellitus is brought to the emergency department because his family notes that he is confused. The family believes he is taking "a pill" to help treat his "sugar." Although his neurologic examination is not focal, he is clearly disoriented. All of his serologic studies are normal except for a blood glucose concentration of 1.7 mmol/L (30 mg/dL). Which of the following statements concerning the current situation is correct?

(A) The patient should be treated with intravenous glucose until his serum glucose concentration is normalized and then be discharged from the emergency department
(B) If the patient has been taking glipizide, the duration of his hypoglycemia is likely to be brief
(C) The patient's insulin concentration is likely to be high
(D) If the patient is on chlorpropamide, he is also at risk for myocardial infarction
(E) The patient should be hospitalized

590. A 26-year-old diabetic man is evaluated for poor control of diabetes. He had taken 30 units of NPH insulin each morning for several years and had consistently negative or trace urine sugars before meals. However, during the last few weeks he increased the dosage to 38 units each morning because of increasing glycosuria detected in the bedtime urine sample. He has gained 2.2 kg (5 lb) during the last month. He has noted increasingly severe hunger pangs and headaches before dinner for the last week, but bedtime urine sugars have not diminished.

The most appropriate management at this point would be to

(A) begin the man on regular insulin at 5 P.M., according to the plasma glucose level at bedtime
(B) increase the dosage of NPH insulin, according to the plasma glucose level at bedtime
(C) decrease the dosage of NPH insulin gradually (initially by 10 percent)
(D) continue the same dosage of insulin but decrease the caloric intake at dinner
(E) switch from ordinary NPH to pork NPH insulin

591. Evidence of continuing ovarian estrogen production in a 29-year-old woman being evaluated for secondary amenorrhea is

(A) normal plasma estrone and luteinizing hormone (LH) levels
(B) normal plasma prolactin level
(C) an increase in plasma estradiol level following administration of human chorionic gonadotropin (hCG)
(D) appearance of menses following a short course of progesterone therapy
(E) normal bone density

592. Which of the following studies is most sensitive for detecting diabetic nephropathy?

(A) Serum creatinine level
(B) Creatinine clearance
(C) Urine albumin
(D) Glucose tolerance test
(E) Ultrasonography

593. Which of the following inhibits growth hormone secretion from the anterior pituitary gland?

(A) Somatostatin
(B) Growth hormone–releasing hormone
(C) Hypoglycemia
(D) Arginine
(E) Serotonin

594. A 7-year-old girl is referred for evaluation of vaginal bleeding for 2 months. The mother says that she has not been exposed to exogenous estrogens. Physical examination reveals height at the 98th percentile, Tanner stage III breast development, and no axillary or pubic hair. No abdominal or pelvic masses are palpated. Neurologic examination is normal. Radiographic and laboratory evaluations reveal the following:

Skull films: normal sella; no intracerebral calcifications
Bone age: 10 years
Urinary 17-ketosteroids: 1.7 μmol (0.5 mg)/g creatinine/24 h
Urinary gonadotropins: undetectable

The appropriate next step in the management of this girl would be

(A) exploratory laparotomy
(B) treatment with medroxyprogesterone acetate
(C) measurement of plasma androstenedione level
(D) abdominal CT scanning and pelvic sonography
(E) karyotype analysis

595. Which of the following inherited chromosomal abnormalities is most likely to allow survival of a patient into adult life?

(A) Trisomy 18
(B) Trisomy 13
(C) 47,XXY
(D) Trisomy 21
(E) 47,XO

596. A 40-year-old man presents with insidious onset of fatigue, headaches, muscle weakness, and paresthesia. Physical examination reveals hypertension, an enlarged tongue, wide spacing of the teeth, and a doughy appearance to the skin. Which of the following laboratory results would be INCONSISTENT with the expected diagnosis?

(A) Serum prolactin = 15 μg/L (15 ng/mL)
(B) Serum glucose = 8.6 mmol/L (155 mg/dL)
(C) Elevated insulin-like growth factor (IGF-I)
(D) Growth hormone concentration = 1 μg/L (1 ng/mL) 1 h after oral administration of 100 g glucose
(E) Serum inorganic phosphorus = 2.0 mmol/L (6.0 mg/dL)

597. Which of the following statements concerning the diagnosis of pheochromocytoma is correct?

(A) Measurement of plasma catecholamines is the preferred initial screening test
(B) Random urine samples are equivalent in diagnostic accuracy to the measurement of catecholamines or catecholamine metabolites in a 24-h urine collection
(C) After collection, the urine should be treated with dilute sodium hydroxide and refrigerated
(D) The ideal time to collect urine is during a period of clinical stability
(E) Strenuous exertion may falsely elevate the level of free urinary catecholamines

598. A 42-year-old man (indicated by the star in the family history below) has renal failure due to Alport's syndrome, which is nephritis associated with sensorineural deafness and is inherited as an autosomal dominant defect. He is being evaluated for a renal transplant from a living related donor. The best candidate for evaluation as a potential kidney donor for this man would be

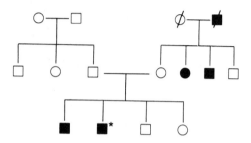

■ Renal failure
/ Deceased

(A) his mother
(B) his father
(C) his unaffected brother
(D) his sister

599. A 42-year-old woman developed severe thirst and polyuria 5 days after transsphenoidal hypophysectomy for Cushing's disease. Her urine volume has been approximately 6 L per day with urine specific gravity of 1.010. The patient has been able to consume large quantities of cold water. Serum electrolytes including glucose are within normal limits. The optimal way to establish the diagnosis in this case is

(A) measurement of plasma arginine vasopressin
(B) measurement of urinary arginine vasopressin
(C) comparison of the urine osmolarity after dehydration before and after vasopressin administration
(D) random comparison of plasma and urine osmolarity
(E) hypertonic saline infusion

600. Peripheral blood cells are obtained from members of a family; the DNA is extracted, treated with restriction endonuclease E run on an agarose gel, transferred to nitrocellulose paper, probed with a 4-kilobase (kb) radiolabeled segment of DNA, and exposed to x-ray film. In the following pattern, solid blocks indicate segments of DNA hybridizing to the probe, and numbers indicate DNA length in kilobases.

What most likely accounts for the fact that only one band appears in the son and only one (different) band appears in the daughter?

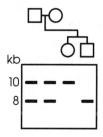

(A) A gene deletion in each child
(B) Chromosome segregation in the offspring
(C) Linkage disequilibrium in the offspring
(D) Parents who are heterozygotes for restriction fragment length polymorphism
(E) Loss of restriction site for endonuclease E in both the children

601. Which of the following statements concerning carbohydrate metabolism during pregnancy is correct?

(A) Diabetic females are relatively protected from ketoacidosis
(B) Insulin resistance occurs
(C) Even tight control of blood glucose fails to reduce the incidence of congenital anomalies among offspring of diabetic patients
(D) Women with diabetic nephropathy should be advised not to become pregnant because of the risk of worsening renal disease and poor fetal outcome
(E) Nondiabetic patients who develop hypoglycemia during pregnancy have the same risk of becoming diabetics later in life as those whose glucose tolerance remains normal

602. A 42-year-old alcoholic man has eaten poorly for the last 10 days but has continued to drink. His family brings him to the emergency room. On neurologic examination he is confused but otherwise normal. Blood glucose concentration is 2.8 mmol/L (50 mg/dL). Intravenous infusion of a bolus of 50% glucose solution is given. His confusion worsens, and he develops horizontal nystagmus, ataxia, and a heart rate of 130 beats per minute.

At this point, the man's physician should

(A) order an immediate CT scan of the head
(B) perform a lumbar puncture
(C) administer another bolus of 50% glucose solution
(D) administer intravenous folic acid, 5 mg
(E) administer intramuscular thiamine, 50 mg

603. A 32-year-old alcoholic man is admitted to the hospital because of acute abdominal pain. Hemorrhagic necrosis of the pancreas is found during emergency laparotomy. Postoperatively, he becomes septic and hyperglycemic. Mechanical ventilation for respiratory failure is required, and attempts to wean him from the ventilator are begun 3 days later. Which of the following daily regimens would provide the most appropriate form of nutrition for this man (assuming that each regimen would include the required amounts of calories, vitamins, and minerals and that the hyperglycemia can be controlled with insulin)?

(A) A defined-formula liquid diet given through a small-bore nasogastric tube
(B) Peripheral intravenous infusion of 3 L of a 25% dextrose solution containing 2% amino acids
(C) Central intravenous infusion of 3 L of a 25% dextrose solution containing 2% amino acids
(D) Peripheral intravenous infusion of 1.5 L of a 25% dextrose solution containing 4% amino acids and mixed with 1 L of a 10% lipid solution
(E) Peripheral intravenous infusion of 1 L of a 12% dextrose solution containing 6% amino acids and mixed with 2 L of a 10% lipid solution

604. A 24-year-old woman with a several-year history of chronic, debilitating, cramping abdominal pain has been evaluated several times for this problem. In each case the possibility of psychogenic causes was raised because of the absence of abdominal tenderness, fever, and leukocytosis during the episodes. The patient has had intermittent vomiting, constipation, arm and chest pain, and difficulty in urination. She also complains of increasing leg weakness. The attacks of abdominal pain are often associated with anxiety, insomnia, and disorientation. Prior workup has also included abdominal angiography, abdominal CT scanning, and endoscopy. Results of all diagnostic studies were normal. The patient's current physical examination and routine laboratory examination, including complete blood count and serum chemistries, are unremarkable. The urinary pyrrole porphobilinogen excretion is elevated. Which of the following is the most appropriate advice for this patient?

(A) The patient's offspring may be at risk only if the father is also a carrier of this disease
(B) Intravenous administration of heme may ameliorate the attacks
(C) Narcotic analgesics should not be used during acute attacks
(D) The patient should avoid aspirin
(E) The patient should avoid prolonged exposure to the sun

605. A 35-year-old man is undergoing a fertility evaluation. He is found to have a low sperm count on three separate ejaculants. The plasma FSH is 10 IU/L. A testicular biopsy is normal. The most likely etiology for the man's infertility is

(A) inherited failure of spermatogenesis
(B) acquired failure of spermatogenesis
(C) hypothalamic disease
(D) history of viral orchitis
(E) blockage of the vas deferens

606. After apical scars are found on chest x-ray in a 48-year-old postmenopausal woman, chemoprophylaxis with isoniazid is begun. Two months later the woman complains of weakness, nausea, and tingling in the feet. Physical examination is unremarkable, and routine blood and urine test results are normal. Four weeks later she has a grand-mal seizure and is admitted to the hospital. Findings on the admission physical include seborrheic dermatitis, glossitis, and absent ankle and knee tendon reflexes; hematologic testing reveals microcytic anemia.

At this point, the woman's physician should

(A) order immediate electroencephalography
(B) order CT scan of the brain
(C) discontinue isoniazid and begin treatment with rifampin
(D) administer intramuscular pyridoxine, 100 mg, then give 50 mg orally daily
(E) administer intramuscular cyanocobalamin, 100 μg, then give 100 μg daily for 1 week

607. A 78-year-old man who lives alone and prepares his own food is found to have numerous ecchymotic areas on the posterior aspect of his lower extremities. On closer examination of the skin, he has hemorrhagic areas around hair follicles; the hairs are fragmented. Splinter hemorrhages are present in the nail beds, and several hematomas are present in the muscles of the arms and legs. Except for the absence of teeth, the rest of the physical examination is unremarkable. Laboratory examination reveals a normal PT, PTT, and CBC, except for a hematocrit of 28 percent (red blood cell indices are normal).

This clinical syndrome is most likely due to a deficiency of

(A) vitamin A
(B) vitamin C
(C) folate
(D) vitamin K
(E) pyridoxine

608. A 20-year-old woman has a history of multiple fractures since childhood, kyphoscoliosis, bluish-gray teeth, and conductive hearing loss. Examination of the face reveals blue sclerae. Several relatives on her mother's side have been similarly affected. She has no history of physical abuse or abnormal serum chemistries. The most likely mechanism of the patient's abnormalities is

(A) excessive deposition of normal collagen fibrils in bone
(B) inability to convert procollagen to collagen
(C) mutation in the gene for type I procollagen
(D) mutation in the gene for type II procollagen
(E) mutation in the gene for type III procollagen

609. A clinical presentation that includes long, thin extremities, dislocation of the ocular lens, and aortic aneurysms is most likely due to a derangement in which of the following molecules?

(A) Procollagen type I
(B) Procollagen type II
(C) Proteoglycan
(D) Elastin
(E) Fibrillin

610. A 25-year-old man with a renal allograft and history of an intracerebral abscess is evaluated for profound polyuria. He is admitted to the hospital for a water deprivation test. No fluids are given after 12 midnight. By 11 A.M. he has lost 1 kg, and urine osmolality has been 120 mosm/kg for the last 3 h. Plasma osmolality is 320 mosm/kg (serum sodium is 155 mmol/L). At 11 A.M. 1 μg desmopressin is given by subcutaneous injection; 45 min later the urine osmolality is measured at 121 mosm/kg. The patient is then allowed to drink.

Treatment of this patient should include

(A) vasopressin tannate in oil
(B) hydrochlorothiazide
(C) desmopressin
(D) chlorpropamide
(E) demeclocycline

611. A person with hypercalcemia due to sarcoidosis would likely have all but which one of the following?

    (A) An abnormal chest x-ray
    (B) Increased absorption of calcium from the gastrointestinal tract
    (C) Hypercalciuria
    (D) Increased serum parathyroid hormone level
    (E) Hypergammaglobulinemia

612. The most likely etiology for the eating disorder anorexia nervosa is

    (A) decreased levels of luteinizing hormone–releasing hormone (LHRH)
    (B) decreased levels of growth hormone
    (C) decreased levels of insulin-like growth factor I (somatomedin C)
    (D) low levels of serum thyroxine
    (E) psychiatric disorder

613. A 45-year-old obese man without known medical problems complains of feeling very sleepy during the day and often falling asleep while listening to friends. The most likely cause of this patient's problem is

    (A) narcolepsy
    (B) upper airway obstruction at night
    (C) glucocorticoid excess
    (D) growth hormone excess
    (E) estrogen excess

614. A 67-year-old man with chronic arthritis is found to have passed a uric acid stone after an episode of renal colic. On workup he is found to have multiple radiolucent stones in the left renal pelvis, uric acid excretion of 5.4 mmol/d (900 mg/d), a serum uric acid concentration of 580 μmol/L (9.8 mg/dL), a serum creatinine concentration of 160 μmol/L (1.8 mg/dL), and monosodium urate crystals in an effusion in the left knee. The drug of choice for long-term therapy in this patient is

    (A) probenecid alone
    (B) probenecid and sodium bicarbonate
    (C) allopurinol
    (D) colchicine
    (E) sulfinpyrazone

615. An obese woman has hypertriglyceridemia without hypercholesterolemia. The most appropriate first step in the treatment of this woman would be

    (A) weight reduction
    (B) nicotinic acid
    (C) gemfibrozil
    (D) clofibrate therapy
    (E) bile acid–binding resin therapy

616. A 68-year-old woman with a history of three vertebral fractures due to osteoporosis is being treated with supplemental calcium, vitamin D, and estrogen therapy. Because of recent myocardial infarction, discontinuation of the estrogen therapy is desired. Which of the following steps would be most appropriate after discontinuing the estrogen?

    (A) Add sodium fluoride
    (B) Double the dose of vitamin D
    (C) Begin etidronate
    (D) Begin calcitonin
    (E) Leave the patient on vitamin D and calcium and undertake measures to decrease the likelihood of falls

617. An X-linked recessive disease characterized by nephrolithiasis, arthritis, self-mutilative behavior, and mental retardation is associated with

    (A) failure to excrete uric acid because of inherited defective renal tubular function
    (B) failure to excrete uric acid because of xanthine oxidase mutation
    (C) uric acid overproduction due to inherited acceleration of purine degradation
    (D) increased urate production due to an inability to convert purine bases to ribonucleotides
    (E) increased urate production due to increased levels of phosphoribosylpyrophosphate

618. In designing a hormone replacement program for patients with coexistent thyroid and adrenal failure,

(A) the dose of glucocorticoid must be increased slowly once thyroid replacement has been initiated

(B) the dose of thyroid hormone must be increased slowly once glucocorticoid replacement has been initiated

(C) mineralocorticoid replacement must also be included if combined therapy is required

(D) thyroid replacement must not be initiated until treatment with glucocorticoid has been instituted

(E) growth hormone replacement must also be included if combined therapy is required

619. A 35-year-old clinically euthyroid woman is seen because of a neck mass. She has no history of prior neck irradiation. A 2-cm, firm nodule is palpated in the left lobe of an otherwise normal gland. Fine-needle aspiration of this lesion reveals sheets of follicular cells. The next appropriate procedure is

(A) subtotal thyroidectomy
(B) levothyroxine suppressive therapy
(C) repeat fine-needle aspiration
(D) follow-up examination in 6 months
(E) radionuclide scan

620. A 20-year-old man presents with weakness. Physical examination reveals mild jaundice and a liver two fingers beneath the right costal margin. Laboratory evaluation is remarkable for the presence of elevated hepatic transaminases (four times normal). Other laboratory results are negative, including serology for hepatitis A, B, and C; ANA; rheumatoid factor; iron; and iron binding. Serum ceruloplasmin is 50 mg/L (5 mg/dL). The patient denies intake of alcohol or exposure to known hepatotoxins. The most appropriate treatment is

(A) liver transplantation
(B) interferon-α
(C) penicillamine
(D) glucocorticoids
(E) desferrioxamine

621. A 45-year-old man who works in the metal smelting industry was involved in an accident in which he was exposed to a great deal of dust and manufacturing by-products. Several days after this episode he developed jaundice, nausea, vomiting, diarrhea, and shortness of breath. Physical examination demonstrated icteric sclerae and tachycardia. Laboratory evaluation revealed hematocrit 32 percent, WBC count 14,000/μL, and platelet count 350,000/μL. Urinalysis disclosed no red cells or white cells per high power field, but there were several granular casts. The urine dipstick was positive for blood and protein. Liver function tests included aspartate aminotransferase (SGOT) level 1.3 μkat/L (80 U/L), alanine aminotransferase (SGPT) level 2 μkat/L (120 U/L), total bilirubin 85.5 μmol/L (5 mg/dL), and direct bilirubin 17.1 μmol/L (1 mg/dL). The ECG revealed T-wave inversion in all leads. Plain x-ray of the abdomen reveals patchy densities. The most appropriate diagnostic measurement would be of

(A) urinary arsenic
(B) serum lead
(C) erythrocyte protoporphyrin
(D) serum cadmium
(E) serum thallium

622. Cholestyramine and colestipol are binding resins that are used to treat patients with hypercholesterolemia. Their serum-cholesterol-lowering effects are thought to be mediated by

(A) causing mild diarrhea and a mild degree of fat malabsorption

(B) binding of intestinal cholesterol, thus decreasing its net absorption from dietary sources

(C) decreasing the intestinal synthesis of very low-density lipoproteins

(D) interrupting the enterohepatic circulation of cholesterol by sequestering bile acids in the intestine

(E) none of the above

623. A 28-year-old woman who is 15 kg (33 lb) over ideal body weight wants to begin dieting. The best initial regimen for weight loss would be

(A) a low-calorie balanced diet
(B) a low-calorie, liquid protein diet ("protein-sparing modified fast")
(C) total starvation
(D) use of amphetamines to curb appetite
(E) an increase in exercise but no dietary changes

624. A 35-year-old woman ingests a hundred 325-mg acetaminophen tablets in a suicide attempt. She is immediately brought to the emergency room by friends. The appropriate therapeutic strategy is

(A) administration of activated charcoal
(B) administration of activated charcoal plus acetylcysteine therapy
(C) chelation therapy
(D) administration of phenytoin (Dilantin)
(E) acetylcysteine therapy

625. The reason for acute renal failure after ingestion of antifreeze is

(A) direct ethanol toxicity on renal tubules
(B) direct ethylene glycol toxicity on renal tubules
(C) toxicity of ethylene glycol metabolites on renal tubules
(D) insufficient renal perfusion due to circulatory collapse induced by ethylene glycol
(E) urinary obstruction due to oxalic acid stones

626. Obese persons are at an increased risk for all the following disorders EXCEPT

(A) hypothyroidism
(B) cholelithiasis
(C) diabetes mellitus
(D) hypertension
(E) hypertriglyceridemia

627. A 45-year-old woman is seen because of headaches, fatigue, and weakness. She takes no medicines. Except for a blood pressure of 150/95, the physical examination is normal. Electrocardiogram discloses prominent QRS voltage consistent with left ventricular hypertrophy and U waves. Serum electrolytes reveal the following: sodium, 148 mmol/L; potassium, 2.9 mmol/L; chloride, 110 mmol/L; and bicarbonate, 35 mmol/L.

Which of the following measurements would be the most helpful in establishing a diagnosis of primary mineralocorticoid excess?

(A) Urinary 17-ketosteroids
(B) Plasma renin activity
(C) Plasma renin following administration of 20 mg furosemide
(D) Plasma aldosterone following saline loading
(E) Abdominal CT scan

628. Which of the following would be the most likely finding in a patient who has taken an overdose of a tricyclic antidepressant?

(A) Elevated hepatic transaminases
(B) Prolongation of the QRS complex on the electrocardiogram
(C) Urinary incontinence
(D) Metabolic alkalosis
(E) Anemia

629. A 25-year-old man complains of diffuse bone pain. Physical examination is remarkable for the presence of an enlarged spleen (9 cm below the left costal margin). CBC discloses pancytopenia. A bone marrow examination reveals normal hematopoiesis; however, large multinucleated, macrophage-like cells engorged with cytoplasmic fibrils are present. Relevant family history includes descent from Eastern European Jewish origin. An appropriate therapeutic intervention in this patient is administration of

(A) penicillamine
(B) desferrioxamine
(C) aglucerase
(D) leuprolide
(E) none of the above

630. Which of the following regimens is best for the preoperative management of a patient with a known pheochromocytoma?

(A) Propranolol alone
(B) Propranolol followed by phenoxybenzamine
(C) Phenoxybenzamine followed by propranolol
(D) Prazosin alone
(E) Propranolol followed by prazosin

631. A person with Cushing's disease undergoes transphenoidal removal of an ACTH-secreting microadenoma. Routine endocrinologic management after recovery from surgery should include administration of

(A) hydrocortisone, 30 mg/d
(B) hydrocortisone, 100 mg/d
(C) hydrocortisone, 30 mg/d, and levothyroxine, 0.1 mg/d
(D) hydrocortisone, 100 mg/d, and desmopressin, 0.2 μg/d
(E) none of the above

632. A 55-year-old postmenopausal woman without prior medical problems presents because of severe hot flashes and vaginal dryness. Before beginning estrogen replacement therapy, counsel concerning the risks and benefits of such therapy should include which of the following statements?

(A) If given for the purpose of hot flashes alone, duration of the therapy can be limited to less than 4 years
(B) The risk of death due to myocardial infarction may be somewhat increased
(C) The risk of metastatic breast cancer is mildly increased
(D) It is unlikely that long-term estrogen therapy will decrease the risk of osteoporotic bone fractures
(E) Progesterone should be given during the last 10 to 13 days of each month of estrogen therapy

633. Match the following statement with the disease it most aptly describes: A disease in which an affected person will bear, on average, both normal and affected offspring in equal proportion, with children of either sex equally likely to be affected, characterized by a delayed age of onset, and in which patients are greater than 90 percent likely to have inherited an abnormal gene from a parent.

(A) Manic depressive psychosis
(B) Myasthenia gravis
(C) Hemophilia A
(D) Neurofibromatosis
(E) Huntington's chorea

634. Which of the following statements is true regarding Cushing's disease caused by bilateral adrenal hyperplasia?

(A) Cortisol production may increase during administration of metyrapone
(B) Urinary 17-hydroxycorticosteroid excretion is usually normal
(C) ACTH secretion increases in response to metyrapone
(D) Administration of dexamethasone, 8 mg/d for 2 days, reduces cortisol production only minimally
(E) Administration of dexamethasone, 2 mg/d for 2 days, is not followed by a reduction in urinary free cortisol excretion

635. Each of the following may be a direct consequence of severe magnesium deficiency EXCEPT

(A) digitalis-induced arrhythmias
(B) hypocalcemia
(C) hypokalemia
(D) hyponatremia
(E) confusion

636. A 65-year-old man who has had mildly symptomatic Paget's disease of the bone for 15 years and has been on etidronate therapy intermittently for the past 2 years presents with a 4-week history of pain and swelling of a well-demarcated area in the right upper leg. The serum alkaline phosphatase, generally under good control, is three times the level measured 1 month ago. The most likely diagnosis at this point is

(A) growth of an arteriovenous shunt
(B) markedly elevated serum calcium
(C) side effect of etidronate therapy
(D) osteogenic sarcoma
(E) aseptic necrosis of the femoral head

637. A 55-year-old woman presents to her physician with mild fatigue. Her past medical history is unremarkable. She is taking no medication. No abnormalities are detected on physical examination. The only abnormality detected on routine blood testing is an elevated calcium (2.96 mmol/L [11.9 mg/dL]) and a serum inorganic phosphorus of 0.65 mmol/L (2 mg/dL). An immunoreactive parathyroid hormone level is undetectable. The most likely etiology for this patient's high serum calcium is

(A) primary hyperparathyroidism
(B) malignancy
(C) hypervitaminosis
(D) hyperthyroidism
(E) familial hypocalciuric hypercalcemia

638. A 28-year-old woman is referred because of failure to menstruate during the 7 months since the delivery of an infant. She is still nursing the baby. Measurement of a random serum prolactin level obtained elsewhere was 310 μg/L. After obtaining a pertinent history and physical examination, your next step in the evaluation of this patient's condition would be which of the following?

(A) Trial of low-dose bromocriptine to assess suppressibility of the hyperprolactinemic state
(B) CT of the head and pituitary gland with contrast
(C) Goldmann visual field assessment
(D) Measurement of serum prolactin levels before and after nursing
(E) Delay in any further evaluation until she stops nursing

639. A 64-year-old man seeks medical attention because of an annoying cough. Physical examination is remarkable only for supraclavicular lymphadenopathy. Chest x-ray shows a parahilar mass and paratracheal lymph node enlargement. Serum and urine chemistries are as follows:

Sodium: 120 mmol/L
Potassium: 4 mmol/L
Bicarbonate: 23 mmol/L
Serum osmolality: 250 mosmol/kg H_2O
Urine osmolality: 600 mosmol/kg H_2O
Urine sodium: 80 mmol/L

The most likely pathophysiologic basis for this man's hyponatremia is

(A) production of a vasopressin-like molecule by tumor tissue
(B) production of authentic vasopressin by tumor tissue
(C) potentiation of vasopressin action on the renal tubule by a tumor product
(D) stimulation of neurohypophyseal vasopressin secretion by a tumor product
(E) central nervous system metastases resulting in loss of vasopressin regulation

640. A 45-year-old woman complains of fatigue and muscle weakness. She also has intermittent headaches. Her physical examination is unremarkable except for a blood pressure of 155/105. Routine laboratory evaluation is unremarkable except for the serum electrolytes, which reveal the following: sodium 152 mmol/L (152 meq/L), potassium 2.5 mmol/L (2.5 meq/L), chloride 110 mmol/L (110 meq/L), and carbon dioxide 37 mmol/L (37 meq/L). The patient is currently taking no medication.

Plasma renin levels fail to increase appropriately upon standing. The next most appropriate test is

(A) measurement of plasma aldosterone after intravenous infusion of saline
(B) measurement of plasma aldosterone after overnight fast
(C) 24-h urine collection for catecholamine metabolite determination
(D) abdominal CT scanning
(E) overnight dexamethasone suppression test

641. Patients who are heterozygous for defective copies of the genes coding for either lipoprotein lipase or apoprotein CII will exhibit which of the following abnormalities?

(A) Excessive chylomicronemia
(B) Excessive amounts of low-density lipoprotein in serum
(C) Excessive amounts of very low-density lipoprotein in serum
(D) Excessive amounts of chylomicron remnant
(E) Excessive amounts of intermediate-density lipoproteins

642. Eight years after surgical resection of a benign nodule in the left lobe of her thyroid gland, a 35-year-old woman presents with a right-sided neck mass. Her thyroid scan is shown below. She is asymptomatic and takes no medication. Which of the following should her physician advise?

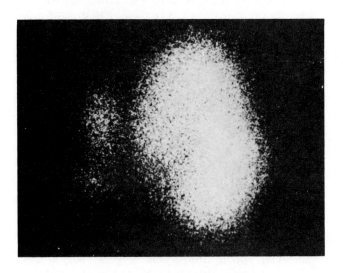

(A) Diagnostic ultrasonography
(B) Surgical exploration of the right side of the neck
(C) Measurement of plasma calcitonin concentration
(D) Reevaluation in 1 year
(E) Exogenous thyroid hormone therapy

643. A 26-year-old pregnant woman has a goiter but is clinically euthyroid. Thyroid function tests reveal a free thyroxine index that is slightly elevated. An ultrasensitive TSH test reveals a level of 0.3 mU/L. The test that would be most appropriate in determining whether the woman is euthyroid or hyperthyroid is

(A) radioactive iodine uptake
(B) technetium thyroid scan
(C) T_3 suppression test
(D) thyrotropin-releasing hormone (TRH) stimulation test
(E) serum T_3 by radioimmunoassay

644. A 32-year-old man sustains a myocardial infarction. He relates a history of early myocardial infarctions in several aunts and uncles. Moreover, it is noted that he has nodular swellings in the Achilles tendon and other tendons in the dorsum of the hand. A serum cholesterol is 10 mmol/L (400 mg/dL). A defect in which of the following proteins is the most likely etiology of this patient's clinical problem?

(A) Apoprotein E
(B) Apoprotein CII
(C) Lipoprotein lipase
(D) Lipoprotein B
(E) LDL receptor

645. A 24-year-old woman develops Graves' disease during the third trimester of pregnancy. The most appropriate treatment would be

(A) subtotal thyroidectomy
(B) propylthiouracil
(C) propylthiouracil and levothyroxine
(D) radioactive iodine
(E) propranolol

646. In a 44-year-old woman with a subnormal serum thyroxine level and a history of treatment at the age of 29 years with radioactive iodine for Graves' disease, the best confirmatory test for suspected primary hypothyroidism is measurement of which of the following?

(A) Serum triiodothyronine (T_3) concentration
(B) Serum reverse triiodothyronine (rT_3) concentration
(C) Serum thyroid-stimulating hormone (TSH) concentration
(D) 24-h radioactive iodine uptake
(E) Thyrotropin-releasing hormone (TRH) stimulation test to measure TSH reserve

647. In persons with congenital adrenal hyperplasia due to inherited defects of adrenal steroid C-21 hydroxylase, excessive androgen production is the result of

(A) autonomous adrenal production of steroids
(B) autonomous pituitary production of ACTH
(C) extraglandular formation from large amounts of nonandrogenic adrenal steroids
(D) failure of production of an adrenal product necessary for negative feedback on pituitary ACTH secretion
(E) positive feedback on pituitary ACTH secretion by abnormal adrenal products

648. A 38-year-old woman with obesity, dermal striae, and hypertension is referred for endocrinologic evaluation of possible cortisol excess. The woman receives a midnight dose of 1 mg of dexamethasone; a plasma cortisol level drawn at 8 A.M. the next day is 386 nmol/L (14 μg/dL). At this point in the evaluation, the most appropriate diagnostic maneuver would be

(A) CT scanning of the pituitary gland
(B) abdominal CT scanning
(C) measurement of 24-h 17-hydroxycorticosteroid excretion in urine
(D) 2-day low-dose dexamethasone suppression test (0.5 mg every 6 h for 48 h)
(E) 2-day high-dose dexamethasone suppression test (2.0 mg every 6 h for 48 h)

649. In a 36-year-old woman who has had insulin-dependent diabetes mellitus since the age of 14, hyperkalemia is being evaluated. On physical examination her blood pressure is 146/96 mmHg. Laboratory evaluation discloses the following:

Fasting plasma glucose: 6 mmol/L
    (110 mg/dL)
Serum creatinine: 194 μmol/L (2.2 mg/dL)
Serum sodium: 135 mmol/L
Serum potassium: 6.2 mmol/L
Serum chloride: 116 mmol/L
Serum bicarbonate: 14 mmol/L

After a short ACTH infusion test, the plasma cortisol concentration increases from 386 to 717 nmol/L (14 to 26 μg/dL). After administration of 80 mg of furosemide and 3 h of upright posture, the plasma renin activity and aldosterone concentration are unchanged from baseline values.

The most appropriate therapeutic regimen to correct the electrolyte imbalance would be

(A) administration of fludrocortisone
(B) administration of furosemide
(C) administration of hydrocortisone and furosemide
(D) hemodialysis
(E) administration of potassium-binding anion-exchange resins

650. A 22-year-old woman who has had diabetes mellitus for 6 years now wishes to become pregnant. She takes 32 units of NPH insulin each morning, and her urine glucose values (done twice daily) are "usually trace or 1+." Her hemoglobin A_{1c} level is 9.8 percent (normal: 5 to 8 percent). She takes oral contraceptive pills. Her physician should advise her that

(A) home glucose monitoring and a daily regimen of multiple subcutaneous injections of regular insulin are necessary now
(B) oral contraceptive agents can falsely elevate HbA_{1c} levels
(C) attempts to achieve better diabetic control can wait until she has become pregnant
(D) the current insulin regimen probably will be adequate until the last trimester of pregnancy
(E) hospitalization will probably be necessary for most of her pregnancy to ensure normal delivery and perinatal survival

651. A 24-year-old man with diabetes since the age of 9 years sees his physician for a routine checkup. He has no complaints and is taking 40 units NPH and 5 units regular insulin each morning as prescribed. Ophthalmoscopic examination reveals the findings in Color Plate E. Based on these findings, his physician should recommend

(A) vitrectomy
(B) photocoagulation
(C) hypophysectomy
(D) more vigorous control of the blood sugar level
(E) follow-up examination in 3 months

652. In a 40-year-old man with long-standing hypogonadism resulting from total surgical castration for bilateral seminomas at the age of 17, the effectiveness of testosterone cypionate therapy can best be monitored by the assessment of

(A) plasma testosterone level
(B) plasma luteinizing hormone (LH) level
(C) plasma testosterone cypionate level
(D) change in muscle mass
(E) frequency of nocturnal erections

653. During a routine checkup, a 67-year-old man is found to have a level of serum alkaline phosphatase three times the upper limit of normal. Serum calcium and phosphorus concentrations and liver function test results are normal. He is asymptomatic. The most likely diagnosis is

(A) metastatic bone disease
(B) primary hyperparathyroidism
(C) occult plasmacytoma
(D) Paget's disease of bone
(E) osteomalacia

654. The most important regulator of serum 1,25(OH)$_2$ vitamin D concentration is

(A) serum calcium
(B) serum magnesium
(C) serum 25OH vitamin D
(D) parathyroid hormone
(E) prolactin

655. Diseases inherited in a multifactorial genetic fashion (i.e., not autosomal dominant, autosomal recessive, or X-linked) and seen more frequently in persons bearing certain histocompatibility antigens include

(A) gluten-sensitive enteropathy
(B) neurofibromatosis
(C) adult polycystic kidney disease
(D) Wilson's disease
(E) cystic fibrosis

656. Which of the following conditions or drugs is LEAST likely to be associated with erectile impotence?

(A) Amitriptyline
(B) Nifedipine
(C) Cimetidine
(D) Peyronie's disease
(E) Elevated serum prolactin

657. A 20-year-old competitive swimmer is examined because of primary amenorrhea. Her height is 170 cm (67 in) and she weighs 50 kg (110 lb). Her breasts are well developed. Findings on pelvic examination are normal, and the pubic hair appears to be normal. Cervical mucus is abundant and demonstrates ferning upon drying. Urine spot and blood tests for pregnancy are negative. She is given 10 mg of medroxyprogesterone acetate twice a day for 5 days, and 3 days later she experiences menstrual bleeding for the first time. The most likely cause of the amenorrhea is

(A) functional hypothalamic amenorrhea
(B) 45,X gonadal dysgenesis
(C) polycystic ovarian disease
(D) chromaphobe adenoma of the pituitary
(E) prolactinoma of the pituitary

658. A 21-year-old woman is examined because of secondary amenorrhea. Cyclic menses had commenced at the age of 14 years. When she was 19 years old she became pregnant and was hospitalized during the sixth month of that pregnancy because of bleeding and hypotension that proved to be the result of a spontaneous abortion with retained placental fragments; she received 10 units of blood, and a dilation and curettage was performed. No menses have occurred during the 2 years since the hospitalization. She now wishes to become pregnant.

Findings on physical examination, including rectopelvic examination, are normal. Results on complete blood counts, SMA-12, and chest x-ray are within normal limits. Serum thyroxine (T_4) concentration is 90 nmol/L (7 μg/dL) and an 8 A.M. plasma cortisol measurement is 470 nmol/L (17 μg/dL). No menstrual bleeding occurs after administration of 10 mg medroxyprogesterone acetate per day for 10 days or cyclic estrogen and progestogen (1.25 mg conjugated estrogens by mouth each day for 3 weeks with 10 mg medroxyprogesterone acetate per day for the last 7 days).

At this point the most appropriate diagnostic study would be

(A) CT scan of the pituitary with contrast
(B) CT scan of the abdomen followed by wedge resection of the ovaries
(C) hysterosalpingogram
(D) metyrapone test
(E) chromosomal analysis

659. A 36-year-old woman has noticed the absence of menses for the last 4 months. A pregnancy test is negative. Serum levels of luteinizing hormone and follicle-stimulating hormone are elevated, and the serum estradiol level is low. These findings suggest

(A) bilateral tubal obstruction
(B) panhypopituitarism
(C) polycystic ovarian disease
(D) premature menopause
(E) exogenous estrogen administration

660. A newborn infant with ambiguous genitalia develops vomiting and profound volume depletion. A diagnosis of congenital adrenal hyperplasia due to C-21 hydroxylase deficiency would be supported by all the following findings EXCEPT

(A) elevated urinary 17-ketosteroid concentration
(B) elevated plasma 11-deoxycortisol concentration
(C) elevated plasma 17-hydroxyprogesterone concentration
(D) elevated plasma androstenedione concentration
(E) elevated urinary pregnanediol and pregnanetriol concentrations

661. In women with gonadal dysgenesis, development of malignancy in the streak gonads is most likely when the karyotype is

(A) $46XX_i$ (isochrome X)
(B) 46,XX
(C) 45,X
(D) 45,X/46,XY mosaicism
(E) 45X,46XX mosaicism

662. The most common presentation of primary hyperparathyroidism is

(A) peptic ulcer
(B) proximal muscle weakness
(C) osteitis fibrosa cystica
(D) calcium kidney stones
(E) asymptomatic hypercalcemia

663. The diagnosis of primary hyperparathyroidism is made in an elderly woman who has osteitis fibrosa cystica and elevated serum levels of calcium (3 mmol/L [12.0 mg/dL]) and creatinine (309 μmol/L [3.5 mg/dL]). The woman is not considered a surgical candidate because of pulmonary disease. The best medical treatment for hyperparathyroidism in this woman would be

(A) plicamycin
(B) estrogen
(C) phosphate
(D) diphosphonate
(E) thiazide

664. A 34-year-old woman has had three hospital admissions during the last year because of nephrolithiasis. The rate of 24-h urinary calcium excretion has been above the normal range on all three occasions and serum calcium concentrations were between 2.5 and 2.8 mmol/L (10.2 and 11.5 mg/dL). The serum phosphorus concentration was 0.77 mmol/L (2.4 mg/dL) and the parathyroid hormone level was 229 nL eq/mL (normal less than 150 nL eq/mL).

The most appropriate management at this time would be

(A) to begin administration of prednisone, 40 mg daily, and taper the dose over a period of 4 weeks
(B) to administer thiazide diuretics to decrease calcium excretion
(C) symptomatic treatment of renal lithiasis only
(D) calcium supplementation to prevent progressive bone loss
(E) surgical exploration of the neck

665. Which of the following conditions is LEAST likely to cause hyperthyroidism associated with low thyroidal radioactive iodine uptake (RAIU)?

(A) Subacute thyroiditis
(B) Struma ovarii
(C) Choriocarcinoma
(D) Ingestion of exogenous levothyroxine
(E) Recent intravenous pyelography

666. Each of the following conditions is characteristic of the presentation of osteomalacia in adults EXCEPT

(A) bowing of the tibia
(B) pseudofractures
(C) long-bone pain
(D) proximal muscle weakness
(E) hypophosphatemia

667. A 61-year-old woman noticed severe sharp pain in her back after lifting a suitcase. A compression fracture of the T11 vertebral body is identified on x-ray examination. Routine laboratory evaluation discloses a serum calcium concentration of 2 mmol/L (8.0 mg/dL), a serum phosphorus concentration of 0.77 mmol/L (2.4 mg/dL), and increased serum alkaline phosphatase activity. The serum parathyroid hormone level was subsequently found to be elevated as well. The most likely diagnosis is

(A) Paget's disease of bone
(B) ectopic parathyroid hormone secretion
(C) primary hyperparathyroidism
(D) postmenopausal osteoporosis
(E) vitamin D deficiency

668. A 60-year-old woman has low-back pain. Radiographic examination reveals diffuse demineralization and a compression fracture of the fourth lumbar vertebra. Serum calcium concentration is 2.8 mmol/L (11.5 mg/dL). Blood count is normal. This clinical picture is most compatible with the presence of which of the following conditions?

(A) Postmenopausal osteoporosis
(B) Paget's disease
(C) Primary hyperparathyroidism
(D) Multiple myeloma
(E) Osteomalacia

669. Which of the following conditions is associated with hypocalcemia but NOT with an increased serum level of parathyroid hormone?

(A) Severe hypomagnesemia
(B) Osteomalacia secondary to vitamin D deficiency
(C) Osteomalacia secondary to vitamin D resistance
(D) Renal failure
(E) Pseudohypoparathyroidism

670. Which of the following conditions is LEAST likely to be associated with a low serum 25(OH) vitamin D level?

(A) Dietary deficiency of vitamin D
(B) Chronic severe cholestatic liver disease
(C) Chronic renal failure
(D) Anticonvulsant therapy with phenobarbital or phenytoin
(E) High-dose glucocorticoid therapy

671. In a person with severe protein starvation, which of the following conditions would be LEAST likely to increase the amount of protein needed to achieve positive nitrogen balance?

(A) Renal failure
(B) Gastrointestinal fistula
(C) Sepsis
(D) Simultaneous caloric malnutrition
(E) Thyrotoxicosis

DIRECTIONS: Each question below contains five suggested responses. For **each** of the five responses listed with every question, you are to respond either YES (Y) or NO (N). In a given item **all, some, or none** of the alternatives may be correct.

672. Anovulatory cycles are characterized by

   (A) elevated levels of plasma progesterone
   (B) dysmenorrhea
   (C) an absent luteal phase
   (D) lack of a normal LH and FSH surge
   (E) irregular uterine bleeding

673. A 15-year-old boy has had hypothyroidism since early childhood. For several years, he has noticed frequent episodes of numbness and tingling of his hands, occasionally accompanied by muscle spasms. Physical examination reveals a positive Chvostek sign, short stature, and short left fourth metacarpals (absent knuckles). The boy's mother is also short and has absent knuckles. Serum calcium concentration is 1.9 mmol/L (7.5 mg/dL).

   Further investigation of the boy's disorder would be expected to reveal

   (A) antibodies to parathyroid and thyroid tissue
   (B) elevated parathyroid hormone concentration
   (C) diminished increase in urinary cyclic AMP in response to administration of parathyroid hormone
   (D) calcification of the basal ganglia
   (E) moniliasis

674. Protein malnutrition commonly occurs in association with energy-deficient diets because

   (A) diets low in carbohydrate and fat cause acute protein malabsorption
   (B) amino acids are diverted from protein synthesis into oxidative metabolism
   (C) normal protein synthesis requires an adequate energy supply
   (D) normal protein metabolism occurs only if fat in the diet is adequate
   (E) it is common for diets to be deficient in both protein and energy

675. A 34-year-old man with alcoholic cirrhosis is admitted to the hospital for evaluation of abdominal swelling, which has become progressively worse over the last 2 weeks. On physical examination, he is noted to be cachectic; the liver is enlarged, ascites and edema are present, and stool is heme-positive. Measurement of which of the following parameters would be useful in determining the extent of the man's *protein* malnutrition?

   (A) Blood ammonia concentration
   (B) Serum albumin and transferrin levels
   (C) Present body weight as a percentage of ideal body weight
   (D) Midarm circumference and triceps skin-fold thickness
   (E) Ratio of 24-h creatinine excretion to height

676. In which of the following situations is total parenteral nutrition (TPN) indicated as the *first* choice to provide partial or complete nourishment?

   (A) A 34-year-old man has an acute exacerbation of Crohn's disease and develops an ileocolic fistula
   (B) A 70-year-old woman has chest and limb injuries and extensive burns following an airplane crash
   (C) A 26-year-old woman has extensive small-bowel resection for life-threatening regional enteritis
   (D) A 53-year-old man scheduled to undergo elective surgery for gallstones will be unable to eat or drink for 5 days
   (E) A 26-year-old woman is unable to swallow because of a relapse of myasthenia gravis

677. Appropriate dietary restrictions have been successful in treating patients who have which of the following inherited metabolic disorders?

(A) Phenylketonuria
(B) Familial lipoprotein lipase deficiency
(C) Hyperprolinemia
(D) Tay-Sachs disease
(E) Galactosemia

678. In a patient with hypercholesterolemia, which of the following may be an appropriate treatment to lower serum cholesterol concentration?

(A) Cholestyramine
(B) Nicotinic acid
(C) Lovastatin
(D) Gemfibrozil
(E) Low-cholesterol diet

679. Disorders associated with premature coronary heart disease include familial

(A) hypercholesterolemia
(B) hyperalphalipoproteinemia
(C) hypertriglyceridemia
(D) combined hyperlipidemia
(E) lipoprotein lipase deficiency

680. Hypertriglyceridemia is frequently encountered in patients with diabetes mellitus. True statements regarding this association include which of the following?

(A) Predisposition to both diseases may be independently inherited
(B) Insulin deficiency is a major factor contributing to the hypertriglyceridemia
(C) Some patients eventually need specific pharmacologic treatment for the hypertriglyceridemia
(D) Acute pancreatitis may occur with uncontrolled diabetes mellitus and elevation of the triglyceride levels
(E) Hypertriglyceridemia may resolve with adequate control of the diabetes

681. A 29-year-old obese man is referred because of hyperlipidemia. He consulted a dermatologist because of tuberous xanthomas in both elbows and yellowish discoloration of the palmar and digital creases. Serum cholesterol and triglyceride levels were 8.4 mmol/L (328 mg/dL) and 3.9 mmol/L (345 mg/dL), respectively. True statements regarding this patient include

(A) he has lipoprotein lipase deficiency
(B) weight loss is an important feature of management to reduce his lipid levels
(C) hypothyroidism or diabetes mellitus, or both, must be excluded by appropriate testing
(D) he is homozygous for a genetic defect of lipid metabolism
(E) clofibrate may be useful in the management of his hyperlipidemia

682. A 24-year-old woman presents because she is concerned that she has too much facial hair. She has irregular menstrual periods but takes no drugs, has no other complaints, and feels well. On examination she is slightly overweight and has a deep voice. There is mild facial cystic acne. There is increased hair on the upper lip and eyebrows, but no other facial hair. Chest hair and pubic hair are normal. The hair on the upper lip is not coarse and there is no frontal balding. Plasma testosterone is 1.7 nmol/L (0.5 ng/dL); plasma dehydroepiandrosterone sulfate is 17 µmol/L (6000 µg/L).

Which of the following disorders could the patient have?

(A) Adrenocortical carcinoma
(B) Polycystic ovaries
(C) Congenital adrenal hyperplasia
(D) Idiopathic hirsuitism
(E) Arrhenoblastoma

683. Which of the following abnormalities may be seen in patients with anorexia nervosa?

(A) Episodic LH release
(B) Elevated serum prolactin
(C) Depressed growth hormone levels
(D) Elevated plasma cortisol
(E) Increased reverse triiodothyronine (rT_3) levels

684. Characteristic manifestations of Nelson's syndrome (pituitary tumor arising after bilateral adrenalectomy) include

(A) hyperpigmentation
(B) erosion of the sella turcica
(C) increased urinary 17-ketosteroid excretion
(D) failure of high doses of dexamethasone to suppress plasma cortisol levels
(E) elevated plasma ACTH levels

685. True statements concerning the "sick euthyroid" syndrome include which of the following?

(A) Thyroid hormone production is usually normal
(B) Values for free thyroxine (T_4) index may be decreased, normal, or increased
(C) Serum total T_4 concentrations are usually normal or decreased
(D) Decreased production of triiodothyronine (T_3) is a consistent feature of the disorder
(E) Although serum levels of thyroid-binding globulin and thyroid-binding prealbumin may be decreased, decreased protein binding of thyroid hormones is caused principally by a circulating inhibitor of binding

686. In a 33-year-old woman who recently had an upper respiratory tract infection, symptoms of thyrotoxicosis develop. Her thyroid gland is exquisitely tender and nodular. The 24-h uptake of radioactive iodine is 2 percent. Appropriate treatment for this woman might include

(A) subtotal thyroidectomy
(B) administration of radioactive iodine
(C) administration of glucocorticoids
(D) administration of propranolol
(E) administration of phenobarbital

687. In a person who has Cushing's syndrome, the diagnosis of functioning adrenal carcinoma would be suggested by

(A) a palpable abdominal mass
(B) markedly increased urinary excretion of 17-ketosteroids
(C) high plasma levels of ACTH
(D) failure to suppress 17-hydroxycorticosteroid secretion with high-dose dexamethasone
(E) a doubling of urinary 17-hydroxycorticosteroid excretion after administration of metyrapone

688. A 52-year-old woman with systemic lupus erythematosus is about to be started on a long-term course of therapy with pharmacologic doses of glucocorticoids. Pretreatment evaluation should include

(A) chest x-ray and tuberculin skin test
(B) ACTH infusion test
(C) thoracic and lumbar spine films
(D) stool test for occult blood
(E) metyrapone test

689. A 30-year-old man, father of three children, has had progressive breast enlargement during the last 6 months. He does not use any drugs. Physical examination is remarkable only for bilateral gynecomastia: testicular size is normal. Evaluation at this time should include

(A) blood sampling for SGOT and serum alkaline phosphatase and bilirubin levels
(B) blood sampling for plasma estradiol, testosterone, and LH levels
(C) a 24-h urine collection for measurement of 17-ketosteroids
(D) chromosomal karyotype
(E) breast biopsy

690. True statements concerning type 1 diabetes mellitus include which of the following?

(A) Direct vertical transmission has been shown by pedigree analysis to occur with a high prevalence

(B) The concordance rate for monozygotic twins less than 40 years of age is over 80 percent

(C) The risk of type 1 diabetes is increased in persons carrying HLA antigens B8, B15, DR3, or DR4

(D) Circulating islet-cell antibodies are usually present in patients with juvenile-onset type 1 diabetes studied either soon before or soon after the onset of symptoms

(E) Mumps virus and coxsackievirus have been identified as possible causative agents in juvenile-onset type 1 diabetes

691. The diagnosis of diabetes mellitus is certain in which of the following situations?

(A) Abnormal oral glucose tolerance in a 24-year-old woman who has been dieting

(B) Successive fasting plasma glucose concentrations of 8, 9, and 8.5 mmol/L (147, 165, and 152 mg/dL) in an asymptomatic, otherwise healthy businesswoman

(C) Hyperglycemic ketoacidosis that developed in an 18-year-old man after surgical reduction of a fractured leg

(D) Persistent asymptomatic glycosuria in a 30-year-old woman

(E) Hyperglycemic hyperosmolar coma that developed in a 73-year-old man after a stroke

692. Characteristics of hyperosmolar coma include

(A) blood glucose concentration of 55 mmol/L (975 mg/dL)

(B) marked elevation of serum free fatty acids

(C) association with thrombosis and bleeding from disseminated intravascular coagulation

(D) occurrence in elderly persons with maturity-onset diabetes

(E) best initial therapeutic response with large volumes of free water and large doses of insulin

693. A 45-year-old woman has had diabetes for the last 8 years and has been treated with either oral hypoglycemic agents or insulin. She has been doing well on human NPH insulin for the last several months. However, in the last week she has developed symptoms of hyperglycemia. Doubling her insulin dosage does not help, and she is admitted to the hospital. Physical examination of this nonobese woman shows no sign of infection, ketoacidosis, or Cushing's syndrome. Following admission, insulin dosage is increased progressively to 240 units daily, but blood glucose concentration never falls below 19 mmol/L (350 mg/dL).

True statements regarding this woman's condition include which of the following?

(A) IgG anti-insulin antibodies are likely to be present in high titer

(B) Cell-surface insulin receptors are likely to be decreased in number

(C) Anti-insulin-receptor antibodies, increased erythrocyte sedimentation rate, and other signs of autoimmune disease are likely to be present

(D) Insulin desensitization procedures should be instituted

(E) Treatment should include high-dose prednisone

694. Which of the following would be associated with a poor prognosis for development of (or progression of) symptomatic renal failure in a 29-year-old woman who has had type 1 diabetes mellitus since the age of 14 years?

(A) Urine albumin excretion of 0.12 to 0.17 g/d on three separate occasions
(B) Urine protein excretion of 0.55 to 0.62 g/d on three separate occasions
(C) Diastolic blood pressure of 110 to 123 mmHg
(D) Nocturia, 3 times per night
(E) Insulin requirement greater than 120 units per day

695. A 40-year-old physician's assistant has had episodic confusion, diaphoresis, and palpitations for the past 4 weeks. She has had several nightmares and three syncopal episodes. Fasting hypoglycemia with inappropriately elevated plasma insulin concentration is documented in the hospital. Plasma C-peptide concentration also is increased. Her physician should

(A) measure plasma insulin antibody levels
(B) measure plasma proinsulin levels
(C) measure plasma or urine sulfonylurea levels
(D) perform abdominal CT scan
(E) consult a surgeon for pancreatic surgery

696. Causes of fasting hypoglycemia due primarily to overutilization of glucose include

(A) carnitine deficiency
(B) hepatoma
(C) insulinoma
(D) congestive heart failure from cor pulmonale
(E) hypopituitarism

697. Testosterone replacement in a patient with Klinefelter syndrome (47,XXY) would be indicated in order to

(A) maintain spermatogenesis
(B) prevent antisocial behavior
(C) maintain sexual potency
(D) cause disappearance of gynecomastia
(E) promote virilization

698. Correctly matched deficiencies of specific trace elements and their recognized features include

(A) zinc deficiency: hyperkeratosis and alopecia
(B) zinc deficiency: gonadal atrophy
(C) copper deficiency: fever
(D) cobalt deficiency: anemia
(E) selenium deficiency: heart failure

699. Increased gonadal production of estrogen is characteristic of

(A) testicular feminization
(B) polycystic ovarian disease
(C) persistent follicle cyst
(D) third trimester of pregnancy
(E) arrhenoblastoma

700. Known causes of ambiguous genitalia include

(A) the sex-chromosome pattern XYY
(B) the mosaic sex-chromosome pattern 45,X/46,XY
(C) single gene mutations that impair androgen action
(D) hypogonadotropic hypogonadism
(E) maternal ingestion of a virilizing drug during pregnancy

701. True statements describing persons who have Klinefelter syndrome include which of the following?

(A) They are 20 times as likely as normal men to develop breast cancer

(B) They may have a normal peripheral-blood karyotype and testes of average size

(C) They have an increased incidence of hypospadias

(D) They almost always are mentally deficient and socially maladjusted

(E) Diagnosis usually is not made until after puberty

702. A 40-year-old woman with known alcoholism is hospitalized because of dizziness and muscle aches. Serum phosphorus concentration is 0.3 mmol/L (0.9 mg/dL) several days after admission. Clinical signs and symptoms associated with hypophosphatemia include

(A) waddling gait

(B) irritability and apprehension

(C) elevated concentration of serum creatine phosphokinase

(D) bacterial infection

(E) congestive cardiomyopathy

703. Correct statements concerning hypervitaminosis D include which of the following?

(A) It may result from prolonged sun exposure

(B) It usually results from a single excessive dose of vitamin D_2 or D_3

(C) Consequences include hypercalcemia, hypercalciuria, and renal impairment

(D) Anephric patients can develop vitamin D toxicity

(E) Serum 1,25(OH) vitamin D levels are elevated

704. A 25-year-old woman presents to her internist complaining of fatigue. Though she does not seem to be depressed, she admits to a diminished appetite and loss of interest in sex. She is also intolerant of the cold and notes that her hair is falling out. She has trouble caring for her 1½-year-old child and recounts a very difficult parturition with a great deal of blood loss. She is on no medicines, has been amenorrheic since the birth of the child, and did not nurse the infant.

Which of the following tests would help to diagnose her problem?

(A) Measurement of growth hormone 1 h after insulin administration

(B) Measurement of plasma cortisol 1 h after insulin administration

(C) Measurement of urinary free cortisol

(D) Thyroid function tests and TSH

(E) ACTH stimulation test

705. Manifestations of hypothyroidism include

(A) diminished QRS voltage on ECG

(B) depressed serum cholesterol

(C) microcytic anemia

(D) increased serum creatine phosphokinase

(E) increased serum lactic dehydrogenase

706. Which of the following would be appropriate in the initial management of patients with diabetic ketoacidosis?

(A) Administer insulin intravenously until the acidosis is reversed

(B) Discontinue insulin therapy when plasma glucose levels approach normal

(C) Increase insulin dosage when plasma ketones rise

(D) Administer 5% glucose solution when the plasma glucose falls below 17 mmol/L (300 mg/dL)

(E) Infuse potassium chloride if the presenting serum potassium level is normal

707. A 25-year-old man presents with a several-month history of fatigue, weakness, anorexia, and nausea. Physical examination reveals a slightly emaciated, thin, tanned man whose baseline blood pressure is 90/60. He complains of extreme lightheadedness during the assessment of orthostatic vital signs. Laboratory evaluation reveals hyponatremia and hyperkalemia. Plasma cortisol level fails to rise significantly 60 min after intramuscular administration of 250 μg cosyntropin.

Which of the following conditions could have caused this clinical picture?

(A) Withdrawal from prolonged (> 1 year) administration of steroids for asthma
(B) Disseminated tuberculosis
(C) Craniopharyngioma
(D) Disseminated cytomegalovirus infection
(E) Esophageal candidiasis requiring long-term high-dose ketoconazole therapy

708. Established complications of oral contraceptive use include

(A) deep venous thrombosis
(B) thromboembolic stroke
(C) hypertension
(D) endometrial cancer
(E) breast cancer

709. In which of the following disorders of incomplete sexual development in the male would testosterone production be normal or high?

(A) Deficiency of 17β-hydroxysteroid oxioreductase
(B) Testicular feminization
(C) Deficiency of 5α-reductase
(D) Deficiency of 17,20-lyase
(E) Reifenstein syndrome

710. In which of the following porphyria syndromes may the diagnosis be made on the basis of a positive Watson-Schwartz reaction in the urine (detection of porphobilinogen)?

(A) Intermittent acute porphyria
(B) Congenital erythropoietic porphyria
(C) Protoporphyria
(D) Porphyria cutanea tarda
(E) Variegate porphyria

711. Correct statements concerning inherited defects of metabolism include which of the following?

(A) Niemann-Pick disease is caused by a deficiency of glucosylceramidase and is associated with a characteristic bone marrow storage cell
(B) The incidence of disease due to hexosaminidase deficiency has been reduced in North America by heterozygote detection programs
(C) Errors in glycogen elongation or branching are incompatible with a normal life expectancy
(D) Early diagnosis of phenylketonuria is possible, but of little therapeutic benefit
(E) Cystinuria, the most common inborn error of amino acid transport, is associated with increased urinary excretion of all dibasic amino acids

Endocrine, Metabolic, and Genetic Disorders

Answers

583. The answer is B. *(Chap 345.)* In persons with symptomatic hemochromatosis, repeated phlebotomy, by removing excessive iron stores, results in marked clinical improvement. Specifically, the liver and spleen decrease in size, liver function improves, cardiac failure is reversed, and skin pigmentation ("bronzing") diminishes. Carbohydrate intolerance may abate in up to half of all affected persons. For unknown reasons there is no improvement in the arthropathy or the hypogonadism (due to pituitary deposition of iron) associated with hemochromatosis. Five-year survival rate is increased from 33 to 90 percent with treatment; prolonged survival may actually increase the risk of hepatocellular carcinoma, which affects one-third of persons treated for hemochromatosis. However, if phlebotomy is begun in the precirrhotic stage, which is possible with effective genetic screening, liver cancer will not develop.

584. The answer is B. *(Chap 337.)* Although non-insulin-dependent diabetes mellitus disease (nonketogenic) is familial, the exact mode of inheritance is not known except for the specific variant known as maturity-onset diabetes of the young (MODY), manifested by mild hyperglycemia without ketosis. Based on family studies, this disease is inherited in an autosomal dominant fashion with almost complete penetrance. Therefore, 50 percent of the children of a diabetic parent with MODY will develop the disease. There is linkage between MODY and mutations in the glucokinase gene located on the short arm of chromosome 7. This abnormality is not present in ordinary nonketotic diabetics. Unlike the case in insulin-dependent diabetes, no HLA relationships have been identified. Moreover, an autoimmune etiology for the disease is not felt to be important, which is also a distinctive feature compared with typical juvenile-onset insulin-dependent diabetes.

585. The answer is A. *(Chap 337. Dineen, N Engl J Med 327:707–713, 1992.)* In the normal postprandial state, food-derived increases in plasma glucose stimulate the secretion of insulin and suppress the secretion of glucagon. At this point, glucose uptake shifts from insulin-independent tissues such as the brain to insulin-dependent tissues such as the liver, muscle, and fat. The decrease in plasma glucagon in concert with the increase in plasma insulin decreases hepatic glucose output by suppression of glycogenolysis and gluconeogenesis (lipolysis is also suppressed). Therefore, muscle cells shift from oxidizing lipids to oxidizing glucose. In non-insulin-dependent diabetes mellitus the ingestion of carbohydrate causes a profound increase in plasma glucose levels. This increase is primarily due to defective suppression of postprandial hepatic glucose release. The reason that the liver releases increased levels of glucose in the diabetic may be accelerated gluconeogenesis, possibly on the basis of the lack of normal suppression of glucagon secretion or hepatic insulin resistance or both. An appropriately timed postprandial subcutaneous injection of insulin may normalize the suppression of hepatic glucose release. The oral hypoglycemic agents, such as the sulfonylureas, are unlikely to have this type of beneficial effect since, while they augment insulin secretion, the timing of such release would not be optimal.

586. The answer is B. *(Chap 60.)*   The genes responsible for X-linked recessive disorders, such as hemophilia A, nephrogenic diabetes insipidus, Duchenne's muscular dystrophy, and testicular feminization, are on the X chromosome. Males, who are XY, will demonstrate the full syndrome whenever they inherit the altered gene from a mother who is heterozygous (or rarely homozygous). Homozygously affected females can only arise from the union of an affected male and a carrier (or homozygous) female. Thus, the disease tends to be seen in uncles and nephews rather than fathers and sons. In fact, an affected father cannot give rise to affected males, since they will inherit his Y chromosome. Assuming marriage to a normal female, all the affected male's female offspring will be carriers, since they will all get the single abnormal gene from their father. A female carrier (having one of her two X chromosomes carrying the mutant allele) will have sons with a 50 percent chance of being affected and daughters with a 50 percent chance of being carriers.

587. The answer is C. *(Chap 397. Gold, Emerg Med Clin North Am 10:249, 1992.)*   Coral snakes rarely bite humans, but when they do the potent neurotoxin can cause death. If it is suspected that a person has been envenomed, antivenin should be given without waiting for systemic manifestations to develop. The bite of a coral snake, though it causes little pain and swelling, produces local numbness and weakness in the region of the bite; ataxia, ptosis, palatal and pharyngeal paralysis, and other neurologic symptoms may follow. If the extremity is not promptly immobilized with a proximal constrictive band after a bite, a significant amount of toxin may be absorbed. Ice, no longer a recommended treatment for snake bite, does not neutralize the toxin. Incision and section or wide surgical debridement are no longer thought necessary.

588. The answer is B. *(Chap 337. The Diabetes Control and Complications Trial Research Group, N Engl J Med 329:977-986, 1993.)*   After many years of uncertainty, the recently reported NIH-sponsored multicenter Diabetes Control and Complications Trial established that intensive therapy was more effective than standard therapy in reducing the development of retinopathy, the progression of retinopathy in patients who already had mild disease, and the occurrence of microalbuminuria and clinical neuropathy. There was, however, an increased likelihood of severe hypoglycemia despite the intensive monitoring practiced in the treated group. Enrollment required the presence of insulin-dependent diabetes mellitus for 1 to 5 years; therefore, these results cannot be definitively generalized to all patients with diabetes, although it is possible that patients with non-insulin-dependent diabetes mellitus might also benefit by strict glucose control. Patients on the intensively treated arm of this trial exhibited better control of blood glucose levels and lower levels of glycosylated hemoglobin. However, return of blood glucose to normal was not achieved. Moreover, patients who undertake such intensive therapy must be highly motivated and capable of withstanding its rigors, both physical and emotional.

589. The answer is E. *(Chap 337.)*   There is no current data to support the notion that the sulfonylureas increase death from heart attacks. Sulfonylureas act by stimulating release of insulin from the pancreatic beta cell. However, while the initial action of such drugs is to increase insulin release, as glucose concentrations fall, insulin levels also decrease because the major stimulus of insulin release (plasma glucose) is no longer present. Therefore, it is unlikely that this patient with hypoglycemia has elevated insulin levels. The newer sulfonylureas, such as glipizide and glyburide, are really no different than agents in longer use such as chlorpropamide and tolbutamide except that they are effective in smaller doses. The hypoglycemic effect of the sulfonylureas is at least 24 h. Though hypoglycemia is less common with these oral agents than with insulin treatment, when hypoglycemia occurs, it requires hospitalization and administration of prolonged glucose infusions to guard against rebound hypoglycemia.

590. The answer is C. *(Chap 337.)* Hypoglycemia is common in patients with type 1 diabetes mellitus, particularly when aggressive efforts are made to bring the fasting glucose concentrations into the normal range and to control postprandial hyperglycemia. Hypoglycemia can worsen diabetic control, in large part by triggering the release of counterregulatory hormones, such as glucagon. This phenomenon of "hypoglycemic hyperglycemia," called the Somogyi effect, should be suspected when wide swings in blood or urine sugar levels occur over a short period of time. Other clues suggesting a Somogyi effect are worsening of diabetic control as insulin dosage is increased and increased hunger and weight gain despite worsening hyperglycemia or glycosuria. By contrast, poor control due to underdosage of insulin usually causes weight loss from caloric wastage in the urine (ketonuria and glycosuria). The correct therapy for the man described in this question is to decrease the morning dose of NPH insulin rather than to administer more or different insulin, to treat the rebound hyperglycemia, or to decrease food intake at supper.

591. The answer is D. *(Chaps 48, 340.)* Progesterone therapy results in secretory differentiation of an estrogen-primed proliferative endometrium, and the endometrium is sloughed following progesterone withdrawal only if it has been stimulated first by estrogen. Thus, in a woman being evaluated for secondary amenorrhea, the appearance of menses following a short course of progesterone is indicative of an estrogen-primed endometrium and is good evidence of ovarian estrogen secretion. Estrone levels do not reflect direct ovarian estrogen secretion because estrone is derived principally from the peripheral conversion of androstenedione, which is secreted from the adrenal glands as well as the ovaries. A woman with amenorrhea caused by hypogonadotropic hypogonadism has deficient ovarian estrogen secretion but may demonstrate an increase in plasma estradiol following human chorionic gonadotropin (hCG) administration. Prolactin secretion is increased by estrogen stimulation, accounting for a slightly higher mean prolactin level in women compared with that in men. However, a normal prolactin level is not evidence of persistent estrogen secretion.

592. The answer is C. *(Chap 337. Nathan, N Engl J Med 328:1676–1685, 1993.)* Nephropathy is a leading cause of death in diabetic patients. Diabetic nephropathy may be functionally silent for 10 to 15 years. Clinically detectable diabetic nephropathy begins with the development of microalbuminuria (30 to 300 mg of albumin per 24 h). The glomerular filtration rate may actually be elevated at this stage. Only after the passage of additional time will the proteinuria be overt enough (0.5 g/L) to be detectable on standard urine dipsticks. Microalbuminuria precedes nephropathy in patients with both non-insulin and insulin-dependent diabetes. An increase in kidney size may also accompany the initial hyperfiltration stage. Once the proteinuria becomes significant enough to be detected by dipstick, a steady decline in renal function occurs with the glomerular filtration rate falling an average of 1 mL per minute per month. Therefore, azotemia begins about 12 years after the diagnosis of diabetes. Hypertension clearly is an exacerbating factor for diabetic nephropathy.

593. The answer is A. *(Chap 331.)* Growth hormone, also known as somatotropin, is secreted by somatotroph cells, which account for 50 percent of the anterior pituitary glands. Release of growth hormone from the anterior pituitary is pulsatile in nature, increasing after meals, with exercise, or during slow-wave sleep. Growth hormone, necessary for normal growth, exerts its effects through mediators such as somatomedins or insulin-like growth factors. In addition to its involvement in growth, somatotropin is also involved in stimulating incorporation of amino acids into protein and inhibiting glucose uptake by tissues. By the latter effect, growth hormone helps to restore low blood sugars to normal and is therefore a counter-regulatory hormone to insulin. Both hypoglycemia and insulin stimulate growth hormone release, as does the presence of free amino acids such as arginine. Hypothalamic secretagogues also control growth hormone release. These molecules include the stimulatory hormone, growth hormone–releasing hormone, and the inhibitory hormone, somatostatin (somatotropin release–inhibitory factor). The former is probably more important, since section of the pathways between the hypothalamus and the anterior pituitary results in inhibition of growth hormone release. Other neurotransmitters influence growth hormone release, including hypothalamus-derived dopamine, which stimulates growth hormone–releasing hormone. Alpha-adrenergic agonists stimulate growth hormone release and alpha-adrenergic blockers inhibit growth hormone increases. Serotonin agonists stimulate growth hormone release, which perhaps accounts for the nocturnal surge in growth hormone secretion.

594. The answer is D. *(Chaps 48, 340.)* In a 7-year-old girl, isosexual precocity that is associated with undetectable levels of gonadotropins and urinary 17-ketosteroid levels appropriate for her chronologic age is most likely due to an estrogen-secreting tumor. Tumor localization procedures, such as abdominal CT scanning and pelvic sonography, should be performed before laparotomy. Plasma androstenedione measurement is unlikely to be helpful if urinary 17-ketosteroid excretion is low or normal. In idiopathic precocious puberty, a diagnosis of exclusion, urinary gonadotropins are either normal for chronologic age or elevated; in addition, if plasma gonadotropins are measured frequently during a 24-h period, the characteristic pubertal nocturnal surge should be seen in patients with idiopathic precocious puberty.

595. The answer is D. *(Chap 62.)* Most autosomal chromosomal trisomies cause death in utero. Among live-born infants with trisomies (21, 18, and 13), trisomies 18 and 13 cause death in infancy. Patients with trisomy 21 (Down's syndrome) may reach adulthood, although with a shortened life expectancy because of an increased incidence of severe infections and complications from associated malformations. On the other hand, sex chromosome trisomies are compatible with intrauterine survival and are usually associated with a normal life expectancy.

596. The answer is D. *(Chap 331.)* Growth hormone excess in adults results in a clinical syndrome known as acromegaly, an insidious disease characterized by bony and soft tissue overgrowth, enlargement of the jaw and tongue, wide spacing of the teeth, and coarsened facial features. Hypertension may occur due to expansion of plasma volume and total body sodium. Laryngeal hypertrophy leads to a hollow sounding voice. A moist, oily, doughy handshake is also characteristic. Because of the slow onset, relatives and friends who see the patient daily may not notice these changes. The diagnosis is more likely to be made by those who have not seen the patient before or for many years.

Laboratory abnormalities include abnormal glucose tolerance, hypercalciuria, hyperphosphatemia, and hyperprolactinemia. The reason for growth hormone excess in virtually all patients with acromegaly is a pituitary adenoma. Useful screening tests for the diagnosis of acromegaly include measurements of glucose-suppressed growth hormone concentrations (60 min after the oral administration of 100 g glucose, growth hormone normally should be suppressed to a value less than 2 μg/L). IGF-I concentrations are elevated secondary to the high levels of growth hormone. Once a laboratory test has confirmed the clinical suspicion of acromegaly, MRI or CT scanning should be undertaken to define the presumptive pituitary adenoma.

597. The answer is E. *(Chap 336.)* Since provocative testing has little role in the diagnosis of pheochromocytoma, the most frequently employed assays include measurement of catecholamines or catecholamine metabolites in a single 24-h urine sample. The three assays used include measurement of vanillylmandelic acid, metanephrines, and unconjugated (or "free") catecholamines. Accuracy of diagnosis depends on collection of a full 24-h urine sample that is treated with acid and refrigerated during and after the collection. The diagnostic yield would be increased if the 24-h urine collection included a time period during which the patient experienced a hypertensive paroxysm. False positive increases in urinary free catecholamine excretion may occur if the patient is taking methyldopa, levodopa, or sympathomimetic amines. Endogenous plasma and urinary catecholamines may also be increased during hypoglycemia, strenuous exercise, and significant central nervous system disease. Urinary metanephrines and vanillylmandelic acid are also falsely positive in situations when endogenous catecholamines may be increased or if the patient is receiving a monoamine oxidase inhibitor. Since plasma catecholamines are highly subject to endogenous variation in catecholamine secretion, they have not been particularly useful as an initial screening test for the diagnosis of pheochromocytoma.

598. The answer is B. *(Chaps 60, 65, 241.)*   Many autosomal dominant disorders vary in the time of onset and severity of expression. Therefore, persons such as the two apparently unaffected siblings who are at risk for development of hereditary nephritis, even in the absence of overt evidence of renal impairment, are poor renal donor candidates. In addition, the mother is clearly a carrier and a poor candidate. The father is the best close relative to evaluate as a potential donor.

599. The answer is C. *(Chap 333.)*   The release of antidiuretic hormone, also known as arginine vasopressin, is stimulated by increased serum osmolarity (as detected by hypothalamic receptors), decreases in plasma volume, hypotension, stress, emesis, and pain, as well as drugs such as vincristine, vinblastine, and cyclophosphamide. Deficiency of antidiuretic hormone release, which may be caused by neoplastic or infiltrative lesions of the hypothalamus, pituitary surgery (in which polyuria develops between 1 and 6 days after the procedure), or severe head injuries, results in diabetes insipidus. Polyuria, excessive thirst, and polydipsia are the cardinal manifestations of this condition. Urine volume is large (more than 6 L per day) and urinary concentrations are generally low with osmolalities below 290 mosm/kg. If patients have access to water, normal function of the thirst center insures that the water intake closely matches the polyuria, so serum sodium may be normal or only mildly elevated. If patients cannot replenish free water, dangerously high levels of serum sodium may be reached. A diagnosis of central diabetes insipidus is usually best established by a dehydration test. Fluids must be withheld long enough to result in stable hourly urinary osmolalities (aiming for an hourly increase of less than 30 mosm/kg for at least 3 h in succession). When the urine osmolality is stable, the patient should be given antidiuretic hormone either by subcutaneous injection or nasal spray. Urine osmolality is determined immediately before the injection of antidiuretic hormone and is then measured on a specimen collected between 30 and 60 min after the injection. In central diabetes insipidus, the urine osmolality should rise by at least 9 percent after the injection of antidiuretic hormone.

600. The answer is D. *(Chap 61.)*   One of the most important techniques for identifying genomic sites responsible for inherited diseases and for prenatal diagnosis is the identification of restriction fragment length polymorphisms (RFLPs). Such RFLP sites are the consequences of variable sequences that may or may not allow a specific restriction endonuclease (an enzyme recognizing a specific, usually four-to-seven-base DNA sequence) to cut at that site. In the Southern blots of the depicted family, the parents are heterozygous for a restriction site that is 2 kb away from one nonpolymorphic site and 8 kb away from another nonpolymorphic site in the other direction (which is the section the probe recognizes). In one of each of the parents' chromosomes the polymorphic site is present; in the other chromosome it is not. Thus, upon digestion of the parents' DNA, both a 10-kb fragment, representing the chromosome that lacks the polymorphic site, and an 8-kb fragment, representing the chromosome that has this site, exist. The son has inherited the chromosome with the site present from both his father and his mother, while the daughter has inherited the chromosome without the sequence that does not allow the extra cut from both parents. If the polymorphic sequence that allows cutting were associated with an autosomal recessive disease (by virtue of its being proximate on the genome), then such a marker could be used to predict the presence of the disease in the son or a fetus with a similar pattern on Southern blotting of DNA.

601. The answer is B.   *(Chap 6.)*   Pregnancy resembles the fasting state in that blood sugar and amino acid levels tend to be low, while free fatty acids, ketones, and triglycerides are increased. If fasting lasts longer than 12 h, plasma glucose may fall to 40 to 45 mg/dL (2.2 to 2.5 mmol/L) and levels of hydroxybutyrate and acetoacetate rise 2 to 4 times higher than in nonpregnant women. Therefore, ketoacidosis in the absence of profound hyperglycemia may occur in pregnant diabetics. However, pregnancy also tends to elicit glucose intolerance due to the development of insulin resistance on the basis of elevation of progesterone, estrogen, prolactin, or human placental lactogen. Most patients with gestational diabetes can be treated with diet; however, following delivery at least 30 percent of women so afflicted will develop diabetes mellitus within 5 years. Though children of pregnant diabetics are at higher risk for infant mortality and congenital anomalies than offspring of normal women, careful glucose control reduces the incidence of such problems. Women with diabetic nephropathy also have a reasonable chance to have a normal pregnancy; no evidence suggests that pregnancy worsens renal function.

602. The answer is E.   *(Chaps 77, 377.)*   Causes of thiamine deficiency in alcoholic persons include poor dietary intake, impaired absorption and storage, and accelerated destruction of thiamine diphosphate. Both the cardiovascular and the neurologic signs of thiamine deficiency (beriberi) can become abruptly evident following the administration of glucose to thiamine-depleted, asymptomatic persons. Nystagmus, ataxia, and confusion, often accompanied by ophthalmoplegia, are strongly suggestive of Wernicke's encephalopathy; cardiovascular involvement may be signaled by tachycardia as an early manifestation of peripheral vasodilation. Thiamine should be administered promptly—and preferably before glucose is given—to any person in whom subclinical thiamine deficiency is suspected.

603. The answer is E.   *(Chap 76.)*   The first decision regarding the administration of a dietary formula is the choice of route. In the case presented, the underlying disorder (hemorrhagic pancreatitis) and recent abdominal surgery are contraindications to enteral therapy. Both lipids and carbohydrates may be infused with amino acids to meet metabolic needs, but several considerations should be taken into account in choosing which mixture to use. First is osmolality—concentrated glucose solutions are hypertonic and cause peripheral vein thrombosis. Another factor is the metabolic state of the patient; both pancreatic insufficiency and hyperglycemia are relative contraindications to using hypertonic glucose solutions. Second, carbohydrate as the sole source of calories raises the metabolic rate and thus the production of carbon dioxide; in a patient being weaned from ventilatory assistance, giving more nonprotein calories as fat reduces CO_2 excretion. Third, lipid infusions provide essential fatty acids, and because lipids do not raise insulin levels or require insulin for metabolism, they may be discontinued abruptly (e.g., if emergency surgery is needed) without risk of hypoglycemia. In summary, a regimen providing 85 percent of nonprotein calories as lipid and 15 percent as glucose is near isotonic and probably optimal in the case described.

604. The answer is B.   *(Chap 346.)*   Acute attacks of abdominal pain that are often precipitated by diet or drugs such as barbiturates, sulfonamides, anticonvulsants, or alcohol and that have no clear-cut etiology despite an aggressive diagnostic workup may be due to acute intermittent porphyria. The porphyrias are inherited or acquired disorders of heme biosynthesis. Acute intermittent porphyria, due to an autosomal dominant mutation, is characterized by a half-normal level of HMB synthase (the enzyme that catalyzes the condensation of four pyrrole porphobilinogen molecules to form the linear tetrapyrrole hydroxymethylbilane, which ultimately undergoes cyclization). Heterozygotes are also prone to a host of sympathomimetic symptoms and psychological problems in addition to recurrent abdominal pain. Peripheral neuropathy, due to axonal degeneration of motor neurons, may also occur. The diagnostic test of choice is demonstration of increased urinary pyrrole porphobilinogen excretion, as well as increased levels of urinary δ-aminolevulinic acid. Usually there is no skin disease, even upon sun exposure. During acute attacks, narcotics may be given without fear of exacerbation of the attack; phenothiazines may also be administered safely. Heme therapy, presumably by including feedback inhibition of early heme biosynthesis, can abrogate attacks. On the other hand, recovery from the severe motor neuropathy may take years.

605. The answer is E. *(Chap 339.)* Evaluation of male infertility begins with the physical examination to ensure that there is no evidence for inadequate androgenization, such as incomplete development of the male hair pattern or of primary sexual organs. Secondly, evidence of hyperestrogenemia, manifested by gynecomastia, should be excluded. A low sperm count could be due to hypothalamic or pituitary dysfunction that results in inappropriately low levels of gonadotropin-releasing hormone or of follicle-stimulating hormone (FSH), which helps to control spermatogenesis. If testicular failure has resulted in impaired spermatogenesis, then the plasma FSH level should be elevated. This patient with a normal plasma FSH and no evidence of testicular dysfunction on biopsy may well have an obstruction of the vas deferens, which may be surgically correctable.

606. The answer is D. *(Chap 77.)* The combination of peripheral neuritis, dermatitis, glossitis, microcytic anemia, and convulsions suggests the presence of pyridoxine deficiency. Naturally occurring pyridoxine deficiency is rare, owing to the widespread distribution of the vitamin in food. Clinical deficiency is frequent, however, because many commonly used drugs act as pyridoxine antagonists. Pyridoxal phosphate is the active cofactor for numerous enzymatic reactions in amino acid metabolism and in heme synthesis; it is also important for normal neuronal excitability. Estrogens inhibit the role of pyridoxine in tryptophan metabolism, and hydrazines such as isoniazid can inhibit various enzymes that use pyridoxine as a cofactor and thereby induce convulsions. Cycloserine and penicillamine act similarly. The appropriate management for persons receiving drugs capable of causing pyridoxine deficiency is dietary supplementation (at least 30 mg of pyridoxine daily); overt deficiency, when present, requires immediate parenteral therapy.

607. The answer is B. *(Chap 77. Revler, JAMA 253:805, 1985.)* Humans, unlike many animals, are incapable of synthesizing ascorbic acid from D-glucose and require exogenous vitamin C. Ascorbic acid functions as a redox agent, and its most important role is in the synthesis of appropriately hydroxylated collagen. Features of scurvy result from defective collagen synthesis and include capillary fragility resulting in ecchymoses (due to impaired collagen formation in blood vessels), poor wound healing, and abnormal hair development. This syndrome is common in edentulous, elderly men who reside alone and ingest a diet deficient in milk, fruits, and vegetables. Resolution of bleeding occurs rapidly after administration of oral ascorbic acid. Vitamin A deficiency tends to produce night blindness and xerophthalmia. Bleeding is seen in vitamin K deficiency but should be accompanied by an elevated prothrombin time caused by impaired synthesis of clotting factors. The anemia of folate deficiency, often seen in concert with scurvy, is macrocytic. Patients with insufficient quantities of available pyridoxine can develop seizures.

608. The answer is C. *(Chap 351.)* Osteogenesis imperfecta, usually transmitted in an autosomal dominant fashion, results in brittle bones because of a generalized decrease in bone mass. Though the clinical course is variable, some patients have multiple fractures in childhood, undergo some remission during puberty, and then begin to suffer fractures again later in life. Associated abnormalities include blue sclerae, brown or translucent bluish-gray discoloration of the teeth, and progressive hearing loss. The family history is usually positive. The most common molecular defect is a mutation in one of the two genes coding for type I procollagen. Some mutations result in a decreased synthesis of proα I collagen genes, whereas other mutations result in the synthesis of structurally abnormal procollagen alpha chains. Most patients with Ehlers-Danlos syndrome have a defect in the synthesis of type III procollagen and those with chondrodysplasia have a defect in the gene for type II procollagen.

Type I collagen is the most abundant of the 18 different collagens thus far identified. It is composed of two identical chains: alpha I and alpha II. After procollagen chains are translated from messenger RNA in ribosomes, they pass into the rough endoplasmic reticulum where hydrophobic signal peptides at the *N* terminus are cleaved (resulting in up to a 50 percent reduction of protein mass). Additional posttranslational modification includes conversion of proline residues to hydroxyproline and hydroxylation of lysine residues. After the requisite number of posttranslational conversions, the protein can then fold into its native triple-helical conformation.

609. The answer is E. *(Chap 351.)* Marfan syndrome, inherited in an autosomal recessive fashion, is characterized by long, thin extremities, reduced vision due to dislocation of the lens (ectopia lentis), and proximal aortic aneurysms. This disease must be distinguished from homocysteinuria which may also cause ectopia lentis, congenital arachnodactyly, and familial aortic aneurysms. Patients with Marfan syndrome are usually tall and have severe chest deformities including pectus excavatum and pectus carinatum. Mitral valve proplapse and dilation of the aortic root are not uncommon and may be detected by echocardiography early in life. Most patients with Marfan syndrome have mutations in the gene for fibrillin, a glycoprotein of 350 kDa. Fibrillin is a major component of elastin-associated microfibrils, abundant in large blood vessels and the lens suspensory ligaments.

610. The answer is B. *(Chap 333.)* The evaluation of polyuric syndromes should include simultaneous measurements of urine and plasma osmolality. Ideally, the plasma osmolality should be elevated so that determination of an inappropriately dilute urine is possible. Such an effort may require an overnight water deprivation test. This test must be carried out carefully to insure that a dangerous level of dehydration does not occur. Once 1 kg of body weight is lost and the plasma osmolality is elevated, the finding of a urine osmolality stable for 3 h at a low level confirms the diagnosis of diabetes insipidus. At that point vasopressin is administered, and the urine osmolality is checked between 30 and 60 min thereafter. In cases of central diabetes insipidus, the rise in urine osmolality exceeds 9 percent, whereas in nephrogenic diabetes insipidus, frequently due to renal dysfunction as in the case presented, there is little, if any, increment. The treatment for nephrogenic diabetes insipidus consists of the administration of diuretics to cause a fall in glomerular filtration rate and a concomitant increase in proximal tubular fluid resorption, decreased distal fluid delivery, and diminished production of dilute urine. This therapeutic strategy should be accompanied by sodium restriction.

611. The answer is D. *(Chaps 356, 357.)* The hypercalcemia of sarcoidosis is usually associated with disseminated disease. Therefore, almost all persons with sarcoidosis who have hypercalcemia also have an abnormal chest x-ray (diffuse fibronodular infiltration or marked enlargement of hilar nodes, or both). This is an important point in the differential diagnosis of hypercalcemia—sarcoidosis is unlikely as a cause of hypercalcemia if the chest x-ray is normal. Hypergammaglobulinemia is another helpful clue to the presence of sarcoidosis. The hypercalcemia of sarcoidosis is thought to be the consequence of increased synthesis of $1,25(OH)_2$ vitamin D_3 and the subsequent increased intestinal absorption of calcium. Elevated serum calcium concentration in sarcoidosis causes a decreased level of serum parathyroid hormone, resulting in marked hypercalciuria.

612. The answer is E. *(Chap 74.)* A host of endocrinologic abnormalities may occur as a consequence of the loss of muscle mass and fat in patients with severe anorexia nervosa. The disease usually begins shortly after puberty and is characterized by profound weight loss due to lack of caloric intake, vomiting after eating, and a high level of physical activity. Other features include cold intolerance due to a secondary defect in regulatory thermogenesis, amenorrhea secondary to an impaired LH and FSH response to LHRH, hypokalemia, low serum immunoglobulins, normal or elevated growth hormone levels, decreased levels of somatomedin C, and low serum triiodothyronine concentrations. Again, all these abnormalities seem to result from, rather than cause, the eating disorder. Most authorities favor a psychiatric etiology on the basis of inadequate familial interpersonal relationships or the need for a patient to establish control in a dominating family. Unfortunately, the benefits of psychiatric intervention and behavior modification have been somewhat marginal. Hospitalization may be required to save the patient's life if the anorexia nervosa is quite severe, meaning that the weight is 35 percent below ideal.

613. The answer is B. *(Chap 73.)* Grossly obese patients are more likely than the nonobese to have high blood pressure, peripheral vascular disease, cerebrovascular disease, diabetes, and hyperlipidemia. The so-called Pickwickian syndrome, characterized by hypersomnolence during the day, is thought to be due to nocturnal upper airway obstruction that leads to hypoxemia and hypercapnia and causes arousal with each episode. This chronic arousal pattern at night causes sleep deprivation and daytime somnolence. The obese habitus, in addition to sleep-induced relaxation of the throat muscles, is believed to cause the aforementioned upper airway obstruction. These patients tend to develop blunted respiratory responses to hypercapnia and hypoxemia as well as ventilation-perfusion mismatches. Progestational agents stimulate the ventilatory response in such patients. Hyperinsulinemia, insulin resistance, diabetes, and hyperlipidemia may all be more common in obesity but are not believed to play a role in the obesity-hypoventilation syndrome or in daytime somnolence.

614. The answer is C. *(Chaps 245, 347.)* Colchicine is useful in the treatment of acute gouty arthritis but not chronic tophaceous gout. However, it can be a useful ancillary drug in treatment of chronic gout at the start of allopurinol therapy to prevent the precipitation of acute gouty arthritis. Chronic gout can be treated either with uricosuric agents (probenecid or sulfinpyrazone) or with an inhibitor of uric acid synthesis (allopurinol). The ideal candidate for uricosuric agents is a patient under the age of 60 years who has normal renal function, a uric acid excretion of less than 700 mg per day, and no history of renal stones. Specific indications for choosing allopurinol over a uricosuric agent include the presence of uric acid nephrolithiasis, high uric acid excretion, and impairment of renal function; hence, allopurinol is the appropriate initial drug in this patient. Combinations of allopurinol and uricosuric agents may be employed when uric acid levels cannot be controlled with either drug alone.

615. The answer is A. *(Chap 344.)* Whether hypertriglyceridemia in an overweight person is due to familial hypertriglyceridemia, multiple lipoprotein-type hyperlipidemia, or sporadic hypertriglyceridemia, the primary mode of therapy should be weight reduction. Dietary saturated fats should be restricted as part of the weight reduction regimen. Hypothyroidism and diabetes mellitus, if present, should be treated, and use of alcohol and oral contraceptives should be avoided. If these measures are inadequate, drug therapy with nicotinic acid or gemfibrozil should be tried. Bile acid–binding resins, such as cholestyramine or colestipol, are used in the treatment of hypercholesterolemia but are not useful for treating hypertriglyceridemia.

616. The answer is D. *(Chap 358. Riggs, N Engl J Med 327:620–627, 1992.)* The best approach to the treatment of osteoporosis is preventive. Measures include encouragement of weight bearing, abstention from cigarettes and alcohol, maintenance of adequate calcium intake, and estrogen replacement therapy at the time of menopause. If the estrogen therapy is to be given solely to prevent osteoporosis, authorities have suggested the use of bone densitometry to identify patients at particular risk. If a woman has already sustained vertebral fractures, it should be recognized that a great deal of bone loss has already occurred. The preferred regimen in such patients is supplemental calcium (1500 mg per day), a small vitamin D supplement, and estrogen therapy. Some patients may have side effects from estrogens, including vaginal bleeding, or contraindications to their use due to thrombotic events. Calcitonin is an acceptable substitute in women who cannot take estrogen. Sodium fluoride stimulates bone formation and increases bone mass, but may not reduce the risk of fractures. Bisphosphonates, such as etidronate, may prevent bone resorption, but their role in this setting has not yet been established.

617. The answer is D. *(Chap 347.)*   Uric acid is the end product of purine metabolism. The serum urate level depends upon dietary ingestion of purines, as well as endogenous sources of purine production. Such sources include de novo purine biosynthesis and "salvage" of purine bases by hypoxanthine phosphoribosyltransferase (HPRT). HPRT catalyzes the addition of phosphated sugars to purine bases to form the ribonucleotides inosine monophosphate and guanosine monophosphate. Increased salvage activity prevents de novo synthesis by reducing phosphoribosylpyrophosphate (PRPP) levels and thereby increasing the concentrations of the inhibitory ribonucleotides. A salvage pathway deficiency due to an increase in PRPP synthetase or to a decrease in HPRT function will cause the overproduction of purines from the 11-step de novo pathway. Therefore, persons deficient in HPRT develop hyperuricemia and nephrolithiasis, as well as gouty arthritis. Complete deficiency of HPRT, known as the Lesch-Nyhan syndrome, is also typified by self-mutilation and choreoathetosis.

618. The answer is D. *(Chap 334.)*   In most instances of hypothyroidism in adults, replacement therapy should be initiated with gradually increasing doses of thyroid hormone. However, in cases of neonatal, infantile, and juvenile hypothyroidism full replacement should be begun immediately to increase the chances of normal intellectual and anatomic development. In patients with secondary hypothyroidism or when coexistent adrenal insufficiency is suspected, it is important that thyroid replacement not be initiated until treatment with glucocorticoid has begun. Adrenocortical insufficiency can be precipitated by an increase in the clearance rate of glucocorticoids engendered by correction of the hypothyroid state.

619. The answer is E. *(Chap 334. Ridgeway, J Clin Endocrinol Metab 74:231, 1992.)*   The finding of a solitary thyroid nodule should raise the suspicion of thyroid carcinoma. However, surgery should be reserved for those patients in whom the diagnosis of thyroid cancer is definite or at least highly probable. Fine-needle aspiration is almost always the procedure of first choice in the evaluation of such solitary nodules. Surgery is indicated in the case of definite lymphoma or carcinoma (papillary, medullary, poorly differentiated, or follicular). If small groups of uniform, colloid-poor cells are seen, these inconclusive results should be met by repeating the fine-needle aspiration. If repeat results are similar, then a trial of levothyroxine suppression should be initiated and follow-up in 6 months planned. If there are sheets of follicular cells reported on pathology from the initial fine-needle aspiration, then the nodule could represent either follicular carcinoma or adenoma. In this situation, a radionuclide scan demonstrating a functioning nodule would be reassuring and merely mandate an evaluation for hyperthyroidism; a "cold" nodule would require subtotal thyroidectomy.

620. The answer is C. *(Chap 348.)*   The hallmark of Wilson's disease is the accumulation of excess copper deposits. The precise reason for this increased deposition of copper is not known, but serum ceruloplasmin levels are low because of secondary inhibition of formation of this protein due to the excess of copper. Whatever the reason, the ability of hepatocytes to store copper is exceeded and this mineral is ultimately released in the blood with subsequent uptake in extrahepatic sites including the brain and Descemet's membrane of the cornea (which produces the characteristic Kayser-Fleischer rings). Liver disease may take the form of acute hepatitis, fulminant hepatitis, cirrhosis, or chronic active hepatitis, as in this patient. Neurologic manifestations such as tremors, spasticity, chorea, drooling, and unusual psychiatric behavior may be primary. The diagnosis can be made because of a depressed serum concentration of ceruloplasmin in the presence of Kayser-Fleischer rings, or a low serum ceruloplasmin in the presence of an elevated hepatic concentration of copper determined on a liver biopsy specimen. The mainstay of therapy for Wilson's disease is orally administered penicillamine, which removes and detoxifies the excess copper deposits. Problems associated with penicillamine treatment include sensitivity as well as the need for lifelong therapy. The one contraindication to the use of penicillamine therapy is fulminant hepatitis (usually accompanied by Coombs-negative hemolytic anemia). This syndrome is almost always fatal if a liver transplant cannot be performed.

621. The answer is A. *(Chap 396.)* Arsenic toxicity may occur after exposure to inorganic arsenic compounds, which are used in insecticides, wood preservatives, and the glass manufacturing industry. Arsine gas is produced by metal smelting and refining, lead plating, and the manufacture of silicon microchips. Both acute and chronic toxicity due to ingestions may be noted. Arsine gas combines with globin to produce severe hemolysis with anemia, hemoglobinuria, and hematuria some 3 to 4 h after ingestion. Additional findings may include gastrointestinal complaints such as nausea, vomiting, and diarrhea as well as malaise, tachycardia, and dyspnea. Massive acute ingestions can lead to cardiovascular collapse, renal failure, delirium, coma, and seizures. Arsenic deposits may be seen on plain radiographs of the abdomen and in hair and nails for long periods after initial exposure. Other laboratory abnormalities may include abnormal results of liver function tests, electrocardiac abnormalities (QT prolongation and T-wave inversion), anemia, leukocytosis, leukopenia, hemoglobinemia, proteinuria, and cellular casts in the urine. Once the acute toxic ingestion is dealt with by induction of vomiting, arsenic chelation must be considered with agents such as dimercaprol. The best way to assess the results of treatment is by insuring that 24-h urine arsenic levels fall to less than 67 nmol.

622. The answer is D. *(Chap 344.)* Cholestyramine and colestipol are bile acid–binding resins that decrease the reabsorption of bile acids from the intestine, thus secondarily decreasing the enterohepatic circulation of cholesterol. The liver responds to the acid depletion by increasing the synthesis of bile acids. The additional cholesterol required for bile acid synthesis is obtained by the liver by increasing the number of receptors for low-density lipoproteins (LDL), which in turn lowers the plasma level of LDL. The most common side effects of these resins are constipation and bloating, although mild steatorrhea may occur when they are used in high doses.

623. The answer is A. *(Chaps 73, 75.)* Weight loss requires caloric deficit: the total number of calories consumed must be exceeded by the total number of calories expended as energy. Notwithstanding the claims for various "fad" diets, there is little evidence to support the efficacy of one type of hypocaloric diet over any other in achieving long-term weight loss. Basically a calorie is a calorie—whether from protein, fat, or carbohydrate. Liquid protein diets have been associated with a variety of adverse developments, including hyperuricemia, hypercholesterolemia, and sudden cardiovascular death. Total starvation diets are simpler to follow and lead to greater weight loss than hypocaloric diets, but adverse effects include increased loss of lean body mass, hypotension, and arrhythmias. Amphetamines act as weak anorexiants but are usually ineffective after several weeks; also, the risks of dependence and abuse are significant. Exercise is a useful adjunct to caloric restriction; it may increase lean body mass and improve the sense of well-being, but moderate exercise does not increase caloric expenditure sufficiently to alter the initial rate of weight loss if caloric restriction is not also undertaken.

624. The answer is B. *(Chap 395. Snilkstein, N Engl J Med 319:1557–1562, 1988.)* Once a significant dose of acetaminophen is ingested, the normal detoxifying pathways, namely sulfation and glucuronidation, become saturated. This process, however, depletes hepatic glutathione, an important protector against oxidative injury. Oxidants cause hepatic necrosis and, if the ingested dose is great enough, fatal hepatic failure. However, one cannot wait for evidence of abnormal transaminases to begin therapy. As is almost certainly the case with this patient given the high number of tablets ingested, a serum acetaminophen level is going to be high and indicate the need for antidote therapy. For patients who arrive within 4 h after the ingestion, initial treatment should include activated charcoal. This strategy does not interfere with the primary therapy, namely *N*-acetylcysteine. The earlier the treatment starts, the better off the patient will be. Therapy with *N*-acetylcysteine, if given orally, should be continued for 72 h.

625. The answer is C. *(Chap 395.)*   Ethylene glycol is an important component of antifreeze as well as hydraulic fluids and windshield cleaners. It is metabolized by alcohol dehydrogenase to glycoaldehyde and then successively oxidized to glycolic acid, glyoxylic acid, and oxalic acid. Ethanol, which is preferentially metabolized by alcohol dehydrogenase compared with ethylene glycol, may be used to prevent buildup of end-stage oxidative metabolites of ethylene glycol. Ethylene glycol is directly responsible for the CNS depression seen in an overdose with this agent. However, its metabolite, glycolic acid, is responsible for the metabolic acidosis, increased anion gap, and renal damage, which is frequently manifested as acute tubular necrosis. Oxalic acid may precipitate as calcium oxalate crystals in various locations including the brain, heart, and kidney. If patients do not suffer from the cardiopulmonary collapse that may acutely accompany a massive overdose, acute tubular necrosis, which occurs 12 to 24 h following ingestion, is usually reversible. In addition to supportive measures and ethanol infusions in cases of severe ingestions, hemodialysis will treat the complications of renal failure and also remove ethylene glycol from the circulation.

626. The answer is A. *(Chap 73.)*   Although only a minority of obese persons have diabetes mellitus, more than 80 percent of type 2 diabetics are obese. Obesity appears to be a major contributory factor to the development of diabetes, largely through its effects on insulin sensitivity. A clear relationship also exists between hypertension and obesity in adults, though the mechanism is unclear. Hypertriglyceridemia is associated commonly with obesity and correlates with the degree of obesity; increased hepatic production of very low-density lipoproteins (VLDL) from free fatty acids is felt to be the major cause of increased triglyceride levels in obese persons, although peripheral defects in VLDL clearance may be present in some. Weight loss can reduce or reverse all these complications. The prevalence of cholelithiasis is increased with increasing adiposity, but the same cannot be said of hypothyroidism—only a small percentage of hypothyroid persons are obese, and an even smaller fraction of obese persons are hypothyroid.

627. The answer is D. *(Chap 335.)*   Primary aldosteronism may be due to an aldosterone-producing adrenal adenoma, bilateral adrenal cortical nodular hyperplasia, or rarely adrenal carcinoma. The diagnosis should be suspected when mild diastolic hypertension, hypokalemia, and metabolic acidosis are present in a patient not taking diuretics. Peripheral edema is uncommon. Plasma renin activity should be suppressed by the chronically elevated aldosterone level, but suppressed renin activity (low after volume depletion maneuvers) also occurs in 25 percent of patients with essential hypertension. To make the diagnosis of primary aldosteronism in a patient with the above clinical features and a low plasma renin, the best test is measurement of plasma aldosterone following an attempt to suppress mineralocorticoid secretion by the infusion of saline. Once failure to suppress aldosterone secretion is demonstrated, then anatomic localization of the adenoma (or documentation of hyperplasia) should be attempted.

628. The answer is B. *(Chap 395.)*   Tricyclic compounds are commonly used in depressed patients and thus frequently employed during suicide attempts. Their primary mode of action may be to block the uptake of synaptic transmitters in the central nervous system, but the side effects are primarily due to their central and peripheral anticholinergic activity, peripheral alpha-blocking activity, and quinidine-like effects on the heart. In mild overdoses, anticholinergic effects, such as mydriasis, urinary retention, confusion, and tachycardia may be seen. In more significant overdoses, cardiac toxicity, seizures, and hypotension may occur. Arrhythmias, including ventricular tachyarrhythmias and bradycardias, are typical. Prolongation of the QRS complex to greater than 100 ms correlates with an increased risk of cardiac arrhythmias and seizures. Treatment includes gastric lavage, supportive care, anticonvulsants if seizures have occurred, and sodium bicarbonate, lidocaine, and phenytoin to treat ventricular tachyarrhythmia. Physostigmine, an acetylcholinesterase inhibitor, may reverse the anticholinergic effects of mild poisoning, but this drug should not be administered during severe poisoning because of the possibility of cardiac toxicity.

629. The answer is C. *(Chap 349. Beutler, N Engl J Med 325:1354, 1991.)* Gaucher's disease, an autosomal recessive syndrome, is caused by a deficiency of the enzyme glucocerebrosidase. Absence of this enzyme results in the accumulation of extremely insoluble glucocerebroside due to failure of lysosome-mediated glycolipid degradation. The gene encoding this enzyme is located on the long arm of chromosome 1. In North America, this disease is most commonly due to a point mutation of cDNA nucleotide 1226, typically found in Jewish persons of Eastern European origin. Though some types of Gaucher's disease can present with dramatic neurologic manifestations or cause death in early life, the most common type is the adult-onset, or type I, variety. The disease is manifested by hepatomegaly and splenomegaly, which may contribute to thrombocytopenia. Hepatic involvement can result in fibrosis and abnormal liver function. Bone involvement—particularly flaring of the distal femur, aseptic necrosis of the femoral heads, and bone infarcts—is a frequent complication. Laboratory abnormalities include pancytopenia, abnormal results of liver function tests, and elevation of serum acid phosphatase. While the diagnosis should be made on the basis of clinical presentation, bone marrow examinations are frequently performed to evaluate the associated hematologic abnormalities. Such an examination will invariably reveal the presence of so-called Gaucher's cells, which are storage macrophages that contain excessive amounts of glucocerebroside, identified as engorgement with a fine, scroll-like pattern. The diagnosis can be confirmed by determination of leukocyte beta-glucosidase activity. While splenectomy is effective in correcting the thrombocytopenia and anemia, the bone disease is, of course, unaffected by this procedure. A major recent change in the therapy of Gaucher's disease has been the availability of aglucerase, the commercially produced modified glucocerebrosidase (mannose-terminated). Therapy with this agent appears to be effective and safe; however, the cost can range to several hundred thousand dollars per year. Other potential therapeutic strategies include allogeneic transplantation or autologous transplantation of stem cells into which a normal glucocerebrosidase gene has been inserted. This gene transfer approach remains to be clinically applied.

630. The answer is C. *(Chap 336. Bravo, N Engl J Med 311:1298, 1984.)* Pheochromocytomas produce and secrete catecholamines, which may lead to paroxysmally high blood pressure. Approximately 80 percent of these tumors are solitary adrenal lesions, but 10 percent are bilateral and 10 percent are extraadrenal. Pheochromocytoma is also associated with familial multiple endocrine neoplasia types IIa and IIb (hyperparathyroidism and medullary carcinoma are the other endocrinologic manifestations). Once the diagnosis is confirmed, usually by documenting excess urinary catecholamine metabolites over a 24-h period plus localization by CT scanning, it is important to prepare the patient for surgery by preventing the effects of catecholamine release by treatment with phenoxybenzamine, a long-acting alpha-adrenergic blocker. Liberal salt intake should also be instituted to help restore the contracted plasma volume to normal prior to surgery. Beta-blockers should not be given before alpha blockade has been established because of the potential for hypertension due to the antagonism of beta-mediated vasodilation in skeletal muscle beds. However, propranolol is useful in treating the reflex tachycardia induced by phenoxybenzamine. While prazosin is an effective agent for the treatment of hypertensive crises associated with pheochromocytoma, its use as a primary agent in the management of this disorder has not been established.

631. The answer is A. *(Chap 331.)* The adrenal glands normally produce hydrocortisone at a rate of approximately 20 to 30 mg/d. As in the treatment of primary adrenal insufficiency, a replacement dose of hydrocortisone, 30 mg/d, should be given to all patients following transsphenoidal removal of an ACTH-secreting microadenoma; treatment should continue until the uninvolved corticotropic cells recover and secrete ACTH at a level sufficient to maintain basal glucocorticoid production. If symptoms of withdrawal from high levels of glucocorticoid develop, a transient increase in glucocorticoid dosage may be necessary. Administration of desmopressin or levothyroxine is required only if diabetes insipidus or hypothyroidism, respectively, develops postoperatively.

632. The answer is A. *(Chaps 13, 340.)* Estrogen replacement in postmenopausal women offers clear-cut benefits in terms of reducing the vasomotor instability, usually characterized by hot flashes, and the vaginal dryness caused by atrophy of the urogenital epithelium and skin. Hot flashes tend to diminish after several years in untreated women; therefore, if vasomotor instability is the sole indication for estrogen therapy, prolonged treatment is usually not required. Routine estrogen therapy, if given in the lowest effective dose possible with or without cycling, will almost certainly decrease the complications of postmenopausal osteoporosis. There is little evidence definitively linking chronic estrogen therapy in the postmenopausal period to the increased frequency of development or the severity of thromboembolic disease, breast cancer, endometrial cancer, or hypertension. In fact, estrogen replacement may decrease the risk of death due to coronary thrombosis. Instead of cycling progestogens, an appropriate therapeutic alternative is to prescribe a low dose of transdermal or oral conjugated estrogen daily for 25 days each month followed by a rest period. Women receiving estrogens should be monitored at yearly intervals to ensure that the drug is being tolerated without side effects.

633. The answer is E. *(Chap 60.)* Autosomal dominant diseases are manifest in the heterozygous state, when only one abnormal gene is present, with the corresponding allele being normal. Consequently, there is a 50 percent chance that offspring of an affected heterozygote will inherit the mutant allele. Furthermore, affected individuals will bear an equal number of normal and affected offspring. There is no sex predilection for such a disease. In many autosomal dominant disorders, the affected person may not have an affected parent. This occurs because mutations leading to such disorders are often spontaneous. The parent in whose germ cell the mutation arose will be clinically normal, as will the parent's other children. However, since the mutation is now present in the reproductive cells of an affected individual, such a patient will transmit the disease to half of his or her children. Some autosomal dominant diseases, such as tuberous sclerosis and achondroplasia, arise in spontaneous mutations in about 80 percent of cases; Marfan syndrome and neurofibromatosis do so in about 30 to 40 percent of cases. On the other hand, Huntington's chorea, adult polycystic kidney disease, and familial hypercholesterolemia have a much lower incidence of occurrence due to spontaneous mutations. Other characteristics of many autosomal dominant disorders, not seen in recessive syndromes, are delayed age of onset and variability of clinical expression. For example, the neurologic abnormalities associated with Huntington's chorea frequently do not present until the fourth or fifth decade. Secondly, the multiple endocrine adenoma-peptic ulcer syndrome may manifest itself with abnormalities in various organs within the same kindred. Hemophilia A is an X-linked recessive disorder and hemochromatosis is autosomal recessive. Myasthenia gravis is inherited in a polygenic fashion, but is more common in patients who harbor an HLA-B8 histocompatibility antigen locus.

634. The answer is C. *(Chap 335.)* The absolute degree of elevation of plasma cortisol concentration is not a reliable criterion in the diagnosis of Cushing's disease. Rather, impaired suppressibility of adrenal cortisol production must be demonstrated by formal dexamethasone testing. Following administration of dexamethasone, 2 mg/d for 2 days, urinary free cortisol excretion may fall in persons with Cushing's disease but not to the degree seen in normal persons (<55 nmol/d [<20 μg/d]). A dexamethasone regimen of 8 mg/d would cause urinary 17-hydroxycorticosteroid excretion to fall to less than 50 percent of baseline in persons with Cushing's disease. Cortisol production never increases in response to metyrapone because this drug inhibits the final enzyme (11β-hydroxylase) in the pathway of cortisol synthesis; however, an exaggerated release of ACTH may follow metyrapone administration and result in a threefold to fivefold increase in urinary excretion of 17-hydroxycorticosteroids (predominantly 11-deoxycortisol). Patients with Cushing's disease characteristically have elevation of urinary 17-ketosteroids in addition to elevation of urinary 17-hydroxycorticosteroids.

635. The answer is D. *(Chap 360.)*   Magnesium deficiency may occur as a result of generalized nutritional insufficiency or lack of supplementation in programs of total parenteral nutrition. Other causes include gastrointestinal malabsorption of any cause, chronic diarrhea, chronic alcoholism, increased renal excretion (due to cisplatin, amphotericin B, aminoglycosides, loop diuretics), and various endocrine disorders (e.g., hyperparathyroidism, hypoparathyroidism, diabetic ketoacidosis, Conn's syndrome, syndrome of inappropriate secretion of vasopressin). Clinical sequelae of severe magnesium deficiency (<0.5 mmol/L [1.0 meq/L]) include anorexia, vomiting, lethargy, paresthesias, muscle cramps, irritability, decreased attention span, and confusion. Hypocalcemia, as a result of diminished responsiveness and release of parathyroid hormone, may be severe enough to produce tetany. About half of patients with hypomagnesemia may become hypokalemic (the mechanism is unclear but secondary hyperaldosteronism may play a role). Low levels of serum calcium, potassium, and magnesium all serve to promote dangerous cardiac arrhythmias, especially in the patient receiving digitalis. Hyponatremia is not a known consequence of hypomagnesemia, although the syndrome of inappropriate secretion of vasopressin may cause a low serum magnesium.

636. The answer is D. *(Chap 361.)*   Known complications of long-standing Paget's disease include high-output cardiac failure due to proliferation of blood vessels in Pagetic bone, pathologic fractures, nephrolithiasis, gait disturbance, and bone pain. However, the most dreaded complication is the development of a secondary osteogenic sarcoma, which occurs in no more than 1 percent of affected patients. These tumors most frequently arise in the femur, humerus, skull, facial bones, and pelvis. Increased pain and swelling in the local area of the tumor or an explosive rise of the serum alkaline phosphatase level may accompany the presentation of sarcoma. These so-called secondary osteosarcomas seem to be relatively unresponsive to chemotherapy; the natural history of such processes is dismal indeed. Etidronate, a bisphosphonate drug that stabilizes the mineralized bone, is generally well-tolerated. Disabling pain over Pagetic lesions may be a consequence of etidronate therapy, but it would not be expected to occur after many months of treatment.

637. The answer is B. *(Chap 357. Burtis, N Engl J Med 322:1106–1112, 1990.)*   Patients who present with hypercalcemia and hypophosphatemia should be thought of as having an excess of parathyroid hormone activity. Patients with nonparathyroid hormone-like mediated hypercalcemia, such as those with excessive levels of vitamin D due to intoxication or sarcoidosis or due to increased bone turnover as in hyperthyroidism, would not be expected to have a low serum phosphate. Secondly, those patients with familial hypocalciuric hypercalcemia, an autosomal dominant trait, often have normal or slightly low levels of immunoreactive parathyroid hormone. Thus, those with hypercalcemia and hypophosphatemia without elevated levels of parathyroid hormone are likely to have the hypercalcemia of malignancy. The clinical setting usually, but not invariably, makes this diagnosis obvious. While the hypercalcemia of malignancy may be due to local bone destruction such as in myeloma and breast cancer, it is now clearly recognized that many solid tumors, including carcinoma of the lung and kidney, may produce a parathyroid hormone–related protein that will not be identified by the currently available assays that detect true parathyroid hormone elaborated from the parathyroid gland. This parathyroid-related protein synthesized by tumors bears striking amino acid homology to that of native parathyroid hormone with regard to amino acids 1 through 13, but is thereafter unique. In fact, it is now recognized that the majority of patients with cancer and hypercalcemia have humoral hypercalcemia, as determined by elevated urinary cyclic AMP excretion.

638. The answer is B. *(Chap 331.)*   A serum prolactin level above 300 μg/L is diagnostic of a pituitary adenoma, even in a nursing woman. In fact, the serum prolactin level only rarely reaches 300 μg/L during pregnancy and declines post partum (with intermittent peaking with each suckling episode). Six months post partum, basal prolactin levels are normal, and the suckling-induced rise is minimal despite continued nursing. Thus, CT or MRI of the pituitary gland is indicated at this time. Suppressive treatment with bromocriptine would be indicated if the diagnosis of a pituitary adenoma is confirmed. Since bromocriptine suppresses all types of hyperprolactinemia, it cannot be used as a diagnostic test of physiologic versus pathologic hyperprolactinemia. Any delay in evaluation could allow further tumor enlargement and the risk of visual impairment resulting from optic nerve compression. Visual field testing should be done if an adenoma is found.

639. The answer is B. *(Chap 333.)*   Patients with lung cancer, particularly small cell carcinoma, frequently present with the syndrome of inappropriate vasopressin (AVP, antidiuretic hormone) secretion. Indeed, more than half of patients with such tumors show evidence of inappropriate secretion of AVP, even when serum sodium concentration remains normal. AVP is produced by the tumor tissue itself and is chemically identical to arginine vasopressin secreted by the neurohypophysis. Central nervous system lesions of infectious, inflammatory, and vascular etiologies can also result in inappropriate AVP secretion, but intracerebral metastases from lung carcinomas are not usually responsible for inappropriate AVP secretion.

640. The answer is A. *(Chap 335.)*   Patients who continually secrete aldosterone inappropriately usually present with diastolic hypertension of moderate severity, headaches, and muscle weakness due to profound hypokalemia. Excessive levels of aldosterone result in increased renal distal tubular exchange of sodium for potassium and hydrogen ions and resultant metabolic alkalosis. Though patients also have expanded extracellular fluid water, they usually do not have edema. It is important to ensure that hyperkalemia and metabolic alkalosis are not due to use of a potassium-wasting diuretic. The diagnosis of hyperaldosteronism is based on (1) diastolic hypertension without edema, (2) failure to increase serum renin level after volume depletion, and (3) failure of aldosterone secretion to decline appropriately after volume expansion. Since this patient's renin failed to rise after she assumed upright posture, she does not have a secondary hypermineralocorticoid state due to elevated plasma renin levels. Instead, she has primary aldosteronism, due either to an aldosterone-producing adrenal adenoma (Conn's syndrome) or to bilateral nodular hyperplasia. Once the requisite biochemical testing is complete, an attempt to localize the aldosterone-producing cells should be made preoperatively by CT scanning or bilateral adrenal vein catheterization with simultaneous adrenal venography or both. If localization of aldosterone secretion can be demonstrated, surgery to remove the adenoma is indicated.

641. The answer is A. *(Chap 344.)*   Dietary triglycerides in cholesterol are packaged by gastrointestinal epithelial cells into large lipoprotein particles called chylomicrons. After secretion into the intestinal lymph and passage into the general circulation, chylomicrons bind to the enzyme lipoprotein lipase located on endothelial surfaces. This enzyme is activated by a protein contained in the chylomicron, apoprotein CII, thereby liberating free fatty acids and monoglycerides, which then pass through the endothelial cells and enter adipocytes or muscle cells. Therefore, complete inactivation of either lipoprotein lipase or apoprotein CII due to inheritance of two defective copies of the relevant gene results in accumulation of chylomicrons (type I lipoprotein elevation), which is due to failure of conversion to the chylomicron remnant particle. Patients with familial lipoprotein lipase deficiency usually present in infancy with recurrent attacks of abdominal pain due to pancreatitis. They also have eruptive xanthomas due to triglyceride deposition. Treatment should consist of a low-fat diet that may be supplemented by medium-chain triglycerides, which are not incorporated into chylomicrons. The absence of functional apoprotein CII, with consequent failure to activate lipoprotein lipase, presents with a similar phenotype, though patients so affected are typically detected at a somewhat later age than patients with familial lipoprotein lipase deficiency.

642. The answer is E. *(Chap 334.)* Surgical treatment of nontoxic goiter is most commonly undertaken for diagnostic purposes (i.e., to rule out malignancy). Enlarged thyroid glands often have a limited functional reserve capacity, and lobectomy can further compromise hormone production. The thyroid scan presented in the question demonstrates adequate concentration and diffuse distribution of the radionuclide throughout the enlarged remnant, and there is little risk of malignancy. Exogenous hormone administration can prevent or improve postsurgical "compensatory" thyroid hyperplasia, which is the likely explanation for the mass in the woman described. Ultrasonography would be useful if the scan showed irregularities of uptake.

643. The answer is D. *(Chap 334.)* Normal pregnancy can simulate thyrotoxicosis in regard to increased heart rate, heat intolerance, and anxiety. The level found in the sensitive TSH test is low, but detectable, and therefore does not confirm hyperthyroidism. The test best able to exclude thyrotoxicosis in this patient would be the thyrotropin-releasing hormone (TRH) stimulation test. Testing radioactive iodine uptake (RAIU) is not always useful in diagnosing hyperthyroidism because of the wide range of normal values in the population and is not advisable in pregnancy. Similarly, the T_3 suppression test, although useful in the diagnosis of thyroid autonomy, requires RAIU tests and therefore would be contraindicated. Technetium thyroid scans are not useful in the diagnosis of hyperthyroidism. A serum T_3 level, in the absence of some measure of thyroid hormone binding capacity, is also not useful in excluding hyperthyroidism.

644. The answer is E. *(Chap 344. Brown, Science 232:34, 1986.)* The most common hyperlipidemic syndrome known to be caused by a single gene defect is familial hypercholesterolemia, an autosomal dominant disorder caused by a mutant LDL receptor. Heterozygotes have a two- to threefold elevation in serum cholesterol due to a reduction in the ability of the liver and other tissues to take up cholesterol-rich LDL lipoprotein particles from the plasma. The clinical features of this syndrome are usually manifest by premature and accelerated coronary atherosclerosis as well as by tendon xanthomas, particularly in the Achilles tendon and tendons near the knee, elbow, and dorsum of the hand. These nodules are caused by deposits of lipid-swollen macrophages. The extremely high LDL levels lead to an enhanced infiltration of cholesterol into the artery wall following episodes of endothelial damage, thereby leading to enhanced atherosclerosis. The presence of very elevated plasma cholesterol levels, the occurrence of tendon xanthomas, and a family history of atherosclerosis or hyperlipidemia is very suggestive of familial hypercholesterolemia.

645. The answer is B. *(Chap 334.)* The most appropriate treatment for Graves' disease in the third trimester of pregnancy is propylthiouracil in the minimal dosages sufficient to control the hyperthyroidism. Because levothyroxine crosses the placenta poorly, hypothyroidism may occur in the fetus if levothyroxine is combined with sufficient doses of propylthiouracil to block thyroid function in the fetus. Subtotal thyroidectomy is usually reserved for treating affected women in the second trimester. Use of radioactive iodine is contraindicated during pregnancy because it crosses the placenta and may have deleterious effects on fetal development. Propranolol can cause fetal hypoglycemia and apnea and should not be used in treating thyrotoxicosis of pregnancy, except in emergencies.

646. The answer is C. *(Chap 334.)* Measurement of serum TSH concentration by radioimmunoassay is useful in the diagnosis of both early and advanced primary hypothyroidism. Because of the exquisitely sensitive feedback relationship between TSH secretion and thyroid hormone levels in plasma, TSH levels in serum are increased in patients with untreated hypothyroidism of thyroidal etiology. In contrast, serum T_3 measurement and radioactive iodine uptake tests are generally poor discriminators of hypothyroidism. The TRH stimulation test is of less value in the diagnosis of hypothyroidism than in the diagnosis of hyperthyroidism. Reverse T_3 measurement, when available, is helpful in separating primary hypothyroidism from the "sick euthyroid" syndrome, since results are subnormal in patients with hypothyroidism but normal or high in association with the "sick euthyroid" syndrome.

647. The answer is D. *(Chap 335.)*   In the various forms of congenital adrenal hyperplasia, including steroid C-21 hydroxylase deficiency, both pituitary and adrenal regulatory mechanisms function appropriately. The enzymatic defect in cortisol production results in an absence of the product (cortisol) necessary for feedback inhibition of ACTH secretion by the pituitary gland. ACTH in turn causes the production of increased amounts of cortisol precursors such as 17-hydroxyprogesterone, which is converted to androgens by the adrenal gland. Therapy with appropriate doses of glucocorticoid causes suppression of pituitary ACTH and adrenal androgen secretion, indicating that inhibiting and stimulating control mechanisms of the hypothalamic-pituitary-adrenal axis can function normally.

648. The answer is D. *(Chap 335.)*   In a single-dose overnight dexamethasone suppression test, which is a screening procedure in the workup of possible cortisol excess, suppression of plasma cortisol concentration to less than 140 nmol/L (5 μg/dL) implies normal hypothalamic-pituitary-adrenal feedback and excludes a diagnosis of Cushing's syndrome. However, failure to suppress plasma cortisol following this procedure is not necessarily diagnostic and must be investigated further. Several factors can affect the validity of screening dexamethasone testing. For example, in 10 to 15 percent of cases obesity interferes with normal suppression of cortisol after the overnight dexamethasone test. However, obese persons uniformly show normal excretion of free cortisol in urine (< 275 nmol/d [< 100 μg/d]). The 2-day low-dose dexamethasone test is necessary to exclude or establish the diagnosis of Cushing's syndrome in all persons with abnormal or equivocal screening tests. The high-dose test, which is reserved for patients with established Cushing's syndrome, serves to delineate the specific cause. Imaging procedures should only be performed once a diagnosis of cortisol excess is established.

649. The answer is B. *(Chap 335.)*   Hyporeninemic hypoaldosteronism occurs most commonly in adults with diabetes mellitus in association with mild renal failure, metabolic acidosis, and hyperkalemia. The defect in aldosterone synthesis is almost certainly caused by hyporeninism, since in these patients aldosterone secretion increases promptly after the administration of ACTH but not after salt restriction or postural changes. Most patients respond to the administration of potent mineralocorticoids (fludrocortisone) or diuretics such as furosemide, or both, but in general mineralocorticoids should not be the sole therapeutic agents in patients with hypertension. Furosemide will treat both the hyperkalemia and the acidosis; this diuretic will be more effective if sodium intake is reduced. Hemodialysis may be useful in emergency situations to correct hyperkalemia. Potassium restriction and enhancement of potassium excretion with anion-exchange resins are both likely to predispose to total-body potassium deficits.

650. The answer is A. *(Chap 337. Coustan, N Engl J Med 319:1663, 1988.)*   The prognosis for pregnancies complicated by diabetes mellitus has improved markedly, and perinatal mortality has decreased to the point that infant survival is similar to that in the population at large. This improved outcome is a result of aggressive treatment of maternal hyperglycemia and of advances in the techniques of fetal surveillance and neonatal care. When mean maternal blood glucose levels exceed 8.3 mmol/L (150 mg/dL) in the third trimester, perinatal mortality is almost six times that associated with mean maternal glucose levels below 5.6 mmol/L (100 mg/dL). Congenital malformations, the leading cause of perinatal mortality in infants of diabetic pregnancies, remain an unresolved problem; such abnormalities are thought to be related to poor glucose control early in the first trimester (during early embryogenesis), a time when many women do not yet know they are pregnant. Optimal care of a diabetic woman wishing to become pregnant requires that a major attempt be made to achieve as normal a mean blood glucose concentration as possible before conception and throughout the duration of pregnancy. Hospitalization may be required for education or treatment of complications but should not be necessary for extended periods of time. Multiple subcutaneous injections of insulin or continuous subcutaneous injection of insulin should be considered to provide "tight" control in all diabetic women wishing to become pregnant.

651. The answer is B. *(Chap 337.)* Dot hemorrhages and several larger lesions near the disk (caused by superficial retinal bleeding) are characteristic changes of background diabetic retinopathy. However, the presence of innumerable, fine, frondlike vessels extending around and partly covering the disk is indicative of the neovascularization of proliferative retinopathy, which requires urgent treatment. The therapy of choice is photocoagulation by xenon arc or ruby or argon laser, which significantly improves visual prognosis in proliferative retinopathy. Hypophysectomy is no longer used to treat proliferative retinopathy because of the morbidity and lack of effectiveness of the procedure. Vitrectomy should be reserved for more advanced cases, such as nonresolving vitreal hemorrhage or retinal detachment.

652. The answer is A. *(Chap 339.)* Testosterone esters are hydrolyzed by esterases in the blood as they are absorbed from the oily depots in which they are administered, and, as a consequence, the esters themselves can rarely be detected in blood. Therefore, effectiveness of therapy with agents such as testosterone cypionate can be monitored by measuring the plasma levels of testosterone itself. In men with recent onset of hypogonadism, plasma LH levels should be suppressed into the normal range by testosterone, but when LH levels have been high for many years, LH secretion becomes semiautonomous and may not return to the normal range for many months or years after the restoration of blood testosterone levels to normal. The frequency of nocturnal erections may or may not reflect plasma testosterone levels on a day-to-day or week-to-week basis, and muscle mass depends on factors in addition to plasma testosterone levels, including exercise level.

653. The answer is D. *(Chap 361.)* Paget's disease of bone is relatively common, and the incidence increases with age. An estimated prevalence of 3 percent in persons over the age of 40 years is a generally accepted figure. Most frequently, the disease is asymptomatic and diagnosed only when the typical sclerotic bones are incidentally detected on x-ray examinations done for other reasons or when an increased alkaline phosphatase activity is recognized on routine laboratory measurements. The etiology is unknown, but increased bone resorption followed by intensive bone repair is thought to be the mechanism causing increased bone density and increased serum alkaline phosphatase activity as a marker of osteoblast activity. Since increased mineralization of bone takes place (although in an abnormal pattern), hypercalcemia is not present unless a severely affected patient becomes immobilized. Hypercalcemia, in fact, would be an expected finding in a patient with primary hyperparathyroidism, bone metastases, or plasmacytoma, the last typically producing no increase in the alkaline phosphatase activity. Osteomalacia resulting from vitamin D deficiency is associated with bone pain and hypophosphatemia; normal or decreased serum calcium concentration produces secondary hyperparathyroidism, further aggravating the defective bone mineralization.

654. The answer is D. *(Chap 357.)* A major function of parathyroid hormone is to act as a trophic hormone to regulate the rate of formation of 1,25(OH)$_2$ vitamin D. The mechanism by which parathyroid hormone exerts this effect may be secondary to its effects on phosphorus metabolism. Other hormones, including prolactin and estrogen, also may play a role in stimulating the production of 1,25(OH)$_2$ vitamin D.

655. The answer is A. *(Chap 60.)* Many common diseases are known to "run in families," yet are not inherited in a simple Mendelian fashion. It is likely that the expression of these disorders depends on a family of genes that can impart a certain degree of risk and then be modified by subsequent environmental factors. The risk of development of disease for a relative of an affected person varies with the degree of relationship; first-degree relatives (parents, siblings, and offspring) have the highest risk, which in itself varies with the specific disease. Many of these multifactorial genetic diseases are inherited in a greater frequency in persons with certain HLA (major histocompatibility system) types. For example, there is a tenfold increased risk of celiac sprue (gluten-sensitive enteropathy) in persons harboring HLA-B8. This genotype also imparts increased risk for chronic active hepatitis, myasthenia gravis, and Addison's disease. The incidence of diabetes mellitus is much higher in those expressing HLA-D3 and HLA-D4. Spondyloarthropathies, psoriatic arthritis (HLA-B27), hyperthyroidism (HLA-DR3), and multiple sclerosis (HLA-DR2) are other examples of diseases with histocompatibility predispositions. On the other hand, Wilson's disease and cystic fibrosis are inherited in an autosomal recessive fashion and adult polycystic kidney disease and neurofibromatosis are among those disorders inherited in an autosomal dominant manner.

656. The answer is B. *(Chap 47.)* The endocrine causes of organic impotence include decreased plasma testosterone and hyperprolactinemia. High serum prolactin, usually due to a pituitary microadenoma, suppresses production of luteinizing hormone–releasing hormone (LHRH). Dopaminergic agonists such as bromocriptine may be useful in reducing prolactin levels and restoring potency. Many antihypertensive agents interfere with the sympathetic nervous system's role in penile erection. Beta blockers are the major offenders in this regard. The angiotensin-converting enzyme inhibitors, calcium channel blockers such as nifedipine, and peripheral vasodilators are not associated with an increased risk of impotence. Histamine (H-2)-receptor antagonists, including cimetidine, cause impotence by both increasing serum prolactin and directly antagonizing the effect of testosterone. Drugs with significant anticholinergic properties, such as tricyclic anti-depressants (including amitriptyline), can prevent erection, which is parasympathetically mediated. Other important causes of impotence include neurogenic disorders and vascular insufficiency (e.g., aortic occlusion, or Leriche syndrome, or distal atherosclerosis). Anatomic abnormalities, such as Peyronie's disease in which penile curvature is associated with fibrosis in the venous sinusoids of the penis, can also cause impotence.

657. The answer is C. *(Chaps 48, 340.)* The fact that withdrawal bleeding occurred after the administration of progestogen indicates that estrogen was being produced. Women with chronic anovulation who react in this way are said to be in the state of "estrus" because of acyclic production of estrogen. This diagnostic response clearly excludes those causes of amenorrhea associated with suppression of ovarian function, including pituitary disease, either functional or organic, and conditions associated with streak gonads. The most likely cause of amenorrhea in such a situation is polycystic ovarian disease (PCOD) in which the ovaries produce androgens that can be converted to estrogens (largely estrone) in extraglandular tissues. In most women with PCOD, menarche occurs at the expected time, and amenorrhea supervenes after a variable time. However, in some women this disorder has an early onset and may cause primary amenorrhea. Other causes of anovulation in the presence of estrogen include estrogen-secreting tumors of the ovary and adrenal tumors.

658. The answer is C. *(Chaps 48, 340.)* Asherman's syndrome, destruction of the endometrium, occurs after vigorous curettage, usually in association with postpartum hemorrhage or therapeutic abortion. The diagnosis is confirmed by hysterosalpingography or by direct visualization of the scarred endometrium using a hysteroscope. Treatment consists of dilation and curettage, followed by the insertion of an intrauterine device for 8 weeks.

659. The answer is D. *(Chaps 48, 340.)* Low circulating levels of estrogens coupled with elevated gonadotropin levels exclude the presence of pituitary disease and indicate primary ovarian failure, which is premature at this patient's age. Bilateral tubal obstruction would cause infertility but not amenorrhea. Polycystic ovarian disease is associated with typical physical findings of weight gain and hirsutism, an earlier age of onset, and elevated circulating levels of estrogens. Exogenous administration of estrogens would lead to suppression of gonadotropin secretion.

660. The answer is B. *(Chaps 335, 342.)* The clinical situation described in the question is characteristic of congenital adrenal hyperplasia due to deficiency of either C-21 hydroxylase or 3β-ol-dehydrogenase. Urinary 17-ketosteroids are elevated in both disorders, whereas urinary pregnanediol and pregnanetriol and plasma 17-hydroxyprogesterone and androstenedione levels are elevated in association with C-21 hydroxylase deficiency. Plasma 11-deoxycortisol is elevated in C-11 hydroxylase deficiency, a disorder producing hypertension owing to overproduction of mineralocorticoids and consequently not associated with vomiting and volume depletion. Congenital adrenal hyperplasia due to C-21 hydroxylase deficiency, the most common cause of ambiguous genitalia in the newborn, results in virilization of females at birth and premature androgenation of males.

661. The answer is D. *(Chap 342.)* Tumors of the streak gonads are unusual in the common forms of gonadal dysgenesis, including those associated with normal karyotypes (46,XX), X-chromosome deletion (45,X), structurally abnormal X chromosomes (46,XX$_i$), and X chromosome mosaicism (45,X/46,XX). However, malignant tumors of the streaks (so-called gonadoblastomas) are common when gonadal dysgenesis is associated with cell lines containing Y chromosomes or fragments of Y chromosomes. Consequently, the gonadal streaks should be resected whenever a Y chromosome is present in a woman with gonadal dysgenesis.

662. The answer is E. *(Chap 357.)* Persons who have hyperparathyroidism can present with manifestations of hypercalcemia—e.g., peptic ulcer, muscle weakness, kidney stones—or symptoms of osteitis fibrosa cystica, a form of bone involvement characteristic of the disease. However, with the widespread application of biochemical screening as a routine tool in patient evaluation, more and more patients are diagnosed early in the course of the disease, when it is manifested only by asymptomatic hypercalcemia. At present, this is the most common source of diagnoses of hyperparathyroidism. A solitary parathyroid adenoma is the most common cause of this entity.

663. The answer is B. *(Chap 357.)* Most patients with primary hyperparathyroidism, even if asymptomatic, should undergo surgery because of its low morbidity and routinely good outcome. Unless contraindicated by a history of thromboembolic phenomena, severe hypertension, or breast cancer, estrogen therapy provides a useful means of controlling hypercalcemia and protecting the skeleton in postmenopausal women who have hyperparathyroidism but are not good operative candidates. Plicamycin, though also of benefit, is administered as weekly intravenous injections and has cumulative toxic effects on the kidneys, liver, and bone marrow; however, it would be a good choice for treatment of hypercalcemic emergencies if saline and furosemide were ineffective or contraindicated. Phosphate promotes the deposition of calcium into the skeleton, but long-term use in persons with renal insufficiency would cause a buildup in serum phosphorus levels and thereby promote soft-tissue calcification. Oral diphosphonate has not been demonstrated to have a sustained effect in controlling the hypercalcemia of primary hyperparathyroidism, perhaps because it retards bone formation as well as bone resorption. Thiazides would exacerbate hypercalcemia by increasing renal calcium reabsorption.

664. The answer is E.   *(Chaps 245, 357.)*   Patients with primary hyperparathyroidism are usually asymptomatic, and mild degrees of hypercalcemia in such patients can usually be managed with adequate hydration. Whether observation alone is appropriate in these patients is controversial, especially when the diagnosis is made at a young age, since surveillance of renal function and bone status is lifelong and cumbersome. On the other hand, definitive treatment is clearly indicated when complications arise. In this patient, hypercalcemia and nephrolithiasis constitute a clear-cut indication for surgical treatment of the hyperparathyroidism. An additional reason would be to prevent bone loss in this young woman that would place her at an increased risk for development of skeletal complications at a later time. Glucorcorticoids are usually ineffective in the management of primary hyperparathyroidism and would affect bone metabolism negatively, besides producing other serious side effects when administered on a long-term basis. Thiazide diuretics or calcium supplementation are contraindicated in this patient because of the risk of inducing hypercalcemia.

665. The answer is C.   *(Chap 334.)*   Radioactive iodine uptake (RAIU) is often a useful test in distinguishing among the various causes of hyperthyroidism. Elevation of RAIU above the normal range usually indicates thyroid hyperfunction (some persons with hyperthyroidism have a normal or low RAIU). Painless thyroiditis is a variant of chronic lymphocytic thyroiditis associated with transient thyrotoxicosis from release of preformed hormone. Radiographic contrast studies, such as intravenous pyelography and oral cholecystography, use organic media that release iodide and thus serve as sources for dilution of administered radioactive iodine; as a result, RAIU may be falsely low for as long as 6 months. *Thyrotoxicosis factitia* is the term used to designate thyrotoxicosis resulting from ingestion of thyroid hormones. Ingestion of liothyronine (T_3) results in a low serum thyroxine (T_4) concentration, while ingestion of levothyroxine leads to elevations of both T_4 and T_3. In either case, feedback of exogenous thyroid hormone decreases TSH secretion and lowers RAIU. Struma ovarii, which is an ovarian tumor with thyroidlike tissue that releases thyroid hormone, is a rare cause of thyrotoxicosis. Measurement of RAIU over the thyroid gland would not, of course, detect the abdominal source of increased RAIU in women affected with struma ovarii. Choriocarcinoma releases factors with TSH-like activity that enhance uptake of radioactive iodine.

666. The answer is A.   *(Chap 358.)*   Osteomalacia and rickets both are characterized by defective mineralization of bone; osteomalacia affects the adult skeleton, and rickets impairs the developing skeleton. Muscle weakness, hypocalcemia, hypophosphatemia, skeletal pain, and pseudofractures are cardinal features of both forms of osteomalacia. Bowing of the tibia, although common in children who have rickets, is not prominent in affected adults.

667. The answer is E.   *(Chap 358.)*   The combination of hypocalcemia, hypophosphatemia, elevated serum parathyroid hormone levels, and bone fractures is consistent with a diagnosis of osteomalacia in this patient. In the absence of other gastrointestinal or renal abnormalities leading to malabsorption or increased renal loss of calcium or phosphorus, vitamin D deficiency is likely to be present. Inadequate intake of vitamin D and calcium together with limited exposure to the sun are frequent in this age group. Postmenopausal osteoporosis is associated with vertebral and hip fractures as well, but laboratory abnormalities are not present. Primary hyperparathyroidism is associated with increased serum calcium concentration, as is ectopic parathyroid hormone secretion (although existence of the latter has been questioned). Paget's disease of bone does not produce hypocalcemia, and it causes typical sclerotic changes on x-ray examination.

668. The answer is C.   *(Chap 358.)*   The presenting findings in both primary hyperparathyroidism and multiple myeloma can include hypercalcemia and vertebral compression fractures. The absence of several key features—anemia, elevated erythrocyte sedimentation rate, abnormal serum protein electrophoresis, and Bence Jones proteinuria—is helpful in eliminating the possibility of multiple myeloma. If doubt remains as to the diagnosis of myeloma, a marrow aspiration should be performed. The presence of hypercalcemia makes unlikely the diagnoses of osteomalacia, which is associated with hypocalcemia, and of osteoporosis and Paget's disease, which are associated with normal blood calcium values.

669. The answer is A. *(Chaps 351, 360.)* In most conditions in which hypocalcemia is present—e.g., osteomalacia, renal failure, and parathyroid hormone-resistance states (pseudohypoparathyroidism)—the concentration of circulating parathyroid hormone (PTH) is increased as assessed by radioimmunoassay. However, the syndrome of hypocalcemia with severe hypomagnesemia (<0.4 mmol/L [< 0.8 meq/L]) is associated with a state of functional hypoparathyroidism. This severe degree of hypomagnesemia, most commonly associated with alcoholism and steatorrhea, may blunt or totally block PTH secretion. Magnesium deficiency also may be associated with reduced peripheral responsiveness to PTH. Correction of hypomagnesemia over several days restores normal parathyroid secretion and responsiveness.

670. The answer is C. *(Chaps 356, 357.)* Measurement of the serum concentration of 25(OH) vitamin D, the major circulating form of vitamin D, can be used to assess the adequacy of dietary intake and absorption of the vitamin. (Vitamin D also is made in the skin in the presence of sunlight.) Once ingested or synthesized, vitamin D is metabolized to 25(OH) vitamin D in the liver. This reaction is not tightly regulated, and an increase in dietary intake or endogenous production of vitamin D is reflected by linear elevations of serum 25(OH) vitamin D levels. Levels are reduced in severe chronic parenchymal and cholestatic liver disease but usually are normal in renal failure. Anticonvulsant drugs and glucocorticoids induce hepatic microsomal enzymes, which metabolize vitamin D and 25(OH) vitamin D into inactive products; this phenomenon, along with other complex effects on calcium metabolism, helps to explain why these drugs cause osteopenia.

671. The answer is A. *(Chaps 72, 76.)* In most malnourished persons, positive nitrogen balance can be achieved by providing 1 g of amino acids per kilogram of ideal body weight. However, in the presence of abnormal protein losses (e.g., from burn exudates, pancreatic secretions, or gastrointestinal fistula) or hypermetabolic states (sepsis, trauma, hyperthyroidism), additional protein intake must be provided. Likewise, daily protein requirements are increased in the presence of caloric deficiency because amino acids are used for oxidative metabolism and gluconeogenesis. Renal insufficiency and hepatic insufficiency are examples of "nitrogen accumulation diseases." When the kidneys are unable to excrete urea, ammonia may be used for the net synthesis of nonessential amino acids; thus, the need for nonessential nitrogen is reduced. In hepatic failure, amino acid catabolism is decreased, so that even normal protein intake may be deleterious.

672. The answer is A-N, B-N, C-Y, D-Y, E-Y. *(Chaps 48, 340.)* The luteal phase of the menstrual cycle follows ovulation and is characterized by an increase in progesterone secretion by the corpus luteum. With anovulatory cycles the corpus luteum does not form, and progesterone levels remain low. Furthermore, with anovulatory cycles the characteristic surge of LH and FSH at midcycle is absent, and menses are usually painless. Irregular estrogen breakthrough bleeding that occurs with anovulatory cycles is the consequence of persistent ovarian estradiol secretion and an absence of luteal-phase progesterone secretion.

673. **The answer is A-N, B-Y, C-Y, D-Y, E-N.** *(Chaps 69, 357.)* Familial hypocalcemia, short stature, and abnormalities of the metacarpal and metatarsal bones are characteristic features of congenital pseudohypoparathyroidism (Albright's hereditary osteodystrophy). The underlying defect is renal resistance to the action of parathyroid hormone due in many patients to a mutation in a guanyl-nucleotide-binding protein. Although plasma levels of parathyroid hormone are elevated, urinary cyclic AMP is low, and there is a diminished response of urinary cyclic AMP to the exogenous administration of the hormone. The basal ganglia are frequently calcified. No antibodies to parathyroid tissue can be demonstrated, and, unlike the situation in idiopathic hypoparathyroidism, the frequency of monilial infection is not increased. Hypothyroidism is common in persons with pseudohypoparathyroidism; it is usually the result of resistance to TSH due to the same defect in membrane adenylate cyclase activity that causes resistance to parathyroid hormone.

674. **The answer is A-N, B-Y, C-Y, D-N, E-Y.** *(Chaps 71, 72.)* Whenever caloric intake is deficient, amino acids are utilized as energy substrates and for gluconeogenesis to maintain an adequate blood level of glucose, especially important for metabolism of the brain. Thus, protein synthesis is compromised when energy requirements are not met by nonprotein calories. Stated in another way, energy undernutrition predisposes to protein starvation even when the protein supply is otherwise adequate. Nevertheless, it should be kept in mind that diets deficient in energy are frequently deficient in protein as well. Carbohydrates have a protein-sparing effect if given in sufficient quantities, but this effect does not hold true for fat. Low carbohydrate and fat diets do not produce a selective protein malabsorption, although generalized malabsorption occurs in patients with severe chronic malnutrition.

675. **The answer is A-N, B-Y, C-N, D-Y, E-Y.** *(Chap 72.)* Several methods are useful in assessing protein undernutrition. Clinically, the ratio of 24-h urinary creatinine excretion to height is the most sensitive and practical measure of muscle mass; it is decreased in the presence of protein malnutrition. Reduced blood levels of proteins synthesized by the liver, such as albumin and transferrin, are also characteristic findings with protein starvation. Anthropometric assessment of mid-arm circumference and triceps skin-fold thickness are measures of the mass of muscle and adipose tissue, respectively. While in many instances calculation of body weight as a percentage of ideal body weight is a good measure of lean body mass plus adipose tissue, the presence of ascites and edema makes this assessment unreliable. Blood ammonia levels may indicate protein overload from intestinal causes (e.g., gastrointestinal bleeding) but are not helpful in assessing protein nutrition. The combination of a careful clinical history and a thorough examination is also a reproducible and valid technique to evaluate nutritional status; however, many cachectic patients are unable to provide a detailed history.

676. **The answer is A-Y, B-Y, C-Y, D-N, E-N.** *(Chap 76.)* As a general rule, when patients cannot eat a normal diet, cannot absorb an oral diet efficiently, or deteriorate in health with oral feeding, total parenteral nutrition (TPN) is needed to provide partial or complete nourishment. Bowel rest, a frequent indication for TPN, is important in treating exacerbations of inflammatory bowel disease, intestinal fistulas, and pancreatitis. While medium-chain triglycerides can be helpful, TPN is the best management for short bowel syndrome (>70 percent resected). Persons who are markedly hypermetabolic from severe trauma, burns, or sepsis, for example, also may be helped by supplemental parenteral nutrition, even when some oral intake is possible. Well-nourished patients who are not expected to be able to eat for 10 to 14 days should receive TPN to avoid excess wasting and malnutrition. It is unclear whether the decrease in negative nitrogen balance that results from administration for a week or less of TPN to otherwise healthy people is of clinical significance. Patients who are unable to swallow for long periods of time (e.g., because of stroke, neuromuscular disorders, or coma) are best treated with enteral feedings.

677. The answer is A-Y, B-Y, C-N, D-N, E-Y. *(Chap 65.)*   Several inborn errors of metabolism can be treated successfully by the appropriate dietary restriction of a substrate or its precursors. Mental retardation and other problems associated with galactosemia and phenylketonuria can be prevented by reduced intake of galactose or phenylalanine, respectively, during childhood. Restriction of neutral fats can prevent pancreatitis in persons with lipoprotein lipase deficiency. Neither hyperprolinemia nor Tay-Sachs disease is treatable by dietary management.

678. The answer is A-Y, B-Y, C-Y, D-N, E-Y. *(Chap 344. Havel, J Clin Invest 81:1653, 1988.)*   Appropriate therapy for patients who have familial hypercholesterolemia should begin with a diet that is low in cholesterol and saturated fats and high in polyunsaturated fats. The administration of nicotinic acid (blocks hepatic cholesterol synthesis) and bile acid–binding resins, such as cholestyramine or colestipol, may be required if diet alone is insufficient therapy. Drugs such as lovastatin that inhibit 3-hydroxy-3-methyl glutaryl coenzyme A, the rate-limiting step in cholesterol biosynthesis, show great promise in treating patients with hypercholesterolemia. Gemfibrozil and clofibrate are used mainly in the treatment of hypertriglyceridemia.

679. The answer is A-Y, B-N, C-Y, D-Y, E-N. *(Chap 344.)*   Genetic analysis of survivors of myocardial infarction indicates that 20 percent of those persons less than 60 years of age have some form of inherited hyperlipidemia. Familial hypercholesterolemia, familial hypertriglyceridemia, and familial combined hyperlipidemia are the three most common primary hyperlipidemias. Inherited in an autosomal dominant manner, these disorders are associated with a fivefold to tenfold increase in the risk of developing premature coronary atherosclerosis. Familial hyperalphalipoproteinemia is characterized by elevated levels of high-density lipoprotein (HDL); it is associated with a slightly increased longevity and confers an apparent protection against myocardial infarction. Familial lipoprotein lipase deficiency is a rare autosomal recessive disorder that leads to marked elevations of serum triglyceride, but not to accelerated atherosclerosis.

680. The answer is A-Y, B-Y, C-Y, D-Y, E-Y. *(Chaps 337, 344.)*   Diabetic patients with insulin deficiency may show massive elevation of the serum level of triglycerides, with the concomitant risk of development of acute pancreatitis, as well as eruptive xanthomas, lipemia retinalis, and hepatomegaly. Adequate insulin replacement restores lipoprotein lipase activity and decreases hepatic production of very low-density lipoproteins by impairing fatty acid mobilization from the adipose tissue. However, hypertriglyceridemia also occurs in well-controlled diabetic patients (generally obese) in whom it may be present as an independently inherited trait as shown by family studies. Specific drug therapy may be required in this group of patients when diet and adequate control of the diabetic state fail to return triglyceride levels to normal.

681. The answer is A-N, B-Y, C-Y, D-Y, E-Y. *(Chap 344.)*   This patient has familial type 3 hyperlipoproteinemia with typical tuberoeruptive and palmar xanthomas. The basic defect in type 3 hyperlipoproteinemia is an abnormal form of apoprotein E (E_2) with a lower affinity for its liver receptor, thus impairing the rate of clearance of chylomicron remnants and intermediate-density lipoprotein (IDL) from the circulation. A "broad beta" pattern is seen on lipoprotein electrophoresis due to excessive amounts of the two lipoproteins. Heterozygotes for the E_2 allele (e.g., E_4/E_2, E_3/E_2) do not have hyperlipidemia. Since the incidence of the E_2/E_2 genotype in the general population is 1 in 100, but the incidence of type 3 hyperlipoproteinemia is only 1 in 10,000, other factors contribute to the expression of the genetic defect. Thus, obesity, hypothyroidism, and diabetes mellitus must be sought and treated accordingly. Clofibrate or gemfibrozil is usually effective when drug therapy is required in these patients.

682.   The answer is A-N, B-Y, C-Y, D-Y, E-N.   *(Chap 69.)*   Hirsutism is a common complaint of women. The evaluation of this problem should include questions regarding the rate of onset of hair growth, menstrual history, and drug intake. Examination should be directed toward sites of androgen-dependent hair (pubic, chest, extremity) and assessment of virilizing features such as clitoromegaly, coarsened voice, acne, and frontal balding. Rapid onset of frank virilization or elevations in serum dehydroepiandrosterone sulfate greater than 22 μmol/L (8100 μg/L) or serum testosterone concentrations > 7 nmol/L (2 ng/mL) suggest the presence of either an adrenal or ovarian tumor. Thus, it is unlikely that the patient had either an adrenal carcinoma or the androgen-producing ovarian tumor called arrhenoblastoma. On the other hand, the patient could have polycystic ovaries (measurement of gonadotropins and pelvic ultrasound might be helpful in this regard), late-onset congenital adrenal hyperplasia (demonstrable by 17-hydroxyprogesterone production after cosyntropin [Cortrosyn] stimulation and treated with synthetic glucocorticosteroids to suppress pituitary ACTH), or idiopathic hirsutism.

683.   The answer is A-N, B-N, C-N, D-Y, E-Y.   *(Chap 74.)*   Anorexia nervosa is an eating disorder usually manifest in teenage girls who markedly restrict nutritional intake and partake in ritualized exercise. Amenorrhea always accompanies this disorder. Presumably because of hypothalamic dysfunction, the episodic pituitary release of LH characteristic of the pubertal state is blunted or absent; basal levels of LH and FSH are low, and the LH response to LHRH is impaired. The skin is dry, scaly, and yellow (due to increased carotene levels). Bradycardia, hypothermia, hypotension, and life-threatening hypokalemia may be present in advanced cases. Growth hormone (GH) levels may be normal or elevated with an acromegalic-type rise in response to injection of thyrotropin-releasing hormone (TRH). Levels of insulin-like growth factor I (IGF-I, somatomedin C) are low, perhaps contributing to the high GH levels because of impaired feedback inhibition. Hypothalamic secretion of corticotropin-releasing hormone is enhanced, resulting in elevated plasma cortisol levels. The thyroid hormone profile is similar to that observed in the "sick euthyroid" state. Decreased activity of the 5'-deiodinase that converts thyroxine (T_4) to triiodothyronine (T_3) and reverse T_3 (rT_3) to diiodothyronine results in reduced serum T_3 and elevated rT_3 concentrations.

684.   The answer is A-Y, B-Y, C-N, D-N, E-Y.   *(Chap 331.)*   The development of a pituitary adenoma in a patient who has undergone bilateral adrenalectomy for the treatment of Cushing's disease is termed *Nelson's syndrome*. This disorder is characterized by hyperpigmentation, erosion of the sella turcica, and high plasma ACTH levels. Because of adrenalectomy, urinary 17-ketosteroid excretion usually is low; plasma cortisol levels are determined by the regimen of replacement therapy.

685.   The answer is A-Y, B-Y, C-Y, D-Y, E-Y.   *(Chap 334.)*   The changes in thyroid hormone economy termed the "sick euthyroid" syndrome may be induced by a variety of illnesses, traumas, and stresses. Depending upon the severity and duration of the stress, these changes lead to alterations in the concentrations of the free and, eventually, the total circulating thyroid hormones. Decreased production of T_3 resulting from inhibition of the peripheral 5'-monodeiodination of T_4 is a consistent feature. A decrease in the protein binding of T_4 and T_3 also occurs, and as a consequence the percentage of free T_4 usually increases. In more seriously ill patients, abnormalities of hormone binding to protein increase still further so that serum T_4 concentrations decrease into the hypothyroid range, most commonly the consequence of an inhibition of thyroid hormone binding to protein. Such inhibition is likely to result from an increase in quantity of a circulating fatty acid.

686.   The answer is A-N, B-N, C-Y, D-Y, E-Y.   *(Chap 334.)*   The woman described has subacute thyroiditis, which seems to have a viral etiology. In more severe cases, the use of glucocorticoids is generally efficacious in treatment, although such therapy is associated with a high rate of recurrence. Hyperthyroidism, when it occurs in association with subacute thyroiditis, is usually transient and is best controlled symptomatically with propranolol or phenobarbital, or both. Subtotal thyroidectomy and therapy with radioactive iodine are never appropriate treatments for subacute thyroiditis.

687. The answer is A-Y, B-Y, C-N, D-Y, E-N. *(Chap 335.)*   Adrenal carcinomas are likely to present as abdominal masses and secrete large amounts of adrenal androgens, which results in markedly elevated urinary 17-ketosteroid excretion. Neoplastic secretion of adrenal steroids characteristically is not suppressed with high doses (2 mg every 6 h) of dexamethasone because it is not regulated by ACTH. Indeed, ACTH levels are usually immeasurably low in persons with adrenal carcinoma. Testing with metyrapone (750 mg every 4 h for a day) usually does not result in an increase in urinary 17-hydroxycorticosteroids or plasma 11-deoxycortisol because of the prolonged suppression of ACTH secretion by the autonomous adrenal tumor. In contrast, patients with pituitary-dependent Cushing's syndrome show a normal response to metyrapone.

688. The answer is A-Y, B-N, C-Y, D-Y, E-N. *(Chap 335.)*   Complications of long-term treatment with high doses of glucocorticoids include the development or acceleration of osteoporosis and depression of immune function. Whether high-dose steroids can induce frank peptic ulceration is not established, but persons with preexisting ulcer disease may have exacerbations while on steroid therapy. Detection of preexisting abnormalities before the start of steroid therapy allows clinicians to institute appropriate treatment concurrently with the institution of steroid therapy. Testing the integrity of the hypothalamic-pituitary-adrenal axis is unwarranted prior to the initiation of chronic high-dose glucocorticoid therapy.

689. The answer is A-Y, B-Y, C-Y, D-N, E-N. *(Chap 341.)*   Pathologic gynecomastia develops when the effective testosterone-to-estrogen ratio is decreased, owing to either diminished testosterone production (as in primary testicular failure) or increased estrogen production. The latter may arise from direct estradiol secretion by a testis stimulated by luteinizing hormone or human chorionic gonadotropin or from an increase in peripheral aromatization of precursor steroids, most notably androstenedione. Elevated androstenedione levels may result from increased secretion by an adrenal tumor (leading to an elevated level of urinary 17-ketosteroids) or decreased hepatic clearance in patients with chronic liver disease. A variety of drugs, including diethylstilbestrol, heroin, digitalis, spironolactone, cimetidine, isoniazid, and tricyclic antidepressants, also can cause gynecomastia. In the case presented in the question, the history of paternity and the otherwise normal physical examination indicate a karyotype is unnecessary, and the bilateral breast enlargement essentially excludes the presence of carcinoma and, thus, the need for biopsy.

690. The answer is A-N, B-N, C-Y, D-Y, E-Y. *(Chap 337. Harrison, Diabetes 38:815, 1989.)*   There is considerable disagreement regarding the genetics of diabetes mellitus, but certain aspects appear to be clear-cut. Genetic factors are probably permissive for the development of type 1 (immune-mediated) and related more directly to the development of type 2 (non-immune-mediated) diabetes. The genetic locus for diabetes appears to be located near the HLA genes on the sixth chromosome. The presence of HLA antigens B8 or B15 increases the risk for developing type 1 diabetes nearly threefold, antigens DR3 and DR4 fourfold to fivefold, and antigen combinations (e.g., B8/B15) up to tenfold. However, homozygosity for a high-risk allele (e.g., DR3/DR3) does not increase the risk further. Evidence implicates positions 45 and 57 of the DQ_β chain as having importance in determining genetic susceptibility to type 1 diabetes. The concordance rate for monozygotic twins under 40 years of age is less than 50 percent. Pedigree analysis has shown a very low prevalence of vertical transmission for type 1 diabetes. The onset of juvenile diabetes has a seasonal variation and may follow mumps, hepatitis, or coxsackievirus infections, among others. These infections in genetically predisposed persons are theorized to produce an immune response with the development of cytotoxic islet-cell antibodies, which complete the destruction of the beta cells. This theory would explain why circulating islet cell antibodies are usually detectable soon after the onset of type 1 diabetes. In some cases anti-islet-cell antibodies have been demonstrated in twins of diabetics destined to develop the disease even before glucose tolerance became abnormal.

691. The answer is A-N, B-Y, C-Y, D-N, E-Y. *(Chap 337.)*   The occurrence of hyperglycemic ketoacidosis or hyperglycemic hyperosmolar coma is diagnostic of diabetes mellitus. Similarly, persistent fasting hyperglycemia (glucose concentration greater than 7.8 mmol/L [140 mg/dL]), even if asymptomatic, has been recommended by the National Diabetes Data Group as a criterion for the diagnosis of diabetes. On the other hand, abnormal glucose tolerance—whether after eating or occurring after a standard "glucose tolerance test"—can be caused by many factors (e.g., anxiety, infection or other illness, lack of exercise, or inadequate diet). Likewise, glycosuria may have renal as well as endocrinologic causes. Therefore, these two conditions cannot be considered diagnostic of diabetes.

692. The answer is A-Y, B-N, C-Y, D-Y, E-N. *(Chap 337.)*   Diabetic, hyperosmolar, nonketotic coma is a medical emergency usually occurring as a complication of maturity-onset diabetes. Typically, affected persons are elderly (often living alone or in a nursing home), have a history of recent stroke or infection, and are unable to drink sufficient water to balance urinary fluid losses. These factors combine to cause sustained hyperglycemic diuresis with profound volume depletion and decreased urine output. Presenting features often include signs of circulatory compromise as well as central nervous system manifestations ranging from confusion or seizures to coma. Ketoacidosis is absent, perhaps because the concentration of portal-vein insulin is high enough to prevent full activation of hepatic ketogenesis. Serum levels of free fatty acids are generally lower than in diabetic ketoacidosis, and although hypertonicity is marked, measured serum sodium concentration is kept from being significantly elevated by the profound hyperglycemia. Infections are common, and disseminated intravascular coagulation can occur as a result of elevated plasma viscosity (both bleeding and in situ thrombosis have been reported). Although administration of free water eventually becomes necessary, the treatment of salt deficits has highest initial therapeutic priority. Several liters of isotonic saline should be given over the first 2 h, followed by half-normal saline, and then a 5% glucose solution when blood glucose levels approach normal. Hypotonic fluids should not be used initially because most of the water enters the intracellular compartment—possibly leading to cerebral edema—rather than remaining in the plasma and interstitial spaces, where it is needed to support the circulation. Insulin also is required but usually in lower doses than in diabetic ketoacidosis.

693. The answer is A-Y, B-N, C-N, D-N, E-Y. *(Chap 337. Flier, Diabetes 41:1207, 1992.)*   Chronic insulin resistance is defined as a need for more than 200 units of insulin per day for several days in the absence of infection or ketoacidosis. This definition was based on the assumption that the normal human pancreas produces this much insulin daily; in fact, normal daily insulin production is probably 30 to 40 units, so that relative resistance is present when more than this amount is required to control blood sugar levels. The most common causes of insulin resistance are obesity and anti-insulin antibodies of the IgG type. Antibodies develop within 60 days of initiation of insulin therapy in nearly all diabetic persons. It is assumed that the binding of insulin by these antibodies is the major cause of severe insulin resistance, but the correlation between antibody titer and resistance is not always close. Uncontrolled hyperglycemia is the major consequence of insulin resistance, though ketoacidosis also may result. A history of discontinuous insulin use is frequent, and concomitant insulin allergy occurs in a minority of affected persons. Most patients require high doses of steroids, which frequently begin to take effect in a few days.

Acanthosis nigricans is a cutaneous disorder associated with two types of insulin resistance: type A, in which young women show accelerated growth, evidence of virilization, and decreased numbers of insulin receptors; and type B, in which older women have anti-insulin-receptor antibodies and other symptoms and signs of autoimmune disease (arthralgias, positive assay for anti-nuclear antibody, and others). The absence of acanthosis nigricans in the woman described in the question makes it unlikely that decreased numbers of insulin receptors or the presence of anti-insulin-receptor antibodies is playing a role in her insulin resistance.

694. The answer is A-Y, B-Y, C-Y, D-N, E-N. *(Chap 337.)* Approximately 40 percent of patients with type 1 diabetes mellitus sustain diabetic nephropathy. Progression of renal disease is markedly accelerated by hypertension, and even mild degrees of hypertension in diabetic patients should be treated aggressively. A hallmark of diabetic nephropathy is the presence of so-called macropro-teinuria (excretion of more than 0.55 g/d), and once this phase is reached there is a steady decline in renal function. So-called microalbuminuria, the excretion of 0.03 to 0.3 g/d of albumin, is also statistically predictive of progression of renal disease. In contrast, nocturia is usually a manifestation of undertreatment of diabetes and is an indication not of renal failure but of an osmotic diuresis. There is no clear-cut relation between insulin requirement and the development of any of the long-term complications of diabetes, including nephropathy; the development of these complications correlates better with the duration rather than the severity of diabetes mellitus.

695. The answer is A-N, B-Y, C-Y, D-N, E-N. *(Chap 338. Grunberger, Ann Intern Med 108:252, 1988.)* Because factitious hypoglycemia due to insulin injection or sulfonylurea ingestion is common, the finding of hyperinsulinemia associated with a low blood sugar concentration can no longer be considered diagnostic of an islet cell tumor (insulinoma). Suspicion of factitious disease should be especially high in medical personnel and in families of diabetics. The alpha and beta subunits of insulin are cleaved from proinsulin in the beta cell and released in equimolar amounts with the connecting (C) peptide; elevation of plasma C-peptide levels signifies endogenous hyperinsuline-mia, because exogenous insulin administration suppresses beta-cell function. Therefore, the triad of fasting hypoglycemia, hyperinsulinemia, and elevated plasma C-peptide levels is consistent with either endogenous hyperinsulinemia or ingestion of a sulfonylurea; documentation of the latter in urine or plasma would be diagnostic. Proinsulin usually is released into the circulation in small quantities. However, in patients with insulinoma, proinsulin concentration frequently exceeds 20 percent of total insulin; ingestion of a sulfonylurea, on the other hand, does not cause a disproportionate elevation of plasma proinsulin levels. Insulin antibody measurements in this case would not be expected to be helpful—antibodies may not develop for several months after the start of insulin injections, and the high C-peptide levels essentially rule out an exogenous source of insulin. However, under some circumstances antibodies to specific species of insulin can be identified and hence establish that exogenous insulin has been taken. Attempts to localize an islet cell tumor by radiologic means should only be done once factitious types of hypoglycemia are excluded.

696. The answer is A-Y, B-Y, C-Y, D-N, E-N. *(Chap 338.)* Hypoglycemia due to overutilization of glucose can be associated either with high or low insulin levels. Hypoglycemia associated with hyperinsulinism can occur in persons who have pancreatic insulinoma or who take exogenous insulin or ingest sulfonylurea drugs. Low plasma insulin levels can be associated with overutilization of glucose; examples include large, solid extrapancreatic tumors (e.g., hepatoma and sarcoma), in which high levels of insulin-like growth factors may play a role, and systemic carnitine deficiency, in which peripheral tissues are unable to use free fatty acids for energy production and the liver cannot synthesize ketone bodies. Underproduction of glucose may occur with acquired liver disease, such as hepatic congestion due to right-sided heart failure or viral hepatitis, or with hormone deficiencies, such as adrenal insufficiency and hypopituitarism.

697. The answer is A-N, B-N, C-Y, D-N, E-Y. *(Chap 339.)* Klinefelter syndrome is frequently not diagnosed in patients until the time of expected puberty or during adult life when incomplete virilization or some other manifestation of androgen deficiency first becomes apparent. Testosterone replacement is likely to promote virilization and to restore potency in these patients. However, if gynecomastia is already present, testosterone replacement therapy does not produce regression of the breast tissue, and it may even aggravate the gynecomastia. Surgical resection of the breast is usually necessary in this situation. Since the basic testicular lesion consists of progressive hyalinization of the seminiferous tubules, spermatogenic function is irreversibly impaired, and no form of hormonal therapy is effective in maintaining spermatogenesis. Even in normal persons, testosterone treatment produces hypospermia because of the inhibition of gonadotropin production. Although antisocial behavior may be a part of Klinefelter syndrome, it is unlikely to be a manifestation of androgen deficiency and is not correctable by testosterone replacement.

698. The answer is A-Y, B-Y, C-N, D-Y, E-Y. *(Chap 78.)* Deficiencies of trace elements (metals present at concentrations less than one microgram per gram of tissue) can be due to dietary deficiency, malabsorption (as in chronic diarrhea), or administration of total parenteral nutrition. Iron, copper, selenium, and zinc form stable complexes with enzymes. Selenium, for example, is a component of glutathione peroxidase and therefore functions as an antioxidant. Selenium deficiency results in myocardial necrosis. Zinc is required in tissues with a high cellular turnover, such as the gonads, and pregnant women and the developing fetus are at particular risk for zinc deficiency. Zinc deficiency dermatitis includes hyperkeratotic lesions and alopecia. Since cobalt is a component of vitamin B_{12}, deficiencies of this metal result in megaloblastic anemia. Copper deficiency may result in anemia, pigmentation abnormalities, hypothermia, and scurvy-like skeletal changes.

699. The answer is A-Y, B-N, C-Y, D-N, E-N. *(Chaps 340, 342.)* In persons with testicular feminization, estradiol secretion by the testes is markedly increased (but not to the level produced by normal ovaries); the mechanism is lack of suppression of luteinizing hormone by testosterone and consequently increased stimulation of gonadal testosterone and estradiol secretion. Ovaries containing follicle cysts may be a source of increased estrogen production, particularly during the postmenopausal years, when gonadotropin levels are very high. The increase in estrogen production characteristic of polycystic ovarian disease is the consequence of peripheral conversion of androstenedione to estrogen and not of direct gonadal production. During the third trimester of pregnancy estrogen production is increased because of formation of estrogen by the placenta rather than by the ovary. Arrhenoblastoma is a virilizing ovarian tumor and does not secrete estrogen.

700. The answer is A-N, B-Y, C-Y, D-N, E-Y. *(Chap 342.)* Ambiguous genitalia results when androgen production (or action) is defective in a male fetus or when androgen production is enhanced in a female fetus. Such aberrations can arise from a variety of causes. The most common cause is congenital adrenal hyperplasia, followed by mixed gonadal dysgenesis, which is a nonfamilial aberration of the sex chromosomes that interferes with normal sexual development, including 45,X/46,XY mosaicism. Examples of single gene mutations leading to abnormal sexual differentiation are the Reifenstein syndrome, in which genetic males have incompletely developed male genitalia because of androgen resistance, and 5α-reductase deficiency, in which testosterone cannot be converted to dihydrotestosterone. The historical use of progestational agents to treat pregnant women presenting with threatened abortion was associated with variable degrees of hypospadias in male offspring. Hypogonadotropic hypogonadism is associated with microphallus in male infants but not with hypospadias or abnormal sexual differentiation. Men whose chromosome pattern is 47,XYY are anatomically normal.

701. The answer is A-Y, B-Y, C-N, D-N, E-Y. *(Chap 342.)* Phenotypic men who have two or more X chromosomes have Klinefelter syndrome. Although the diagnosis of Klinefelter syndrome may be suspected prepubertally owing to the increased length of the lower body segment, most affected persons first present postpubertally with signs of decreased testosterone production and small testes. The risk of breast cancer is 20 times that of normal men (and one-fifth that of women), presumably the consequence of long-term estrogen stimulation of the breast. Mosaic chromosome patterns (46XY/47,XXY) are found in 10 percent of affected persons, 70 percent of whom display the mosaicism only in the testes, which may be normal in size. Hypospadias is not increased in incidence in affected persons. Although mental deficiency and social maladjustment occur with increased frequency in persons with Klinefelter syndrome, most patients with the disorder have normal mental and social competence.

702. The answer is A-Y, B-Y, C-Y, D-Y, E-Y. *(Chap 359.)* Persistent hypophosphatemia is character- ized by varying degrees of anorexia, dizziness, bone pain, proximal muscle weakness, cardiomy- opathy, and waddling gait. Severe hypophosphatemia may result in rhabdomyolysis, which is her- alded by a sharp elevation in serum creatine phosphokinase concentration. A consequence of reduced levels of 2,3-diphosphoglycerate and ATP in erythrocytes is reduced tissue oxygenation. Leukocyte dysfunction resulting in defective phagocytosis makes the hypophosphatemic patient more susceptible to bacterial and fungal infection. Nervous system dysfunction, manifested by irritability and apprehension progressing to obtundation, may occur upon refeeding. Persons with alcoholism may develop severe hypophosphatemia shortly after hospitalization, probably related to the combined effects of glucose administration and phosphorus deficiency due to diminished intake. Correction of phosphorus deficits leads to prompt reversal of the abnormalities.

703. The answer is A-N, B-N, C-Y, D-Y, E-N. *(Chaps 356, 357.)* Vitamin D toxicity generally occurs after chronic ingestion of large doses of vitamin D_2 or D_3 (usually in excess of 50,000 to 100,000 IU daily for months). Ingestion of a single large dose of vitamin D_2 or D_3 does not cause acute toxicity because excessive quantities are stored in body fat and released slowly into the blood- stream. Some vitamin D metabolites, such as $1,25(OH)_2$ vitamin D, could conceivably cause tox- icity after a single overdose. Hypervitaminosis D has not been reported following prolonged sun exposure, partly because the vitamin is released slowly from the skin after conversion from pre- vitamin D. Hypervitaminosis D causes hypercalcemia, hypercalciuria, and soft-tissue calcification, particularly in the kidneys. It is believed that high circulating levels of 25(OH) vitamin D directly stimulate intestinal calcium absorption and bone resorption, since toxicity can occur in anephric persons.

704. The answer is A-Y, B-Y, C-N, D-Y, E-Y. *(Chap 331.)* The enlarged pituitary gland of pregnancy is particularly vulnerable to ishchemic necrosis (Sheehan's syndrome) should hypotension occur in the postpartum period. Symptoms and signs of panhypopituitarism even several years after a difficult childbirth are consistent with this condition. Continued amenorrhea, decreased libido, cold intolerance typical of hypothyroidism, and loss of hair should therefore prompt an evaluation for anterior pituitary hypofunction. Lowering the blood sugar by giving a small amount of IV insulin normally triggers release of counterregulatory hormones, including growth hormone and cortisol. The urinary free cortisol itself is not helpful, since a normal or low value is compatible with a stressless period and not just panhypopituitarism. Since the patient probably has central hypothyroidism, the TSH will be inappropriately low in the face of low peripheral hormone. The response to ACTH stimulation should be blunted because the adrenal glands are not "primed" to respond to the pituitary release. Treatment of panhypopituitarism consists of hydrocortisone and thyroid hormone. Growth hormone injections are rarely required.

705. The answer is A-Y, B-N, C-N, D-Y, E-Y. *(Chap 334.)* Hypothyroidism should be suspected in the setting of certain laboratory findings not clearly associated with an obvious explanation. In addition to an increased ratio of preejection period to left ventricular ejection time on cardiac systolic time intervals, decreased QRS amplitude on electrocardiographic examination is common. Elevated creatine phosphokinase and lactic dehydrogenase serum values may mimic a myocardial infarction. Hypothyroidism is also typically associated with macrocytic red blood cell indices, due either to coexistent pernicious anemia or to unknown causes. Serum cholesterol is elevated in many patients with primary hypothyroidism.

706. The answer is A-Y, B-N, C-N, D-Y, E-N. *(Chap 337. Siperstein, Endocrinol Metab Clin North Am 21:915, 1992.)* Insulin must be supplied to the patient with diabetic ketoacidosis to inhibit production of ketone bodies that can cause life-threatening levels of acidosis. While low-dose insulin infusions are now commonly employed, it is generally believed appropriate to use 25 to 50 units/h until the acidosis is reversed. Since there are no known toxic effects of excess insulin in the carefully monitored patient, such an approach will saturate insulin receptors and circumvent the problem of insulin resistance. Insulin therapy should be directed to the pH and the calculated anion gap, not to the plasma ketone value. Tests for ketones measure acetone and acetoacetate but fail to measure β-hydroxybutyrate, which is converted to acetoacetate as tissue oxygenation is restored. Thus, plasma ketones may increase as the patient improves clinically and not mandate an increase in the insulin dosage. When the plasma glucose approaches normal levels, some glucose should be added to the intravenous solutions to prevent cerebral edema. However, since plasma glucose falls more rapidly than plasma ketones, insulin therapy should not be discontinued as glucose levels return to normal; the pH and anion gap remain the most important determinants. Potassium should be given if the admission serum potassium is normal or low, since total body potassium is invariably low and serum potassium will fall as a consequence of insulin therapy. However, it is recommended that potassium initially be given in the form of potassium phosphate because of the severe phosphate depletion associated with ketoacidosis.

707. The answer is A-N, B-Y, C-N, D-Y, E-Y. *(Chap 335.)* Weakness, hypotension, weight loss, nausea, and vomiting are each present in over 80 percent of patients with adrenal insufficiency, as documented by a failure of exogenously administered ACTH to effect a rise in the serum cortisol level. Hyperpigmentation, resulting from the melanocyte-stimulating hormone released in excess along with ACTH in cases of primary adrenal failure, is not seen in cases of secondary failure that occur because of suppressed ACTH. The best example of the latter condition is long-term steroid administration, which depresses ACTH release. Any cause of panhypopituitarism, such as a brain tumor's invasion of the sellar region, could also lead to adrenal failure on a secondary basis. Measurement of serum ACTH will distinguish between primary and secondary adrenal insufficiency. Destruction of the adrenal glands may occur as a consequence of infection with mycobacteria, cytomegalovirus, histoplasmosis, coccidioidomycosis, or cryptococcosis. Noninfectious causes of adrenal gland failure include bilateral tumor metastasis, bilateral hemorrhage, amyloidosis, sarcoidosis, autoimmune disease, and administration of certain medications (e.g., rifampin, ketoconazole, and phenytoin).

708. The answer is A-Y, B-Y, C-Y, D-N, E-N. *(Chap 340.)* Death rates associated with oral contraceptive use in women under age 40 are lower than those in women using no contraception. The increased death rate in those not taking oral contraceptives is probably due to the higher pregnancy rate and the consequent risks associated with pregnancy. However, even with the low estrogen dose in current contraceptive pills, there are risks. The most serious are due to the tendency toward hypercoagulability induced by these agents and the increased relative risk for deep venous thrombosis, pulmonary embolism, and thromboembolic stroke. Smoking and advanced age both increase the incidence of these complications. Five percent of women taking oral contraceptives develop significant hypertension, which is possibly due to an estrogen-induced rise in angiotensinogen synthesis. Rare complications involving the liver include peliosis hepatitis (blood-filled venous lakes) and cholestatic jaundice. There is no convincing evidence to implicate the oral contraceptive as a cause of increased risk of breast cancer (though such agents should not be used in the known or suspected presence of an estrogen-responsive neoplasm); its use may be associated with a decreased risk of endometrial and ovarian cancer.

709. **The answer is A-N, B-Y, C-Y, D-N, E-Y.** *(Chap 342. Griffin, N Engl J Med 336:611, 1992.)* Congenital deficiencies of the enzymes catalyzing the final two steps in testosterone biosynthesis, namely 17,20-lyase and 17β-hydroxysteroid oxioreductase, result in ambiguous genitalia due to lack of embryologic exposure to testosterone. LH levels are high owing to the deficiency of testosterone, but adrenal hyperplasia does not occur because glucocorticoid production is normal. Defects in testosterone synthesis proximal to these two enzymes also lead to ambiguous genitalia in males, but ACTH levels are high, and associated salt loss or hypertension will occur. In 5α-reductase deficiency, testosterone formation is normal, but an inability to convert this compound to dihydrotestosterone impairs development of external genitalia (although partial virilization may occur at puberty). Severe androgen receptor defects cause testicular feminization and phenotypical females who have a male genotype. Less severe defects of the androgen receptor can lead to a male with cryptorchidism, severe hypospadias, and gynecomastia (Reifenstein syndrome). In cases of defective or insufficient androgen receptor, levels of testosterone tend to be elevated, since the hypothalamic-pituitary axis cannot recognize the presence of the testosterone and continues to secrete LH in large quantities.

710. **The answer is A-Y, B-N, C-N, D-N, E-Y.** *(Chap 346.)* The porphyrias represent disorders of heme biosynthesis. The biochemical abnormalities and clinical manifestations depend on the step that is blocked and accumulation of precursor metabolites. Congenital erythropoietic porphyria is a rare autosomal recessive disorder due to a defect in the enzyme uroporphyrinogen II cosynthase, which is expressed solely in maturing erythroid cells. Porphobilinogen is preferentially converted to uroporphyrinogen I and then to coproporphyrinogen I. These latter metabolites account for the red urine observed in children with this disorder, but excretion of porphobilinogen is normal. Intermittent acute porphyria, characterized by attacks of recurrent neurologic and psychiatric dysfunction, is an autosomal dominant deficiency of porphobilinogen deaminase, the enzyme that converts porphobilinogen to uroporphyrinogen I. Thus, urinary levels of porphobilinogen are high during attacks. Hereditary coproporphyria is a similar disease caused by partial deficiency of coproporphyrinogen oxidase. A deficiency of protoporphyrinogen oxidase, the next-to-last enzyme involved in heme synthesis, leads to variegate porphyria manifested by attacks of neuropsychiatric dysfunction and photosensitivity and overexcretion of the proximal metabolite, porphobilinogen. Porphyria cutanea tarda, which is inherited or acquired deficiency of hepatic uroporphyrinogen decarboxylase, is not associated with excess porphobilinogen production, probably because aminolevulinic acid synthase activity is not enhanced. Mild skin photosensitivity is the major manifestation of protoporphyria, which is due to a deficiency of ferrochelatase, the final enzyme in heme biosynthesis. Protoporphyrins may accumulate in erythrocytes, but urinary porphobilinogen is normal.

711. **The answer is A-N, B-Y, C-N, D-N, E-Y.** *(Chaps 349, 350, 352, 353.)* In Niemann-Pick disease accumulation of sphingomyelins occurs usually because of sphingomyelinase deficiency. Organomegaly and neurologic involvement are clinical features, but there is highly variable expression depending on the subtype. The most common lysosomal storage disease, adult Gaucher's, is characterized by splenomegaly, pancytopenia, hepatic dysfunction, and bone pain. Accumulation of glucosylceramides presumably accounts for the clinical manifestations and for the distinctive Gaucher cell observed on bone marrow examinations. Tay-Sachs disease, caused by a deficiency of hexosaminidase A with concomitant accumulation of sphingolipids, presents as rapidly progressive neurologic deterioration during infancy and with a characteristic macular cherry-red spot. Heterozygote detection programs (enzyme assays in Ashkenazi Jews) have reduced the incidence of this disease in North America.

Diseases of glycogen metabolism can result in disorders whose pathophysiology is based either on hepatic hypoglycemia, as in von Gierke disease (glucose-6-phosphatase deficiency), or on muscle-energy deficiency, as in McArdle disease (muscle phosphorylase deficiency). Muscle-energy diseases generally result in painful cramping or myoglobinemia after exercise, so strenuous exercise should be avoided. These diseases are otherwise compatible with a normal life.

A defect in the phenylalanine hydroxylase enzyme complex leads to accumulation of phenylalanine in blood and urine with associated brain damage. The plasma phenylalanine concentration does not usually rise until the institution of protein feedings but is abnormal by the fourth day of life. A diet low in phenylalanine, if instituted during the first month of life, can avert mental retardation. Screening all newborns for blood phenylalanine concentration has been beneficial in this regard.

Excessive urinary excretion of the dibasic amino acids cysteine, lysine, arginine, and ornithine due to impaired tubular reabsorption is the pathophysiologic hallmark of cystinuria, the most common inborn error of amino acid transport. Due to the insolubility of cysteine, the primary clinical manifestation of this disorder is cysteine nephrolithiasis.

Dermatologic Disorders

DIRECTIONS: Each question below contains five suggested responses. Select the **one best** response to each question.

712. A 7-year-old girl is brought to the local emergency room after having a generalized seizure during which she lost consciousness. No history of head trauma can be elicited from her family and friends. A paternal uncle is mentally retarded and has had seizures. On examination, numerous brown spots—each greater than 3 cm and similar to those in Color Plate F—are present on the torso and extremities; one spot is 5 cm in size. Many smaller lesions (1 mm or less) are noted, especially in the axillary areas. The most likely diagnosis is

   (A) Peutz-Jeghers syndrome
   (B) Gardner's syndrome
   (C) neurofibromatosis
   (D) xeroderma pigmentosum
   (E) hemochromatosis

713. A 21-year-old woman is hospitalized for the treatment of a painful ulcer that has been present on her right lower leg for the last 4 weeks. The lesion began as a painful, reddish-purple nodule, then rapidly broke down and enlarged (see Color Plate G). Bacterial cultures did not yield a significant pathogen, and a 2-week course of oral dicloxacillin, 250 mg four times daily, was not helpful. The lesion border now is undermined with a violaceous rim; biopsy is consistent with pyoderma gangrenosum. The lesion described is associated with all the following disorders EXCEPT

   (A) ulcerative colitis
   (B) regional enteritis
   (C) multiple myeloma
   (D) rheumatoid arthritis
   (E) pernicious anemia

714. A 55-year-old Japanese businessman visiting the United States has been in excellent health until 6 months ago, when he first noted mild upper abdominal fullness after meals. On examination the man is noted to have hyperpigmented, heaped-up velvety lesions (as shown in Color Plate H) confined to the neck, axillae, and groin. All the following conditions have been associated with the skin findings presented EXCEPT

(A) Cushing's syndrome
(B) massive obesity
(C) acromegaly
(D) adenocarcinoma of the stomach
(E) Addison's disease

715. A 35-year-old man began intensive induction chemotherapy with daunorubicin and cytosine arabinoside for acute myeloid leukemia 3 weeks ago. He is febrile and profoundly neutropenic. The skin lesion seen on Color Plate I is noted. The cause of this lesion could be any of the following EXCEPT

(A) *Pseudomonas aeruginosa*
(B) *Escherichia coli*
(C) *Staphylococcus aureus*
(D) *Candida*
(E) *Aspergillus*

716. A 17-year-old girl complains of pain during chewing and tender lesions on the sides of her fingers. Shallow yellow-to-gray ulcerations with erythematous halos are present on her tongue, hard palate, and buccal mucosa. On the dorsal and lateral surfaces of her fingers are oval vesicles with a surrounding ring of erythema (as shown in Color Plate J). Her 5-year-old sister had a similar eruption last week and is now well. The most likely diagnosis is

(A) bullous erythema multiforme
(B) herpes simplex
(C) hand-foot-and-mouth disease
(D) Behçet's syndrome
(E) gonococcemia

717. For the last 2 days, a 24-year-old woman has had fever and pain in the left wrist, right ankle, and left knee. Nine painful skin lesions are present on the distal extremities, predominantly about the joints (as shown in Color Plate K). The most likely diagnosis is

(A) herpes simplex
(B) meningococcemia
(C) gonococcemia
(D) erythema multiforme
(E) anthrax

Questions 718–719

A 26-year-old man from Cape Cod sees his physician because of a 3-week history of an expanding, slightly burning ring of redness (as shown in Color Plate L) that first surrounded a red papule on the posterior neck. He complains of headaches, generalized muscle aches, anorexia, and malaise. On examination, he is noted to be febrile (38.3°C [101°F]); his rash is slightly raised and slightly tender and displays central clearing but no scaling, even after vigorous scraping.

718. Which of the following vectors has been strongly associated with the type of rash described above?

(A) Kissing bug
(B) Spider
(C) Flea
(D) Tick
(E) Housefly

719. After 6 weeks of observation without treatment, the rash and systemic signs and symptoms disappear. Two months later, however, the man develops acute arthritis of his shoulders and knees. Joint and bone x-rays are normal, and serologic studies for systemic lupus erythematosus and rheumatoid arthritis are negative. The man's joint complaints resolve without therapy in a week, but during the next 3 months he has three similar episodes of asymmetric arthritis of the knees, elbows, and shoulders, each episode lasting 5 to 7 days and responding to therapy with aspirin. Between episodes, he has been entirely asymptomatic, and neither joint deformities nor persistent synovitis has occurred.

Appropriate therapies could include all the following EXCEPT

(A) intravenous penicillin G
(B) oral doxycycline
(C) oral amoxicillin and probenecid
(D) intravenous ceftriaxone
(E) oral chloroquine

720. A homosexual male develops a violaceous nodule on his right forearm (as shown in Color Plate M). Biopsy reveals spindle cell infiltration in the dermis with erythrocyte-containing vascular channels. Which of the following statements about this man's condition is true?

(A) It is caused by retroviral infection of dermal mesenchymal cells
(B) Extracutaneous involvement is uncommon
(C) The entity is seen most frequently in association with intravenous drug abuse
(D) Interferon-α is a useful treatment modality
(E) Standard cytotoxic chemotherapy is absolutely contraindicated because of the low response rate and enhancement of immunosuppression

721. A 24-year-old man is concerned because of the appearance of several light brown spots on his trunk (Color Plate N). The lesions (limited to the chest, back, abdomen, and upper arms) are flat and sharply marginated and have a fine scale that is easily scraped off. The most appropriate diagnostic study is

(A) Giemsa stain of scraped material (Tzanck preparation)
(B) bacterial culture of the lesions
(C) fungal culture of the lesions
(D) microscopic examination of potassium hydroxide–treated scrapings
(E) examination of the serum for anticardiolipin antibody

722. A 39-year-old pediatrician presents with severe scaling of the hands with vesicle formation (see color Plate O). She reports a long-standing history of similarly dry, somewhat painful lesions that have undergone a series of remissions and exacerbations. She denies a history of asthma, hay fever, or skin problems as a child. She also notes that the small vesicles on the sides of her fingers are quite pruritic. The most likely diagnosis is

(A) herpes zoster
(B) atopic dermatitis
(C) asteatotic eczema
(D) dyshidrotic eczema
(E) lichen planus

723. For 25 years, a 55-year-old man has had recurrent episodes of nonpruritic red patches on both elbows, typically covered with thick, white scales (see Color Plate P). He has one brother with a similar condition. Both siblings state that their lesions are exacerbated by stress. Physical examination reveals similar lesions on the lower legs. A biopsy of such a lesion would reveal

(A) an increased number of mitotic figures in skin cells
(B) neutrophils at the tips of follicular openings
(C) degeneration of the basal cell layer
(D) infiltration of neutrophils in small dermal vessels
(E) patchy infiltration of upper dermis with atypical lymphocytes that have convoluted nuclei

724. A 45-year-old woman presents with a pruritic diffuse rash over her trunk and lower legs (see Color Plate Q). The remainder of her physical examination is unremarkable. She has no known past medical history. Detailed questioning reveals that she was seen at an outpatient clinic last week because of dysuria. Trimethoprim-sulfamethoxazole was prescribed. Which of the following statements concerning the patient's rash is correct?

(A) The basis for this reaction is drug-induced IgE release from mass cells
(B) The patient would likely have a similar reaction to penicillin
(C) If untreated, this reaction is likely to progress to skin necrosis
(D) This rash represents an example of the most common form of drug-induced eruption
(E) Topical steroids should be prescribed

725. A 65-year-old man presents with several lesions on both thighs as well as a similar lesion in his mouth. He noted pruritus in these areas several weeks ago. The patient is generally well and on no medications. Each of the lesions (see Color Plate R) is approximately 1 to 4 cm in size. Thumb pressure fails to cause extension of the lesion. The most likely diagnosis is

(A) pemphigus vulgaris
(B) bullous pemphigoid
(C) herpes zoster
(D) impetigo
(E) dermatitis herpetiformis

726. A 67-year-old man presents with a history of headache for 5 days and 2 days of swelling of the right part of the forehead and right eye (see Color Plate S). A Tzanck preparation of the lesion reveals multinucleate giant cells on Giemsa stain. The patient was admitted to the hospital and begun on intravenous acyclovir. The most important next step would be

(A) ophthalmologic consultation
(B) administration of systemic corticosteroids to prevent postherpetic neuralgia
(C) administration of antistaphylococcal antibiotics to prevent secondary bacterial infection
(D) application of iodine-containing solution to prevent secondary bacterial infections
(E) CT scan of the brain

727. A 20-year-old woman presents with a 2-week history of facial rash, fever of 39°C (102.2°F), and progressive malaise. In addition to her dermatologic findings (Color Plate T), physical examination also reveals swollen and tender knees and wrists bilaterally. Additional skin lesions that may be found in patients with this disorder include

(A) silvery scales on elbows and knees
(B) ulcerative lesions of the lower extremities
(C) hemorrhagic bullae
(D) hyperkeratosis
(E) vesicles in a dermatomal distribution

728. A 25-year-old homosexual man presents with a diffuse maculopapular rash over his trunk, head, neck, palms, and soles. Generalized lymphadenopathy is also present. He has a history of 4 weeks of anal pain. Which of the following tests is likely to identify the etiologic agent?

(A) Antinuclear antibody
(B) Blood culture
(C) Serum rapid plasma reagin (RPR)
(D) Skin biopsy
(E) Serum HIV antibody

729. A 35-year-old man is noted to have multiple telangiectatic lesions on the lips, face, feet, and nail beds. When the skin is stretched over an individual lesion, an eccentrically placed central area with radiating vessels is noted. The patient states that many members of his family have similar lesions. Which of the following is likely in this patient?

(A) Consumptive coagulopathy
(B) Gastrointestinal bleeding
(C) Renal failure
(D) Joint diffusions
(E) No clinical problems

DIRECTIONS: Each question below contains five suggested responses. For **each** of the five responses listed with every question, you are to respond either YES (Y) or NO (N). In a given item **all, some, or none** of the alternatives may be correct.

730. A 35-year-old woman visits her doctor for her yearly checkup. Physical examination is unremarkable except for white patches (as shown in Color Plate U) involving her face, hands, torso, anus, and genitalia. The white spots have been present for 2 years. This dermatologic condition has been associated with which of the following diseases?

(A) Alopecia areata
(B) Pernicious anemia
(C) Addison's disease
(D) Hyperthyroidism
(E) Hypothyroidism

731. A 35-year-old man has had recurrent diarrhea for at least 5 years. About 7 years ago many reddish-brown macules appeared on his torso and extremities (see Color Plate V). Rubbing these lesions gently results in the formation of a wheal. He also has been bothered by severe generalized itching, which is made worse when he takes aspirin for his frequent headaches. He has lost 11.4 kg (25 lb) in the last few months. Reasonable measures in his management would include

(A) reassurance that his disease is likely to disappear spontaneously
(B) bone survey and liver scan for evaluation of systemic involvement
(C) prescription of oral cromolyn for diarrhea
(D) prescription of codeine for his headaches
(E) genetic counseling

732. An 18-year-old man (pictured in Color Plate W) presents because of unsightly facial inflammation. Correct statements concerning this patient include which of the following?

(A) Closed comedones (whiteheads) are less commonly associated with the inflammatory lesions than are open comedones (blackheads)
(B) Glucocorticoids, although not indicated except in the most severe cases, would likely result in improvement
(C) Vigorous scrubbing of the face, which will eliminate surface oils, is indicated
(D) Systemic antibiotic therapy is unlikely to be helpful
(E) Patients on systemic retinoic acid may experience very dry skin and hypertriglyceridemia

Questions 733–734

A 55-year-old female noted the onset of skin fragility on the back of her hands 6 months ago. Occasional tense blisters are noted at these sites (see Color Plate X). The blisters heal with the formation of tiny inclusion cysts (milia). Increased facial hair on the upper cheeks and a violaceous color periocularly is noted. The skin appears entirely normal in non-sun-exposed areas. She has smoked two packs of cigarettes per day for 20 years and has consumed a six-pack of beer daily for years.

733.   Laboratory findings might include

    (A)   elevated AST (SGOT)
    (B)   elevated serum iron
    (C)   elevated urinary uroporphyrin and coproporphyrin
    (D)   elevated immunoglobulin E
    (E)   anemia

734.   Effective treatments might include

    (A)   oral ferrous sulfate
    (B)   serial phlebotomy
    (C)   oral estrogens
    (D)   oral hexachlorobenzene
    (E)   oral chloroquine

735.   Known cutaneous reactions to specific drugs include

    (A)   aspirin-induced photosensitivity
    (B)   phenytoin-induced skin necrosis
    (C)   propylthiouracil-induced vasculitis
    (D)   thiazide-induced photosensitivity
    (E)   gold-induced hyperpigmentation

Dermatologic Disorders

Answers

712. The answer is C. *(Chaps 54, 369.)* Flat, brown spots, called *café au lait spots,* are areas of increased pigmentation produced by clones of genetically programmed melanocytes. Café au lait spots, which can vary in size from several millimeters up to 1 cm in diameter, occur in both neurofibromatosis (von Recklinghausen's disease) and Albright's disease (polyostotic fibrous dysplasia with precocious puberty in females), as well as in some normal persons. One or two spots at least 0.5 cm in diameter appear in 25 percent of normal children, but three or more spots of the same size occur in only 0.6 percent. About 9 percent of college-age persons have at least one spot 1.5 cm in size or greater. Of those persons with neurofibromatosis, 95 percent have at least one spot 1.5 cm or larger, and 78 percent have six or more spots. Because persons with Albright's disease rarely have more than four macules, the presence of six or more spots 1.5 cm or greater in size, especially in the presence of axillary freckling, is strongly suggestive of neurofibromatosis. Furthermore, the café au lait spots in Albright's disease tend to be larger and more irregular than those in neurofibromatosis.

713. The answer is E. *(Chap 54.)* Pyoderma gangrenosum is most closely associated with ulcerative colitis and regional enteritis. Its association with rheumatoid arthritis also is well recognized, and it can accompany a variety of hematologic disorders, such as acute and chronic myelogenous leukemia, myeloma, myeloid metaplasia, and polycythemia vera. Bacterial cultures and skin biopsies should be done in an evaluation for sepsis, vasculitis, or leukemia cutis. However, diagnosis of pyoderma gangrenosum is based on the lesion's morphology, not histological analysis.

714. The answer is E. *(Chap 54.)* Acanthosis nigricans is a skin disease associated with a number of disorders. The skin, which is thrown up into folds, appears velvety and hyperpigmented (brown to black) grossly and papillomatous microscopically. The lesions appear on the flexural areas of the neck, axillae, groin, antecubital fossae, and occasionally around the areolae, periumbilical and perianal areas, lips, buccal mucosa, and over the surfaces of the palms, elbows, knees, and interphalangeal joints. The disorder may be hereditary or appear in association with obesity or an endocrinopathy (acromegaly, polycystic ovary syndrome, diabetes mellitus, Cushing's syndrome, but *not* adrenal insufficiency). Drugs such as nicotinic acid also can produce the condition. When acanthosis nigricans develops in a nonobese adult, neoplasia, particularly gastric adenocarcinoma, must be suspected.

715. The answer is C. *(Chaps 54, 115.)* Patients who are profoundly neutropenic are at risk of developing disseminated infections due to skin flora such as *Staphylococcus aureus* and *Staphylococcus* *epidermidis,* as well as enteric gram-negative rods, *Candida,* and *Aspergillus.* Although *Pseudomonas aeruginosa* is the classic etiologic agent, blood stream infection with any of these organisms, except those typically inhabiting the skin, can produce the centrally necrotic lesion termed *ecthyma gangrenosum.* This lesion, which represents a localized necrotizing vasculitis due to invasion with microorganisms, may begin as an erythematous papule.

716. The answer is C. *(Chaps 54, 154.)* Although hand-foot-and-mouth disease usually affects children under the age of 10 years, especially preschoolers, the disease has been noted in adults with or without contact with affected children. The responsible agent is a coxsackievirus. The differential diagnosis includes aphthous ulcers, herpangina, herpes simplex, and erythema multiforme. Characteristically, the prodromal phase of hand-foot-and-mouth disease features malaise and upper-respiratory-tract symptoms; then, acute ulcerative stomatitis, mild pyrexia, and vesiculation of hands, feet, and buttocks occur. Vesicles in the oral cavity rapidly become ulcerated; tongue, gums, buccal mucous membrane, palate, and pharynx can all be involved. The cutaneous vesicles frequently are oval in shape and have an erythematous halo. Recovery occurs without specific treatment in 7 to 10 days.

717. The answer is C. *(Chaps 54, 110.)* The skin lesions of disseminated gonococcal infection occur on the distal extremities, usually around joints, and appear within a week of the onset of joint symptoms. The lesions, which may number as many as 20 (average: 4 or 5), often are painful, and each crop of new lesions is associated with a temperature rise. Lesions begin as a red macule or purpuric spot and then develop into a papule, a vesicle, and, finally, a pustule. Organisms rarely are cultured from the skin lesions; they can be demonstrated occasionally on Gram stain and more regularly with immunofluorescent techniques. Herpes simplex typically occurs as grouped vesicles. Skin lesions of meningococcemia consist of red macules that quickly become petechial or purpuric; migratory polyarthralgias and tenosynovitis are atypical. Erythema multiforme requires "iris" lesions for diagnosis. Anthrax consists of a single pimple or papule on exposed parts of the body; the lesion rapidly enlarges, developing into a vesicle that is surrounded by edema and later undergoes hemorrhagic necrosis, ulceration, and eschar formation.

718. The answer is D. *(Chaps 54, 137. Steere, N Engl J Med 321:586, 1989.)* An expanding erythematous rash not associated with scaling is characteristic of erythema chronicum migrans. The disease first appears weeks to months after a tick bite. The lesion begins as a red macule at the site of the bite; the borders of the lesion then expand to form a red ring, with central clearing, as wide as 20 to 30 cm or more in diameter. Occasionally, secondary rings may occur within the original one. The lesion may itch or burn and may be accompanied by fever, headache, vomiting, fatigue, and regional adenopathy.

719. The answer is E. *(Chaps 54, 137. Steere, N Engl J Med 321:586, 1989.)* Acute recurrent arthritis not associated with joint damage should suggest the possibility of Lyme arthritis. The spirochete *Borrelia burgdorferi* is the causative agent. The arthritis is sometimes monoarticular, often asymmetric and migratory; the knee joints most commonly are involved. Attacks are separated by gradually lengthening intervals: 1 to 3 weeks at first, later as much as 1 to 3 years. Acute attacks, which may be associated with fever, sometimes are preceded by a few days to several weeks by erythema chronicum migrans. For the arthritis characteristic of stage 3 Lyme disease, 100 mg of doxycycline twice daily or amoxicillin and probenecid, each 500 mg four times a day, are effective. Alternatively, or in the case of therapeutic failures, intravenous penicillin or ceftriaxone may be given. Chloroquine is a disease-modifying agent used for rheumatoid arthritis, which is not the diagnosis in this case because of the short-lived, intermittent nature of the man's symptoms.

720.   The answer is D.   *(Chaps 54, 279.)*   AIDS-associated Kaposi's sarcoma, which is present in this man, is a much more fulminant disease than the variant of the disease seen in elderly, non-HIV-infected patients. There is no evidence to implicate direct HIV-induced transformation as the etiology. For unknown reasons, the disease is much more common in homosexuals with AIDS than in heterosexuals with AIDS. While the lesions begin as papules or plaques on the face and upper extremities, they typically evolve into nodules and may be present in any location, most commonly the lungs, lymph nodes, and gastrointestinal tract. Treatment strategies include watchful waiting in low-volume, cosmetically acceptable disease; electron-beam (superficial) radiation therapy for local disease that requires palliation; and carefully administered chemotherapy (VP-16, doxorubicin, vinblastine, and bleomycin have activity) for disseminated disease. A promising approach involves the use of interferon-α, which is associated with a 30 percent rate of complete remission in those with Kaposi's sarcoma and relatively well-preserved circulating helper T cells (CD4+ cells).

721.   The answer is D.   *(Chaps 50, 51.)*   A very common asymptomatic fungus infection of the skin caused by the dermatophyte *Pityrosporum orbiculare* (tinea versicolor) is often the source of a patient's concerns regarding cancer or serious infectious disease. However, this infection is easily treated by scrubbing off the scales with soap and water and with short applications of selenium sulfide (2.5%) for 12 nights. Antifungal creams, including imidazoles such as miconazole, can also be used. Lesions are sharply marginated macules with fine scaling that is easily scraped off with the edge of a microscopic glass slide. The scrapings, examined microscopically after treatment with potassium hydroxide, will reveal hyphae and spores commonly referred to as "spaghetti and meatballs." Tinea versicolor has a predilection for sites in the upper trunk and upper arms; lesions rarely appear on the face.

722.   The answer is D.   *(Chap 51.)*   Hand eczema is one of the most common chronic skin disorders. This condition may or may not be associated with atopic dermatitis (based on a family history of atopy, presence of other forms of allergy such as asthma or allergic rhinitis, or a history of childhood or infantile eczema). Excessive exposure to water and detergents (such as might be experienced by pediatricians who frequently wash their hands) may initiate or aggravate this disorder. Typically, the hands are dry and cracked, but redness and swelling may also accompany the lesions. A common variant of hand dermatitis, exhibited by the patient in this question, is dyshidrotic eczema, which is characterized by multiple highly pruritic vesicles on the sides of the fingers. Lichen planus is a papulosquamous disorder in which the primary lesions are pruritic and characterized by a violaceous hue. Herpes zoster presents with grouped vesicles on an erythematous base. Asteatotic eczema develops most commonly on the lower legs of elderly persons during dry seasons and is characterized by fine cracks, with or without erythema. Therapy of hand dermatitis requires avoidance of frequent washing or harsh soaps, treatment of secondary staphylococcal and streptococcal infection if present, and application of topical steroids.

723.   The answer is A.   *(Chap 51.)*   Psoriasis is a very common skin disorder that typically involves the elbows, knees, gluteal cleft, and scalp. Traumatized areas may also be involved (Kobner phenomenon). The lesions are characterized by erythematous, sharply demarcated papules and rounded plaques covered by a silvery scale. Histologically, the epidermis shows intraepidermal collections of neutrophils (microabscesses of Munro), but capillaries are usually not filled with neutrophils, a finding more characteristic of leukocytoclastic vasculitis. Infiltration of the dermis with lymphocytes that have convoluted nuclei would suggest cutaneous T-cell lymphoma (mycosis fungoides). The dermatopathology of psoriasis is characterized by inflammation and alteration of the cell cycle manifested by a marked thickening of the epidermis, increased keratinocyte mitotic figures and inflammatory cells in the dermis (usually lymphocytes and monocytes), and neutrophils in the upper dermis. Though treatment depends on the type, location, and extent of disease, localized application of glucocorticoids in conjunction with keratolytic agents such as salicylic acid may be used. If psoriasis is widespread, B spectrum ultraviolet light alone or in combination with coal tar (Goeckerman regimen) may be required.

724. The answer is D. *(Chap 52.)* Morbilliform or maculopapular eruptions are arguably the most common type of drug-induced reaction. Such rashes may be asymptomatic or associated with moderate to severe itching or fever. The pathogenesis is unclear but is almost certainly distinct from the IgE-mediated immediate reactions that can produce urticaria, laryngeal edema, and bronchospasm. The typical morbilliform reaction exemplified by this patient usually begins within 1 week of initiation of the offending drug and may last between 1 and 2 weeks thereafter. Such skin reactions are particularly common in patients taking ampicillin, amoxicillin, allopurinol, or trimethoprim-sulfamethoxazole. The optimal treatment is discontinuation of the drug and avoidance of the drug in the future. Such reactions are self-limited and tend not to progress to toxic epidermal necrolysis or skin necrosis, which is seen after warfarin administration in patients with protein C deficiency.

725. The answer is B. *(Chap 53.)* Bullous pemphigoid is a blistering skin disease of the elderly. Extensive blisters may appear after a prodrome of urticarial or eczematous eruption over the lower abdomen, groin, and flexor service of the extremities. Oral mucosal involvement is seen in about 10 to 40 percent of patients. Unlike pemphigus vulgaris, there is no ethnic or racial association. Nikolsky's sign (extension of the blister on pressure by the examining finger) is negative. Light microscopic examination of a lesional biopsy would reveal subepidermal bullae; immunofluorescent studies would demonstrate IgG deposits along the basement membrane zone. Bullous pemphigoid is believed to be an autoimmune disease; 70 percent of patients' serum contains circulating IgG autoantibodies capable of binding the epidermal basement membrane of normal human skin. These autoantibodies and their subsequent deposition in the skin are believed to activate complement, leading to the blister-producing inflammatory cell infiltrate. The mainstay of treatment is systemic glucocorticoids. However, minimal disease may be managed with topical steroids alone. Azothioprine is useful if alternative systemic therapy is required.

726. The answer is A. *(Chaps 59, 144.)* Herpes zoster, caused by the varicella zoster virus, which resides in ganglia after primary infection, usually produces a vesicular eruption limited to the dermatome innervated by the corresponding sensory ganglia. Frequently the characteristic rash, grouped vesicles on an erythematous base, is preceded by several days of pain and paresthesia in the involved area. The most common site of involvement is in thoracic dermatomes, but trigeminal, lumbar, and cervical regions may also be affected. Immunosuppressed persons may display dissemination of zoster, which certainly mandates systemic therapy. Nasociliary branch involvement is not uncommon in ophthalmic zoster and may be heralded by vesicular lesions on the side or tip of the nose. Given the possibility of associated conjunctivitis, keratitis, scleritis, or iritis, an ophthalmologist should always be consulted. Though the risk of postherpetic neuralgia is significant in patients over age 60, it is unclear if early use of steroids prevents this complication. While it is reasonable to undertake measures to contain bacterial superinfection, including the use of antibacterial compresses, administration of prophylactic systemic antibiotics is not indicated.

727. The answer is C. *(Chap 53.)* Systemic lupus erythematosus is a systemic multiorgan disease that involves connective tissue and blood vessels. Fever and skin lesions are the most common manifestations, while arthritis and renal pulmonary disease are also typical. The characteristic rash, as exemplified by the patient in this question, is an erythematous, confluent, macular eruption in a butterfly pattern on the face with fine scaling. Other possible skin lesions include erythematous urticarial lesions on the face and arms, hemorrhagic bullae during acute flares, and discoid plaques, which would typify chronic discoid lupus erythematosus. Lupus vasculitis may also present with palpable purpura. Skin biopsy reveals an atrophic epidermis with liquefaction necrosis at the dermal-epidermal junction, edema of the dermis, and a lymphocytic infiltrate. Fibrinoid degeneration of the connective tissue and blood vessel walls may also be noted. Immunofluorescent studies demonstrate staining for immunoglobulins in a granular or globular pattern along the dermal-epidermal junction.

728. The answer is C. *(Chap 54.)* The rash of secondary syphilis is a maculopapular squamous eruption characterized by scattered reddish-brown lesions with a thin scale. The eruption often involves the palms and the soles, which is an important clue in the differential diagnosis. This rash can resemble atypical pityriasis rosea or erythema multiforme. The nontreponemal serologic tests such as the Venereal Disease Research Laboratory (VDRL) or RPR tests are positive. Patients usually give a history of a chancre at the site of the primary infection—in a heterosexual male usually the penis, but possibly the anus or pharynx. Treatment for both HIV-positive and HIV-negative adults is 2.4 million units of benzathine penicillin by intramuscular injection. If this treatment is successful, the nontreponemal serologic tests should become negative.

729. The answer is B. *(Chap 54.)* The shape and configuration of the dilated blood vessels are important features in distinguishing among the various types of telangiectasias. For example, linear telangiectasias are seen on the face of patients with actinically damaged skin. Broad telangiectasias are seen in scleroderma, especially that associated with the CREST variant of this disease. Periungual telangiectasias may be seen in systemic lupus, scleroderma, and dermatomyositis. Finally, spiderlike telangiectasias are characteristic of hereditary hemorrhagic telangiectasia (Osler-Rendu-Weber disease). These lesions are inherited in an autosomal dominant fashion and the major symptoms are recurrent epistaxis and gastrointestinal bleeding. These mucosal abnormalities are actually arteriovenous communications and tend to bleed easily. A consumptive coagulopathy is noted in hereditary Kasabach-Merritt arteriovenous malformation but not in Osler-Rendu-Weber disease.

730. The answer is A-Y, B-Y, C-Y, D-Y, E-Y. *(Chap 54.)* The photographed skin lesions are depigmented macules of vitiligo. Vitiliginous macules are completely lacking in pigment and are histologically devoid of melanocytes. This disorder is believed to be transmitted as an autosomal dominant trait with incomplete penetrance. Although the majority of cases of vitiligo are not associated with other disease processes, an association has been described between vitiligo and several disorders, including diabetes mellitus, pernicious anemia, hyperthyroidism, hypothyroidism, Addison's disease, alopecia areata, and hypoparathyroidism. The polyglandular autoimmune syndromes, which may involve several of the aforementioned endocrine abnormalities, are also associated with vitiligo.

731. The answer is A-N, B-Y, C-Y, D-N, E-Y. *(Chap 54.)* Urticaria pigmentosa is a disorder of mast cells. The development of a wheal on gentle stroking of a pigmented macule (Darier's sign) is a useful diagnostic maneuver. Prognosis is said to worsen with age of onset: half the patients who develop multiple lesions by 4 years of age are disease-free by adolescence. Onset in adulthood is more ominous, with active lesions persisting indefinitely; systemic mastocytosis, which may have a fatal outcome, occurs frequently in affected adults. Symptomatic improvement has been reported with oral cromolyn. Affected persons should be warned to avoid substances and environmental factors known to cause mast-cell degranulation (e.g., cold, heat, trauma, or the ingestion of alcohol, aspirin, or morphine-opium alkaloid drugs). Although the disorder is usually an isolated event, familial disease occurs, indicating autosomal dominant inheritance in some cases.

732. **The answer is A-N, B-N, C-N, D-N, E-Y.** *(Chap 51.)* Acne vulgaris is a self-limited disease mainly of young adults that causes inflamed cysts (comedones), which sometimes result in scarring. Closed comedones, or whiteheads, seen as white lesions of 1 to 2 mm, are often accompanied by inflammatory papules, pustules, or nodules as a consequence of the extrusion of oily and keratinous cyst debris. On the other hand, blackheads, or open comedones, which are filled with easily expressible dark material, do not usually cause serious problems. Vigorous facial scrubbing is contraindicated since this trauma could lead to rupture of comedones. Other predisposing factors include the use of systemic glucocorticoids, phenytoin, isoniazid, or phenobarbital. Treatment strategies include oral tetracycline or erythromycin therapy to decrease cyst colonization. Severe acne may be treated with a 20-week course of oral retinoic acid therapy, which may prevent formation of comedones by altering the pattern of epidermal desquamation. Pregnant patients should avoid retinoic acid given the teratogenic nature of this compound; this drug also causes extremely dry skin and hypertriglyceridemia.

733. **The answer is A-Y, B-Y, C-Y, D-N, E-N.** *(Chaps 55, 346.)* Porphyria cutanea tarda results from a derangement in the synthesis of heme usually induced by an ingestion (e.g., of alcohol or estrogens). There is decreased activity of the enzyme uroporphyrinogen decarboxylase. Laboratory findings usually include elevation of hematocrit, serum iron, hepatic transaminases, and urinary uro- and coproporphyrins. The elevation of porphyrins in the circulation leads to the development of phototoxic tense blisters in sun-exposed areas, which heal with miliary formation. Increased facial hair, increased skin fragility in sun-exposed areas, and periocular violaceous skin coloration are also frequently found.

734. **The answer is A-N, B-Y, C-N, D-N, E-Y.** *(Chaps 55, 346.)* Porphyria cutanea tarda should be treated by removal of inciting agents. The use of phlebotomies or chelation therapy will reduce the potentially dangerous buildup of iron stores. Intermittent low doses of antimalarials, such as chloroquine and hydroxychloroquine, may also be useful.

735. **The answer is A-N, B-N, C-Y, D-Y, E-Y.** *(Chap 52.)* It is well recognized that drugs can produce virtually any cutaneous reaction. Drug-induced urticaria, for example, may be induced via IgE release, immune complexes, or nonimmunologic means. Aspirin, penicillin, and blood products are commonly associated with urticaria, but virtually any drug can cause this particular reaction. Photosensitivity reactions may be due to phototoxicity, which is predictable, dose-related, and tends to produce sunburnlike changes, or to photoallergy, in which an immune response plus light is required to produce a wide variety of skin manifestations. The list of drugs producing photosensitivity is long and includes chlorpromazine, tetracycline, and thiazides. Hyperpigmentation is either secondary to drug-induced melanocyte stimulation (estrogens) or to direct skin deposition as in the case of the phenothiazines or heavy metals, including arsenic, gold, silver, bismuth, and mercury. Immune-complex formation is probably the mechanism of drug-induced palpable purpura as a manifestation of vasculitis. In addition to propylthiouracil, which can cause splenomegaly and lymphadenopathy plus cutaneous lesions, other drugs able to produce vasculitis include allopurinol, thiazides, penicillin, and phenytoin. Phenytoin is associated with a particular hypersensitivity reaction that occurs 1 to 3 weeks after starting the drug. It is characterized by purpuric eruption accompanied by fever, edema, lymphadenopathy, and hepatitis. Some patients, usually women, develop a sharply demarcated erythematous eruption 3 to 10 days after warfarin or heparin therapy has been started. The eruption progresses to hemorrhagic bullae and skin necrosis. Such a phenomenon is seen in patients with protein C deficiency. In such patients, the warfarin-induced drop in low baseline levels of this vitamin K–dependent antithrombotic protein leads to hypercoagulability and thrombosis of dermal vessels.

Disorders of the Nervous System and Muscles

DIRECTIONS: Each question below contains five suggested responses. Select the **one best** response to each question.

736. The function of the muscle spindle is to furnish the central nervous system with information concerning

    (A) muscle tension
    (B) muscle length
    (C) muscle tone
    (D) joint flexion
    (E) joint extension

737. For the last 5 weeks, a 35-year-old woman has had episodes of intense vertigo lasting several hours. Each episode is associated with tinnitus and a sense of fullness in her right ear; during the attacks, she prefers to lie on her left side. Examination during an attack shows that she has fine rotary nystagmus, which is maximal on gaze to the left. There are no ocular palsies, cranial-nerve signs, or long-tract signs. An audiogram shows a high-tone hearing loss in the right ear, with recruitment but no tone decay.

    The most likely diagnosis in the case described is

    (A) labyrinthitis
    (B) Ménière's disease
    (C) vertebral-basilar insufficiency
    (D) acoustic neuroma
    (E) multiple sclerosis

738. A 58-year-old man with diabetes presents with severe bilateral burning pain in both feet. Neurologic examination reveals a sensory neuropathy in a stocking-glove distribution. The drug of choice in this situation is

    (A) desipramine
    (B) fluoxetine
    (C) mexiletine
    (D) fentanyl
    (E) fenoprofen

739. A 25-year-old woman presents to the emergency department with a severe, throbbing headache of the right supraorbital area for the past hour. She also complains of nausea and photophobia. She has had similar attacks in the past, often brought on by menstruation. About 45 min ago she took 400 mg of ibuprofen. Which of the following would be the best therapeutic choice at this time?

    (A) Meperidine, 50 mg intramuscularly
    (B) Codeine, 60 mg orally
    (C) Naproxen, 750 mg orally
    (D) Sumatriptan, 6 mg subcutaneously
    (E) Verapamil, 300 mg orally

740. A 29-year-old woman who uses oral contraceptives comes to the emergency room because when she looked in the mirror this morning, her face was twisted. It felt numb and swollen. Eating breakfast, she found that her food tasted different and she drooled out of the right side of her mouth when she swallowed. Neurologic examination discloses only a dense right facial paresis equally involving the frontalis, orbicularis oculi, and orbicularis oris. Finger rubbing is appreciated as louder in the right ear than in the left. The physician should

(A) instruct the patient in using a patch over the right eye during sleep
(B) recommend that she discontinue use of oral contraceptives
(C) order brainstem auditory evoked potentials to assess her hearing asymmetry
(D) inform her that her chances of substantial improvement within several weeks are only about 40 percent
(E) order an echocardiogram to rule out mitral valve prolapse as a source of emboli

741. The distinctive tetrad of symptoms of the narcolepsy-cataplexy syndrome includes all the following EXCEPT

(A) uncontrollable daytime sleepiness
(B) sudden brief episodes of loss of muscle tone
(C) paralysis upon falling asleep
(D) confusional episodes
(E) hallucinations at the onset of sleep or wakening

742. A 45-year-old man presents with a daily headache. He describes two attacks per day over the past 3 weeks. Each attack lasts about an hour and awakens the patient from sleep. The patient has noted associated tearing and reddening of his right eye as well as nasal stuffiness. The pain is deep, excruciating, and limited to the right side of the head. The neurologic examination is nonfocal. The most likely diagnosis of this patient's headache is

(A) migraine headache
(B) cluster headache
(C) tension headache
(D) brain tumor
(E) giant cell arteritis

743. A 25-year-old woman who was the driver of a car struck by another car in the rear while she was stopped at a red light presents to the emergency department with neck pain, as well as discomfort in the axilla, upper arm, elbow, dorsal forearm, and index and middle fingers. Coughing exacerbates the pain. Neurologic examination reveals weakness in the right second and third fingers, forearm, and wrist. The right triceps reflex is diminished. The most likely diagnosis in this case is

(A) syringomyelia
(B) cervical sprain
(C) thoracic outlet syndrome
(D) cervical disk herniation
(E) brachial plexopathy

744. A man brought into an emergency department is unresponsive and is displaying posturing. Pupils are 4 mm in size and react to light. No eye movements occur with head turning (oculocephalic maneuver) or with ice-water irrigation of the ear canals. The most likely diagnosis is

(A) brain death
(B) hysteria-conversion coma
(C) brainstem hemorrhage
(D) drug ingestion
(E) bilateral internal carotid artery occlusion

745. A patient with previous spells of diplopia, ataxia, dysarthria, and dizziness becomes acutely comatose. The most likely cause is

(A) basilar artery thrombosis
(B) subarachnoid hemorrhage
(C) carotid occlusion
(D) cerebellar hemorrhage
(E) pontine hemorrhage

746. A 75-year-old woman complains of dizziness and lightheadedness while walking. The patient has had long-standing diabetes and is taking an oral hypoglycemic agent. She has no other medical problems. She lives alone. Physical examination reveals visual activity of 20/80 in both eyes, and sensory neuropathy in a stocking-glove distribution. On close questioning she denies any symptoms of "herself spinning or the world spinning." She has no apparent anxiety or depression. Orthostatic vital signs are normal. A head tilt maneuver reveals no nystagmus. The most likely diagnosis in this case is

(A) dysequilibrium of aging
(B) benign positional vertigo
(C) Ménière's disease
(D) brainstem stroke
(E) neoplasm of the central nervous system

747. A 35-year-old woman complaining of trouble with her "peripheral vision" is subjected to visual field examination. Testing one eye at a time, she is asked to focus on a central target while the examiner's fingers are moved in from various directions. She is unable to distinguish objects brought laterally toward the midline, encompassing about half the visual field in each eye. Which of the following lesions would most likely account for these findings?

(A) Open-angle glaucoma
(B) Closed-angle glaucoma
(C) Multiple sclerosis
(D) Pituitary tumor
(E) Embolic occlusion of the posterior cerebral artery

748. Evoked-potential testing is most useful in diagnosing

(A) brainstem involvement in stroke
(B) a clinically occult lesion in multiple sclerosis
(C) large hemispheral strokes
(D) spinal cord compression
(E) shearing of white matter tracts after head injury

749. A 25-year-old weight lifter comes to the emergency department frightened by recent headaches. He recently read a newspaper article about cerebral aneurysms. He reports 5 to 10 sudden, severe headaches, all occurring during coitus, each lasting about 1 h. The physician should

(A) recommend that the patient seek psychiatric help for his sexual dysfunction
(B) perform a CT scan with contrast and schedule four-vessel cerebral angiography to search for an aneurysm or arteriovenous malformation
(C) inform the patient that coital headache is a benign clinical syndrome that may be helped by administration of propranolol, 20 mg three times a day
(D) tell the patient to report back to the emergency department for a cerebrospinal fluid examination and CT scan without contrast to search for subarachnoid blood
(E) determine whether other members of his family have a history of migraine

750. A 60-year-old male diabetic complains of the acute onset of diplopia. He denies headache, fever, stiff neck, or other symptoms. The only abnormality on neurologic examination pertains to the eye movements. The patient's right eyelid is ptotic. The pupil is deviated downward and outward. The patient cannot move the eye upward, downward, or inward. There is, however, no anisocoria, and normal pupillary responses are present bilaterally. The appropriate course of action at this time is

(A) administration of high-dose steroids
(B) administration of a topical ophthalmic beta-adrenergic blocker
(C) cerebral angiography
(D) visual field testing
(E) reexamination in 1 month

751. Presbycusis, the hearing loss associated with aging, may affect 33 percent of people who are age 75 or older. The most common cause of this problem is

(A) fixation of middle ear bones
(B) tympanic membrane failure
(C) loss of neuroepithelial cells
(D) vascular lesions in central auditory pathways
(E) exposure to ototoxins, such as furosemide

752. While wrestling with his young son, a 32-year-old man suddenly develops a severe headache, then lapses into unconsciousness. Examination in the emergency department reveals retinal hemorrhages, nuchal rigidity, and normal eye movements on passive head rotation. The best initial diagnostic measure would be

(A) lumbar puncture
(B) skull x-rays
(C) CT scan of the head
(D) radionuclide brain scan
(E) bilateral carotid and vertebral angiography

753. Depression may be mistaken for dementia because of the hypokinetic state, poor attention span, and loss of impulse control common to both conditions. However, a major distinguishing feature of dementia would be

(A) anorexia
(B) headache
(C) multiple somatic complaints
(D) impaired performance on memory tests
(E) prominent release reflexes

754. Bradykinesia, a decreased ability to initiate volitional movements, as well as constant impedance to the examiner's efforts to extend the arm would most likely be due to lesions in which of the following structures?

(A) Anterior horn cell of the spinal cord
(B) Descending corticospinal fibers
(C) Basal ganglia
(D) Internal capsule
(E) Cerebral cortex

755. A 70-year-old man complains of pain and stiffness in both shoulders and hips. Examination reveals atrophic shoulder girdle and gluteal musculature. Reflexes and cerebellar function are intact. There is no sensory loss. The serum creatine kinase level is normal. Temporal artery biopsy is negative. The most appropriate therapeutic strategy at this time is

(A) prednisone, 60 mg daily
(B) prednisone, 10 mg daily
(C) potassium repletion
(D) naproxen, 750 mg twice daily
(E) reassurance; no treatment required

756. A 65-year-old man with advanced pancreatic cancer complains of increasing abdominal pain. He is taking codeine 60 mg every 4 h. Examination reveals an alert man with a benign abdomen and normal neurologic function. The best step at this point would be to

(A) add phenytoin
(B) add indomethacin
(C) increase the dose of codeine
(D) add sustained-release morphine sulfate and use the codeine as circumstances require (prn)
(E) refer the patient for a celiac block

757. A 55-year-old woman presents because of intermittent, brief, extreme stabbing pains in her lips and right cheek. The pain can be brought on by touching her face. The results of examination of the structures of the face and cranial nerves are entirely normal. Appropriate initial treatment for this condition would be

(A) ergotamine
(B) amitriptyline
(C) propranolol
(D) carbamazepine
(E) referral to an otolaryngologist for nerve block

758. During evaluation of a patient with a gait disorder, it is noted that the patient is unable to accurately identify the direction of examiner-initiated movement of the great toe. Pain and temperature sense in the same distribution are intact. This abnormality reflects a lesion in which of the following structures?

(A) Posterior column on the same side as the affected toe
(B) Spinothalamic tract on the same side as the affected toe
(C) Thalamic nucleus on the same side as the affected toe
(D) Lower sensory neuron on the same side as the affected toe
(E) Frontal cortex on the opposite side from the affected toe

759. A patient being evaluated for aphasia is unable to repeat sentences correctly or to name objects properly. However, the patient's speech is effortless and melodic. There are frequent errors in word choice and obvious difficulties in comprehension. The remainder of the patient's neurologic examination is normal. Damage in which area of the brain would account for this type of aphasia?

(A) Posterior temporal and parietal lobes, dominant hemisphere
(B) Frontal and parietal lobes, dominant hemisphere
(C) Prefrontal and frontal regions, dominant hemisphere
(D) Posterior parietal and temporal lobes, nondominant hemisphere
(E) Parietal and occipital lobes, nondominant hemisphere

760. A patient is evaluated for anisocoria. The right pupil is small and round compared with the left pupil in room light; this difference is magnified when the room is darkened. The right pupil responds briskly to light, constricts when pilocarpine is placed in the eye, and dilates when atropine is placed in the eye. Minimal dilation is produced by 4% cocaine. This patient has a lesion in the

(A) right optic nerve
(B) right iris
(C) right third nerve
(D) right sympathetic chain
(E) left occipital lobe

761. Which of the following would help to exclude the diagnosis of seizure in a patient with sudden loss of consciousness?

(A) A brief period of tonic-clonic movements at the time of falling
(B) An aura of a strange odor prior to falling
(C) Sudden return to normal mental function upon awakening, though feeling physically weak
(D) Urinary incontinence
(E) Laceration of the tongue

762. A 55-year-old man who lost his job approximately 5 months ago complains of profound difficulty in sleeping at night. He recently found a new job but has continued to experience difficulty in sleeping. He notes that he falls asleep more easily while watching television early in the evening and feels sleepy outside of the house. He is quite preoccupied with his inability to sleep at night. General physical examination and routine laboratory screening are unremarkable. He denies use of alcohol, coffee, or other drugs. What is the most appropriate approach?

(A) Administration of benzodiazepine
(B) Administration of stimulants
(C) Administration of estrogen
(D) Administration of tricyclic antidepressants
(E) No therapy

763. CT of the brain is preferred over MRI (with gadolinium enhancement) in which of the following situations?

(A) Chronic renal failure
(B) Suspected acute subarachnoid hemorrhage
(C) Suspected demyelinating diseases
(D) Screening for metastatic neoplasms
(E) Suspected posterior fossa lesions

764. A physician confronted with a comatose patient with a severe head injury would be best advised to

(A) perform a skull and neurologic examination, obtain a CT scan of the head, and recommend burr holes if the pupils are enlarged
(B) stabilize the neck, administer mannitol and steroids, and obtain a CT scan
(C) treat hypotension, ensure airway patency, perform a skull and neurologic examination, and obtain a CT scan
(D) treat hypoxia and hypotension, raise the head, and obtain a CT scan
(E) stabilize the neck, obtain neck and skull x-rays, and recommend burr holes if the pupils are enlarged

765. A 65-year-old man presents with severe right-sided eye and facial pain, nausea, vomiting, colored halos around lights, and loss of visual acuity. His right eye is quite red and his pupil is dilated and fixed. Which of the following diagnostic tests would confirm the diagnosis?

(A) CT scan of the head
(B) MRI scan of the head
(C) Cerebral angiography
(D) Tonometry
(E) Slit-lamp examination

766. A 35-year-old woman presents with an apparent seizure. She was feeling well when she noted that her right thumb began suddenly to retract repetitively followed by right hand movements. Within 1 min her right arm and the right side of her face also began to contract. About 2 min later the patient developed diffuse convulsive motor activity and loss of consciousness lasting about 5 min. After recovery of consciousness the patient was amnestic for the event and also had about 6 h of weakness in her right arm. Which of the following is the most likely cause of this type of seizure?

(A) Herpes encephalitis
(B) Temporal lobe epilepsy
(C) Juvenile myoclonic epilepsy
(D) Abscess or tumor in the left motor strip
(E) Cerebral embolism

767. A 19-year-old man has had an 8-year history of recurrent episodes of loss of conscious activity that last for seconds to several minutes. Sometimes he has as many as 100 such lapses. The patient regains awareness of his environment very quickly. There is no major motor manifestation during the episodes, nor is there any period of confusion after the episodes. The patient's neurologic examination is totally normal. Which of the following drugs would be the most effective for this patient's problem?

(A) Phenytoin
(B) Carbamazepine
(C) Phenobarbital
(D) Ethosuximide
(E) Primidone

768. A patient who complains of imbalance is found to walk with a wide-based gait and to sway forward and backward upon standing. Balance cannot be maintained when standing with the feet together when the eyes are open or closed. No limb ataxia or nystagmus can be elicited. These findings are most consistent with a lesion or lesions in the

 (A) vestibular apparatus
 (B) midline cerebellar zone
 (C) intermediate cerebellar zone
 (D) lateral cerebellar zone
 (E) left frontal cortex

769. Which of the following brain tumors tends to occur in immunosuppressed persons, arise in periventricular regions, and respond both clinically and radiographically to corticosteroid therapy?

 (A) Glioblastoma
 (B) Ependymoma
 (C) Meningioma
 (D) Medulloblastoma
 (E) B-cell lymphoma

770. A 59-year-old chronic alcoholic has loss of consciousness and shaking of his entire body for approximately 5 min. He is somewhat confused after this episode and is brought to the emergency department, where another such episode occurs. The patient develops incontinence during the event and is again confused after the episode. A CT of the brain and a lumbar puncture are negative. No major metabolic abnormalities were detected on blood testing. Appropriate therapy for this condition is

 (A) phenytoin, 1000 mg given in a slow IV push
 (B) diazepam, 10 mg IV bolus
 (C) phenobarbital, 400 mg given over 30 min
 (D) carbamazepine, 600 mg orally daily
 (E) no specific anticonvulsant therapy

771. A patient who is being treated for temporal lobe epilepsy (complex partial seizures) and who is having recurrent seizures on his chronic regimen of carbamazepine is given phenobarbital as a second drug. However, the seizures increase in frequency. What is the probable reason for the apparent deleterious effect of adding phenobarbital?

 (A) Intracerebral bleeding from worsening bone marrow suppression
 (B) Decreased carbamazepine level
 (C) Decreased stability of CNS neuronal membranes
 (D) Hypokalemia
 (E) Increased intracranial pressure

772. A person who has right hemiparesis from stroke would be LEAST likely to display

 (A) left facial weakness
 (B) left-gaze paresis
 (C) inability to calculate
 (D) left-right confusion
 (E) ignoring of the deficit

773. For the last several days a college student has had back pain in the midlumbar area, difficulty in starting urination, and paresthesias in the feet. On examination, temperature is 38.3°C (101°F); straight leg raising produces pain, slight hip weakness is present, and Babinski signs are absent. The physician should

 (A) perform a lumbar puncture
 (B) obtain spine films and a bone scan
 (C) obtain blood cultures and start antibiotic therapy
 (D) obtain urinalysis and retroperitoneal ultrasound
 (E) arrange for emergency MRI or CT scan of the spine

774. A 65-year-old man with a long-standing history of hypertension complains of recurrent 30-min episodes of right arm weakness occasionally associated with difficulty speaking. Results of his neurologic examination at this time are normal. Cerebral angiography reveals an 80 percent stenosis of the left internal carotid artery. The most appropriate therapy at this point would be

(A) intravenous heparin with plan to convert to oral warfarin
(B) oral warfarin
(C) aspirin
(D) ticlopidine
(E) carotid endarterectomy

775. A 54-year-old man with long-standing hypertension presents to the emergency department with severe occipital headache and dizziness. He has noted several hours of nausea and vomiting. Neurologic examination reveals inability to stand. His eyes are deviated to the right side and he has mild left-sided facial weakness. Assuming that blood is seen on CT scanning, which is the most appropriate therapeutic strategy at this time?

(A) Intravenous high-dose dexamethasone
(B) Intravenous mannitol
(C) Intravenous nitroprusside
(D) Surgical removal of clot
(E) Cerebral angiography

776. For the last 6 weeks, a 64-year-old woman has had a headache and difficulty reading. Her husband has noted a mild but progressive intellectual decline in his wife during this period. On examination, she has grasping reactions and myoclonic jerks when loud noises occur. CT scan and cerebrospinal fluid examination are normal. The most likely diagnosis is

(A) multiple sclerosis
(B) Alzheimer's disease
(C) bilateral subdural hematoma
(D) Creutzfeldt-Jakob disease
(E) subacute sclerosing panencephalitis

777. The most common presenting finding or symptom of multiple sclerosis is

(A) internuclear ophthalmoplegia
(B) transverse myelitis
(C) cerebellar ataxia
(D) optic neuritis
(E) urinary retention

778. A 45-year-old woman presents with a generalized tonic-clonic seizure, the first of her life. MRI evaluation reveals a midline mass along the falx cerebri. The mass enhances with gadolinium, which documents the existence of tumor vessels supplied by the external carotid artery. The optimal therapy would be

(A) surgery
(B) radiation
(C) radiation plus surgery
(D) radiation plus surgery plus chemotherapy
(E) radiation plus chemotherapy

779. The most common cause of death in patients with intracerebral metastatic lesions from carcinoma is

(A) intractable seizures
(B) infection
(C) radiation toxicity
(D) progressive intracerebral metastases
(E) systemic tumor

780. A 28-year-old woman complains of horizontal diplopia. Examination shows only a lag in adduction of the left eye with nystagmus in the abducting right eye. The most appropriate workup would include

(A) electroencephalography and CT scan with contrast infusion
(B) cerebral angiography and formal visual-field testing
(C) lumbar puncture and evoked potentials
(D) electronystagmography and electroencephalography
(E) none of the above

781. A comatose patient is being evaluated by caloric stimulation of the vestibular apparatus. Cold-water irrigation of the right external auditory canal leads to deviation of both eyes to the right for 2 min followed by a slow drift back to the midline. This finding is most consistent with a lesion in the

   (A) right labyrinth
   (B) midbrain
   (C) medulla
   (D) pons
   (E) cerebral hemispheres

782. A 68-year-old woman presents with an 18-month history of progressive loss of recent memory and inattentiveness. At this time she is having difficulty speaking, her judgment appears to be impaired, and she occasionally evidences paranoid behavior. In addition to neurofibrillary tangles, the neuropathologic findings in this condition include plaques made up of

   (A) low-density lipoprotein
   (B) unesterified cholesterol
   (C) beta-amyloid protein
   (D) immunoglobulin proteins
   (E) protease inhibitor

783. A 68-year-old man develops a rest tremor of his right hand and arm. The patient moves slowly and has a diminished range of facial expressions. He has no postural abnormalities. Which of the following drugs would be most appropriate at this time?

   (A) Deprenyl
   (B) Levodopa
   (C) Carbidopa-levodopa (Sinemet)
   (D) Bromocriptine
   (E) Benztropine

784. A 69-year-old man is brought to the doctor by his wife because she complains that he has been "talking strangely." The patient enunciates words slowly and with difficulty. The melody of speech is abnormal. The speech is agrammatic in the sense that many prepositions and articles are omitted. When a word can be discerned, it is usually appropriate for the conversation and the patient appears to comprehend what is said to him. The lesion accounting for this problem is most likely to be in the

   (A) left frontal lobe
   (B) right frontal lobe
   (C) left parietal lobe
   (D) right parietal lobe
   (E) bilateral temporal lobes

785. Initial therapy for persons with increased intracranial pressure would include

   (A) beta-adrenergic blockers
   (B) phenytoin
   (C) mechanical ventilation to achieve high airway pressures
   (D) hyperosmolar dehydration
   (E) intravenous fluids

786. A 50-year-old woman presents to her primary care physician complaining of intermittent unprovoked attacks of severe shortness of breath, palpitations, shaking, diffuse numbness, and an intense fear of dying or going crazy. These attacks are not precipitated by any obvious anxiety-provoking situation. Moreover, the patient is particularly loathe to leave her house without a companion. General physical examination and routine laboratory studies, which include normal electrolytes, thyroid function tests, electrocardiography, and continuous cardiac rhythm monitoring, have convinced the physician that there is no clear-cut organic cause for this problem. The patient is not on chronic medicine and does not abuse alcohol. The most appropriate therapy for this patient is

   (A) diazepam
   (B) flurazepam
   (C) imipramine
   (D) lithium
   (E) fluphenazine

787. A previously active 25-year-old woman presents with profound fatigue. She had an upper respiratory infection about 6 months ago from which she has never recovered. She now complains of intermittent headaches, sore throat, muscle and joint aches, and occasional feverishness. Her fatigue is so severe that she is unable to work. She now complains of excessive irritability, confusion, and inability to concentrate. Her physician has documented the presence of fever to 38.6°C (101.5°F) orally and the presence of palpable anterior cervical adenopathy both now and approximately 2 months ago. The patient has undergone an extensive workup, which included complete blood count, serum chemistry analysis, HIV serology, EBV serology, CMV serology, and a CT scan of the head, all of which were either negative or not consistent with an acute infection. The patient had no past psychiatric or medical problems. Appropriate therapy at this time would be

(A) acyclovir
(B) corticosteroids
(C) vitamin B_{12} injections
(D) intravenous immunoglobulin
(E) ibuprofen

788. A 59-year-old man who has alcoholic cirrhosis but has been abstinent for 10 years has progressive dysarthria, tongue dystonia, shuffling gait, and fast tremor that worsens as his hand moves toward a target. These symptoms are most likely caused by

(A) Wilson's disease
(B) acquired hepatocerebral degeneration
(C) Wernicke's disease
(D) Marchiafava-Bignami disease
(E) paraneoplastic syndrome

789. The most likely diagnosis for a patient with impotence and urinary incontinence who, over years, sustains a tremor at rest, bradykinesia, rigidity, severe orthostatic hypotension, and anhidrosis is

(A) autonomic form of the Landry-Guillain-Barré syndrome
(B) Shy-Drager syndrome
(C) guanethidine intoxication
(D) micturition syncope
(E) Parkinson's disease

790. A 65-year-old man with long-standing schizophrenia is admitted to the general medical service because of an atypical pneumonia. The patient has been on chlorpromazine for at least 10 years. In addition to findings related to his pneumonia and thought disorder, he also repetitively smacks his lips and thrusts his tongue as well as exhibits a bizarre, stooped posture. Which of the following would be the best approach to reverse these troublesome neurologic symptoms?

(A) Administration of benztropine
(B) Administration of oxazepam
(C) Administration of propranolol
(D) Administration of levodopa-carbidopa (Sinemet)
(E) Reduction of the dose of chlorpromazine

791. A 27-year-old male intravenous drug abuser hospitalized for the treatment of *S. aureus* endocarditis develops diarrhea, rhinorrhea, sweating, and muscle twitching on the third hospital day. Physical examination includes vital signs that disclosed temperature 38°C (100.4°F), respiratory rate 28, blood pressure 160/90, and pulse 120. The patient also complains of intense, diffuse pain. Based on the available data, the best approach would be

(A) administration of oral methadone
(B) administration of intravenous naloxone
(C) administration of intravenous propranolol
(D) administration of oral oxazepam
(E) echocardiography to assess valve patency

792. Lower brachial plexus injuries commonly occur during certain surgical procedures or in association with apical lung tumors. These injuries most typically cause

    (A) weakness of thumb abduction and apposition
    (B) ulnar hand numbness and a "claw hand" deformity
    (C) ulnar hand numbness and inability to flex the elbow
    (D) weakness of shoulder abduction and a patch of numbness over the triceps
    (E) wrist drop and numbness over the dorsal hand between the thumb and index finger

793. A 42-year-old man, who has had difficulty concentrating on his job lately, comes to medical attention because of irregular, jerky movements of his extremities and fingers. A sister and an uncle died in mental institutions, and his mother became demented in middle age. The most likely diagnosis is

    (A) alcoholic cerebral degeneration
    (B) Huntington's chorea
    (C) Wilson's disease
    (D) Hallervorden-Spatz disease
    (E) Gilles de la Tourette's disease

794. A 72-year-old woman presents with brief, intermittent, excruciating episodes of lancinating pain in the lips, gums, and cheek. These intense spasms of pain may be initiated by touching the lips or movement of the tongue. Results of physical examination are normal. MRI of the head is also normal. The most likely cause of this patient's pain is

    (A) acoustic neuroma
    (B) meningioma
    (C) temporal lobe epilepsy
    (D) trigeminal neuralgia
    (E) facial nerve palsy

795. A 30-year-old patient presenting with a gradual decline in mental function is found to have a large lesion on CT examination of the brain. Biopsy reveals glioblastoma multiforme. Physical examination of the skin reveals large, cream-brown cutaneous macules and numerous subcutaneous nodules. Gene mutations in which of the following account for this clinical syndrome?

    (A) Rb protein
    (B) Neurofibromin
    (C) Hexosaminidase A
    (D) KALIG-1
    (E) Amyloid precursor protein

796. A 67-year-old woman appears to have parkinsonian rigidity but no tremor. In addition, she is completely unable to look down and has difficulty looking up. No improvement is seen after treatment with carbidopa-levodopa (Sinemet). The most likely diagnosis is

    (A) atypical parkinsonism
    (B) postencephalitic parkinsonism
    (C) drug-induced parkinsonism and oculogyric crisis
    (D) striatonigral degeneration
    (E) progressive supranuclear palsy

797. Syringomyelia is characterized by all the following EXCEPT

    (A) thoracic scoliosis
    (B) ataxia
    (C) muscle atrophy in the hands
    (D) loss of pain sensation in the shoulders
    (E) preservation of sense of touch

798. A 45-year-old man complains of severe right arm pain. He gives a history of having slipped on the ice and severely contusing his right shoulder approximately 1 month ago. At this time he has sharp, knifelike pain in the right arm and forearm. Physical examination reveals a right arm that is more moist and hairy than the left arm. There is no specific weakness or sensory change. However, the right arm is clearly more edematous than the left and the skin appears somewhat atrophic in the affected limb. The patient's pain is most likely due to

(A) subclavian vein thrombosis
(B) brachial plexus injury
(C) reflex sympathetic dystrophy
(D) acromioclavicular separation
(E) cervical radiculopathy

799. An 18-year-old man is brought to the emergency department because of a bicycle accident. He was riding with a group of friends who noted that the patient's bike hit a rock, the bike tumbled, and the patient's head hit the pavement. Unconsciousness lasted for about 30 s. It is now approximately 1 h since the accident. At this time the patient is alert, though he has thrown up once and complains of difficulty in concentration and blurred vision. Furthermore, he is complaining of a severe frontal headache. Physical examination is notable for the absence of blood at the tympanic membranes and at the mastoid processes and a completely nonfocal neurologic examination. Skull x-rays and an MRI scan are normal. The most appropriate course of action at this point is to

(A) obtain a neurosurgical consultation
(B) admit the patient to the hospital for observation
(C) administer phenytoin and admit the patient to the hospital for observation
(D) perform an electroencephalogram
(E) discharge the patient home in the care of his friends

800. A 30-year-old man comes to the emergency department because for the last 3 days he has had progressive weakness of his legs, sensory loss ascending from his toes to the level of his umbilicus, and urinary retention. Examination reveals a central scotoma, absent knee and ankle jerks, and diminished pinprick sensation in the legs and abdomen up to the umbilicus. Cerebrospinal fluid contains 40 lymphocytes per cubic millimeter and a protein concentration of 0.72 g/L (72 mg/dL).

This clinical picture is LEAST consistent with which of the following diagnoses?

(A) Acute idiopathic polyneuritis
(B) Acute necrotizing myelitis
(C) Postvaccinal myelitis
(D) Postinfectious myelitis
(E) Multiple sclerosis

801. A 70-year-old man is brought in by his wife because of increased drowsiness and generally confused thinking over the past 2 months. Prior to a seemingly minor motor vehicle accident about 2 months ago, the patient had been running a small business without difficulty. There are no focal or lateralizing signs on neurologic examination. A noncontrast CT scan of the brain is normal except that there are no cortical sulci and the ventricles are small. The most likely diagnosis is

(A) Alzheimer's disease
(B) metabolic encephalopathy
(C) subdural hematoma
(D) cerebrovascular accident
(E) depression

802. The bone most commonly fractured in association with an epidural hematoma is

(A) frontal
(B) parietal
(C) temporal
(D) occipital
(E) sphenoidal

803. A patient presents with a rapidly progressive dementia associated with prominent myoclonic jerks that are provoked by her being startled, as well as signs and symptoms of cerebellar dysfunction and emotional lability. Routine cerebrospinal fluid analysis is unremarkable. MRI shows minimal cortical loss. The electroencephalogram discloses periodic sharp wave complexes on a generalized slow background. This disease is caused by

(A) slow-virus infection
(B) deposition of fibrillary amyloid
(C) deposition of aluminum
(D) proteinaceous infectious particle
(E) spirochetes

804. A 60-year-old, mildly obese woman complains of a very bothersome burning pain on the anterolateral aspect of her right thigh from the groin almost as far distally as the knee. Examination shows reduction of sensation to touch and pinprick in the affected area. There is no loss of muscle strength and reflexes are normal. The most likely diagnosis is

(A) ruptured intervertebral disk
(B) femoral hernia
(C) nutritional neuropathy
(D) compression of the lateral femoral cutaneous nerve
(E) disruption of the lumbosacral plexus

805. The major pathologic feature of idiopathic inflammatory polyneuropathy (Guillain-Barré syndrome) is

(A) loss of anterior horn cells
(B) destruction of axons
(C) inflammation of sensory ganglia
(D) wallerian degeneration
(E) segmental demyelination

806. Cataracts, frontal baldness, testicular atrophy, and muscle weakness and wasting occur in association with

(A) myotonic dystrophy
(B) limb-girdle dystrophy
(C) pseudohypertrophic dystrophy
(D) facioscapulohumeral dystrophy
(E) myotonia congenita

807. The form of muscular dystrophy most likely to be encountered in persons older than 50 years of age is

(A) facioscapulohumeral dystrophy
(B) oculopharyngeal dystrophy
(C) myotonic dystrophy
(D) Duchenne's dystrophy
(E) limb-girdle dystrophy

808. Delayed relaxation of a muscle after voluntary contraction is characteristic of certain dystrophic diseases and periodic paralysis. This phenomenon is called

(A) myokymia
(B) myoedema
(C) myotonia
(D) contracture
(E) fibrillation

809. A 65-year-old woman with diabetes mellitus has a 3-month history of sacral pain. In the last month a burning pain progressively developed over the lateral aspect of her left foot and was followed by loss of sensation and weakness of plantar flexion and dorsiflexion. Electromyography showed fibrillations in left gastrocnemius, extensor hallucis, and quadriceps muscles. Nerve conduction was normal in the legs. A myelogram showed normal results. Now she complains that her knee "gives out" while walking; she has an absence of left knee and ankle jerks.
    Her physician should

(A) inform the patient that normal results on her myelogram make a diabetic neuropathy the most likely diagnosis
(B) arrange for a pelvic examination and schedule a CT scan of the pelvis to search for a malignancy compressing or infiltrating the lumbar-sacral plexus
(C) arrange for a repeat myelogram because of new quadriceps weakness
(D) arrange for a CT scan of the head to search for an expanding mass over the right sensorimotor strip that would affect the foot and leg
(E) reexamine her at 2-month intervals to determine progression of her condition

810. The weakness associated with myasthenia gravis is due to which of the following disorders in the neuromuscular junction?

(A) Reduced acetylcholine in presynaptic vesicles
(B) Presynaptic block in release of acetylcholine
(C) Presence of antibodies against presynaptic membranes
(D) Degradation and blockage of postsynaptic receptors
(E) Damage of postsynaptic membranes by T lymphocytes

811. A 49-year-old man with long-standing hypertension presents with right-sided weakness involving the face, arm, and leg, which has evolved over the past 6 h. Neurologic examination is remarkable only for a right-sided hemiparesis without associated aphasia, papilledema, or sensory loss. A CT scan done after several days would most likely reveal

(A) small infarction in the left internal capsule
(B) large infarction in the left cerebral cortex
(C) left internal capsule hemorrhage
(D) left cerebral cortical hemorrhage
(E) normal findings

812. A 54-year-old woman with metastatic breast cancer and extensive bony involvement presents with headache and diplopia. Neurologic examination reveals no evidence for increased intracranial pressure and the only new abnormalities are slight disorientation and inability to abduct the right eye. Head CT without contrast is negative. Lumbar puncture reveals a mononuclear pleocytosis and elevated protein, but the results, including those of cytologic examination, are otherwise unremarkable. Of the following studies, which is most likely to establish a diagnosis?

(A) Contrast CT of the head
(B) MRI of the head
(C) CT of the right orbit, performed with bone windows
(D) Retinal angiography
(E) Repeat lumbar puncture

813. A 27-year-old man seeks advice because he has noticed fasciculations in his calf muscles. He has no other complaints. Examination shows that muscle bulk and strength, tendon and plantar reflexes, and sensory function are all normal. He should undergo

(A) muscle biopsy
(B) sural nerve biopsy
(C) myelography
(D) electromyography
(E) none of the above

814. Which of the following statements concerning porphyric neuropathy is true?

(A) It is rarely associated with confusion or seizures
(B) It predominantly involves the sensory system
(C) It is symmetric, and weakness is often more proximal than distal
(D) It causes elevated protein concentration in cerebrospinal fluid
(E) It is associated with inflammation of nerves

815. A patient has a total right hemianesthesia at the time of cerebral infarction. One year later he complains of constant severe burning pain with occasional sharp jabs of pain in the left side of his face and left arm. The chronic pain syndrome is most likely

(A) part of a biologic depressive syndrome secondary to a right parietal lobe stroke
(B) caused by a lesion in the spinal cord affecting the right spinothalamic tract
(C) a sequela of thalamic infarction
(D) secondary to a shoulder-hand syndrome involving the side affected by the stroke
(E) tic douloureux

816. A 55-year-old man is evaluated for weakness. Over the past few months he has noted slowly progressive weakness and cramping of his left leg. Lately he has also had some trouble swallowing foods. He is awake and alert. Findings on the neurologic examination are normal except for marked atrophy with fasciculations in the muscles of both legs, hyperactive reflexes in the upper and lower extremities, a diminished gag reflex, and a positive extensor plantar response. Which of the following represents the most likely diagnosis?

(A) Cervical spondylosis
(B) Guillain-Barré syndrome
(C) Lambert-Eaton syndrome
(D) Vitamin-B_{12} deficiency
(E) Amyotrophic lateral sclerosis

817. Duchenne's muscular dystrophy is characterized by

(A) autosomal dominant inheritance
(B) onset in second decade of life
(C) normal cardiac muscle
(D) universal elevation of serum creatine kinase
(E) the requirement in prenatal diagnosis of family studies for analysis of restriction fragment length polymorphisms (RFLPs)

818. A 68-year-old, previously healthy woman develops a lilac-colored rash in a butterfly distribution about the eyes, on the bridge of the nose, and on the cheeks. She has a similar rash on her knuckles. She has had an associated muscle weakness manifested by difficulty arising from a chair or climbing stairs. She takes no medicines. Other than the rash and proximal muscle weakness, the woman's examination is unremarkable. The most appropriate subsequent procedure would be

(A) barium enema, upper-GI series, intravenous pyelography, mammography, and chest x-ray
(B) hemogram, serum chemistries, Pap smear, urinalysis, mammography, and chest x-ray
(C) biopsy of an affected muscle
(D) electromyography (EMG)
(E) glucocorticoid treatment

819. Which of the following statements correctly characterizes Wernicke's encephalopathy?

(A) The most prominently affected area is the frontal cortex, bilaterally
(B) Most patients present with the triad of encephalopathy, ophthalmoplegia, and ataxia
(C) In the absence of response to glucose, thiamine should be administered
(D) After the patient responds to emergent treatment, profound amnesic psychosis may supervene
(E) Intake of alcohol is required to produce the full-blown syndrome

820. Which of the following disorders is LEAST likely to produce a sensory level on neurologic examination?

(A) Myelopathy due to vitamin-B_{12} deficiency
(B) Neoplastic cord compression
(C) Vertebral dislocation and cord compression
(D) Acute myelitis
(E) Spinal epidural abscess

DIRECTIONS: Each question below contains five suggested responses. For **each** of the five responses listed with every question, you are to respond either YES (Y) or NO (N). In a given item **all, some or none** of the alternatives may be correct.

821. Progressive gait disability in elderly persons may be due to

(A) normal-pressure hydrocephalus
(B) cervical spondylosis
(C) subdural hematoma
(D) carotid stenosis
(E) subacute combined degeneration

822. Which of the following elements would be involved in the appreciation of pain due to an injurious stimulus?

(A) Spinocerebellar tract
(B) Spinothalamic tract
(C) Dorsal horn of the spinal cord
(D) Red nucleus
(E) Nucleus ventralis posterolateralis

823. A patient complains of hearing loss in the right ear. A 256-Hz tuning fork is placed in the middle of the forehead; the patient reports that he hears the tone in his right ear. He also notes better perception of a tone when the tuning fork is placed in contact with the right mastoid process than when it is placed outside of his right ear. Lesions in which of the following structures could account for these findings?

(A) Eighth nerve
(B) Central auditory pathways
(C) Cochlea
(D) External auditory canal
(E) Middle ear

824. Useful tests for myasthenia gravis would include which of the following?

(A) Repetitive motor-nerve stimulation
(B) Single-fiber electromyography
(C) Muscle biopsy
(D) Nerve conduction studies
(E) Curare challenge testing

825. Which of the following would be consistent with a diagnosis of low back strain in a patient with low back pain?

(A) Limitation of flexion of the spine
(B) Scoliosis or straightening of the normal lordosis as noted on x-ray films
(C) Urinary retention and obstipation
(D) Sudden onset while bending over shoveling snow
(E) Absence of ankle reflex with radiating pain

826. A lesion in the corticospinal tract rather than in an anterior horn neuron projecting to muscle cells is suggested by

(A) spasticity
(B) marked atrophy
(C) fasciculations
(D) involvement of individual muscles
(E) presence of an extensor plantar reflex

827. The tremor associated with Parkinson's disease is characterized by

(A) worsening with voluntary movement
(B) occurrence with flexed posture
(C) occurrence at a rate of 5 Hz
(D) association with rigidity
(E) abolition by moderate intake of alcohol

828. Treatment can reverse or cease progression of which of the following causes of dementia?

(A) Alzheimer's disease
(B) Binswanger's disease
(C) Creutzfeldt-Jakob disease
(D) Chronic subdural hematoma
(E) Infection by HIV

829. Peripheral nerve damage caused by diabetes may result in

    (A) relapsing weakness
    (B) distal sensory neuropathy
    (C) incontinence
    (D) footdrop
    (E) ophthalmoplegia

830. Chronically progressive spinal cord disease with sensory and motor signs evolving over years may be due to

    (A) spinocerebellar degeneration
    (B) multiple sclerosis
    (C) cervical spondylosis
    (D) lumbar disk disease
    (E) amyotrophic lateral sclerosis

831. A person with long-standing alcoholism develops bilateral lateral-rectus (sixth-nerve) palsies. Diagnostic considerations would include

    (A) brainstem hemorrhage
    (B) subdural hematoma
    (C) orbital fractures
    (D) neurosyphilis
    (E) Wernicke's encephalopathy

832. A 60-year-old man comes to the emergency room with sudden onset of a neurologic deficit. After examining the patient the physician orders cerebral angiography. Results show occlusion of the left vertebral artery from its origin to where it joins the basilar. The right vertebral artery, basilar artery, and both carotid arteries are patent. Examination in the emergency room probably disclosed

    (A) left hemiparesis sparing the face
    (B) deviation of the uvula to the right on phonation
    (C) left appendicular ataxia
    (D) left internuclear ophthalmoplegia
    (E) diminished pain and temperature sensation in the right arm and leg

833. Which of the following may occur ipsilateral to a disease process within the cavernous sinus?

    (A) Ptosis
    (B) Numbness of the brow
    (C) Numbness of the chin
    (D) Marked decrease in visual acuity
    (E) Inability to elevate the eye

834. Favorable prognostic factors for a patient's remaining seizure-free when anticonvulsants are stopped after 2 years on therapy include

    (A) a normal EEG before drug withdrawal
    (B) complex partial seizures with secondary generalization
    (C) simple partial seizures
    (D) requirement of a single drug for seizure control
    (E) few seizures prior to becoming seizure-free

835. Correct statements concerning the use of lithium in psychiatry include

    (A) lithium is effective for treating acute manic/hypomanic episodes but has no role in prophylaxis against future attacks
    (B) hyperthyroidism is an important long-term complication
    (C) nephrogenic diabetes insipidus is common
    (D) gastrointestinal complaints and thirst are common side effects
    (E) during acute mania, lithium can be administered with behavior control as the sole end point

836. True statements regarding hypokalemic periodic paralysis include

    (A) it is inherited in an autosomal recessive fashion
    (B) patients exhibit myotonia between attacks
    (C) proximal musculature is involved more than distal musculature
    (D) deranged renal handling of potassium accounts for the pathogenesis
    (E) prophylactic administration of potassium is effective

DIRECTIONS: Each group of questions below consists of five lettered headings followed by a set of numbered items. For each numbered item select the **one** lettered heading with which it is **most** closely associated. Each lettered heading may be used **once, more than once, or not at all.**

Questions 837–840

For each clinical syndrome described below, select the most likely site of disk protrusion.

(A)   L2-L3 interspace
(B)   L3-L4 interspace
(C)   L4-L5 interspace
(D)   L5-S1 interspace
(E)   S1-S2 interspace

837.   Sciatica, inability to walk on toes, and depressed ankle tendon reflex

838.   Sciatica, weakness of foot inversion, and hallux extensor weakness

839.   Sciatica, footdrop, and normal reflexes

840.   Hip flexion weakness, knee extension weakness, and diminished knee tendon reflex

Questions 841–845

For each of the following conditions, select the region of the brain most likely affected by a pathologic process.

(A)   Frontal lobe
(B)   Temporal lobe
(C)   Dominant parietal lobe
(D)   Nondominant parietal lobe
(E)   Occipital lobe

841.   Wernicke's aphasia

842.   Apathy and lack of initiative and spontaneity

843.   Acalculia

844.   Inability to recognize faces

845.   Dense homonymous hemianopia

Questions 846–850

For each abnormality of eye movement listed below, select the associated lesion.

(A)   Lesion in the low pons surrounding the left abducens (sixth-nerve) nucleus, including the left pontine gaze center
(B)   Lesion in the right frontal lobe
(C)   Lesion in the left upper pons affecting the medial longitudinal fasciculus
(D)   Unilateral left labyrinthine dysfunction
(E)   Midbrain lesion affecting the rostral interstitial nucleus of the medial longitudinal fasciculus

846.   Absence of vertical gaze

847.   Inability to move the eyes to the left of midline

848.   Tendency to keep the eyes to the right of midline

849.   Saw-toothed jerk nystagmus with slow phase to the left and quick corrective movements to the right

850.   Inability to adduct the left eye past the midline and nystagmus in the right eye when abducted

Disorders of the Nervous System and Muscles

Answers

736. The answer is B. *(Chap 21.)* Muscle spindles are bundles of small striated muscle fibers encased in a connective-tissue capsule around which are coiled specialized sensory nerve endings. Dispersed throughout each muscle, spindles send subliminal afferent impulses that aid the central nervous system in monitoring changes in muscle length. Joint capsule receptors are responsible for conscious proprioception; muscle tension is monitored by Golgi tendon organs.

737. The answer is B. *(Chap 18.)* The symptoms and signs described in the question are most consistent with Ménière's disease. In this disorder, paroxysmal vertigo due to labyrinthine lesions is associated with nausea, vomiting, rotary nystagmus, tinnitus, high-tone hearing loss with recruitment, and, most characteristically, fullness in the ear. Labyrinthitis would be an unlikely diagnosis in the case presented because of the hearing loss and multiple episodes. Vertebral-basilar insufficiency and multiple sclerosis typically are associated with brainstem signs. Acoustic neuroma only rarely causes vertigo as its initial symptom, and the vertigo it causes is mild and intermittent.

738. The answer is A. *(Chap 11. Max, N Engl J Med 326:1250–1256, 1992.)* There are few viable therapeutic options for the pain of diabetic neuropathy, which can be quite severe. Due to the chronic nature of the pain, narcotic analgesics such as fentanyl are not optimal choices. Nonsteroidal anti-inflammatory drugs such as fenoprofen also seem to have little role in this condition. On the other hand, tricyclic antidepressant drugs (e.g., desipramine), used at doses lower than required for the treatment of depression, are quite helpful in neuropathic pain syndromes, including diabetic neuropathy and postherpetic neuralgia. The tricyclics are effective in both patients who are depressed and those who are not. Relief can usually be obtained at doses lower than those associated with troublesome anticholinergic side effects. Fluoxetine (Prozac) is not effective. Such a finding supports the notion that the positive effect of tricyclics in neuropathic pain is due to a blocking of neuroepinephrine uptake. Patients with severe lancinating neuropathic pain may also respond to anticonvulsants such as phenytoin and carbamazepine. The antiarrhythmic drug mexiletine is particularly useful in pain secondary to traumatic peripheral nerve damage.

739. The answer is D. *(Chap 14. Welch, N Engl J Med 329:1476–1483, 1993.)* While the pathophysiology of migraine remains unclear, electrical stimulation of midline dorsal raphe in the brainstem leads to characteristic pain. Pharmacologically, serotonin-mediated neurotransmission appears critical to the generation of migrainous pain. Sumatriptan and dihydroergotamine each work by blocking 5-hydroxytryptamine receptors (type I, especially D subtype). While nonsteroidal anti-inflammatory agents such as ibuprofen and naproxen are helpful in patients with mild to moderate migraine, presumably by reducing inflammatory stimuli due to cyclooxygenase inhibition leading to reduced prostaglandin generation, the patient in the question has too severe an attack to benefit from additional use of this class of agents. Secondly, the use of narcotic analgesics as a primary therapy is no longer recommended; sumatriptan will relieve a migraine headache in approximately 75 percent of patients within 1 h of treatment. Unfortunately, because of its short half-life (with either oral or subcutaneous administration) headache recurs in up to one-third of patients. Suma-triptan-associated side effects are usually mild to moderate and highly reversible; they include reactions at the injection site, flushing sensations, and neck pain or stiffness. Although up to 5 percent of patients treated with sumatriptan experience chest tightness or pressure, myocardial ischemia is exceedingly rare. Nonetheless, this drug should not be given to those with a history of myocardial infarction, ischemic heart disease, or Prinzmetal's angina. Both beta-adrenergic antagonists and calcium-channel blocking drugs are effective prophylactic agents useful in patients with frequent migraines.

740. The answer is A. *(Chap 380.)* The abrupt appearance of an isolated peripheral facial palsy, which may include ipsilateral hyperacusis resulting from involvement of fibers to the stapedius and loss of taste on the anterior two-thirds of the tongue resulting from involvement of the fibers of the chorda tympani, is most often idiopathic, i.e., Bell's palsy. If the patient is unable to close the eye, artificial tears may be helpful during the day to prevent drying, and the eye should be patched at night to prevent corneal abrasion. Excellent recovery occurs in 80 percent of such cases. Oral contraceptives and mitral valve prolapse are not associated with causes of such a clinical picture. Evoked potentials are not helpful diagnostically.

741. The answer is D. *(Chap 29.)* Narcolepsy is uncontrollable daytime sleepiness, and cataplexy is sudden, brief loss of muscle tone. Sleep paralysis and hypnagogic hallucinations are common in persons with narcolepsy. A properly performed sleep electroencephalogram is useful in supporting a diagnosis of narcolepsy—REM sleep occurs much earlier in sleep than normal in affected persons. (False positive tests can occur if the subject has recently been sleeping, awakens briefly, and then falls asleep again for the test.) Confusion and epileptic disorders are not part of the narcolepsy-cataplexy syndrome.

742. The answer is B. *(Chap 14.)* Cluster headaches, which can cause excruciating hemicranial pain, are notable for their occurrence during characteristic episodes. Usually attacks occur during a 4 to 8 week period in which the patient experiences one to three severe, brief headaches daily. There may then be a prolonged pain-free interval before the next episode. Men between the ages of 20 and 50 are most commonly affected. The unilateral pain is usually associated with lacrimation, eye reddening, nasal stuffiness, ptosis, and nausea. During episodes alcohol may provoke the attacks. Even though the pain due to brain tumors may awaken a patient from sleep, the typical history and the normal neurologic examination do not mandate evaluation for a neoplasm of the central nervous system. Acute therapy for a cluster headache attack is oxygen inhalation, although intranasal lidocaine and subcutaneous sumatriptan may also be effective. Prophylactic therapy with either prednisone, lithium, methysergide, ergotamine, or verapamil can be administered during an episode to prevent further cluster headache attacks.

743. The answer is D. *(Chap 15.)*   Herniation of a lower cervical disk may be due to trauma, especially in the setting of neck hyperextension. If the disk herniates laterally, it will generally compress the nerve route exiting the lower of the two vertebrae that account for the intervertebral space. For example, if the disk between the fifth and sixth cervical vertebrae herniates, the full syndrome would be characteristic of a C6 radiculopathy: pain in the trapezius, shoulder, radial forearm, and thumb; absent biceps reflex; and preserved triceps reflex. A C7 radiculopathy caused by a disk protruding between the sixth and seventh cervical vertebrae would produce the following: pain in the shoulder blade, pectoral and medial axillary region, upper arm, elbow, dorsal forearm, and index and middle fingers; paresthesia and sensory loss in the second and third fingers or tips of all the fingers; weakness in forearm and wrist extension, as well as hand grip; and a preserved biceps but a diminished triceps reflex. Coughing and sneezing often exacerbate the pain caused by a herniated cervical disk. Unlike the aforementioned lateral disk syndromes, a disk that herniates centrally may be painless yet cause symptoms in the lower extremities.

744. The answer is D. *(Chap 26.)*   In a comatose person, reactive pupils and the absence of eye movements in response to head turning or ice-water irrigation of the ear canals signify metabolic suppression of brainstem neurons. The major distinction that must be made is between true unresponsiveness and a "locked-in" stroke state, in which eye movements also may be obliterated. In brain death, pupils are unreactive. A person unresponsive because of a conversion reaction cannot voluntarily suppress the nystagmus induced by caloric irrigation, although tonic eye movements can be suppressed by gaze fixation. Pontine hemorrhage is associated with small pupils. Bilateral infarcts in a carotid distribution may cause coma, but oculocephalic movements are normal.

745. The answer is A. *(Chap 26.)*   Patients with basilar artery stenosis frequently have spells of ischemic brainstem dysfunction prior to a catastrophic stroke caused by arterial thrombosis. Timely anticoagulation and allowing a higher blood pressure can arrest the progression of this potentially fatal stroke. Acute coma can occur in association with each of the cerebrovascular accidents mentioned except carotid occlusion. Subarachnoid hemorrhage causes an acute increase in intracranial pressure that reduces blood flow to the brain. Unilateral cortical infarction does not cause coma, but damage to brainstem structures via infarction or compression will cause coma.

746. The answer is A. *(Chap 18. Froehling, JAMA 271:385–388, 1994.)*   Evaluation of the "dizzy" patient relies on a combination of careful history taking and neurologic examination. It is important to try to get a sense of whether or not the patient has true vertigo, which is usually manifest as the sensation that either the world or the patient is spinning. Some elderly patients complain of dizziness while ambulating or standing without true vertigo, although they may have some mild lightheadedness. Typically such patients have peripheral neuropathy, myelopathy, parkinsonian rigidity, cerebellar ataxia, or poor vision. Such patients actually have multiple sensory-defect dizziness, also known as *benign dysequilibrium of aging*. Unlike patients with benign paroxysmal positional vertigo, they should not display excess nystagmus on head-tilt testing. Central lesions are unlikely given a normal neurologic examination except for the peripheral neuropathy and other sensory deficits.

747. The answer is D. *(Chap 19.)*   Knowledge of visual pathway anatomy is necessary to understand visual field defects. Monocular visual field loss often results from retinal fiber loss, corresponding to lesions visible upon ophthalmoscopic examination. Retinal fibers traveling in the optic nerve change direction at the optic chiasm so that the right brain appreciates left visual space and the left brain appreciates right visual space. Therefore, a discrete vertical midline characterizes all visual pathway disorders due to lesions at or posterior to the chiasm. Because chiasmal lesions interrupt the central fibers that mediate temporal vision (with peripheral fibers mediating more midline vision), a pituitary tumor or craniopharyngioma (which typically impinges centrally) results in loss of visual fields in the bitemporal regions. If a lesion exists well posterior to the optic chiasm, such as loss of visual cortex in the one occipital lobe due to a posterior cerebral artery embolism, a complete loss of visual perception in one field will result. For example, destruction of the right visual cortex will lead to complete left homonymous hemianopia with loss of temporal vision in the left eye and medial vision in the right eye.

748. The answer is B. *(Chap 366.)*   The testing of evoked potentials is of greatest utility in detecting subclinical spinal cord and optic nerve lesions. Up to two-thirds of persons who have multiple sclerosis have neurologic deficits evident on visual or peroneal somatic evoked potentials but *not* on physical examination. Such a "second lesion" frequently establishes the diagnosis of multiple sclerosis. Evoked potentials may be abnormal in the other conditions listed in the question.

749. The answer is C. *(Chap 14.)*   Errors made in the investigation of patients with sudden onset of severe headache can result in catastrophic subarachnoid hemorrhage from a ruptured aneurysm. Patients frequently have "warning" bleeding that causes severe headache and brings them for medical attention. Sudden headache during physical exertion is a presentation of ruptured intracranial aneurysm. A careful cerebrospinal fluid examination is the most sensitive test, but a noncontrast CT scan may show the subarachnoid blood and make the lumbar puncture unnecessary. A patient with a reasonable suspicion for aneurysmal bleeding should not be sent home to wait for other symptoms because the next symptom is often a catastrophic subarachnoid hemorrhage. In the patient described, however, the repeated onset of headache with coitus is characteristic of a benign coital headache syndrome. If faced with only a single sudden coital headache, then an investigation for a cerebral aneurysm would be appropriate. The family history of migraine is usually not helpful for the diagnosis of coital headache.

750. The answer is E. *(Chap 19.)*   Isolated lesions of the third nerve with pupillary sparing are common and are usually due to microinfarction in association with diabetes or hypertension. As such, older patients with such a third nerve palsy can be followed expectantly in the absence of signs of subarachnoid hemorrhage or other more diffuse processes. More detailed reinvestigation would be mandated if recovery is not complete, as it usually is, within a 3-month period. The third nerve is a midline structure that contains both sympathetic motor and visceral nuclei. It innervates the ipsilateral medial rectus, inferior rectus, and inferior oblique muscles as well as the contralateral superior rectus muscle. A central nucleus innervates both levator palpebrae superioris muscles. Moreover, axons from visceral nuclei project ipsilateral parasympathetic outflow to the pupillary sphincter and ciliary ganglion, which control pupillary reflexes as well as accommodation. Therefore, a midbrain infarction (involving the nucleus of the oculomotor nerve), if complete, would produce a unilateral third nerve palsy, characterized by ipsilateral ptosis and inability to turn the eye upward, downward, and inward. Bilateral ptosis and paralysis of the contralateral superior rectus muscle would result. Pupillary involvement would also be complete. More distal lesions could produce either single or multiple extraocular muscle abnormalities with or without pupillary derangement. It is also important to recognize that the third nerve may be impinged along its extracranial extent. Particularly noteworthy is compression against the tentorial edge, which may occur during profound intracranial hypertension with temporal lobe herniation. In herniation the pupillary fibers are affected first, which causes pupillary dilation and unresponsiveness to light. Cavernous sinus thrombosis may also affect the third nerve; this process typically affects the fourth and sixth nerves.

751. The answer is C. *(Chap 20.)*   The primary evaluation of a patient with hearing impairment is the determination of whether the loss is sensorineural (lesions in the inner ear, eighth nerve, or central auditory pathways) or conductive (lesions in the external auditory canal or middle ear). The demonstration that bone conduction is better than air conduction suggests a conductive hearing loss. About a third of persons over age 70 require a hearing aid because of presbycusis, which is manifested by a loss of discrimination for particular sounds and difficulty in understanding speech in noisy environments. This is usually due to sensorineural deafness, with lesions either in the neuroepithelial cells (hair cells), neurons, or the stria vascularis of the peripheral auditory system. Though of lesser magnitude, degeneration of central auditory pathways may also be a problem in those with presbycusis. Hearing aids are the mainstay of treatment for those with this condition; however, cochlear implants, by providing a neural prosthesis, may aid patients with profound sensorineural deafness.

752. The answer is C. *(Chap 368.)*   The clinical picture presented in the question suggests acute subarachnoid hemorrhage, either from a ruptured saccular aneurysm or from an arteriovenous malformation. A CT scan of the head, done initially without infusion of contrast material, would be more likely than the other procedures listed to demonstrate the presence of blood in the subarachnoid space and possibly in the ventricles as well. In addition, a CT scan also can detect the presence of hydrocephalus and intracerebral hematoma, two conditions that, in the presence of coma, may require surgical intervention. Skull films are not likely to be informative in this case, although in the presence of a large arteriovenous malformation they may show intracranial calcification. The finding of retinal hemorrhages, a sign of acute intracranial hemorrhage, renders lumbar puncture as a means of establishing the presence of intracranial bleeding less useful, and the procedure is possibly dangerous in this instance. A radionuclide scan would have little to offer in this set of circumstances, and angiography would be premature.

753. The answer is E. *(Chap 25.)*   Grasp or suck responses, though not diagnostic of dementia, do indicate a loss of neurons and thus support the diagnosis of dementia. Somatic complaints, including headache, are common in both dementia and depression, although they tend to be more persistent in depression. Memory may be impaired in persons with depression because of lack of attention to tasks, as well as in persons with dementia; immediate recall is usually poor in severe depression, whereas it is often good in dementia.

754. The answer is C. *(Chap 21.)*   Lesions in the basal ganglia, rather than resulting in the clasp-knife spasticity and hyperreflexia of upper motor neuron lesions or the hypotonia of lower motor neuron lesions, may result in a host of movement disorders including akinesia or bradykinesia, lead-pipe rigidity, chorea, irregular and variable continuous movements, dystonia (increased muscle tone that causes fixed abnormal postures), myoclonus (brief involuntary random muscular contractions), asterixis (quick arrhythmic movements), hemiballismus (violent flinging motion of an arm), tremor, or tics (stereotyped, purposeless, and irregularly repetitive movements). These so-called extrapyramidal syndromes do not involve the characteristic weakness of muscles or muscle groups typical of lesions of the corticospinal tracts. It is possible that these extrapyramidal syndromes may coexist with lesions in the corticospinal tract or cerebellum, which makes precise delineation of the abnormality difficult. Other degenerative conditions, such as Shy-Drager syndrome, have many elements of Parkinson's disease (bradykinesia, bland facial expression, rest tremor, and muscular rigidity), but postural hypotension, abnormal eye movements, and Babinski's signs may also occur. In addition to dopamine, other important neurotransmitters in the basal ganglia include gamma-aminobutyric acid, enkephalin, and substance P.

755. The answer is D. *(Chap 23.)* Polymyalgia rheumatica typically occurs in elderly patients and is characterized by complaints of weakness, stiffness, and pain in the proximal musculature. There may be an associated inflammatory arthritis, elevated erythrocyte sedimentation rate, or accompanying temporal arteritis. Inflammatory myositis is ruled out by the presence of normal creatine kinase levels; a muscle biopsy would show atrophy without evidence of inflammation. Unless temporal arteritis is also present, nonsteroidal anti-inflammatory agents are the treatment of choice; low-dose prednisone may be administered if the initial agents fail.

756. The answer is D. *(Chap 11.)* The patient is already on maximal doses of a relatively weak narcotic analgesic that also has quite a few side effects. Increasing the dose of codeine or adding a nonsteroidal anti-inflammatory drug such as indomethacin is likely to be of little benefit. Neuropathic pain, unlike the somatic pain afflicting the patient, might be managed with the help of an anticonvulsant such as phenytoin. Since the patient has not yet failed an adequate trial of narcotics, referral for a nerve-altering intervention is premature. One should now institute a sustained release preparation of morphine, with another narcotic to be taken in between doses of morphine until a sufficient level of analgesia is achieved.

757. The answer is D. *(Chaps 14, 380.)* A disease of middle-aged and elderly patients, particularly women, paroxysmal facial pain (tic douloureux, trigeminal neuralgia) is usually of idiopathic origin. It may occur in association with multiple sclerosis, herpes zoster, or a tumor. Brief, intense, lancinating pains brought on by manipulation of trigger zones in the lips or face, without motor or sensory paralysis, characterize this disorder. The treatment of first choice is the anticonvulsant carbamazepine, which is effective in most patients. In cases of nonresponse or intolerance to carbamazepine, radiofrequency ablation of the gasserian ganglion of the trigeminal nerve may be beneficial.

758. The answer is A. *(Chap 24.)* Peripheral nerve trunks contain fibers of various sizes. Small fibers mediate sensations of pain and temperature and larger fibers are involved in touch, vibration, and joint position sense. Therefore, a lesion in a peripheral nerve would be expected to affect all such functions. The different fibers segregate near the dorsal roots. The smaller fibers cross and ascend in the contralateral side through the spinal cord to the brainstem and to the ventral posterior lateral nucleus of the thalamus, ultimately projecting to the parietal cortex. The larger fibers that mediate tactile and position sense project upward in the posterior columns of the spinal cord and synapse initially in the cuneate nuclei of the lower medulla; a secondary neuron crosses to ascend in the medial lemniscus and synapses in the ventral posterolateral nucleus of the thalamus with ultimate projections to the parietal cortex. Therefore, loss of joint position without loss of pain sensation would reflect a lesion in the ipsilateral posterior column, contralateral brainstem, thalamus, or parietal cortex.

759. The answer is A. *(Chap 28. Domasio, N Engl J Med 326:531–539, 1992.)* Patients with Wernicke's aphasia usually have damage in an area of the posterior temporal and parietal regions, which are supplied by the lower division of the middle cerebral artery. Not only are spoken and written communication affected, but auditory and visual understanding may also be deranged. At first glance, speech with lesions in this area appears to be effortless and well-woven together. However, because of problems in finding words, the content is often unintelligible, as there are frequent errors in word choice and substitution of incorrect phonemes (e.g., "trable" for "table"). Patients rarely have associated motor defects with lesions in this location, but problems in sensory processing are possible depending on the degree of parietal lobe disease. As in true Broca's aphasia, these patients have difficulty in repeating sentences and in naming things properly. Patients with Wernicke's aphasia may experience paranoid ideation and become agitated and hostile.

760. The answer is D. *(Chaps 14, 380.)*   The features described are consistent with sympathetic denervation of the right eye, the so-called Horner pupil. This lesion, frequently produced by pulmonary neoplasms of the superior sulcus, is usually associated with ipsilateral ptosis and anhidrosis. Pupillary light responses should be normal, as should the response to mydriatics (substances causing pupillary dilation [e.g., anticholinergics]) and miotics (drugs causing pupillary constriction [e.g., cholinergics, beta-adrenergic blockers]). However, since the sympathetic nerve endings are depleted, cocaine is unable to cause local release of sympathomimetic substances and is a poor mydriatic. An oculomotor palsy would also produce ipsilateral ptosis, but a dilated pupil that is poorly reactive to light on that side would be the cause of anisocoria.

761. The answer is C. *(Chap 17.)*   Patients with loss of consciousness resulting from a seizure usually have mental confusion, headache, and drowsiness postictally, whereas the patient with a brief syncopal spell recovers fully as soon as the blood pressure returns to normal. Auras, urinary incontinence, and a laceration of the tongue are clues that the cause of the loss of consciousness was a seizure. Moreover, syncope rarely occurs during recumbency.

762. The answer is A. *(Chap 29.)*   Chronic or long-term insomnia, by definition, lasts for months or years and is usually reflective of a psychiatric or chronic medical condition, drug use (including caffeine or alcohol), or a primary sleep disorder. Psychophysiologic insomnia is characterized by preoccupation with an inability to sleep at night. The problem is often triggered by a stressful event, but may persist for long periods of time due to the acquisition of poor sleep habits. Patients are often aroused by their own failed efforts to sleep. They more readily sleep at unusual times or places. This patient does not have narcolepsy since excessive daytime sleep and cataplexy are not included in his syndrome. Narcolepsy may be treated with stimulants such as methylphenidate. Moreover, he has no findings suggestive of sleep apnea syndromes, which might benefit from the use of conjugated estrogens. Instead, rigorous attention to sleep hygiene, such as making sure the bedroom is only used for sleep and removing distracting stimuli at bedtime, is most appropriate. Benzodiazepine hypnotics may be helpful during the initiation of treatment by serving to allow behavioral therapy, which is probably the most specific way to treat this problem.

763. The answer is B. *(Chap 365. Adelman, N Engl J Med 328:708–716, 1993.)*   MRI of the central nervous system, especially with the use of gadolinium vascular enhancement, is generally preferred over CT. Severe reactions to gadolinium are much less common than with radiographic contrast agents. The only real disadvantage is that MRI requires a longer scanning time and is more sensitive to motion artifacts. However, CT scanning is still preferred in emergency departments when acute hemorrhage is suspected, both because of the shorter scanning time in patients whose condition is unstable and because it is actually more sensitive in detecting blood within the first several hours of the insult. MRI is particularly useful for the early evaluation of stroke, particularly strokes in the posterior fossa, which are poorly seen on CT scanning. Gadolinium-enhanced MRI scanning is highly sensitive for detection of metastatic tumor and primary brain tumors as well for meningitis. However, gadolinium-enhancement of meninges does not distinguish between infectious and neoplastic causes. Finally, MRI is particularly sensitive for the detection of fairly subtle developmental abnormalities, such as Arnold-Chiari malformations.

764. The answer is C. *(Chap 376.)*   Treatment of hypotension, control of the airway, and a search for lesions that raise intracranial pressure are the first priorities in managing persons with severe head trauma. Skull x-rays have been largely replaced by CT scans because contusions and hemorrhages are better seen by CT scanning. Although stabilization of the neck is very important, the other treatment choices mentioned in the question are not.

765. The answer is D. *(Chap 19.)*   The patient in question is suffering from acute angle-closure glaucoma, the result of obstruction of outflow of aqueous humor at the iris. The buildup of intraocular pressure can be confirmed by measurement and requires urgent treatment by the use of hyperosmotic agents. Permanent treatment requires laser or surgical iridotomy. Angle-closure glaucoma is less common than primary open-angle glaucoma, which is asymptomatic and usually detectable only through measurements of intraocular pressure at routine eye examination.

766. **The answer is D.** *(Chap 367.)* It is important to classify seizures based on whether or not they begin in a focal area of the brain, remain localized or secondarily generalize, or whether they are generalized from their earliest manifestation. This patient exhibited the classic "Jacksonian march," with repetitive shaking of contiguous ipsilateral body parts, caused by a demonstrable progression of epileptiform discharges in the contralateral motor cortex usually due to a focus from a tumor or abscess. This patient, therefore, had a simple partial seizure with secondary generalization. In this case the focus was obvious; in some cases the focal features can only be discerned on the basis of a postictal deficit (e.g., Todd's paralysis of an extremity). Juvenile myoclonic epilepsy begins in adolescence and is characterized by postawakening myoclonic seizures marked by sudden, brief muscle contractions involving one body part or the entire body. Complex partial seizures, also referred to as temporal lobe epilepsy (typical of herpes simplex encephalitis), involve episodic changes in behavior with loss of attachment to the environment and are typically associated with a minor automatism, such as lip-smacking or picking at clothes.

767. **The answer is D.** *(Chap 367.)* Different types of seizures respond better to certain classes of anticonvulsant drugs. For example, generalized tonic-clonic seizures may be treated successfully with phenytoin, carbamazepine, phenobarbital, or valproic acid. Carbamazepine and phenytoin are also effective for the treatment of partial seizures, though those with complex partial seizures may require more than one type of drug at a time. Partial absence seizures, such as depicted in the question, are best treated with ethosuximide or valproic acid, although clonazepam (a benzodiazepine) may also be effective. Side effects of ethosuximide include ataxia, lethargy, GI irritation, skin rash, and bone marrow suppression.

768. **The answer is B.** *(Chap 22.)* Alcoholic cerebellar degeneration is an example of a disease primarily of the midline area of the cerebellum (vermis). A characteristic cerebellar gait disorder will be manifested by a wide-based walk and stance and inability to stand with the feet together even with the eyes open. Patients complain of imbalance and frequently try to hold on to other objects as they walk. However, unlike more diffuse cerebellar disease, there is no associated limb ataxia or nystagmus.

769. **The answer is E.** *(Chap 369. Fine, Ann Intern Med 119:1093–1104, 1993.)* Lymphoma of the brain (usually diffuse large cell) is increasingly common as a sporadic tumor and occurs frequently in immunosuppressed patients, especially in those with AIDS. Its clinical sensitivity to corticosteroids can mistakenly suggest a diagnosis of multiple sclerosis, and its complete disappearance or dramatic improvement on CT scan after steroid therapy is baffling. Radiosensitivity is a well-known feature of most primary CNS lymphomas, which are almost always of B-cell origin.

770. **The answer is E.** *(Chap 367.)* When a patient presents with a generalized tonic-clonic seizure, it is important to consider alcohol as a potential etiology. Persons who heavily abuse alcohol may have seizures due to cerebral contusion or subdural hematoma caused by trauma, metabolic abnormalities, central nervous system infection, or alcohol withdrawal. Seizures occurring during alcohol withdrawal or during binge drinking usually are brief tonic-clonic seizures that occur in a flurry of several over a short period of time. Once other causes for seizures in alcoholics are ruled out, it is not necessary to administer chronic antiepileptic treatment. First, such seizures tend to be self-limited and will abate once withdrawal is completed or binge drinking is stopped. Second, use of anticonvulsant medicines in this typically noncompliant group of patients with a host of other medical problems is fraught with the dangers of severe side effects.

771. The answer is B. *(Chap 367.)* Antiepileptic drugs commonly have a host of side effects. For example, phenytoin has a narrow therapeutic index and is associated with neurologic symptoms including ataxia and nonneurologic symptoms such as gum hyperplasia, lymphadenopathy, hirsutism, and osteomalacia. Carbamazepine is notable for causing bone marrow suppression and gastrointestinal irritation as well as ataxia, dizziness, and vertigo. Phenobarbital enhances the metabolism of many other drugs via liver enzyme induction. In fact, carbamazepine levels, potentially increased by erythromycin, are decreased by phenobarbital. Especially if the phenobarbital is not destined to have a major therapeutic effect in this patient with complex partial seizures, induction of a reduced carbamazepine level may actually lead to worse control. It may be necessary to increase the carbamazepine dose to achieve a therapeutic level in order to give the combination therapy an adequate trial. The bone marrow suppression of carbamazepine may produce a dose-dependent mild-to-moderate depression in the white count, but is not notable for causing severe thrombocytopenia.

772. The answer is E. *(Chap 368.)* Before assuming that a stroke is due to hemispheral disease, clinicians should search for contralateral brainstem signs. Right hemiparesis with either left facial weakness or left-gaze paresis indicates a pontine stroke, which generally is due to basilar artery branch disease. Inability to calculate (acalculia) and left-right confusion with dysgraphia are part of the Gerstmann syndrome of left parietal stroke and may occur with right hemiparesis. Minimizing or ignoring the deficit is most typical of a right-brain lesion and is associated with a left hemiparesis.

773. The answer is E. *(Chaps 374, 381.)* Spinal epidural abscess, a neurologic emergency, is currently best diagnosed by MRI or CT, which would demonstrate the site of impingement. Lumbar puncture would show a high protein content and cell count but would not establish the diagnosis and may in fact be harmful. Babinski signs are absent in the case described because lumbar pain indicates an abscess overlying the cauda equina, which is made up of peripheral nerves, rather than the spinal cord.

774. The answer is E. *(Chap 368. Gilman, N Engl J Med 326:1671–1676, 1992.)* Transient ischemic attacks (TIA) are caused by either low flow in large vessels such as the internal carotid artery, embolism from an arterial or cardiac source, or lacunar (small penetrating vessel) atherosclerosis. As exemplified in this case, a low-flow TIA is usually brief and recurrent and is frequently due to a tightly stenotic atherosclerotic lesion at the internal carotid artery. Hypoperfused distal branches of the middle cerebral artery cause hip, shoulder, or arm weakness and possible aphasic symptoms, depending on the amount of territory involved. Transient recurrent monocular blindness (amaurosis fugax) may also be a manifestation of an internal carotid artery occlusion. Embolic TIAs tend to be of longer duration than the low-flow TIA previously described. Lacunar TIAs occur because of blockage of one of the intracerebral penetrating vessels arising from the middle cerebral, basilar, or vertebral arteries. Based on the carotid angiography performed in this case, it is apparent that the patient in fact did have a low-flow TIA due to a tightly stenotic lesion of the internal carotid artery. Heparin may be useful for impending stroke due to this pathophysiology, warfarin may be appropriate after embolic phenomena, and antiplatelet agents may have prophylactic value for secondary strokes. However, the procedure of choice in this case is carotid endarterectomy. If the lesion had not been tightly stenotic (less than 70 percent stenosis), the value of such surgery would have been less clear.

775. The answer is D. *(Chap 368.)* There are four major hypertensive hemorrhage syndromes. The most common site for bleeding is the internal capsule adjacent to the basal ganglia, which generally produces contralateral hemiplesia with eye deviation away from the side of the weakness. As the blood expands within the brain, stupor and coma may occur rapidly. Thalamic hemorrhage results in hemiplegia due to pressure on the adjacent internal capsule, as well as in a prominent sensory deficit. The eyes typically deviate downward and inward and the pupils are unequal. Pontine hemorrhages produce rapid onset of deep coma, quadriplegia, and pinpoint pupils that do react to light.

Cerebellar hemorrhages develop over several hours and are manifested by nausea, vomiting, vertigo, dizziness, and occipital headache. The eyes tend to deviate away from hemorrhage; there may be an ipsilateral sixth nerve palsy, blepharospasm, or ocular bobbing. Cerebellar findings tend to be limited. It is important to recognize this lesion since it is treatable up until the point of coma from brainstem compression. While osmotic therapy to reduce intracranial pressure may be helpful, the most important therapy for such infratentorial clots is surgical removal. Neurosurgical therapy for acute supratentorial clots such as might be caused by a thalamic or capsular hemorrhage is more controversial because of the difficulty in safely reaching these central areas.

776. The answer is D. *(Chap 375.)*   Very few diseases cause rapid dementia, noticeable in a period of weeks. Among them are depression, metabolic encephalopathy, encephalitis, poisoning, Binswanger's disease (white-matter infarction), and Creutzfeldt-Jakob disease. (Alzheimer's disease has a more insidious onset.) Creutzfeldt-Jakob disease is a slow-virus infection that causes a spongiform change in the cerebral cortex; it is characterized by rapid dementia, startle myoclonus, and, frequently, signs of occipital and cerebellar disease. CT scan and cerebrospinal fluid examination are nearly always normal in affected persons; after a period of time electroencephalography shows rapid, synchronous sharp waves, a diagnostic finding.

777. The answer is D. *(Chap 373.)*   Optic neuritis is the initial symptom in approximately 40 percent of persons who eventually are diagnosed as having multiple sclerosis. This rapidly developing ophthalmologic disorder is associated with partial or total loss of vision, pain on motion of the involved eye, scotoma affecting macular vision, and a variety of other visual-field defects. Ophthalmoscopically visible optic papillitis occurs in about half of cases.

778. The answer is A. *(Chap 369. Black, N Engl J Med 324:1555–1564, 1991.)*   Meningiomas are the most common type of benign brain tumor and account for 15 percent of primary CNS neoplasms. They may grow to an extremely large size before detection. Meningiomas most commonly present in women in the fifth or sixth decades. They may arise around the midline between the cerebral hemispheres, in the olfactory groove, along the sphenoidal ridge, the foramen magnum, and tentorium of the cerebellum. The neoplastic cells arise from pia or arachnoid tissue, though up to seven histologic subtypes have been identified. Cytogenetic analysis typically reveals abnormalities of chromosome 22. If possible, based on the site, meningiomas should be totally surgically removed. Parasagittal tumors are usually resectable and have low recurrence rates. Chemotherapy has no role, and radiation is reserved for postsurgical treatment for the rare malignant meningiomas and for those symptomatic patients whose tumors cannot be completely excised. Meningiomas represent a stark contrast to primary high-grade malignant astrocytoma (glioblastoma), whose median survival, even with trimodality therapy, is little more than a year.

779. The answer is E. *(Chap 369.)*   The most common tumors of the central nervous system by far are those derived from metastatic systemic cancer. The most common sources of intracerebral metastases are cancer of the lung in men and breast cancer in women. Melanoma, though a less common tumor, has a definite predilection for spread to the central nervous system. As patients fare better from the standpoint of their primary neoplasms compared with historical controls, such as the case for ovarian cancer or sarcoma, the incidence of intracerebral metastases rises. Headache, focal neurologic deficits, and seizures are common ways in which those with intracerebral metastases may present. Treatment usually consists of a combination of glucocorticoids and radiation therapy. However, patients with solitary lesions, particularly if they are asymptomatic in the presence of minimal systemic disease (particularly if there has been a disease-free interval of greater than 1 year), should be considered for surgical resection. Though most patients with metastatic cancer to the brain improve clinically and by radiographic evaluation after treatment, their 1-year survival is less than 20 percent. The presence of intracerebral metastases is actually a marker for advanced systemic disease, since the vast majority of patients die not from complications of therapy or the intracerebral tumor itself, but rather from advanced recurrent systemic malignancy.

780. The answer is C. *(Chap 373.)* By far the most common cause of unilateral internuclear ophthalmoplegia is multiple sclerosis. Preferred diagnostic tests for multiple sclerosis are lumbar puncture to check particularly for an elevated immunoglobulin G fraction and evoked potentials to search for an occult second lesion in the nervous system (the demonstration of a second lesion makes the diagnosis of multiple sclerosis definite). The workup can be performed on an outpatient basis. MRI may also reveal occult white matter lesions.

781. The answer is E. *(Chap 26.)* Bilateral conjugate eye movement to the side of the caloric stimulation indicates integrity of the brainstem pathways from the medulla to the midbrain (where the third nerve originates), as do full conjugate oculocephalic motions (doll's eye maneuvers). The absence of the rapid corrective phase manifested by nystagmus-like leftward gazing indicates a bilateral hemispheric lesion. Failure of an eye to adduct properly in the initial phase of the caloric response indicates a lesion in the ipsilateral third nerve (midbrain) or in the medial longitudinal fasciculus producing an internuclear ophthalmoplegia. In the former case, the pupil would be dilated and the eye abducted at rest.

782. The answer is C. *(Chap 370. Yankner, N Engl J Med 325:1849–1857, 1991.)* Alzheimer's disease is the most common cause of dementia in the elderly. It is a highly prevalent disease, affecting as many as 45 percent of those who are over age 85. In a relatively small percentage of the cases, the disease occurs in a familial pattern, thought due to autosomal dominant inheritance with linkage to either chromosome 21 or 19. The clinical beginnings of the disease tend to be subtle. Initial symptoms usually are limited to loss of recent memory. Psychiatric symptoms may then supervene and could include depression, anxiety, delusions, or paranoid behavior. An extrapyramidial component exists such that patients walk in a shuffling manner with short steps. Radiographic evaluation usually reveals neuronal atrophy. Neuropathologically, the disease is characterized by neurofibrillary tangles, which may contain an abnormally phosphorylated form of a microtubular protein known as tau, as well as spherical deposits known as senile plaques. A protein known as beta-amyloid can be found in these plaques. Certain families with inherited Alzheimer's disease have been found to harbor a point mutation in the amyloid precursor protein. From a neurotransmitter standpoint, acetylcholine, a neurotransmitter important in memory formation, is synthesized at abnormally low levels. The current model for the pathogenesis of Alzheimer's disease is that altered cleavage of the amyloid precursor protein generates the so-called beta-amyloid protein, which then binds to a protease inhibitor–enzyme complex, in turn preventing the normal inactivation of extracellular proteases. It is these abnormally activated extracellular proteases that may mediate the neuronal degeneration characteristic of Alzheimer's disease. Therapeutic strategies that could inhibit the generation of beta-amyloid are of potential therapeutic interest.

783. The answer is A. *(Chap 371. Standaert, Med Clin North Am 77:169, 1993.)* Parkinson's disease is a chronic degenerative disease of middle-aged and elderly persons that is characterized pathologically by a decrease in dopaminergic transmission in the caudate nucleus and putamen. Early manifestations of the disease include a unilateral rest tumor with a frequency of 4 to 5 per second. The tremor may progress to involve structures on both sides of the body with eventual postural imbalance, profound restriction of movement, and eventual degeneration to a chair-bound existence. Total paralysis is highly uncharacteristic and tendon reflexes as well as sensory examination are normal. The early stage of the disease can be treated with deprenyl, a monoamine oxidase inhibitor that slows disease progression. Treatment of more progressive Parkinson's disease requires dopamine replacement in the form of levodopa. Levodopa is given in combination with a dopa-decarboxylase inhibitor (carbidopa), which prevents bloodstream destruction of levodopa, but is unable to pass through the blood-brain barrier. Carbidopa in combination with levodopa in a ratio of 1:4 or 1:10 (Sinemet) is available. Though costly, dopamine-receptor agonists such as bromocriptine may be used to lower the required dose of Sinemet. Anticholinergic drugs such as benztropine or trihexyphenidyl may be useful adjunctive therapy, but must be used carefully because of the side effects of confusion, glaucoma, urinary retention, and progression of dementia.

Amantadine, which causes release of dopamine from presynaptic terminals, may also be useful early in the disease. Unfortunately, as the disease progresses, the therapeutic index of the levodopa-carbidopa combination decreases. If levodopa-induced hallucinations occur, clozapine may be helpful, although neutropenia may occur.

784. The answer is A. *(Chap 28.)* Most lesions that lead to aphasia, a disturbance in the production or comprehension of speech and language, occur in the dominant cerebral hemisphere. Ninety percent of people are right-handed; the left hemisphere is dominant in 95 percent of right-handed people, and in 50 percent of those who are left-handed. Broca's, or major motor, aphasia denotes a syndrome in which the praxis of speech is severely disturbed. This problem usually results from a large lesion in the posterior frontal lobe along the insula and sylvian fissure, not simply Broca's area in the inferior frontal lobe. Patients have great difficulty in articulation, grammar, and writing, though comprehension and fluency are relatively well preserved. Emboli of the superior division of the left middle cerebral artery are the most common cause of this syndrome.

785. The answer is D. *(Chap 26.)* Hyperosmolar dehydration with mannitol or an equivalent agent reduces abnormally elevated intracranial pressure (ICP). Using intravenous fluids to support blood pressure, especially if they are hypoosmolar, would exacerbate cerebral edema and raise ICP still further. Similarly, high airway pressures are transmitted by way of the thoracic venous system and cerebrospinal fluid to the intracranial cavity and thus may worsen ICP elevation. The administration of phenytoin or beta blockers would be ineffective.

786. The answer is C. *(Chap 389. Shader, N Engl J Med 328:1398–1405, 1993.)* Anxiety symptoms are extraordinarily common in medical patients. Such symptoms may occur as a consequence of a primary psychiatric problem or be due to drug therapy or medical illness. There are several different subcategories of anxiety disorders, including posttraumatic stress disorder, phobic disorders (e.g., agoraphobia, social phobias, or simple phobias), obsessive-compulsive disorder, generalized anxiety disorder, and panic disorder. The most important feature of panic disorders is the sudden onset of overwhelming feelings of terror and fear, associated with multiple symptoms including dyspnea, palpitations, and faintness. Attacks usually occur away from home and tend to be recurrent. This disorder may well have a genetic basis, insofar as panic disorder occurs to a greater degree in first-degree relatives. In addition to the elicitation of often complex medical workups for these dramatic symptoms, the morbidity of panic disorder often stems from its association with agoraphobia and the house-bound situation to which patients restrict themselves. Major depression, substance abuse, and suicide may complicate panic disorders. As in the case of patients presenting with a generalized anxiety disorder, it is important to rule out a host of medical conditions. The list of such medical disorders is long, but includes angina, carcinoid syndrome, hyperthyroidism, menopausal symptoms, mitral valve prolapse, pheochromocytoma, porphyria, pneumothorax, pulmonary embolus, and temporal lobe epilepsy. Complications also include the use or abuse of drugs such as alcohol, amphetamines, aminophylline, anticholinergics, antihistamines, caffeine, cocaine, glucocorticoids, monosodium glutamate, salicylates, and thyroid replacement drugs. The currently accepted theories concerning the etiology of panic disorder center on the genetic susceptibility to an environmental event that triggers adrenergic overload. While tricyclic antidepressants, monoamine oxidase inhibitors, and benzodiazepines are each effective in the treatment of panic disorder, the drug of first choice is usually a low dose of a tricyclic such as imipramine. The newer serotonin reuptake–inhibitor antidepressants such as fluoxetine and sertraline may also be effective. It is important to maintain patients with panic disorder on long-term medication because the relapse rate is very high if these medicines are discontinued. The only benzodiazepine approved for use in panic disorder is alprazolam; however, clonazepam is also useful, especially in view of its longer half-life. In fact, the benzodiazepines may be used to prevent the episodes while the tricyclic dose is being increased over the 1 to 2 weeks required to achieve full therapeutic efficacy.

787.   The answer is E.   *(Chap 388.)*   Although a viral cause has been postulated, no clear-cut etiology has been demonstrated for the chronic fatigue syndrome. Furthermore, while several subtle immunologic abnormalities have been documented in certain patients with this syndrome, there is no definitive diagnostic test. The diagnosis of chronic fatigue syndrome rests on the Centers for Disease Control's working definition. Definitive diagnosis is based on the presence of both of the major criteria: persistent or relapsing fatigue that does not resolve with bedrest and is severe enough to reduce the average daily activity by 50 percent; and exclusion of other chronic conditions, including preexisting psychiatric diseases. Physical examination must include two of the following three physical findings by a doctor on at least two occasions 1 month apart: low-grade fever, pharyngitis, or palpable lymphadenopathy. Finally, at least six of the common symptoms must be present. These symptoms include mild fever or chills, sore throat, painful lymph nodes in the cervical chains, muscle weakness, muscle discomfort, fatigue following minimal exercise, new headaches, arthralgias, neuropsychological symptoms, and sleep disturbance. Patients who do not have the required physical findings need to fulfill eight of the symptom criteria. Since there is certainly no specific therapy for this disease, treatment requires understanding patients and the avoidance of unproven therapies such as acyclovir, vitamin B_{12}, intravenous gammaglobulin, and steroids. Treatment should be symptom-directed. As such, nonsteroidal anti-inflammatory agents, decongestants, and antidepressants may be helpful depending on symptoms. Finally, life-style modification including a graded exercise program, minimal caffeine intake, and avoidance of complete rest is advisable.

788.   The answer is B.   *(Chap 377.)*   Acquired hepatocerebral degeneration is a neurologic syndrome composed mainly of extrapyramidal signs. A well-known consequence of chronic liver disease, this disorder simulates Wilson's disease in many ways, including the presence of neuropathologic lesions in the cortex, basal ganglia, and other deep nuclei. Many cases become evident after a bout of hepatic encephalopathy, but others occur insidiously in persons who never have had encephalopathy.

789.   The answer is B.   *(Chap 373.)*   The combination of autonomic insufficiency and parkinsonian symptoms is known as the Shy-Drager syndrome. The autonomic form of the Landry-Guillain-Barré syndrome causes acute autonomic paralysis but does not cause the parkinsonian symptoms of tremor at rest, bradykinesia, and rigidity. A number of antihypertensive agents cause orthostatic hypotension, but none cause parkinsonism. Micturition syncope is a condition in which syncope occurs because of vagal surge at the time of release of intravesicular pressure.

790.   The answer is E.   *(Chap 389. Michels, N Engl J Med 329:552–560, 628–638, 1993.)*   The outlook for patients with schizophrenic disorders has improved with use of antipsychotic medications such as phenothiazines, which include chlorpromazine, fluphenazine, and thioridazine. In particular, these medicines are useful for treatment of the "positive" symptoms of schizophrenia, such as hallucinations and psychotic agitation. However, they are less useful against the "negative" symptoms typified by social withdrawal. In general, antipsychotic medications block dopamine neurotransmission in nigrostriatal structures. This dopamine blockade can induce extrapyramidal side effects that mimic Parkinson's disease. Although many of the antipsychotics have intrinsic anticholinergic action, which can result in dry mouth, hypotension, and urinary retention, the addition of benztropine, another anticholinergic medicine used in the treatment of Parkinson's disease, may be effective in treating these extrapyramidal side effects. A particularly notable side effect of antipsychotic medicines is akathisia, which is characterized by an obligatory movement of the extremities and motor restlessness. Akathisia may respond to the institution of beta-blocking drugs or antiparkinsonian agents, but would most likely benefit from a decrease in the dose of neuroleptic agent. The most common serious side effect of neuroleptic medicines is tardive dyskinesia, manifest by involuntary repetitive movements of musculature such as tongue thrusting and lip-smacking. Involuntary limb movements and postural dystonia may also be part of this syndrome. While it is possible that newer antipsychotic medications such as clozapine may have a role in the treatment or the amelioration of tardive dyskinesia, currently the best approach is to lower the dose of the neuroleptic agent. Of course, such reductions might not be possible without exacerbation of the underlying thought disorder.

791. The answer is A. *(Chap 391.)*   Abusers of opiate analgesics fall into two major groups: (1) medical abusers, subdivided into those with chronic pain syndromes and health professionals; and (2) street abusers. Once persistent opiate abuse is established, the medical consequences are quite severe and include a 25 percent death rate within 10 to 20 years due to suicide, homicide, accidents, or infectious diseases. At this time the mortality is escalating because of the epidemic of AIDS among intravenous drug abusers with up to 60 percent of such persons serologically positive for HIV infection. If addicted persons are deprived of access to opiates, they will experience a withdrawal syndrome beginning 8 to 16 h after the last dose with the highest intensity of symptoms within 36 to 72 h. Withdrawal symptoms tend to be opposite those attributable to the acute effects of narcotics. They include nausea, diarrhea, coughing, lacrimation, rhinorrhea, profuse sweating, muscle twitching, and "goose bumps" due to piloerection, as well as mild elevations in temperature, respiratory rate, and blood pressure. Though the acute withdrawal symptoms usually abate within 8 days, a more prolonged though milder withdrawal-type syndrome may persist for up to 6 months and certainly could contribute to relapse, which is incredibly common in this group. Treatment of withdrawal requires readministration of opiates. Though any opiate will be effective, it is standard to use a long-acting drug such as methadone, with the usual starting dose being 10 to 25 mg given twice daily orally. One nonopiate approach to treatment withdrawal is the use of clonidine, which decreases the autonomic dysfunction characteristic of the withdrawal syndrome.

792. The answer is B. *(Chap 383.)*   Lower brachial plexus injuries predominantly produce C8 and T1 deficits. Typically, ulnar border sensory loss affects the hand, and a Horner's syndrome may develop from damage to sympathetic nerve roots exiting at C8. Wasting of the intrinsic hand muscles leads to a "claw hand" deformity.

793. The answer is B. *(Chap 370. Martin, N Engl J Med 315:1267, 1986.)*   Huntington's chorea, which is inherited as an autosomal dominant trait, is characterized by dementia and choreiform movements. The motor disorder may include grimacing, respiratory spasms, speech irregularity, and a dancing, jangling quality of the gait. Laboratory workup is normal except that atrophy of the caudate nucleus may be seen on a carefully evaluated CT or MRI scan. Through the use of DNA linkage analysis, patients can be tested before disease development, if this is appropriate from a psychosocial standpoint. The disease-specific gene is located on the short arm of chromosome 4.

794. The answer is D. *(Chap 380.)*   Brief paroxysms of severe, sharp pains in the face without demonstrable lesions in the jaw, teeth, or sinuses are called tic douloureux, or trigeminal neuralgia. The pain may be brought on by stimuli applied to the face, lips, or tongue or by certain movements of these structures. Aneurysms, neurofibromas or meningiomas impinging on the fifth cranial nerve at any point during its course typically present with trigeminal neuropathy, which would cause sensory loss on the face or weakness of the jaw muscles or both; neither of these symptoms is demonstrable in this patient. The treatment for this idiopathic condition is carbamazepine or phenytoin, if the former is not tolerated. In cases where drug treatment is not successful, surgical therapy, including the commonly applied percutaneous retrogasserian rhizotomy, may be effective. A possible complication of this procedure is partial facial numbness with a risk of corneal anesthesia, which increases the potential for ulceration.

795. The answer is B. *(Chaps 364, 378.)*   Neurofibromatosis type 1 is an autosomal dominant condition carried on the long arm of chromosome 17. It is characterized by tumors involving the sheaths of peripheral nerves and associated with café au lait spots (tanned cutaneous flat lesions). The neurofibromas are rarely symptomatic, although they may occasionally entrap nerve roots. In addition to sarcomatous degeneration, central nervous system tumors including optic glioma, glioblastoma, and meningioma may occur in patients with neurofibromatosis. Mutations in the gene encoding the protein neurofibromin account for this disease. The structure of this protein suggests that it may have GTPase activating properties and as such may be a tumor-suppressor gene. Neurofibromatosis type II, in which bilateral acoustic neuromas are found in addition to multiple neurofibromas, is believed to be caused by mutations in the gene that encodes the protein merlin, a 587-amino acid cytoskeletal protein. Other neurologic disorders known to be caused by gene mutations include ocular retinoblastoma, due to mutations in the Rb protein on chromosome 13; hexosaminadase A mutations, which account for Tay-Sachs disease; and KALIG-1 mutations, which give rise to Kallman's syndrome.

796. The answer is E. *(Chap 371.)*   Several illnesses produce parkinsonian symptoms—rigidity, bradykinesia, and masked facies—but at the same time are not associated with tremor and do not respond to typical antiparkinsonism drugs. The most common of these diseases is progressive supranuclear palsy, which is characterized by vertical ophthalmoplegia, speech difficulty (hypophonia), and anxiety. No form of therapy has been consistently successful in controlling the symptoms of this disorder.

797. The answer is B. *(Chap 381.)*   The most characteristic symptom of syringomyelia is loss of pain sense with preservation of touch. This phenomenon occurs most commonly over the shoulders in a capelike distribution. Tissue loss in the central gray matter of the spinal cord, where pain fibers cross to join the contralateral spinothalamic tract, is the neuropathologic process involved. Other characteristic features of syringomyelia include thoracic scoliosis and muscle atrophy of the hands. Ataxia does not occur unless the syrinx extends into the brainstem.

798. The answer is C. *(Chap 380.)*   Pain, loss of function (without clear-cut sensory or motor deficits), and a localized autonomic impairment is known as reflex sympathetic dystrophy (also as shoulder-hand syndrome or causalgia). Precipitating events in this unusual syndrome include myocardial infarction, shoulder trauma, or limb paralysis. In addition to the neuropathic-type pain, autonomic dysfunction, possibly due to neuroadrenergic and cholinergic hypersensitivity, produces localized sweating, changes in blood flow, and abnormal hair and nail growth, as well as edema or atrophy of the affected limb. Treatment is difficult; however, anticonvulsants such as phenytoin and carbamazepine may be effective as in other conditions in which neuropathic pain is a major problem.

799. The answer is E. *(Chap 376. White, N Engl J Med 327:1507–1511, 1992.)*   Concussion, the transient loss of consciousness consequent to blunt impact to the skull, is believed to occur because of electrophysiologic dysfunction of the upper midbrain due to sudden movement of the brain within the skull. About 3 percent of those with concussions will also have an associated intracranial hemorrhage, but the absence of a skull fracture decreases the risk. Amnesia for events just prior to the trauma is common, as are a single episode of emesis, severe bilateral frontal headache, faintness, blurred vision, and problems in concentration. However, minor injuries are characterized by an absence of neurologic signs, normal skull x-ray, and normal CT or MRI scan. In the absence of persistent confusion, behavioral changes, decreased alertness, or focal neurologic signs, patients may be discharged to be observed by responsible individuals. Several more worrisome clinical syndromes may accompany more severe head injury. Such symptoms are characterized by

(1) delirium and wishing not to be moved; (2) severe memory loss; (3) focal deficit; (4) global confusion; (5) repetitive vomiting and nystagmus; (6) drowsiness; and (7) diabetes insipidus. Positive findings on CT scan or EEG would be common with these types of postconcussive syndromes, neurosurgical evaluation would be required, and prophylactic phenytoin, glucocorticoids, and haloperidol could be considered.

800. The answer is A.   *(Chap 381.)*   Neuromyelitis optica (Devic's disease) usually occurs in association with necrotizing myelitis but also is seen in persons who have multiple sclerosis and postinfectious and postvaccinal myelitis. Neuromyelitis optica is characterized by both transverse myelitis and optic neuritis; affected persons can display such signs and symptoms as progressive sensorimotor deficits, central scotoma, and elevated protein concentration and cell count in cerebrospinal fluid. In the case presented in the question, the presence of optic nerve involvement and the finding of a sensory level on the trunk rule out acute idiopathic polyneuritis, although analysis of cerebrospinal fluid is not inconsistent with polyneuritis in its early stages. A diagnosis of acute spinal epidural abscess is made less likely by the presence of optic neuritis.

801. The answer is C.   *(Chap 376.)*   The cause of chronic subdural hematoma may be a trivial or inapparent injury, such as might be sustained by a sudden deceleration experienced in a motor vehicle accident. Symptoms are relatively nonspecific, usually characterized by an intermittent headache accompanied by some degree of personality change, drowsiness, or confusion. This condition is easily confused with drug intoxication, stroke, dementia, and depression. For the patient in the question, however, the lack of focal findings argues against stroke and the rapidity of onset would be unusual for dementia. The CT scan does not define the hematomas because they have become isodense with the passage of time (2 to 6 weeks since injury); however, the absence of sulci and the small size of the ventricles coupled with the clinical scenario are highly suggestive of bilateral subdural hematomas. Surgical evacuation of the hematomas is the treatment of choice.

802. The answer is C.   *(Chap 376. White, N Engl J Med 327:1507–1511, 1992.)*   Epidural bleeding may cause rapidly deteriorating mental status after an initial lucid interval following head trauma. Such hematomas occur in 1 to 3 percent of all head injuries. The typical profile of a patient with an acute epidural hematoma is an alcoholic who sustains severe trauma and fractures the squamous portion of his temporal bone, thereby tearing the origin of dural vessels arising from the middle meningeal artery. Therefore, the most common location of an epidural hematoma is overlying the lateral temporal convexity. These hematomas expand rapidly because of the force of arterial bleeding, strip the dura from the attached inner table of the skull, and produce a characteristic bulge-type clot on CT scan. This dramatically evolving picture requires neurosurgical intervention, usually in the form of clot evacuation.

803. The answer is D.   *(Chap 375.)*   Rapidly progressive dementia with myoclonus is the hallmark of Creutzfeldt-Jakob disease. While most cases are sporadic, a small percentage are familial with an autosomal dominant pattern of inheritance. In addition to dementia, myoclonus, and cerebellar signs, the electroencephalogram shows a characteristic pattern as described above. CT or MRI scanning is usually not specifically helpful except that the degree of dementia is out of proportion to the degree of radiographic brain loss. Definitive diagnostic accuracy requires a brain biopsy, which would show vascular degeneration, neuronal loss, and glial hypertrophy without significant inflammation. White Creutzfeldt-Jakob disease was formerly thought to be a disease of viral etiology, it is now accepted that the cause is deposition of a proteinaceous infectious particle (prion) devoid of nucleic acid that is encoded by a gene present on the short arm of human chromosome 20. The function of this protein is at present unknown, but certain mutations in this gene have been found in families with hereditary Creutzfeldt-Jakob disease.

804. The answer is D. *(Chap 383.)* Entrapment of the lateral femoral cutaneous nerve, which can occur where it enters the thigh beneath the inguinal ligament near the anterior superior iliac spine, causes a sensory neuropathy known as "meralgia paresthetica." Symptoms of this disorder, which typically occurs in obese persons, include pain and decreased tactile sensation over the lateral aspect of the thigh. Treatment is infiltration with a local anesthetic or, if this procedure proves ineffective, surgical sectioning of the nerve.

805. The answer is E. *(Chap 383.)* The inflammatory response in Guillain-Barré syndrome strips myelin between the nodes of Ranvier in peripheral nerves. This phenomenon explains both the slowing of nerve conduction and the potential for recovery. Axons are only destroyed in extensively involved areas as a secondary phenomenon. To date, no convincing evidence has emerged to support the contention that the central nervous system is involved in Guillain-Barré syndrome.

806. The answer is A. *(Chap 385.)* Myotonia, muscle wasting, cataracts, testicular atrophy, and frontal baldness characterize the hereditary disorder myotonic dystrophy. Onset usually is in early adulthood. In affected persons, mental retardation is common, atrial arrhythmia is a frequent complication, and diabetes mellitus is more prevalent than in the general population. Myotonic dystrophy is the type of muscular dystrophy most commonly observed in hospitalized patients.

807. The answer is B. *(Chap 385.)* Oculopharyngeal dystrophy is a dominantly inherited disease occurring in families of French-Canadian or middle-European ancestry. Because it causes late-onset progressive ptosis and difficulty with swallowing, it may be difficult to distinguish from myasthenia gravis, which is not a dystrophic muscle disease. Proximal weakness and ophthalmoplegia suggest the presence of a progressive external ophthalmoplegia.

808. The answer is C. *(Chap 385.)* Myotonia is the phenomenon in which brief, persistent contractions of a muscle occur after voluntary contraction or, sometimes, percussion. Myokymia is continuous, small-muscle movement that is frequently difficult to distinguish from fasciculations. Fibrillation is the electromyographically detected spontaneous firing of muscle fibers and is not visible except in the tongue. Myoedema is a poorly defined sign similar to myotonia in which a ridge of percussed muscle remains contracted for 5 to 8 s. It was once thought to be related to hypoalbuminemia, but this relationship probably does not exist.

809. The answer is B. *(Chap 15.)* Malignancy in the pelvis not infrequently causes compression or infiltration of nerves exiting the spinal cord en route to the leg. This results in stepwise progression of sensory and motor deficits in areas supplied by the involved nerve roots or trunks. Continuous pain in the distribution of a specific nerve or root is also common. In this patient the neurologic deficits began in an S1 distribution but then progressed to L5 and, finally, L4 roots, suggesting an expanding paravertebral mass. Isolated, spontaneous activity of muscle fibers called *fibrillations* is characteristic of denervation. Nerve conduction will be normal in the leg if the lesion is proximal to the measuring electrodes, i.e., in the pelvis. An expanding cortical mass might also cause progressive numbness in the foot and leg and might be missed on a CT scan that does not take cuts all the way up to the vertex. Back pain and neuropathic pain would not occur with a cortical lesion, and the reflexes under such circumstances should be hyperactive.

810. The answer is D. *(Chap 386.)* More than three-quarters of patients with myasthenia have circulating antibodies against components of the postsynaptic membrane, including acetylcholine receptors. Antibody action leads to an unfolding, or "simplification," of the membrane and, consequently, a reduced number of acetylcholine receptors. As a result, existing acetylcholine in the synapse is less effective in producing muscle contraction.

811. The answer is A. *(Chap 368. Fisher, Neurology 32:871, 1982.)*   A pure motor hemiparesis on one side (with ipsilateral face and body involvement) and no other cortical deficits (aphasia or cortical sensory loss) suggests an internal capsular lesion. The major differential diagnosis in this setting is between a hypertensive hemorrhage or an internal capsular lacunar infarct. Both entities may present with a fluctuating course over hours; however, hemorrhages tend to produce some manifestation of increased intracranial pressure. Lacunar infarctions result from atherothrombotic and hyalinization changes in the penetrating branches of the circle of Willis, middle cerebral artery stem, and vertebrobasilar system. Other than the internal capsule, common locations for lacunar infarctions include the thalamus, where they produce pure sensory deficit, and the base of the pons, where they produce hemiparesis and dysarthria with a clumsy hand. CT scanning can document most supratentorial lacunar infarctions, whose size usually ranges from 0.5 to 2 cm.

812. The answer is E. *(Chap 369.)*   Typical symptoms of neoplastic meningitis include headache, confusion, radiculopathy, and cranial nerve abnormalities in patients with a variety of tumors, including non-Hodgkin's lymphoma, leukemia, melanoma, breast cancer, lung cancer, and stomach cancer. Given these symptoms, especially in the face of a negative CT, MRI, or both, the diagnosis of leptomeningeal metastases from breast cancer is quite likely. A single lumbar puncture is a relatively insensitive test; repeat examinations of cerebrospinal fluid are often required to establish the diagnosis of cancer that has spread to the meninges. Especially in cases where the cancer cells are "caked" onto the inferior portion of the brain, eradication by chemotherapy alone (usually methotrexate, thiotepa, or cytosine arabinoside) is difficult and radiation therapy should be administered as well.

813. The answer is E. *(Chaps 21, 382.)*   Fasciculations may occur in a variety of metabolic and toxic disorders, including amyotrophic lateral sclerosis, progressive bulbar palsy, ruptured intervertebral disk, and peripheral neuropathy. However, they should not be viewed with alarm in the absence of weakness, muscle atrophy, or loss of tendon reflexes. The best treatment a physician could offer a person who is asymptomatic except for fascicular twitches is reassurance and, if appropriate, advice to reduce coffee intake.

814. The answer is C. *(Chap 383.)*   Although porphyric neuropathy may occur without involvement of the central nervous system, with acute paralysis there is frequently a history of confusion or coma. Predominantly a motor neuropathy, porphyric neuropathy can cause significant sensory loss in some persons. In this respect it may simulate inflammatory polyneuropathy, though inflammation does not occur. Curiously, protein concentration in CSF is usually normal in affected persons.

815. The answer is C. *(Chaps 11, 24.)*   One of the most distressing sequelae of thalamic damage is a chronic pain syndrome (Déjerine-Roussy syndrome) that occurs months to a few years after the initial lesion. The findings of total hemianesthesia and loss of all sensory modalities in the face, arm, and leg are characteristic of thalamic infarction. Lesions of the spinothalamic tract may also cause neuropathic pain syndromes, but hemianesthesia of the face does not occur with spinal cord lesions. Parietal lobe lesions usually affect the cortical senses (i.e., two-point discrimination, graphesthesia, or stereognosia) rather than cause a total hemianesthesia. Depression is not commonly associated with burning pain. Tic douloureux is not associated with sensory loss.

816. The answer is E.   *(Chap 372. Prados, Neurology 43:751, 1993.)*   Amyotrophic lateral sclerosis (ALS) is an untreatable disease that results in progressive loss of upper and lower motor neuron function. Other components of the nervous system remain intact, including the neurons required for ocular motility. Limb weakness and cramping is the first symptom, followed by muscular atrophy, fasciculations, and loss of function of cranial nerve musculature. Early in the disease, upper-tract signs may predominate, resulting in spasticity. Pneumonia due to failure of clearance of secretions is usually the terminal event. Treatable causes of motor neuron disease, such as cervical spondylosis (no bulbar involvement) and lead poisoning, should be excluded whenever the diagnosis of ALS is considered. Guillain-Barré syndrome produces an ascending, rapidly developing paralysis. Vitamin-B_{12} deficiency should lead to abnormalities in posterior column function. Lambert-Eaton syndrome is a paraneoplastic neuromuscular disorder that would not feature upper-tract signs.

817. The answer is D.   *(Chap 385. Koenig, Cell 50:509, 1987.)*   Duchenne's muscular dystrophy is an X-linked recessive disorder in which affected boys develop progressive weakness of limb girdle muscles beginning at age 5 or earlier. By age 12 walking is impossible and patients usually succumb to respiratory failure by age 25. Most muscular tissues, including cardiac, are involved. An abnormally high creatine kinase level is found in all patients before disease onset and in many female carriers. The responsible gene has been identified. This 2000-kb gene codes for a product termed *dystrophin*, a 400-kDa protein localized to the muscle plasma membrane. Since about 60 percent of patients have an exon deletion or duplication in the dystrophin gene, it is possible to test directly for these genetic abnormalities in utero, thus obviating the need for more cumbersome family studies to determine RFLPs for linkage.

818. The answer is B.   *(Chap 384. Dalakas, N Engl J Med 325:1487, 1991.)*   This patient displays the characteristic heliotropic rash, with knuckle involvement and proximal muscle weakness typical of dermatomyositis. Although a biopsy could be done, the disease is patchy and the absence of a lymphocytic infiltration would not rule out the diagnosis. EMG will be diagnostic in about 40 percent of affected persons. Since the diagnosis is straightforward and dermatomyositis is frequently associated with malignancy in those over age 60, it is quite reasonable to screen for cancer. In addition to the common epithelial malignancies, myeloproliferative disorders can be heralded by dermatomyositis. However, an unfocused radiologic diagnostic attack should definitely be suspended in favor of the simple and cost-effective tests outlined in choice B. Although steroids will probably be symptomatically beneficial even in those with malignancies, their use should probably be delayed until the screening is completed. If an early neoplasm can be found and treated, the dermatomyositis could respond without the need for resorting to the dangers of high-dose glucocorticoid therapy.

819. The answer is D.   *(Chap 377. Charness, N Engl J Med 321:442, 1989.)*   Wernicke's encephalopathy is a consequence of thiamine (vitamin B_1) deficiency. Though most commonly observed in chronic alcoholics in this country, well-documented cases have occurred in prisoners-of-war in whom alcohol played no role. Certain areas in the thalamus, hypothalamus, midbrain, floor of the fourth ventricle, and cerebellar vermis are prone to destruction as a consequence of thiamine deficiency. While most patients present with some form of abnormal mental functioning, the classic triad of ophthalmoplegia, confusion, and ataxia is rarely encountered. Based on autopsy series, many patients frequently go undiagnosed. When the diagnosis is suspected, thiamine should be administered before glucose, since the latter substance can precipitate worsening of the disease. Thiamine will relieve the ocular palsies within hours, although improvement in ataxia and in apathy and confusion takes longer. Many of those who recover from the acute encephalopathy will be left with a profound defect in memory and learning known as *Korsakoff's psychosis*.

820. The answer is A. *(Chap 381.)* The finding of a clear sensory level above which pinprick is felt but below which sensation is absent is the *sine qua non* of spinal cord disease. The segmental level at which sensory loss begins also gives the corresponding cord level of the lesion. Other typical signs of spinal cord disease, such as hypertonicity and hyperreflexia, may be absent in acute lesions; bladder function, however, is invariably affected if the lesion is severe. Myelopathy due to deficiency of vitamin B_{12} only rarely gives a vague sensory level on the trunk.

821. The answer is A-Y, B-Y, C-N, D-N, E-Y. *(Chap 22.)* Normal-pressure hydrocephalus and cervical spondylosis typically present with gait difficulty: short steps (sometimes mistaken for parkinsonism), and leg stiffness and slowness of step, respectively. Subacute combined degeneration may produce spasticity of gait as part of its lateral column (corticospinal) damage. Subdural hematoma generally does not cause isolated gait difficulty, and carotid stenosis causes either transient ischemic attacks or strokes but not a progressive syndrome of any sort.

822. The answer is A-N, B-Y, C-Y, D-N, E-Y. *(Chaps 11, 24.)* Owing to release of substances from damaged tissue (e.g., histamines, prostaglandins) or from the circulation (e.g., bradykinin), sensory stimuli activate free nerve endings in the skin. Such nerves terminate in the segmental dorsal horn of the spinal cord. Substance P and other neurotransmitters released from terminals stimulate transmission via long axons composing the spinothalamic tract that terminate in the thalamic nucleus ventralis posterolateralis (VPL). VPL fibers project to the cerebral somatosensory cortex. Descending pathways that mediate analgesia project from the periaqueductal gray region in the midbrain to the medullary midline raphe nuclei. Raphe nuclei neurons in turn project to dorsal horn nuclei, where painful afferent impulses may be modified. This system contains many opiate receptors. Another descending pain inhibitory pathway, which projects from the pontine locus ceruleus to the dorsal horn of the spinal cord, mediates its effects by alpha-adrenergic signals.

823. The answer is A-N, B-N, C-N, D-Y, E-Y. *(Chap 20.)* Localization of the tone in the affected ear when the tuning fork is placed in the midline position (Weber's test) suggests unilateral conductive loss (external or middle ear), while perception in the unaffected ear would suggest sensorineural hearing loss. A tone heard louder by bone conduction compared with air conduction (Rinne's test) also suggests conductive rather than sensorineural hearing loss. Assuming that the patient's bone conduction is normal (since he did perceive the tone when the fork was at the mastoid process) and that only his air conduction was diminished, we can presume that the lesion is either in the external auditory canal or the middle ear. A common cause of conductive hearing loss in the elderly is otosclerosis (stapes footplate fusion), which is potentially treatable by surgical reconstructive procedures involving the middle ear.

824. The answer is A-Y, B-Y, C-N, D-N, E-N. *(Chaps 366, 386.)* Conventional electromyography (EMG) and nerve conduction studies as well as muscle biopsy procedures are not useful in an evaluation of myasthenia gravis because it is not a disease of muscle or nerve. (Electron microscopy of muscle can show unfolding of the postsynaptic muscle membrane, but this procedure is not commonly done.) Curare testing to precipitate myasthenic weakness is dangerous, undependable, and mainly of historical interest. Single-fiber EMG measures the timing of firing of two fibers in the same motor unit. The timing between pairs is inconsistent in myasthenia, giving rise to "jitter" in the oscilloscope tracing; this finding is virtually diagnostic of myasthenia. Repetitive stimulation of motor nerves to observe a decremental response also is a useful procedure in testing for myasthenia gravis.

825. The answer is A-Y, B-Y, C-N, D-Y, E-N. *(Chap 15.)* Low back pain without ruptured disk or other nerve damage is common. It requires bed rest, administration of muscle relaxants, and time for recovery. It is often precipitated by lifting while the spine is flexed or laterally rotated. X-rays may show the nonspecific signs of paravertebral muscle spasm, i.e., straightening of the normal lumbar lordosis or scoliosis. Because of pain and spasm the patient cannot flex the spine normally. Signs of nervous system damage distinguish the patient with a more serious disorder. Bowel and bladder difficulty accompany damage to sacral roots or the spinal cord. Perineal sensation and rectal tone should be tested along with individual muscle strength, stretch reflexes, Babinski reflexes, and dermatomal sensation. Abnormal results on any of these tests suggest that there is nerve injury in addition to muscular strain.

826. The answer is A-Y, B-N, C-N, D-N, E-Y. *(Chap 21.)* The distinction between upper motor neuron and lower motor neuron lesions is critical in clinical medicine. Lesions proximal to the anterior horn cells (in general, the cerebral motor cortex or the corticospinal tract) produce the characteristic upper motor neuron syndrome of spasticity, increased reflexes, and an extensor plantar response (Babinski's sign). On the other hand, atrophy of muscles in a paretic limb suggests lower motor neuron disease. Such disorders, which may affect individual muscles, will be accompanied by fascicular twitches, which are manifestations of the hyperactivity of the diseased motor unit(s).

827. The answer is A-N, B-Y, C-Y, D-Y, E-N. *(Chaps 21, 371.)* Rest tremor, frequently associated with Parkinson's disease, occurs at a rate of 4 to 5 beats per second. The rest tremor of Parkinson's disease is associated with flexed posture, slowness of movement, rigidity, postural instability, and suppression by willful activity. Many tremors that worsen during movement are exaggerations of the normal physiologic tremor. The essential-familial tremor is a faster action tremor (about 8 Hz) responsive to moderate doses of alcohol or beta-adrenergic blockade.

828. The answer is A-N, B-Y, C-N, D-Y, E-N. *(Chaps 25, 370.)* It is important to search for treatable causes of dementia among the long list of conditions that account for this progressive and debilitating loss of cognitive function. Alzheimer's disease is by far the most common cause of dementia in this country. The diagnosis of this entity is based on the hallmark of progressive deterioration in mental and social functioning. Cases of vascular dementia—exemplified by multi-infarct dementia, which is usually the result of bilateral carotid disease—can be approached by anticoagulation and other strategies to lessen the risk of further small strokes. Patients with hypertension may develop another form of (theoretically treatable) vascular dementia known as Binswanger's disease (subcortical arteriosclerotic encephalopathy), which involves atherosclerosis-induced loss of subcortical white matter and ventricular enlargement. A host of chronic infections, some of which are treatable (e.g., syphilis, tuberculosis, and Whipple's disease), should be excluded during the workup of a patient with dementia. However, the courses of the dementias associated with human immunodeficiency virus or with slow-virus infection (Creutzfeldt-Jakob disease) have not yet been conclusively shown to be modified by treatment, though zidovudine may be somewhat effective in management of the AIDS-dementia complex. Mass lesions, such as those caused by tumors, hematoma, or hydrocephalus, are partially remediable and should be excluded by anatomic imaging of the brain. Other potentially treatable causes of dementia that can be excluded by appropriate studies include the following: vasculitis, hypothyroidism, vitamin-B_{12} deficiency, thiamine deficiency, nicotinic acid deficiency, adrenal insufficiency, Cushing's syndrome, chronic hypoglycemia, hypoparathyroidism, hyperparathyroidism, Wilson's disease, dialysis, and toxicities of drugs, alcohol, heavy metals, and organic metals.

829. The answer is A-N, B-Y, C-Y, D-Y, E-Y. *(Chap 383.)* Acute mononeuropathy involving the oculomotor or peroneal nerves should prompt an investigation for diabetes. A neuropathy that is progressive, distal, and primarily sensory is most characteristic of diabetes but may also occur with an occult neoplasm. The autonomic neuropathy of diabetes usually coexists with the sensory type, but the latter may be mild. Relapsing neuropathy is more typical of idiopathic polyneuritis.

830. **The answer is A-Y, B-Y, C-Y, D-N, E-N.** *(Chaps 372, 373.)*   Several disorders produce chronic, progressive spinal cord disease with sensory and motor involvement. Syndromes of spinocerebellar degeneration may involve the motor and sensory spinal cord systems in addition to causing ataxia. Multiple sclerosis usually causes a relapsing illness but can cause a progressive, usually cervical myelopathy in elderly women. Cervical spondylosis, or bony compression of the cervical cord by osteophytic bars, is another common cause of myelopathy in the elderly. Lumbar disk compression of the cauda equina, which is made up of peripheral nerves, does not cause spinal cord signs. Amyotrophic lateral sclerosis is a disease of spinal cord motor neurons and corticospinal tracts, but has no sensory signs.

831. **The answer is A-N, B-Y, C-N, D-N, E-Y.** *(Chaps 19, 377, 380.)*   Bilateral lateral-rectus palsies that develop acutely in alcoholic persons should suggest Wernicke's encephalopathy, which requires prompt treatment with thiamine. Bilateral sixth-nerve malfunction may be a falsely localizing sign from increased intracranial pressure, as in subdural hematoma, but does not occur as an isolated disturbance from intrinsic brainstem diseases (e.g., hemorrhage). Orbital fractures usually entrap the fourth nerve, less commonly the sixth; only rarely would the palsy be bilateral. Although neurosyphilis can cause cranial nerve palsies from adhesive meningitis, palsy of oculomotor-related nerves is a rarity.

832. **The answer is A-N, B-Y, C-Y, D-N, E-Y.** *(Chap 368.)*   Unilateral occlusion of a vertebral artery typically results in Wallenberg's lateral medullary syndrome. With an infarct on the left, this is likely to include damage to the left ninth and tenth cranial nerves, the left inferior cerebellar peduncle, and the spinothalamic fibers subserving pain and temperature on the right side. Vertigo and nystagmus are common since the lower vestibular complex may be affected. Horner's syndrome is also common with a smaller pupil and ptosis *ipsilateral* to the lesion. Only rarely is the medullary pyramid involved (Babinski-Nageotte syndrome), which results in a *contralateral* hemiparesis sparing the face; hypoglossal weakness may then be present ipsilateral to the lesion. Lesions of the median longitudinal fasciculus producing internuclear ophthalmoplegia occur in the pons and midbrain in the territory of branches of the basilar artery.

833. **The answer is A-Y, B-Y, C-N, D-N, E-Y.** *(Chap 380.)*   Cranial nerves III, IV, and VI all pass through the cavernous sinus, so that complete ophthalmoplegia, including ptosis, may result from a disease process there. Since the supraorbital and maxillary divisions of the fifth nerve, but not the mandibular branch, pass through the cavernous sinus, the brow and cheek may be numb, but not the chin. The optic nerve will be involved only if the process extends superiorly.

834. **The answer is A-Y, B-N, C-Y, D-Y, E-Y.** *(Chap 367. Callahan, N Engl J Med 318:942, 1988.)*   Although many patients with epilepsy require anticonvulsants for life, about half will remain seizure-free long enough to warrant a trial without medications, many of which bear imposing side effects. Favorable prognostic factors for remaining seizure-free include few seizures before control is attained, control on single first-choice drug therapy, history of simple partial seizures or primary generalized seizures, absence of a structural lesion, and a normal EEG before drug withdrawal. Even if a patient has had a long seizure-free interval (> 2 years) and has a good chance of remaining seizure-free without anticonvulsants, the drug should be tapered over 3 to 6 months. Moreover, the patient and the physician should be aware of the consequences of relapse and be willing to accept the risk.

835. The answer is A-N, B-N, C-Y, D-Y, E-N. *(Chap 389.)* Lithium has revolutionized the treatment of bipolar affective disorders. It is effective both during acute mania and in the prevention of recurrent attacks. Although side effects—particularly gastrointestinal upset, mild tremor, and thirst—are common, the drug is safe if used carefully. Lithium dosage should be titrated to serum levels: control of mania should be achieved at a level between 0.8 and 1.4 mmol/L and maintenance levels should be between 0.6 and 1.0 mmol/L. Lithium intoxication is manifested by depression of mental status; treatment is mainly supportive. Other important long-term side effects include hypothyroidism (by inhibiting secretion of thyroid hormone) and renal complications. Effects on the renal tubules produce nephrogenic diabetes insipidus with polyuria, polydipsia, and impaired urinary concentrating ability in about 25 percent of patients on the drug.

836. The answer is A-N, B-Y, C-Y, D-N, E-N. *(Chap 387.)* Hypokalemic periodic paralysis is an autosomal dominant condition in two-thirds of cases; sporadic cases account for one-third of the incidence. It preferentially affects males. The pathogenesis of this disorder is unknown, but it is believed to involve excessive flux of potassium from blood into muscle during attacks. Furthermore, since attacks can occur when the potassium level is normal, factors other than hypokalemia alone must be important. Attacks generally involve proximal limb muscles. Between attacks the results of physical examination are normal except for persistent eyelid myotonia. Acute attacks can be managed successfully with oral or intravenous potassium and in most patients can be essentially abolished with the chronic administration of acetazolamide. Administration of potassium salts does not diminish the frequency of attacks.

837–840. The answers are 837-D, 838-C, 839-C, 840-A. *(Chap 15.)* In the assessment of uncomplicated disk protrusion, it is important to keep in mind that many lesions cause sciatica and that a protruding disk generally impinges on the nerve root that exits just below it (e.g., an "L5-S1 disk" most often compresses the S1 root). Walking on the toes requires a powerful gastrocnemius muscle, which is innervated by L5 and S1. When weakness in this maneuver is coupled with a depressed ankle reflex, an S1 compression is likely (protrusion of the L5-S1 disk). Compression of the L5 root by an L4-L5 disk does not affect knee or ankle reflexes but causes anterior tibial weakness (footdrop), extensor hallicus longus weakness, and weakness of foot inversion. The knee reflex is affected by an L3 or L4 radicular lesion (L2-L3 or L3-L4 disks, respectively), but hip flexors are affected by L2 and L3 only. These are the major lower extremity disk syndromes. In complex cases, several nerve roots are involved by protrusion of a single disk.

841–845. The answers are 841-B, 842-A, 843-C, 844-E, 845-E. *(Chaps 27, 28.)* Persons with large lesions of one or both of the frontal lobes or lesions of the central white matter and the anterior region of the corpus callosum may exhibit several clinical syndromes. Some affected persons develop what is known as the apathetic-akinetic-abulic state, which is characterized by decreased initiative and spontaneity combined with diminished speech and motor activity. Other syndromes include motor abnormalities, impaired intelligence, and personality changes.

Wernicke's aphasia occurs as a result of a lesion in the dominant temporal lobe. Affected persons are unable to read, write, or comprehend the speech of others. Quadrantic homonymous anopsia also may be associated with Wernicke's aphasia.

A lesion of the dominant parietal lobe can cause Gerstmann's syndrome. This syndrome is considered representative of an agnosia in that both the formulation and use of symbolic concepts are defective. As a result, affected persons are unable to write and calculate and to differentiate right from left.

Inability to recognize faces (prosopagnosia) results from a lesion in the visual association areas of the occipital lobe. This disorder can arise from either unilateral or, more frequently, bilateral involvement of the occipitotemporal regions. Visual acuity is intact in affected persons. A destructive lesion in one occipital lobe that destroys all terminal fibers in the geniculocalcarine pathway required for visual sensation would result in dense homonymous hemianopia.

846–850. The answers are 846-E, 847-A, 848-B, 849-D, 850-C. *(Chap 19.)* Eye movement abnormalities occur as a result of a number of nervous system abnormalities. The pontine gaze center controls ipsilateral horizontal gaze. The medial longitudinal fasciculus (MLF) connects the gaze centers and the oculomotor nuclei. A lesion of the MLF, typically caused by multiple sclerosis, results in an internuclear ophthalmoplegia—failure of adduction of the eye on the side of the lesion accompanied by contralateral nystagmus. Lesions of the frontal lobe gaze center cause a gaze preference to the side of the lesion, but the eyes can usually be made to cross the midline. The rostral interstitial nucleus of the MLF controls vertical gaze. Labyrinthine disorders cause vertigo and nystagmus, though nystagmus is also caused by a number of brainstem and cerebellar lesions.

Bibliography

Aaltonen LA, Peltomaki P, Leach FS, et al: Clues to the pathogenesis of familial colorectal cancer. *Science* 260:812–816, 1993.

Adelman RR, Warachs S: Magnetic resonance imaging. *N Engl J Med* 328:708–716, 1993.

Agarwal N, Pitchumoni CS: Assessment of severity in acute pancreatitis. *Am J Gastroenterol* 86:1385–1391, 1991.

Allen JN, Pacht ER, Gadek JE, et al: Acute eosinophilic pneumonia as a reversible cause of noninfectious respiratory failure. *N Engl J Med* 321:569–574, 1989.

Anderson HV, Willerson JT: Thrombolysis in acute myocardial infarction. *N Engl J Med* 329:703–709, 1993.

Andriole GL: Serum prostate-specific antigen: The most useful tumor marker. *J Clin Oncol* 10:1205–1207, 1992.

Arbuthnott J, Bergdoll MS, Best GJ, et al (eds): International symposium on toxic shock syndrome. *Rev Infect Dis* 11(suppl 1):S1–S333, 1989.

Armitage JO: Drug therapy. Treatment of non-Hodgkin's lymphoma. *N Engl J Med* 328:1023–1030, 1993.

Baer GM, Fishbein DB: Rabies post-exposure prophylaxis: *N Engl J Med* 316:1270–1271, 1987.

Baker DG, Schumacher HR: Acute monoarthritis. *N Engl J Med* 329:1013–1020, 1993.

Balow JE, Austin HA, Tsokos GC, et al: Lupus nephritis. *Ann Intern Med* 106:79–94, 1987.

Barlogie B, Epstein J, Selvanayagam P, et al: Plasma cell myeloma: New biological insights and advances in therapy. *Blood* 73:865–879, 1989.

Barnes PF, Bloch AB, Davidson PT, et al: Tuberculosis in patients with human immunodeficiency virus infection. *N Engl J Med* 324:1644–1650, 1991.

Barnes PF, DeCock KM, Reynolds TN, et al: A comparison of amoebic and pyogenic abscess of the liver. *Medicine* 66:472–483, 1987.

Bennet WM, Debroe ME: Analgesic nephropathy. A preventable renal disease. *N Engl J Med* 320:1269–1271, 1989.

Berkman N, Kramer MR: Diagnostic tests in pleural effusion: An update. *Postgrad Med J* 69:12–18, 1993.

Beutler E: Gaucher's disease. *N Engl J Med* 325:1354–1360, 1991.

Beutler E: Glucose 6-phosphate dehydrogenase deficiency. *N Engl J Med* 324:169–174, 1991.

Bishop JM: The molecular genetics of cancer. *Science* 235:305–311, 1987.

Black P McL: Brain tumors. *N Engl J Med* 324:1555–1564, 1991.

Black RE: Epidemiology of traveler's diarrhea and relative importance of various pathogens. *Rev Infect Dis* 12(suppl 1):S73–S79, 1990.

Bochner BS, Lichtenstein LM: Anaphylaxis. *N Engl J Med* 324:1785–1790, 1991.

Bone RC, Balk R, Slotman G, et al: Adult respiratory distress syndrome: Stage and importance of development in multiple organ failure. *Chest* 101:320–326, 1992.

Bothwell TH, Charlton RW: A general approach to the problems of iron deficiency and iron overload in the population at large. *Semin Hematol* 19:54–69, 1982.

Bravo EL, Gifford RW: Pheochromocytoma: Diagnosis, localization and management. *N Engl J Med* 311:1298–1303, 1984.

Brooks PM, Day RO: Non-steroidal anti-inflammatory drugs: Differences and similarities. *N Engl J Med* 324:1716–1725, 1991.

Brown MS, Goldstein JL: A receptor-mediated pathway for cholesterol homeostasis. *Science* 232:34–47, 1986.

Buckley RH, Schiff RI: The use of intravenous immune globulin in immunodeficiency diseases. *N Engl J Med* 325:110–117, 1991.

Burtis WJ, Brady TG, Orloff JJ, et al: Immunochemical characterization of circulating parathyroid hormone-related protein in patients with humoral hypercalcemia of cancer. *N Engl J Med* 322:1106–1112, 1990.

Calhoun DA, Oparil S: Treatment of hypertensive crisis. *N Engl J Med* 323:1177–1183, 1991.

Callahan N, Garrett A, Goggin T: Withdrawal of anticonvulsant drugs in patients free of seizures for two years: A prospective study. *N Engl J Med* 318:942–946, 1988.

Carbone DP, Minna JD: The molecular genetics of lung cancer. *Adv Intern Med* 37:153–171, 1991.

Centers for Disease Control: Policy guidelines in the prevention and management of pelvic inflammatory disease. *MMWR* 4022–4025, 1992.

Caroff SN, Mann SC: Neuroleptic malignant syndrome. *Med Clin North Am* 77:185–202, 1993.

Centers for Disease Control: Prevention and control of influenza. *MMWR* 40:1–2, 1991.

Charness ME, Simon RP, Greenberg DA, et al: Ethanol and the nervous system. *N Engl J Med* 321:442–454, 1989.

Cherubin CE, Eng RH: Quinolones for the treatment of infections due to *Salmonella*. *Rev Infect Dis* 13:343–344, 1991.

Chu KC, Smart CR, Tarone RE: Analysis of breast cancer mortality and stage distribution by age for the Health Insurance Plan clinical trial. *J Natl Cancer Inst* 80:1125–1132, 1988.

Coe FL, Parks JH, Asplin JR: The pathogenesis and treatment of kidney stones. *N Engl J Med* 327:1141–1152, 1992.

Cohn JN, Levine TB, Olvari MT, et al: Plasma nor-

epinephrine as a guide to prognosis in patients with chronic congestive heart failure. *N Engl J Med* 311:819–823, 1984.

Collins FS: Cystic fibrosis: Molecular biology and therapeutic implications. *Science* 256:774–779, 1992.

Coustan DR: Pregnancy in diabetic women. *N Engl J Med* 319:1663–1665, 1988.

Crawford ED, Eisenberger MA, McLeod DG, et al: A controlled trial of leuprolide with and without flutamide in prostatic carcinoma. *N Engl J Med* 321:419–424, 1989.

Crook JE, Moertel CG, Gunderson LL, et al: Effective surgical adjuvant therapy for high-risk rectal carcinoma. *N Engl J Med* 324:709–715, 1991.

Crossley IR, Williams R: Spontaneous bacterial peritonitis. *Gut* 26:325–331, 1985.

Dalakas MC: Polymyositis dermatomyositis and inclusion body myositis. *N Engl J Med* 325:1487–1498, 1991.

The Diabetes Control and Complications Trial Research Group: The effect of intensive treatment of diabetes on the development and progression of long-term complications in insulin-dependent diabetes mellitus. *N Engl J Med* 329:977–986, 1993.

Dinarello CA, Cannon JG, Wolff SM: New concepts on the pathogenesis of fever. *Rev Infect Dis* 10:168–189, 1988.

Dineen S, Gerich J, Rizza R: Carbohydrate metabolism in non-insulin-dependent diabetes mellitus. *N Engl J Med* 327:707–713, 1992.

Domasio AR: Aphasia. *N Engl J Med* 326:531–539, 1992.

Drew WL: Diagnosis of cytomegalovirus infection. *Rev Infect Dis* 10:S468–S476, 1988.

Dubois RM: Idiopathic pulmonary fibrosis. *Ann Rev Med* 44:441–450, 1993.

Early Breast Cancer Trialists' Collaborative Group: Systemic treatment of early breast cancer by hormonal, cytotoxic, or immune therapy: 133 randomized trials involving 31,000 recurrences and 24,000 deaths among 75,000 women. *Lancet* 339:71–85, 1992.

Emmanuel D, Cunningham I, Jules-Elysee K, et al: Cytomegalovirus pneumonia after bone marrow transplantation successfully treated with the combination of ganciclovir and high-dose intravenous immune globulin. *Ann Intern Med* 109: 777–782, 1988.

Ernst CB: Abdominal aortic aneurysm. *N Engl J Med* 328:1167–1172, 1993.

Eschbach JW, Abdulhadi MH, Browne JK, et al: Recombinant erythropoietin in anemic patients with end-stage renal disease. *Ann Intern Med* 111: 992–1000, 1989.

Estey EH, Kurzrock R, Kantarjian HM, et al: Treatment of hairy cell leukemia with 2-chlorodeoxy-adenosine (2-CdA). *Blood* 79:882–887, 1992.

Fang G-D, Fine M, Orloff J, et al: New and emerging etiologies for community acquired pneumonia with implications for therapy. *Medicine* 69:307–316, 1992.

Farley MM, Stephens DS, Brachman PS Jr, et al: Invasive *Haemophilus influenzae* disease in adults. *Ann Intern Med* 116:806–812, 1992.

Feinstein DI: Lupus anticoagulant, anticardiolipin, antibodies, fetal loss, and systemic lupus erythematosus. *Blood* 80:859–862, 1992.

Field M, Rao MC, Chang EB: Intestinal electrolyte transport and diarrheal disease. *N Engl J Med* 321:879–883, 1989.

Fine H, Mayer RJ: Primary central nervous system lymphoma. *Ann Intern Med* 119:1093–1104, 1993.

Fisher B, Redmond C, Poisson R, et al: Eight-year results of a randomized clinical trial comparing total mastectomy and lumpectomy with or without irradiation in the treatment of breast cancer. *N Engl J Med* 320:822–828, 1989.

Fisher CM: Lacunar strokes and infarcts: A review. *Neurology* 32:871–876, 1982.

Fitzpatrick TB, Johnson RA, Polano MK, et al: *Color Atlas and Synopsis of Clinical Dermatology,* 2/e. New York, McGraw-Hill, 1992.

Flier JS: Syndromes of insulin resistance: From patient to gene and back again. *Diabetes* 41:1207–1219, 1992.

Fowler NO: Tuberculous pericarditis. *JAMA* 266:99–103, 1991.

Frank BB: Clinical evaluation of jaundice: A guideline of the patient care committee of the American Gastroenterological Association. *JAMA* 262: 3031–3034, 1989.

Frank MM: Complement in the pathophysiology of human disease. *N Engl J Med* 316:1525–1530, 1987.

Froehling DA, Silverstein MD, Mohr DN, et al: Does this dizzy patient have a serious form of vertigo? *JAMA* 271:385–388, 1994.

Fujita S: Obstructive sleep apnea syndrome: Pathophysiology, upper-airway evaluation, and surgical treatment. *Ear Nose Throat J* 72:67–72, 75–76, 1993.

Fuster V, Badimon L, Badimon JJ, Chesebro JH: Mechanisms of disease: Pathophysiology of coronary artery disease and the acute coronary syndromes. *N Engl J Med* 326:242–250, 310–318, 1992.

Gilman S: Advances in neurology, part II. *N Engl J Med* 326:1671–1676, 1992.

Gold BS, Barish RA: Venomous snakebites: Current concepts in diagnosis, treatment, and management. *Emerg Med Clin North Am* 10:249–267, 1992.

Goodgame RW: Gastrointestinal cytomegalovirus disease. *Ann Intern Med* 119:924–935, 1993.

Graham DY, Lew GM, Klein PD, et al: Effect of treatment of *Helicobacter pylori* infection on the long-term recurrence of gastric or duodenal ulcers. *Ann Intern Med* 116:705–708, 1992.

Greenberger PA, Patterson R: Allergic bronchopulmonary aspergillosis. Model of bronchopulmonary disease with defined serologic, radiologic, pathologic and clinical findings from asthma to fatal destructive lung diseases. *Chest* 91:165S–171S, 1987.

Greene WC: The molecular biology of human immunodeficiency virus type 1 infection. *N Engl J Med* 321:308–316, 1991.

Griffin JE: Androgen resistance: The clinical and molecular spectrum. *N Engl J Med* 336:611–618, 1992.

Grossman W: Diastolic dysfunction in congestive heart failure. *N Engl J Med* 325:1557–1564, 1991.

Grunberger G, Weiner JL, Silverman R, et al: Factitious hypoglycemia due to surreptitious administration of insulin: Diagnosis, treatment, and long-term follow-up. *Ann Intern Med* 108:252–257, 1988.

Haber DA, Mayer RJ: Primary gastrointestinal lymphoma. *Semin Oncol* 15:154–169, 1988.

Hainer BL: Cat-scratch disease. *J Fam Pract* 25:497–503, 1987.

Hainsworth JD, Greco FA: Treatment of patients with cancer of an unknown primary site. *N Engl J Med* 329:257–263, 1993.

Harris ED, Jr: Rheumatoid arthritis: Pathophysiology and implications for therapy. *N Engl J Med* 322:1277–1289, 1990.

Harris JR, Lippman ME, Veronesi U, et al: Breast cancer. *N Engl J Med* 327:319–328, 390–398, 473–480, 1992.

Harrison LC, Campbell IL, Allison J, et al: MHC molecules and beta-cell destruction. Immune and nonimmune disorders. *Diabetes* 38:815–818, 1989.

Havel RJ: Lowering cholesterol, 1988. Rationale, mechanism, and means. *J Clin Invest* 81:1653–1660, 1988.

Heyman MR, Schiffer CA: Platelet transfusion therapy for the cancer patient. *Semin Oncol* 17:198–209, 1990.

Hinson JR, Marini JF: Principles of mechanical ventilation in respiratory failure. *Ann Rev Med* 43:341–361, 1992.

Hirsch MS, D'Aquila RT: Therapy for human immunodeficiency virus infection. *N Engl J Med* 328:1686–1695, 1993.

Hoffman GS, Kerr GS, Leavitt RY, et al: Wegener's granulomatosis: An analysis of 158 patients. *Ann Intern Med* 116:488–498, 1992.

Hoofnagle JH: Type D (delta): hepatitis. *JAMA* 261:1321–1325, 1989.

Hook EW, Marra CM: Acquired syphilis in adults. *N Engl J Med* 326:1060–1069, 1992.

Hooper DC, Wolfson JS: Fluoroquinolone antimicrobial agents. *N Engl J Med* 324:384–394, 1991.

Horning SJ, Carrier EK, Rouse RV, et al: Lymphomas presenting as histologically unclassified neoplasms: Characteristics and response to treatment. *J Clin Oncol* 7:1281–1287, 1989.

Isselbacher KJ, Braunwald E, Wilson JD, Martin JB, Fauci AS, Kasper DL: *Harrison's Principles of Internal Medicine, 13/e. New York, McGraw-Hill, 1994.*

Ihde DC: Chemotherapy of lung cancer. *N Engl J Med* 327:1434–1441, 1992.

Jarcho JA, McKenna W, Pare JAP, et al: Mapping a gene for familial hypertrophic cardiomyopathy to chromosome 14q1. *N Engl J Med* 321:1372–1378, 1989.

Kaye BR: Rheumatologic manifestations of infection with human immunodeficiency virus (HIV). *Ann Intern Med* 11:158–167, 1989.

Kaye D, Abrutyn E: Prevention of bacterial endocarditis 1991. *Ann Intern Med* 114:803–804, 1991.

Kazazian HH Jr: The thalassemia syndromes: Molecular basis and prenatal diagnosis in 1990. *Semin Hematol* 27:209–228, 1990.

Kinzler KW, Nilbert MC, Vogelstein B, et al: Identification of a gene located at chromosome 5q21 that is mutated in colorectal cancers. *Science* 251:1366–1370, 1991.

Kirchoff LV: American trypanosomiasis (Chagas' disease): A tropical disease now in the United States. *N Engl J Med* 329:639–644, 1993.

Koenig M, Hoffman EP, Bertelson CJ, et al: Complete cloning of the Duchenne muscular dystrophy (DMD) cDNA and preliminary genomic organization of the DMD gene in normal and affected individuals. *Cell* 50:509–517, 1987.

Koh HK: Cutaneous melanoma. *N Engl J Med* 325:171–182, 1991.

Krockta WP, Barnes WC: Sexually transmitted diseases. Genital ulceration with regional adenopathy. *Infect Dis Clin North Am* 1:217–233, 1987.

Kuntz RE, Tosteson AN, Berman AD, et al: Predictors of event-free survival after balloon aortic valvuloplasty. *N Engl J Med* 325:17–23, 1991.

Kupin WL, Narins RG: The hyperkalemia of renal failure: Pathophysiology, diagnosis, and therapy. *Contrib Nephrol* 102:1–22, 1993.

Lawly TJ, Bielory L, Gascon P, et al: A prospective clinical and immunologic analysis of patients with serum sickness. *N Engl J Med* 311:1407–1413, 1984.

Luzzatto G, Schafer AI: The prethrombotic state in cancer. *Semin Oncol* 17:147–159, 1990.

Lynn RB, Friedman LS: Irritable bowel syndrome. *N Engl J Med* 329:1940–1945, 1993.

Malech HL, Gallin JI: Neutrophils in human diseases. *N Engl J Med* 317:687–694, 1987.

Mandel JS, Bond JH, Church TR, et al: Minnesota Colon Cancer Control Study: Reducing mortality from colorectal cancer by screening for fecal occult blood. *N Engl J Med* 328:1365–1371, 1993.

Marks AR, Choong CY, Sanfilippo AJ, et al: Identification of high-risk and low-risk subgroups of patients with a mitral valve prolapse. *N Engl J Med* 320:1031–1036, 1989.

Martin JB, Gusella JF: Huntington's disease: Pathogenesis and management. *N Engl J Med* 315: 1267–1276, 1986.

Max MB, Lynch SA, Muir J, et al: Effects of desipramine, amitriptyline, and fluoxetine on pain and diabetic neuropathy. *N Engl J Med* 326:1250–1256, 1992.

McCarthy DM: Sucralfate. *N Engl J Med* 325:1017–1025, 1991.

McFadden ER Jr., Gilbert IA: Asthma. *N Engl J Med* 327:1928–1937, 1993.

Michels R, Marzuk PM: Progress in psychiatry. *N Engl J Med* 329:552–560, 628–638, 1993.

Michet CJ: Vasculitis and relapsing polychondritis. *Rheum Dis Clin North Am* 16:441–444, 1990.

Mitchelson F: Pharmacologic agents affecting emesis: A review (part 1). *Drugs* 43:443–463, 1992.

Modell JH: Drowning. *N Engl J Med* 328:253–256, 1993.

Naclerio RM: Allergic rhinitis. *N Engl J Med* 325:860–869, 1991.

Narins RG, Jones ER, Stom MC, et al: Diagnostic strategies in disorders of fluid, electrolyte, and acid-base homeostasis. *Am J Med* 72:496–520, 1982.

Nathan DM: Long-term complications of diabetes mellitus. *N Engl J Med* 328:1676–1685, 1993.

National Cholesterol Education Panel: Report of the National Cholesterol Education Panel on detection, evaluation, and treatment of high blood cholesterol in adults. *Arch Intern Med* 148:36–69, 1988.

National Institutes of Health–University of California Expert Panel for Corticosteroids as Adjunctive Therapy for *Pneumocystis* Pneumonia: Consensus statement on the use of corticosteroids as adjunctive therapy for *Pneumocystis* pneumonia in AIDS. *N Engl J Med* 323:1500–1504, 1990.

Neu HC: Ciprofloxacin: A major advance in quinolone chemotherapy. *Am J Med* 82(4A):1–2, 1987.

Oates JA, Wood AJJ: Adenosine and superventricular tachycardia. *N Engl J Med* 325:1621–1629, 1991.

Okuda H: Hepatocellular carcinoma: Recent progress. *Hepatology* 15:948–963, 1992.

Pantaleo G, Graziosi C, Fauci AS: New concepts in the immunopathogenesis of human immunodeficiency virus infection. *N Engl J Med* 328:327–335, 1993.

Peppercorn MA: Advances in drug therapy for inflammatory bowel disease. *Ann Intern Med* 812:50–60, 1990.

Perrillo RP, Schiff ER, Davis GL, et al: A randomized controlled trial of interferon, alpha-2b alone and after steroid withdrawal for treatment of chronic hepatitis B. *N Engl J Med* 323:295–301, 1990.

Pizzo PA: Management of fever in patients with cancer and treatment-induced neutropenia. *N Engl J Med* 328:1323–1332, 1993.

Podolsky DL: Inflammatory bowel disease. *N Engl J Med* 325:928–937, 1008–1016, 1991.

Popp RL: Medical progress: Echocardiography (two parts). *N Engl J Med* 323:101–108, 165–172, 1990.

Posner JB: Paraneoplastic syndromes. *Neurol Clin* 9:919–936, 1991.

Prados J, Finison L, Andres PL, et al: The natural history of amyotrophic lateral sclerosis and the use of natural history controls in therapeutic trials. *Neurology* 43:751–755, 1993.

Pras E, Aksentijevich I, Gruberg L, et al: Mapping of a gene causing familial Mediterranean fever to the short arm of chromosome 16. *N Engl J Med* 326:1509–1513, 1992.

Ransohoff DF, Miller GL, Forsythe SB, et al: Outcome of acute cholecystitis in patients with diabetes mellitus. *Ann Intern Med* 106:829–832, 1987.

Reed SL, Wessel DW, Davis CE: *Entamoeba histolytica* infection and AIDS. *Am J Med* 90:269–271, 1991.

Reeders S: Multilocus polycystic disease. *Nat Genetics* 1:235–237, 1992.

Relman DA, Schmidt TM, MacDermott RP, Falkow S: Identification of the uncultured bacillus of Whipple's disease. *N Engl J Med* 327:293–301, 1992.

Resnick NM, Valla SV, Laurine E: The pathophysiology of urinary incontinence among institutionalized elderly persons. *N Engl J Med* 320:1–7, 1989.

Revler JB, Broudy VC, Cooney TG: Adult scurvy. *JAMA* 253:805–807, 1985.

Rich S: Primary pulmonary hypertension. *Prog Cardiovasc Dis* 31:205–238, 1988.

Ridgway EC: Clinician's evaluation of a solitary thyroid nodule. *J Clin Endocrinol Metab* 74:231–235, 1992.

Rigel DS, Rivers JK, Koff AW, et al: Dysplastic nevi: Markers for increased risk from melanoma. *Cancer* 63:386–389, 1989.

Riggs BL, Melton LJ III: The prevention and treatment of osteoporosis. *N Engl J Med* 327:620–627, 1992.

Robertson MJ, Ritz J: Biology and clinical relevance of natural killer cells. *Blood* 76:2421–2438, 1990.

Rosen FS, Cooper MD, Wedgewood RJP: The primary immunodeficiencies. *N Engl J Med* 311: 235–242, 300–310, 1989.

Roth BJ, Nichols CR: Testicular cancer. *Semin Oncol* 19:117–118, 1992.

Schreiber AD: Paroxysmal nocturnal hemoglobinuria revisited. *N Engl J Med* 309:723–725, 1983.

Sears DA: Anemia of chronic disease. *Med Clin North Am* 76:567–579, 1992.

Shader RI, Greenblatt DJ: Use of benzodiazepines in anxiety disorders. *N Engl J Med* 328:1398–1405, 1993.

Shapiro ED, Berg AT, Austrian R, et al: The protective efficacy of polyvalent pneumococcal vaccine. *N Engl J Med* 325:1453–1460, 1991.

Simon HB: Hyperthermia. *N Engl J Med* 329:483–487, 1993.

Siperstein MD: Diabetic ketoacidosis and hyposmolar coma. *Endocrinol Metab Clin North Am* 21:415–432, 1992.

Slamon DJ, Godolphin W, Jones CA, et al: Studies of the HER-2/neu proto-oncogene in human breast and ovarian cancer. *Science* 244:707–712, 1989.

Sneller MC, Strober W, Isenstein E, et al: New insights into common variable immunodeficiency. *Ann Intern Med* 118:720–730, 1993.

Snilkstein MJ, Knapp GL, Kulig KW, Rumack BH: Efficacy of oral *N*-acetylcysteine in the treatment of acetaminophen overdose: Analysis of the national multi-center study. *N Engl J Med* 319:1557–1562, 1988.

SOLVD Investigators: Effect on survival in patients with induced left ventricular ejection fractions and congestive heart failure. *N Engl J Med* 325:293–302, 1991.

Spach DH, Liles WC, Campbell GL, et al: Tick-borne diseases in the United States. *N Engl J Med* 329:936–947, 1993.

Stabler SP, Allen RH, Savage DG, et al: Clinical spectrum and diagnosis of cobalamin deficiency. *Blood* 76:871–881, 1990.

Standaert DG, Stern MB: Update on the management of Parkinson's disease. *Med Clin North Am* 77:169–183, 1993.

Standards and guidelines for cardiopulmonary resuscitation (CPR) in emergency cardiac care (ECC). *JAMA* 255:2905–2989, 1986.

Steere AC: Lyme disease. *N Engl J Med* 321:586–596, 1989.

Stockley RA: Alpha-1 antitrypsin and the pathogenesis of emphysema. *Lung* 165:61–77, 1987.

Swenerton K, Jeffrey J, Stuart G, et al: Cisplatin-cyclophosphamide versus carboplatin-cyclophosphamide in advanced ovarian cancer: A randomized phase III study of the National Cancer Institute of Canada clinical trials group. *J Clin Oncol* 10:718–726, 1992.

Talpaz M, Kantarjian H, Kurzrock R, et al: Interferon-alpha produces sustained cytogenetic response in chronic myelogenous leukemia. *Ann Intern Med* 114:532–538, 1991.

Terblanche J, Burroughs AK, Hobbs KE: Controversies in the management of bleeding esophageal varices. *N Engl J Med* 320:1469–1475, 1989.

Thaler M, Pastakia B, Shawker TH, et al: Hepatic candidiasis in cancer patients: The evolving picture of the syndrome. *Ann Intern Med* 108:88–100, 1988.

Third International Study of Infarct Survival Collaborative Group: 1515-3: A randomized comparison of streptokinase 'vs' tissue plasminogen activator 'vs' antistreplase and of aspirin plus heparin 'vs' aspirin alone among 41,299 cases of suspected myocardial infarction. *Lancet* 339:753–770, 1992.

Thompson CE, Damon LE, Ries CA, et al: Thrombotic microorganiopathies in the 1980s. Clinical Features. *Blood* 80:1890–1895, 1992.

Tompkins LS: Use of molecular methods in infectious diseases. *N Engl J Med* 327:1290–1297, 1992.

Trier JS: Celiac sprue. *N Engl J Med* 325:1709–1719, 1991.

Urba WJ, Longo DL: Hodgkin's disease. *N Engl J Med* 326:678–687, 1992.

Vogelstein B, Fearon ER, Hamilton SR, et al: Genetic alterations during colorectal-tumor development. *N Engl J Med* 319:525–532, 1988.

Vokes EE, Weichselbaum RR, Lippman SM, et al: Head and neck cancer. *N Engl J Med* 328:184–194, 1993.

Walt RP: Drug-therapy: Misoprostol for the treatment of peptic ulcer and anti-inflammatory-drug-induced gastroduodenal ulceration. *N Engl J Med* 327:1575–1580, 1992.

Warrell RP Jr, DeThé H, Wang Z-Y, et al: Acute promyelocytic leukemia. *N Engl J Med* 329:177–189, 1993.

Warshaw AL, Fernandez-del Castillo C: Pancreatic carcinoma. *N Engl J Med* 326:455–465, 1992.

Wayne AS, Kevy SV, Nathan DG: Transfusion management of sickle cell disease. *Blood* 81:1109–1123, 1993.

Weinberg RA: Tumor suppressor genes. *Science* 254:1138–1146, 1991.

Weinberger SE: Recent advances in pulmonary medicine. *N Engl J Med* 328:1389–1397, 1993.

Welch KMA: Drug therapy of migraine. *N Engl J Med* 329:1476–1483, 1993.

Wheat LJ, Connolly-Stringfield PA, Baker RL, et al: Disseminated histoplasmosis in AIDS: Clinical findings, diagnosis, treatment, and review of the literature. *Medicine* 69:361–374, 1990.

White RJ, Likavech MJ: The diagnosis in initial management of head injury. *N Engl J Med* 327:1507–1511, 1992.

Whitley RJ, Gnann JW Jr: Acyclovir: A decade later. *N Engl J Med* 327:782–789, 1992.

Willard JE, Lange RA, Hillis LD: The use of aspirin in ischemic heart disease. *N Engl J Med* 327:175–181, 1992.

Williams GH: Converting enzyme inhibitors in the treatment of hypotension. *N Engl J Med* 319:1517–1525, 1989.

Wolff SM: Monoclonal antibodies and the treatment of gram-negative bacteremia and shock. *N Engl J Med* 324:486–488, 1991.

Wrenn KD, Solvis SM, Minion GE, et al: The syndrome of alcoholic ketoacidosis. *Am J Med* 91:119–128, 1991.

Yankner BA, Mesulam M-M: Beta-amyloid and the pathogenesis of Alzheimer's disease. *N Engl J Med* 325:1849–1857, 1991.

APPENDIX: LABORATORY VALUES OF CLINICAL IMPORTANCE

INTRODUCTORY COMMENTS

All laboratory appendices should be interpreted with caution because normal values differ widely among clinical laboratories. The values given in this appendix are meant primarily for use with this text. In preparing this Appendix, the editors have taken into account the fact the system of international units (SI, système international d'unités) is now used in most countries and in virtually all medical and scientific journals, including most in the United States.[1] However, most clinical laboratories in the United States continue to report values in traditional units. Therefore, a system has been adopted that utilizes both systems for this Appendix and for the text itself. Values in SI units appear first, and *traditional units appear in parentheses* after the SI units. This dual system is also used for the most part in the text. In those instances in which the numbers remain the same but only the terminology is changed (mmol/L for meq/L or IU/L for mIU/L, only the SI units are given. In all other instances in the text the SI unit is followed by the traditional unit in parentheses. The SI base units, SI derived units, other units of measure referred to in this Appendix and SI prefixes are listed in Tables A-1 to A-3 at the end of this Appendix. Conversions from one system to another can be made as follows:

$$mmol/L = \frac{mg/dL \times 10}{atomic\ weight}$$

$$mg/dL = \frac{mmol/L \times atomic\ weight}{10}$$

ASCITIC FLUID

See Chapter 43.

BODY FLUIDS AND OTHER MASS DATA

Body fluid, total volume: 50 percent (in obese) to 70 percent (lean) of body weight
   Intracellular: 0.3–0.4 of body weight
   Extracellular: 0.2–0.3 of body weight
Blood:
   Total volume:
      Males: 69 mL/kg of body weight
      Females: 65 mL/kg of body weight
   Plasma volume:
      Males: 39 mL/kg of body weight
      Females: 40 mL/kg of body weight
   Red blood cell volume:
      Males: 30 mL/kg of body weight (1.15–1.21 L/m² of body surface area)
      Females: 25 mL/kg of body weight (0.95–1.00 L/m² of body surface area)

[1] Young DS: Implementation of SI units for clinical laboratory data. Ann Intern Med 106:114–129, 1987

CEREBROSPINAL FLUID[2]

		Conversion Factor (CF) C × CF = SI
Osmolarity	292–297 mmol/kg water (292–297 mOsmol/L)	—
Electrolytes:		
Sodium	137–145 mmol/L (137–145 meq/L)	—
Potassium	2.7–3.9 mmol/L (2.7–3.9 meq/L)	—
Calcium	1–1.5 mmol/L (2.1–3.0 meq/L)	0.5
Magnesium	1–1.2 mmol/L (2.0–2.5 meq/L)	0.5
Chloride	116–122 mmol/L (116–122 meq/L)	—
CO_2 content	20–24 mmol/L (20–24 meq/L)	—
P_{CO_2}	6–7 kPa (45–49 mmHg)	0.1333
pH	7.31–7.34	—
Glucose	2.2–3.9 mmol/L (40–70 mg/dL)	0.05551
Lactate	1–2 mmol/L (10–20 mg/dL)	0.1110
Total protein:	0.2–0.5 g/L (20–50 mg/dL)	0.01
Prealbumin	2–6 percent	—
Albumin	56–75 percent	—
Alpha$_1$ globulin	2–7 percent	—
Alpha$_2$ globulin	4–12 percent	—
Beta globulin	8–16 percent	—
Gamma globulin	3–12 percent	—
IgG	0.01–0.014 g/L (1–1.4 mg/dL)	0.01
IgG index[3]	<0.65	
IgA	0.001–0.003 g/L (0.1–0.3 mg/dL)	0.01
IgM	0.0001–0.00012 g/L (0.01–0.012 mg/dL)	0.01
Ammonia	15–47 µmol/L (25–80 µg/dL)	0.05872
Creatinine	44–168 µmol/L (0.5–1.9 mg/dL)	88.40
Myelin basic protein	<4 µg/L	—
CSF pressure	50–180 mmH₂O	—
CSF volume (adult)	100–160 mL	—
Leukocytes:		
Total	<4 per mL	—
Differential:		
Lymphocytes	60–70 percent	—

[2] Since cerebrospinal fluid concentrations are equilibrium values, measurements of the same parameters in blood plasma obtained at the same time is recommended. However, there is a time lag in attainment of equilibrium, and cerebrospinal levels of plasma constituents that can fluctuate rapidly (such as plasma glucose) may not achieve stable values until after a significant lag phase.

[3] $IgG\ index = \dfrac{CSF\ IgG\ (mg/dL) \times serum\ albumin\ (g/dL)}{Serum\ IgG\ (g/dL) \times CSF\ albumin\ (mg/dL)}$

		Conversion Factor (CF) C × CF = SI
Monocytes	30–50 percent	—
Neutrophils	None	—

CHEMICAL CONSTITUENTS OF BLOOD

See also function tests, especially metabolic and endocrine.

	Conversion Factor (CF) C × CF = SI
Acetoacetate, plasma: <100 μmol/L (<1 mg/dL)	97.95
Albumin, serum: 35–55 g/L (3.5–5.5 g/dL)	10
Aldolase: 0–100 nkat/L (0–6 U/L)	16.67
Alpha$_1$ antitrypsin, serum: 0.8–2.1 g/L (85–213 mg/dL)	0.01
Alpha fetoprotein (adult), serum: <30 μg/L (<30 ng/mL)	—
Aminotransferases, serum:	
Aspartate (AST, SGOT): 0–0.58 μkat/L (0–35 U/L)	0.01667
Alanine (ALT, SGPT): 0–0.58 μkat/L (0–35 U/L)	0.01667
Ammonia, whole blood, venous: 47–65 μmol/L (80–110 μg/dL)	0.5872
Amylase, serum: 0.8–3.2 μkat/L; 60–180 U/L	0.01667
Arterial blood gases:	
[HCO$_3^-$]: 21–28 mmol/L (21–30 meq/L)	—
P$_{CO_2}$: 4.7–5.9 kPa (35–45 mmHg)	0.1333
pH: 7.38–7.44	—
P$_{O_2}$: 11–13 kPa (80–100 mmHg)	0.1333
Ascorbic acid (vitamin C), serum: 23–57 μmol/L (0.4–1.0 mg/dL)	56.78
Barbiturates, serum: normal, nondetectable	
Phenobarbital, "potentially fatal" level: approximately 390 μmol/L (9 mg/dL)	43.06
Most short-acting barbiturates, "potentially fatal" levels: approximately 150 μmol/L (35 mg/dL)	4.419
Base, total, serum: 145–155 mmol/L (145–155 meq/L)	—
β-Hydroxybutyrate, plasma: <300 μmol/L (<3 mg/dL)	96.05
Bilirubin, total, serum (Malloy-Evelyn): 5.1–17 μmol/L (0.3–1.0 mg/dL)	17.10
Direct, serum: 1.7–5.1 μmol/L (0.1–0.3 mg/dL)	17.10
Indirect, serum: 3.4–12 μmol/L (0.2–0.7 mg/dL)	17.10
Bromides, serum: nondetectable	
Toxic levels: >17 mmol/L (>17 meq/L)	—
Calciferols (vitamin D), plasma:	
1,25-Dihydroxyvitamin D [1,25(OH)$_2$D]: 40–160 pmol/L (16 to 65 pg/mL)	0.2400
25-Hydroxyvitamin D [25(OH)D]: 20–200 nmol/L (8–80 ng/mL)	2.496
Calcium, ionized: 1.1–1.4 mmol/L (4.5–5.6 mg/dL)	0.2495
Calcium, plasma: 2.2–2.6 mmol/L (9–10.5 mg/dL)	0.2495
Carbon dioxide content, plasma (sea level): 21–30 mmol/L (21–30 meq/L)	—
Carbon dioxide tension (P$_{CO_2}$), arterial blood (sea level): 4.7–6.0 kPa (35–45 mmHg)	0.1333
Carbon monoxide content, blood: symptoms with over 20 percent saturation of hemoglobin	
Carotenoids, serum: 0.9–5.6 μmol/L (50–300 μg/dL)	0.01863

	Conversion Factor (CF) C × CF = SI
Ceruloplasmin, serum: 270–370 mg/L (27–37 mg/dL)	10
Chlorides, serum (as Cl$^-$): 98–106 mmol/L (98–106 meq/L)	—
Cholesterol: see Table A-4	
Complement, serum:	
C3: 0.55–1.20 g/L (55–120 mg/dL)	0.01
C4: 0.20–0.50 g/L (20–50 mg/dL)	0.01
Copper, serum: 11–22 μmol/L (70–140 μg/dL)	0.1574
Creatine phosphokinase, serum (total):	
Females: 0.17–1.17 μkat/L (10–70 U/L)	0.01667
Males: 0.42–1.50 μkat/L (25–90 U/L)	0.01667
Creatinine, serum: <133 μmol/L.(1.5 mg/dL)	88.40
Digoxin serum:	
Therapeutic level: 0.6–2.8 nmol/L (0.5–2.2 ng/mL)	1.281
Toxic level: >3.1 nmol/L (>2.4 ng/mL)	1.281
Ethanol, blood:	
Mild to moderate intoxication: 17–43 mmol/L (80–200 mg/dL)	0.2171
Marked intoxication: 54–87 mmol/L (250–400 mg/dL)	0.2171
Severe intoxication: >87 mmol/L (>400 mg/dL)	0.2171
Fatty acids, free (nonesterified), plasma: 180 mg/L (<18 mg/dL)	10
Ferritin, serum:	
Women: 10–200 μg/L (10–200 ng/ml)	—
Men: 15–400 μg/L (15–400 ng/ml)	
Fibrinogen, plasma: see "Hematologic Evaluations: Platelets and Coagulation"	—
Fibrinogen split products: see "Hematologic Evaluations: Platelets and Coagulation"	—
Folic acid, red cell: 340–1020 nmol/L cells (150–450 ng/mL cells)	2.266
Gastrin, serum: 40–200 ng/L (40–200 pg/mL)	—
Globulins, serum: 20–30 g/L (2.0–3.0 g/dL)	10
Glucose (fasting), plasma:	
Normal: 4.2–6.4 mmol/L (75–115 mg/dL)	0.05551
Diabetes mellitus: >7.8 mmol/L on more than than one occasion (>140 mg dL)	0.05551
Glucose, 2 h postprandial, plasma:	
Normal: <7.8 mmol/L (<140 mg/dL)	0.05551
Impaired glucose tolerance: 7.8–11.1 mmol/L (140–200 mg/dL)	0.05551
Diabetes mellitus: >11.1 mmol/L on more than one occasion (>200 mg/dL)	0.05551
Hemoglobin, blood (sea level):	
Male: 140–180 g/L (14–18 g/dL)	10
Female: 120–160 g/L (12–16 g/dL)	10
Hemoglobin A$_{1c}$: up to 6 percent of total hemoglobin	—
Immunoglobulins, serum:	
IgA: 0.9–3.2 g/L (90–325 mg/dL)	0.01
IgD: 0–0.08 g/L (0–8 mg/dL)	0.01
IgE: <0.00025 g/L (<0.025 mg/dL)	0.01
IgG: 8.0–15.0 g/L (800–1500 mg/dL)	0.01
IgM: 0.45–1.5 g/L (45–150 mg/dL)	0.01
Iron, serum: 9–27 μmol/L (50–150 μg/dL)	0.01791
Iron-binding capacity, serum: 45–66 μmol/L (250–370 μg/dL)	0.01791
Saturation: 0.2–0.45 (20–45 percent)	
Lactate dehydrogenase, serum:	
200–450 units/mL (Wrobleski)	—
60–100 units/mL (Wacker)	—

	Conversion Factor (CF) C × CF = SI
0.4–1.7 μkat/L (25–100 units/L)	0.01667
Lactic dehydrogenase isoenzymes, serum (agarose):	
Fraction 1 (of total): 0.14–0.25 (14–26 percent)	0.01
Fraction 2: 0.29–0.39 (29–39 percent)	0.01
Fraction 3: 0.20–0.25 (20–26 percent)	0.01
Fraction 4: 0.08–0.16 (8–16 percent)	0.01
Fraction 5: 0.06–0.16 (6–16 percent)	0.01
Lactate, venous plasma: 0.6–1.7 mmol/L (5–15 mg/dL)	0.1110
Lead, serum: <1.0 μmol/L (<20 μg/dL)	0.04826
Lipids: see Table A-4	—
Lipids, triglyceride, serum: see "Triglycerides"	—
Lipoprotein: see Table A-4	—
Lithium, serum:	
Therapeutic level: 0.6–1.2 mmol/L (0.6–1.2 meq/L)	—
Toxic level: >2 mmol/L (2 meq/L)	—
Magnesium, serum: 0.8–1.2 mmol/L (2–3 mg/dL)	0.4114
Osmolality, plasma: 285–295 mmol/kg serum water (285–295 mosmol/kg serum water)	—
Oxygen content:	
Arterial blood (sea level): 17–21 volume percent	—
Venous blood, arm (sea level): 10–16 volume percent	—
Oxygen percent saturation (sea level):	
Arterial blood: 0.97 mol/mol (97 percent)	0.01
Venous blood, arm: 0.60–0.85 mol/mol (60–85 percent)	0.01
Oxygen tension (P_{O_2}) blood: 11–13 kPa (80–100 mmHg)	0.1333
pH, blood: 7.38–7.44	—
Phenytoin, plasma:	
Therapeutic level: 40–80 μmol/L (10–20 mg/L)	3.964
Toxic level: >120 μmol/L (>30 mg/L)	3.964
Phospatase, acid, serum: 0.90 nkat/L (0–5.5 U/L)	—
Phosphatase, alkaline, serum: 0.5–2.0 μkat/L (30–120 U/L)	—
Phosphorus, inorganic, serum: 1.0–1.4 mmol/L (3–4.5 mg/dL)	0.3229
Potassium, serum: 3.5–5.0 mmol/L (3.5–5.0 meg/L)	—
Proteins, total, serum: 55–80 g/L (5.5–8.0 g/dL)	10
Protein fractions, serum:	
Albumin: 35–55 g/L [3.5–5.5 g/dL (50–60 percent)]	10
Globulin: 20–35 g/L [2.0–3.5 g/dL (40–50 percent)]	10
Alpha$_1$: 2–4 g/L [0.2–0.4 g/dL (4.2–7.2 percent)]	10
Alpha$_2$: 5–9 g/L [0.5–0.9 g/dL (6.8–12 percent)]	10
Beta: 6–11 g/L [0.6–1.1 g/dL (9.3–15 percent)]	10
Gamma: 7–17 g/L [0.7–1.7 g/dL (13–23 percent)]	10
Pyruvate, venous, plasma: 60–170 μmol/L (0.5–1.5 mg/dL)	113.6
Quinidine, serum:	
Therapeutic range: 4.6–9.2 μmol/L (1.5–3 mg/L)	3.082
Toxic range: 15.4–18.5 μmol/L (5–6 mg/L)	3.082

	Conversion Factor (CF) C × CF = SI
Salicylate, plasma: 0 mmol/L	—
Therapeutic range: 1.4–1.8 mmol/L (20–25 mg/dL)	0.07240
Toxic range: >2.2 mmoi/L (>30 mg/dL)	0.07240
Sodium, serum: 136–145 mmol/L (136–145 meq/L)	—
Steroids: see "Metabolic and Endocrine Tests"	—
Triglycerides: <1.8 mmol/L (<160 mg/dL)	0.01129
Urea nitrogen, serum: 3.6–7.1 mmol/L (10–20 mg/dL)	0.3570
Uric acid, serum:	
Men: 150–480 μmol/L (2.5–8.0 mg/dL)	59.48
Women: 90–360 μmol/L (1.5–6.0 mg/dL)	59.48
Vitamin A, serum: 0.7–3.5 μmol/L (20–100 μg/dL)	0.03491
Vitamin B$_{12}$, serum: 148–443 pmol/L (200–600 pg/mL)	0.7378
Zinc, serum: 11.5–18.5 μmol/L (75–120 μg/dL)	0.1530

CIRCULATION FUNCTION TESTS

Arteriovenous oxygen difference: 30–50 mL/L
Cardiac output (Fick): 2.5–3.6 L/m^2 of body surface area per minute
Contractility indexes:
Maximum left ventricular dp/dt: 1650 ± 300 mmHg/s
Maximum $(dp/dt)/p$: 44 ± 8.4 s^{-1}
(dp/dt)/DP at DP = 40 mmHg: 37.6 ± 12.2 s^{-1} (DP = diastolic press.)
Mean normalized systolic ejection rate (angiography): 3.32 ± 0.84 end-diastolic volumes per second
Mean velocity of circumferential fiber shortening (angiography) 1.66 ± 0.42 circumferences per second
Ejection fraction, stroke volume/end-diastolic volume (SV/EDV):
Normal range: 0.55–0.78; average: 0.67
End-diastolic volume: 75 ± 15 mL/m^2
End-systolic volume: 25 ± 8 mL/m^2
Left ventricular work:
Stroke work index: 30–110 (g·m)/m^2
Left ventricular minute work index: 1.8–6.6 [(kg·m)/m^2]/min
Oxygen consumption index: 110–150 mL
Pulmonary vascular resistance: 20–120 (dyn·s)/cm^5 (2–12 kPa·s/L)
Systemic vascular resistance: 770–1500 (dyn·s)/cm^5 (77–150 kPa·s/L)

GASTROINTESTINAL TESTS

See also "Stool Analysis."

Absorption tests:
D-Xylose absorption test: After an overnight fast, 25 g xylose is given in aqueous solution by mouth. Urine collected for the following 5 h should contain 5–8 g (33–53 mmol) (or >20 percent of ingested dose). Serum xylose should be 25–40 mg/100 mL 1 h after the oral dose (1.7–2.7 mmol/L).
Vitamin A absorption test: A fasting blood specimen is obtained and 200,000 units of vitamin A in oil is given by mouth. Serum vitamin A levels should rise to twice fasting level in 3–5 h.
Bentiromide test (pancreatic function): 500 mg bentiromide (chymex) orally; p-aminobenzoic acid (PABA) measured in plasma and/or urine
Plasma: >3.6 (±1.1) μg/mL at 90 min
Urine: >50 percent recovered as PABA in 6 h
Gastric juice:
Volume:
24 h: 2–3 L
Nocturnal: 600–700 mL
Basal, fasting: 30–70 mL/h

	Conversion Factor (CF) C × CF = SI
Reaction:	
pH: 1.6–1.8	
Titratable acidity of fasting juice: 4–9 μmol/s (15–35 meq/h)	0.261
Acid output:	
Basal:	
Females (mean ± 1 SD): 0.6 ± 0.5 μmol/s (2.0 ± 1.8 meq/h)	0.2778
Males (mean ± 1 SD): 0.8 ± 0.6 μmol/s (3.0 ± 2.0 meq/h)	0.2778
Maximal (after subcutaneous histamine acid phosphate 0.004 mg/kg body weight and preceded by 50 mg promethazine or after betazole 1.7 mg/kg body weight or pentagastrin 6 μg/kg body weight):	
Females (mean ± 1 SD): 4.4 ± 1.4 μmol/s (16 ± 5 meq/h)	0.2778
Males (mean ± 1 SD): 6.4 ± 1.4 μmol/s (23 ± 5 meq/h)	0.2778
Basal acid output/maximal acid output ratio: 0.6 or less	
Gastrin, serum: 40–200 ng/L (40–200 pg/mL)	—
Secretin test (pancreatic exocrine function: 1 unit/kg of body weight, intravenously	
Volume (pancreatic juice): >2.0 mL/kg in 80 min	—
Bicarbonate concentration: >80 mmol/L (80 meq/L)	—
Bicarbonate output: >10 mmol in 30 min (10 meq in 30 min)	—

METABOLIC AND ENDOCRINE TESTS

	Conversion Factor (CF) C × CF = SI
Adrenocorticotropin (ACTH) plasma, 8 A.M.: <18 pmol/L (<80 pg/mL)	0.2202
Adrenal cortex function tests: see Chap. 335	—
Adrenal medulla function tests: see Chap 336	—
Adrenal steroids, plasma:	
Aldosterone, 8 A.M.: <220 pmol/L (patient supine, 100 meq Na and 60–100 meq K intake) (<8 ng/dL)	27.74
Cortisol:	
8 A.M.: 140–690 nmol/L (5–25 μg/dL)	27.59
4 P.M.: 80–330 nmol/L (3–12 μg/dL)	27.59
Dehydroepiandrosterone (DHEA): 7–31 nmol/L (2–9 μg/L)	3.467
Dehydroepiandrosterone sulfate (DHEA sulfate): 1.3–6.7 μmol/L (500–2500 μg/L)	0.002714
11-Deoxycortisol (compound S): <30 nmol/L (<1 μg/dL)	28.86
17-Hydroxyprogesterone:	
Women: follicular phase, 0.6–3 nmol/L (0.20–1 μg/L); luteal phase, 1.5–10.6 nmol/L (0.5–3.5 μg/L)	3.026
Men: 0.2–9 nmol/L (0.06–3 μg L)	3.026
Adrenal steroids, urinary excretion:	
Aldosterone: 14–53 nmol/d (5–19 μg/d)	2.774
Cortisol, free: 55–275 nmol/d (20–100 μg/d)	2.759
17-Hydroxycorticosteroids: 5.5–28 μmol/d (2–10) mg/d)	2.759
17-Ketosteroids:	
Men: 24–88 μmol/d (7–25 mg/d)	3.467
Women: 14–52 μmol/d (4–15 mg/d)	3.467
Angiotensin II, plasma, 8 A.M.: 10–30 nmol/L (10–30 pg/mL)	—

	Conversion Factor (CF) C × CF = SI
Arginine vasopressin (AVP), plasma:	
Random fluid intake: 1.5–5.6 pmol/L (1.5–6 ng/L)	0.92
Calcitonin, plasma: <50 ng/L (<50 pg/mL)	—
Catecholamines, urinary excretion:	
Free catecholamines: <590 nmol/d (<100 μg/d)	5.911
Epinephrine: <275 nmol/d (<50 μg/d)	5.458
Metanephrines: <7 μmol/d (<1.3 mg/d)	5.458
Vanillylmandelic acid (VMA): <40 μmol/d (<8 mg/d)	5.046
Glucagon, plasma: 50–100 ng/L (50–100 pg/mL)	—
Gonadal function tests: see Chaps. 339 and 340	—
Gonadal steroids, plasma:	
Androstenedione:	
Women: 3.5–7.0 nmol/L (1–2 ng/ml)	3.492
Men: 3.0–5.0 nmol/L (0.8–1.3 ng/ml)	3.492
Estradiol:	
Women: 70–220 pmol/L (20–60 pg/mL), higher at ovulation	3.671
Men: <180 pmol/L (<50 pg/mL)	3.671
Progesterone:	
Women: luteal peak >16 nmol/L (7 ng/mL)	3.180
Men, prepubertal girls, preovulatory women, and postmenopausal women: <6 nmol/L (<2 ng/mL)	3.180
Testosterone:	
Women: <3.5 nmol/L (<1 ng/mL)	3.467
Men: 10–35 nmol/L (3–10 ng/mL)	3.467
Prepubertal boys and girls: 0.17–0.7 nmol/L (0.05–0.2 ng/mL)	3.467
Gonadotropins, plasma:	
Women, mature, premenopausal, except at ovulation:	
FSH: 5–20 IU/L (5–20 mIU/mL)	—
LH: 5–25 IU/L (5–25 mIU/mL)	—
Ovulatory surge:	
FSH: 12–30 IU/L (12–30 mIU/mL)	—
LH: 25–100 IU/L (25–100 mIU/mL)	—
Postmenopausal:	
FSH: 12–30 IU/L (12–30 mIU/mL)	—
LH: >50 IU/L (>50 mIU/mL)	—
Men, mature:	
FSH: 5–20 IU/L (5–20 mIU/mL)	—
LH: 5–20 IU/L (5–20 mIU/mL)	—
Children of both sexes, prepubertal:	
FSH: <5 IU/L (<5 mIU/mL)	—
Growth hormone, after 100 g glucose by mouth: <5 μg/L (<5 ng/mL)	—
Human chorionic gonadotropin, β subunit (β-hCG), plasma:	
Men and nonpregnant women: <3 IU/L (<3 mIU/mL)	—
Insulin, serum or plasma, fasting: 43–186 pmol/L (6–26 μU/mL)	7.175
Insulin-like growth factor 1 (somatomedin C, IGF-1/SM-C): see Chap. 332	—
Oxytocin: random 1–4 pmol/L (1.25–5 ng/L)	0.80
Ovulatory peak in women: 4–8 pmol/L (5–10 ng/L)	
Pancreatic islet function tests: see Chap. 337	—
Parathyroid function tests: see Chap. 357	—
Pituitary function tests: see Chaps. 331 to 333	—
Pregnancy tests: see Chap. 340	—

	Conversion Factor (CF) C × CF = SI

Prolactin, serum: 2–15 μg/L (2–15 ng/mL) — —

Renin-angiotensin function tests: see Chap. 335 — —

Semen analysis: see Chap. 339 — —

Thyroid function tests:

Dynamic tests of thyroid function: see Chap. 334 — —

Radioactive iodine uptake, 24 h: 5–30 percent (range varies in different areas due to variations in iodine intake) — —

Resin T_3 uptake: 0.25–0.35 (25–35 percent) (varies among laboratories; for calculation of indexes of resin T_3 uptake, see Chap. 334) — 0.01

Reverse triiodothyronine (rT_3), plasma: 0.15–0.61 nmol/L (10–40 ng/dL) — 0.01536

Thyroid-stimulating hormone (TSH): 0.4–5 mU/L (0.4–5 μU/mL) — —

Thyroxine (T_4), serum radioimmunoassay: 64–154 nmol/L (5–12 μg/dL) — 12.86

Triiodothyronine (T_3), plasma: 1.1–2.9 nmol/L (70–190 ng/dL) — 0.01536

PULMONARY FUNCTION TESTS

See Table A-7.

RENAL FUNCTION TESTS

Clearances (corrected to 1.72 m² of body surface area):

Measures of glomerular filtration rate:

Inulin clearance (C1):

Males (mean ± 1 SD): 2.1 ± 0.4 mL/s (124 ± 25.8 mL/min) — 0.01667

Females (mean ± 1 SD): 2.0 ± 0.2 mL/s (119 ± 12.8 mL/min) — 0.01667

Endogenous creatinine clearance: 1.5–2.2 mL/s (91–130 mL/min) — 0.01667

Urea: 1.0–1.7 mL/s (60–100 mL/min) — 0.01667

Measures of effective renal plasma flow and tubular function:

p-Aminohippuric acid clearance (Cl_{PAH}):

Males (mean ± 1 SD): 10.9 ± 2.7 mL/s (654 ± 163 mL/min) — 0.01667

Females (mean ± 1 SD): 9.9 ± 1.7 mL/s (594 ± 102 mL/min) — 0.01667

Concentration and dilution test:

Specific gravity of urine:

After 12-h fluid restriction: 1.025 or more — —

After 12-h deliberate water intake: 1.003 or less — —

Protein excretion, urine: <0.15 g/d (<150 mg/d) — 0.01

Males: 0–0.06 g/d (0–60 mg/d) — 0.01

Females: 0–0.09 g/d (0–90 mg/d) — 0.01

Specific gravity, maximal range: 1.002–1.028 — —

Tubular reabsorption, phosphorus: 79–94 percent of filtered load — —

HEMATOLOGIC EVALUATIONS

See also "Chemical Constituents of Blood." — —

Bone marrow See Table A-6. — —

	Conversion Factor (CF) C × CF = SI

Carboxyhemoglobin:

Nonsmoker: 0–0.023 (0–2.3 percent) — 0.01

Smoker: 0.021–0.042 (2.1–4.2 percent) — 0.01

Erythrocyte:

Count: 4.15–4.90 × 10^{12}/L (4.15–4.90 × 10^6/mm³) — —

Distribution width (Coulter): 0.13–0.15 (13–15 percent) — —

Glucose-6-phosphate dehydrogenase: 12.1 ± 2 IU/gHb (WHO) — —

Life span:

Normal survival: 120 days — —

Chromium-labeled, half-life ($t^{1/2}$): 28 days — —

Mean corpuscular hemoglobin (MHC): 28–33 pg/cell (28–33 pg/cell) — —

Mean corpuscular hemoglobin concentration (MCHC): 320–360 g/L (32–36 g/dL) — —

Mean corpuscular volume (MCV): 86–98 fL (86–98 mm³) — —

Ham's test (acid serum): negative — —

Haptoglobin, serum: 0.5–2.2 g/L (50–220 mg/dL) — 0.01

Hematocrit:

Males: 0.42–0.52 (42–52 percent) — —

Females: 0.37–0.48 (37–48 percent) — —

Hemoglobin:

Plasma: 0.6–3 μmol/L (1–5 mg/dL) — 0.6206

Whole blood:

Males: 8.1–11.2 mmol/L (13–18 g/dL) — 0.6206

Females: 7.4–9.9 mmol/L (12–16 g/dL) — 0.6206

Hemoglobin A_2 (HbA$_2$): 0.015–0.035 (1.5–3.5 percent) — 0.01

Hemoglobin, fetal (HbF): <0.02 (<2 percent) — 0.01

Hemoglobin H prep: negative — —

Leukocytes:

Alkaline phosphatase (LAP): 0.2–1.6 μkat/L (13–100 U/L) — —

Count: 4.3–0.3X10⁹/L (4.3–10.8 × 10³/mm³) — —

Differential:

Neutrophils: 0.45–0.74 (45–74 percent) — —

Bands: 0–0.04 (0–4 percent) — —

Lymphocytes: 0.16–0.45 (16–45 percent) — —

Monocytes: 0.04–0.10 (4–10 percent) — —

Eosinophils: 0–0.07 (0–7 percent) — —

Basophils: 0–0.02 (0–2 percent) — —

Lysozyme (muramidase):

Serum: 5–25 mg/L (5–25 μg/mL) — —

Urine: <2 mg/L (<2 μg/mL) — —

Methemoglobin: <2 mg/L (<2 μg/mL) — —

Osmotic fragility:

Slight hemolysis: 0.45–0.39 percent — —

Complete hemolysis: 0.33–0.30 percent — —

Plasma iron turnover: 20–42 mg/d or 0.45 mg/kg of body weight per day — —

Platelets and coagulation parameters:

Alpha$_2$ antiplasmin: 70–130 percent — —

Antithrombin III: 80–80–120 percent — —

Bleeding time:

Duke method: <4 min — —

Simplate: <7 min — —

Clot retraction, qualitative: apparent in 60 min, complete <24 h, usually <6 h — —

Euglobulin lysis time: >2 h — —

Factor II: 60–100 percent — —

	Conversion Factor (CF) C × CF = SI		Conversion Factor (CF) C × CF = SI

Factor V: 60–100 percent
Factor VII: 60–100 percent
Factor IX: 60–100 percent
Factor X: 60–100 percent
Factor XI: 60–100 percent
Factor XII: 60–100 percent
Factor XIII: 60–100 percent
Fibrinogen: 200–400 mg/dL
Fibrin split products: <10 μg/mL
Plasminogen: 2.4–4.4 CTA U/mL
Protein C (antigenic assay): 58–148 percent
Protein S (antigenic assay): 58–148 percent
Partial thromboplastin time (activated PTT): comparable with control
Prothrombin time (quick one-stage): control ± 1 s
Protamine paracoagulation (3P) test: negative
Platelets: 130,000–400,000 per microliter
Thrombin time: control ± 3 s
von Willebrand's antigen: 60–150 percent
Protoporphyrin, free erythrocyte (FEP): 0.28–0.64 μmol/L of red blood cells (16–36 μg/dL of red blood cells) — 0.0177
Red cells: see "Erythrocytes"
Schilling test: 7–40 percent of orally administered vitamin B_{12} excreted in urine
Sedimentation rate:
  Westergren, <50 years of age:
    Males: 0–15 mm/h
    Females: 0–20 mm/h
  Westergren, >50 years of age:
    Males: 0–20 mm/h
    Females: 0–30 mm/h
Sucrose hemolysis: negative
Viscosity
  Plasma: 1.7–2.1
  Serum: 1.4–1.8
White blood cells: see "Leukocytes"

URINE ANALYSIS

See also "Metabolic and Endocrine Tests"
Acidity, titratable: 20–40 mmol/d (20–40 meq/d) —
Ammonia: 30–50 mmol/d (30–50 meq/d) —
Amylase: 35–260 Somogyi units/h —
Amylase/creatinine clearance ratio [(Cl_{am}/Cl_{cr}) × 100]: 1–5 —
Bentiromide (pancreatic function): 50 percent excreted in 6 h as *p*-amino benzoic acid (PABA) after 500 mg oral bentiromide —
Calcium (10 meq/d or 200-mg/d calcium diet): <3.8 mmol/d (<7.5 meq/d) 0.5
Catecholamines: <600 nmol/d (<100 μg/d) 5.911
Copper: 0–0.4 μmol/d (0–25 μg/d) 0.01574
Coproporphyrins (types I and III): 150–460 nmol/d (100–300 μg/d) 1.527
Creatine, as creatinine:
  Adult males: <380 pmol/d (<50 mg/d) 7.625
  Adult females: <760 pmol/d (<100 mg/d) 7.625
Creatinine: 8.8–14 mmol/d (1.0–1.6 g/d) 8.840
Glucose, true (oxidase method): 0.3–1.7 mmol/d (50–300 mg/d) 0.5551
5-Hydroxyindoleacetic acid (5-HIAA): 10–47 μmol/d (2–9 mg/d) 5.230
Lead: <0.4 μmol/d (<80 μg/d) 0.004826
Protein: <0.15 g/d (<150 mg/d) 0.1
Porphobilinogen: none —
Potassium: 25–100 mmol/d [25–100 meq/d (varies with intake)] —
Sodium: 100–260 mmol/d [100–260 meq/d (varies with intake)] —
Urobilinogen: 1.7–5.9 μmol/d (1–3.5 mg/d) 1.693
Vanillylmandelic acid (VMA): <40 μmol/d (<8 mg/d) 5.046
D-Xylose excretion: 5 to 8 g within 5 h after oral dose of 25 g —

STOOL ANALYSIS

Bulk:
  Wet weight: <197.5 (115 ± 41) g/d —
  Dry weight: <66.4 (34 ± 15) g/d —
Alpha$_1$ antitrypsin: 0.98 (±0.17) mg/g dry weight stool —
Coproporphyrin: 600–1500 nmol/d (400–1000 μg/d) 1.527
Fat (on diet containing at least 50 g fat): <6.0 (4.0 ± 1.5) g/d when measured on a 3-day (or longer) collection
  Percent of dry weight: 0.30 (<30.4 percent) 0.01
  Coefficient of fat absorption: >0.95 (>95 percent) 0.01
Fatty acid:
  Free: 0.01–0.10 (1–10 percent of dry matter) 0.01
  Combined as soap: 0.005–0.12 (0.5–12 percent of dry matter) 0.01
Nitrogen: <1.7 (1.4 ± 0.2) g/d —
Protein content: minimal —
Urobilinogen: 68–470 μmol/d (40–280 mg/d) 1.693
Water: 0.65 (approximately 65 percent) 0.01

TABLE A-1 SI and other units

Quantity	Name of unit	Symbol for unit	Derivation of units
SI BASE UNITS			
Length	meter	m	
Mass	kilogram	kg	
Time	second	s	
Thermodynamic temperature	Kelvin	K	
Amount of substance	mole	mol	
SI DERIVED UNITS			
Area	square meter	m^2	
Force	newton	N	$(m \cdot kg)/s^2$
Pressure	pascal	Pa	$N \cdot m^2$
Work, energy	joule	J	$N \cdot m$
Celsius temperature	degree Celsius	°C	K
OTHER UNITS RETAINED FOR USE			
Time	minute	min	
	hour	h	
	day	d	
Volume	liter	L	

TABLE A-3 SI prefixes and their symbols

Factor	Prefix	Symbol for prefix
10^9	giga	G
10^6	mega	M
10^3	kilo	k
10^2	hecto	h
10^1	deka	da
10^{-1}	deci	d
10^{-2}	centi	c
10^{-3}	milli	m
10^{-6}	micro	μ
10^{-9}	nano	n
10^{-12}	pico	p
10^{-15}	femto	f
10^{-18}	alto	a

TABLE A-4 Classification of total cholesterol and LDL-cholesterol values

	Total plasma cholesterol	LDL-cholesterol	Conversion factor (C to SI)
Desirable	<5.20 mmol/L (<200 mg/dL)	<3.36 mmol/L (<130 mg/dL)	0.02586
Borderline high	5.20–6.18 mmol/L (200–239 mg/dL)	3.36–4.11 mmol/L (130–159 mg/dL)	0.02586
High	≥6.21 mmol/L (≥240 mg/dL)	≥4.14 mmol/L (≥160 mg/dL)	0.02586

SOURCE: The Expert Panel. Report of the National Cholesterol Education Program Expert Panel on Detection, Evaluation, and Treatment of High Blood Cholesterol in Adults. Arch Intern Med 148:36, 1988

TABLE A-2 Radiation derived units

Quantity	Old unit	SI unit	Name for SI unit (and abbreviation)	Conversion
Activity	curie (Ci)	Disintegrations per second (dps)	becquerel (Bq)	$1\ Ci = 3.7 \times 10^{10}\ Bq$ 1 mCi = 37 mBq 1 μCi = 0.037 MBq or 37 GBq $1\ Bq = 2.703 \times 10^{-11}\ Ci$
Absorbed dose	rad	joule per kilogram (J/kg)	gray (Gy)	1 Gy = 100 rad 1 rad = 0.01 Gy $1\ mrad = 10^{-3}\ cGy$
Exposure	roentgen (R)	coulomb per kilogram (C/kg)	—	1 C/kg = 3876 R $1\ R = 2.58 \times 10^{-4}\ C/kg$ 1 mR = 258 pC/kg
Dose equivalent	rem	joule per kilogram (J/kg)	sievert (Sv)	1 Sv = 100 rem 1 rem = 0.01 Sv 1 mrem = 10 μSv

TABLE A-5 Normal values of echocardiographic measurements in adults

	Range, cm	Mean, cm	Number of subjects
Age (years)	13 to 54	26	134
Body surface area (m^2)	1.45 to 2.22	1.8	130
RVD—flat	0.7 to 2.3	1.5	84
RVD—left lateral	0.9 to 2.6	1.7	83
LVID—flat	3.7 to 5.6	4.7	82
LVID—left lateral	3.5 to 5.7	4.7	81
Posterior LV wall thickness	0.6 to 1.1	0.9	137
Posterior LV wall amplitude	0.9 to 1.4	1.2	48
IVS wall thickness	0.6 to 1.1	0.9	137
Mid IVS amplitude	0.3 to 0.8	0.5	10
Apical IVS amplitude	0.5 to 1.2	0.7	38
Left atrial dimension	1.9 to 4.0	2.9	133
Aortic root dimension	2.0 to 3.7	2.7	121
Aortic cusps' separation	1.5 to 2.6	1.9	93
Percentage of fractional shortening[†]	34 to 44%	36%	20
Mean rate of circumferential shortening (Vcf)[‡], or mean normalized shortening velocity	1.02 to 1.94 circ/s	1.3 circ/s	38

* RVD = right ventricular dimension; LVID = left ventricular internal dimension; d = end diastole; s = end systole; LV = left ventricle; IVS = interventricular septum.

† $\dfrac{LVIDd - LVIDs}{LVIDd}$

‡ $\dfrac{LVIDd - LVIDs}{LVIDd \times ejection\ time}$

SOURCE: From H. Feigenbaum, Echocardiography, in *Heart Disease*, 4th ed, E Braunwald (ed). Philadelphia, Saunders, 1992.

TABLE A-6 Differential nucleated cell counts of bone marrow

	Normal, mean%*	Range, %[†]		Normal, mean%*	Range, %[†]
Myeloid:	56.7		Erythroid:	25.6	
Neutrophilic series:	53.6		Pronormoblasts	0.6	0.2–1.3
Myeloblast	0.9	0.2–1.5	Basophilic normoblasts	1.4	0.5–2.4
Promyelocyte	3.3	2.1–4.1	Polychromatophilic	21.6	17.9–29.2
Myelocyte	12.7	8.2–15.7	normoblasts		
Metamyelocyte	15.9	9.6–24.6	Orthochromatic normoblasts	2.0	0.4–4.6
Band	12.4	9.5–15.3	Megakaryocytes	<0.1	
Segmented			Lymphoreticular	17.8	
Eosinophilic series	3.1	1.2–5.3	Lymphocytes	16.2	11.1–23.2
Basophilic series	<0.1	0–0.2	Plasma cells	2.3	0.4–3.9
			Reticulum cells	0.3	0–0.9

* From MM Wintrobe et al, *Clinical Hematology*, 8th ed. Philadelphia, Lea & Febiger, 1981.
[†] Range observed in 12 healthy men.

TABLE A-7 Summary of values useful in pulmonary physiology

	Symbol	Typical values	
		Men	Women

PULMONARY MECHANICS

	Symbol	Men	Women
Spirometry—volume-time curves:			
Forced vital capacity	FVC	$\geq$4.0 L	$\geq$3.0 L
Forced expiratory volume in 1 s	FEV_1	>3.0 L	>2.0 L
FEV_1/FVC	FEV_1%	>60%	>70%
Maximal midexpiratory flow	MMF (FEF 25–27)	>2.0 L/s	>1.6 L/s
Maximal expiratory flow rate	MEFR (FEF 200–1200)	>3.5 L/s	>3.0 L/s
Spirometry—flow-volume curves:			
Maximal expiratory flow at 50% of expired vital capacity	V_{max} 50 (FEF 50%)	>2.5 L/s	>2.0 L/s
Maximal expiratory flow at 75% of expired vital capacity	V_{max} 75 (FEF 75%)	>1.5 L/s	>1.0 L/s
Resistance to airflow:			
Pulmonary resistance	RL (R_L)	<3.0 (cmH$_2$O/s)/L	
Airway resistance	Raw	<2.5 (cmH$_2$O/s)/L	
Specific conductance	SGaw	>0.13 cmH$_2$O/s	
Pulmonary compliance:			
Static recoil pressure at total lung capacity	Pst TLC	25 ± 5 cmH$_2$O	
Compliance of lungs (static)	CL	0.2 L/cmH$_2$O	
Compliance of lungs and thorax	C(L + T)	0.1 L/cmH$_2$O	
Dynamic compliance of 20 breaths per minute	C dyn 20	0.25 ± 0.05 L/cmH$_2$O	
Maximal static respiratory pressures:			
Maximal inspiratory pressure	MIP	>90 cmH$_2$O	>50 cmH$_2$O
Maximal expiratory pressure	MEP	>150 cmH$_2$O	>120 cmH$_2$O

LUNG VOLUMES

	Symbol	Men	Women
Total lung capacity	TLC	6–7 L	5–6 L
Functional residual capacity	FRC	2–3 L	2–3 L
Residual volume	RV	1–2 L	1–2 L
Inspiratory capacity	IC	2–4 L	2–4 L
Expiratory reserve volume	ERV	1–2 L	1–2 L
Vital capacity	VC	4–5 L	3–4 L

GAS EXCHANGE (SEA LEVEL)

	Symbol	Men	Women
Arterial O$_2$ tension	Pa$_{O_2}$	12.7 ± 0.7 kPa (95 ± 5 mmHg)	
Arterial CO$_2$ tension	Pa$_{CO_2}$	5.3 ± 0.3 kPa (40 ± 2 mmHg)	
Arterial O$_2$ saturation	Sa$_{O_2}$	0.97 ± 0.02 (97 ± 2%)	
Arterial blood pH	pH	7.40 ± 0.02	
Arterial bicarbonate	HCO$_3^-$	24 + 2 meq/L	
Base excess	BE	0 ± 2 meq/L	
Diffusing capacity for carbon monoxide (single breath)	DL$_{CO}$	0.42 mLCO/s/mmHg (25 mL CO/min/mmHg)	
Dead space volume	V$_D$	50 ± 25 mL	
Physiologic dead space; dead space-tidal volume ratio (rest)	V$_D$/V$_T$	$\leq$35% V$_T$	
(exercise)		$\leq$20% V$_T$	
Alveolar-arterial difference for O$_2$	A-aD$_{O_2}$	$\leq$2.7 kPa $\leq$20 kPa ($\leq$20 mmHg)	

Color Plates

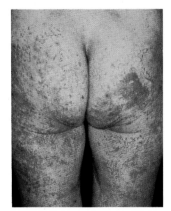

A (QUESTION 381)

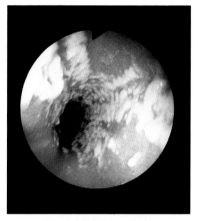

B (QUESTION 382)

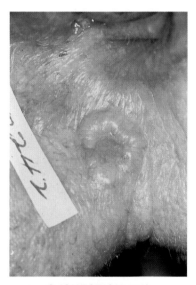

C (QUESTION 493)

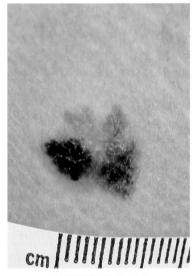

D (QUESTION 494)

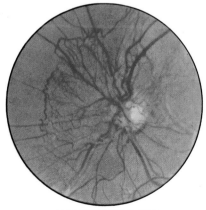

E (QUESTION 651)

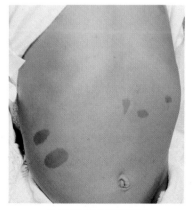

F (QUESTION 712)

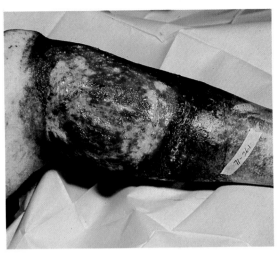

G (QUESTION 713)

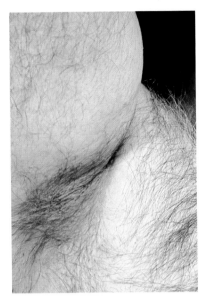

H (QUESTION 714)

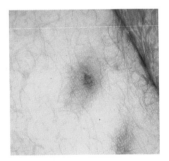

I (QUESTION 715)

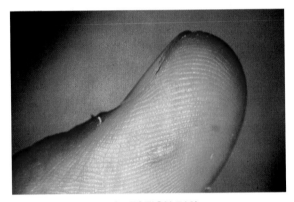

J (QUESTION 716)

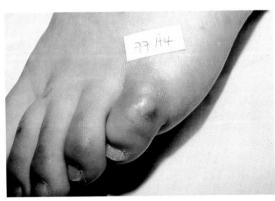

K (QUESTION 717)

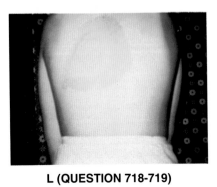

L (QUESTION 718-719)

(From Steere AC et al: Ann Intern Med 86:685, 1977; with permission)

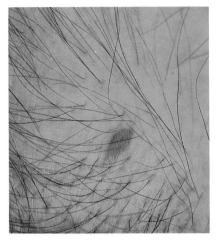

M (QUESTION 720)

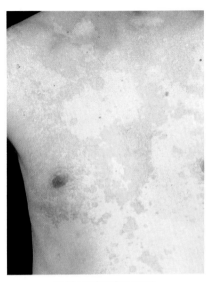

N (QUESTION 721)

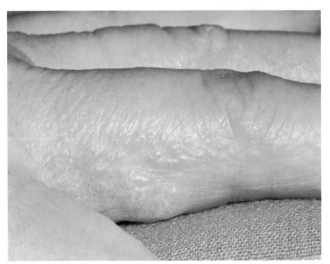

O (QUESTION 722)

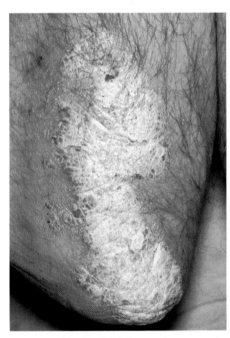

P (QUESTION 723)

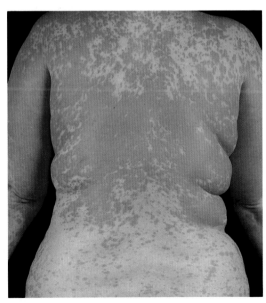

Q (QUESTION 724)

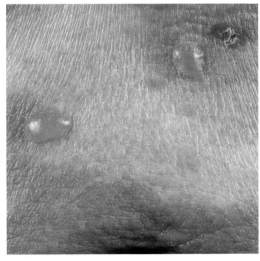

R (QUESTION 725)

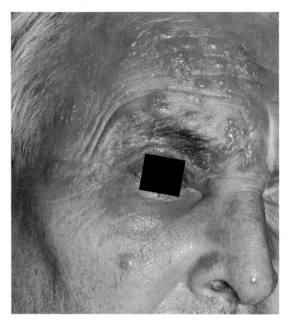

S (QUESTION 726)

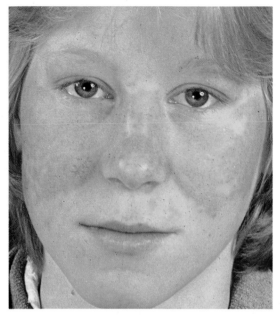

T (QUESTION 727)

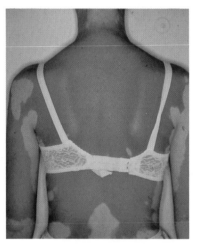

U (QUESTION 730)

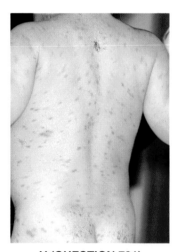

V (QUESTION 731)

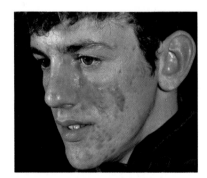

W (QUESTION 732)

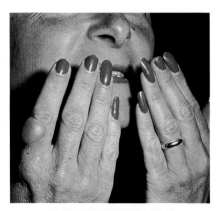

X (QUESTION 733-734)